Pediatric Neuroimaging

Second Edition

Pediatric Neuroimaging

Second Edition

A. James Barkovich, M.D.
Professor of Radiology
Chief, Pediatric Neuroradiology
Department of Radiology
University of California, San Francisco
San Francisco, California

Raven Press ☙ New York

Raven Press Ltd., 1185 Avenue of the Americas, New York, New York 10036

Made in the United States of America

Library of Congress Cataloging-in-Publication Data

Barkovich, A. James, 1952–
    Pediatric neuroimaging/A. James Barkovich.—2nd ed.
        p.   cm.
    Includes bibliographical references and index.
    ISBN 0-7817-0179-1
    1. Nervous system—Magnetic resonance imaging.   2. Nervous system—
Ultrasonic imaging.   3. Pediatric diagnostic imaging.   4. Pediatric
neurology—Diagnosis.   I. Title.
    [DNLM: 1. Nervous System Diseases—in infancy & childhood.
2. Nervous System Diseases—diagnosis.   3. Magnetic Resonance
Imaging—in infancy & childhood.   4. Tomography, X-Ray Computed—in
infancy & childhood.   WS 340 B256p 1995]
RJ488.5.M33B37   1995
618.92'8047548—dc20
DNLM/DLC
for Library of Congress   94-9720
                                                                                CIP

9 8 7 6 5 4 3 2 1

*To my mother and father, who gave me my motivation,
to my wonderful wife Karen, who allows me my dedication,
and to my sons, Matthew, Krister, and Emil, who are my inspiration*

Contents

Preface to the First Edition

New techniques for pediatric brain and spine diagnoses have rapidly developed over the past ten years. Computed tomography, ultrasound, and magnetic resonance imaging have opened a new window to the pediatric central nervous system. Through the use of these imaging modalities, an increased understanding of the pathological processes that occur in the pediatric brain has emerged. However, in spite of the wealth of new concepts that have evolved from these new resources, there has been a notable lack of textbooks on the subject, particularly in dealing with CT and MR. In this book, I attempt, at least in part, to fill the gap of knowledge that exists in pediatric neuroimaging.

This book strongly emphasizes CT and MR in pediatric neurodiagnosis. The reasons for this are twofold. First, there are a number of good textbooks available which focus on plain film and sonographic evaluation of the pediatric central nervous system. Second, and more important, I feel that CT and MR, particularly MR, are the best modalities by far for imaging the pediatric brain. In those areas where ultrasound and plain film radiology are important adjuncts or are of primary importance in diagnosis, they have been included. Specifically, this includes the diagnosis of intracranial pathology in premature infants.

Readers will note that this is not an encyclopedic work on diseases of the pediatric central nervous system. Those disease processes that are well covered in other texts, or are extremely uncommon, are de-emphasized here. Instead, I have attempted to cover subjects that are encountered in everyday practice. Furthermore, I have emphasized concepts that are crucial to proper imaging techniques and image interpretation. Embryology, normal development, and pathophysiology are explained. Once these basic concepts are understood, interpretation of images is greatly facilitated. Finally, an attempt was made to present the information in a concise and straightforward manner that will make reading this book an enjoyable learning experience.

Preface

When I first began work on this Second Edition, I did not realize the degree of the growth and development of pediatric neuroimaging in the past six years. As I progressed, I was amazed at the number of publications dealing with pertinent topics in the literature of many medical specialties. Modern neuroimaging, magnetic resonance in particular, has proved to be a method of unraveling some of the mysteries of the developing brain. As a result, pediatric neuroimaging plays an important role not only in neonatology, child neurology, and pediatric neurosurgery, but in pediatric dermatology, pediatric endocrinology, pediatric oncology, and obstetrics as well.

As was the case in the First Edition, most of the illustrations in the book are of magnetic resonance studies. The reasons for this are twofold. First, it is my belief that MR is the imaging study of choice in most children with neurological disorders. Second, cranial sonography, which is extensively used in preterm and term neonates, is already covered by a number of textbooks; thus, I did not feel that extensive coverage of sonography was necessary. I have included cranial sonograms in those sections of this book where I believe it is appropriate. Furthermore, I have included discussions of nuclear medicine studies (cisternograms, shunt studies, SPECT, PET), CT, and plain skull films in situations where they are useful.

The enlarged scope of pediatric neuroradiology made the focus of this Second Edition a little different from that of the First Edition, although I have tried to keep the book basically simple and stress concepts where possible. Coverage has been expanded in the chapters on destructive and metabolic disorders. The chapters on developmental brain anomalies and tumors have been reorganized and expanded to include the orbits and skull.

An understanding of the concepts of basic neuroembryology, normal brain development, and neuropathophysiology are essential for the proper interpretation of pediatric neuroimaging studies; therefore, normal development of the brain, skull, and spine are emphasized. When complicated concepts are discussed, the ideas and facts that underlie the concepts are introduced first to simplify understanding. Pathophysiology is included for those disorders in which it aids in the understanding of the imaging findings. In addition, disorders with similar imaging appearances and similar embryological bases are grouped.

This book will serve as a textbook that can be read by the aspiring resident or fellow and as a reference book that can be used by the practicing physician in daily practice.

Acknowledgments

Special thanks to David Norman, Hans Newton, Alisa Gean, Nancy Fishbein, and Rebecca Smith-Bindman, who helped with proofreading; and to Liz Howell, who organized the morass of chapter pages and figures into a book.

Pediatric Neuroimaging
Second Edition

CHAPTER 1

Techniques and Methods in Pediatric Imaging

Modern imaging modalities, such as computed tomography and magnetic resonance, have greatly advanced both the understanding and the diagnosis of pathology of the central nervous system. To maximize the information gained from these studies, high-quality images must be obtained. Modern CT technology has resulted in short (less than 2 sec) imaging times. Spiral scanners and cine-CT obtain images in fractions of a second. As a result, motion is minimized and high-quality images are generally obtained. Although the use of fractional echoes and new "fast scan" techniques has decreased the time needed for acquisition of MR images, patient motion is still occasionally a problem, especially if sedation is inadequate. Moreover, the imaging parameters for the acquisition of optimal images in the pediatric patient differ from those of the adult because standard adult imaging sequences do not consider the changing chemical composition of the developing brain. The purpose of this chapter is to outline techniques for safely obtaining high-quality imaging studies in pediatric patients. In addition, all the techniques we currently use in the CT and MR evaluation of infants and children are described. These techniques will be referred to throughout the remainder of the book.

SEDATION

The most important factor in obtaining high-quality MR images in children is adequate sedation. In the absence of adequate sedation, motion artifact will obscure important diagnostic information. In general, sedation is not necessary for CT scanning when modern scanners (less than 2-sec imaging times) are being used. It is important for the technologist to watch the patient during the CT exam and to scan while the patient is not moving. In those difficult cases where sedation is required, the protocols outlined in this section are applicable. In certain institutions, the use of newer, very fast scanners, such as "spiral CT" (1) and Cine-CT have made sedation for CT entirely unnecessary.

Many different drugs can be and have been used safely for pediatric sedation (2–9). No attempt to recommend any particular regimen is made here, nor to list comprehensively all available or useful drugs. A few safe, proven regimens are listed. However, it is recommended that any protocols used by the readers, whether or not they are listed here, be discussed with and approved by local anesthesiologists or pediatricians who are experienced in sedating pediatric patients.

Sedation can be administered by many routes: oral, rectal, intramuscular (IM), or intravenous (IV). The oral, rectal, and intramuscular routes have an advantage in that they do not require any special skills for administration of the sedative. However, absorption of many drugs is somewhat erratic from the muscle and gastrointestinal tract and a large dose of drug is irrevocably in the patient if he/she has a complication. The recommendation of the American Academy of Pediatrics is that infants be

1

kept NPO for at least 4 hours prior to deep sedation; older children should be NPO for at least 6 hours (10).

Sodium pentobarbital (Nembutal) is a useful drug for intramuscular or rectal sedation of pediatric patients (3), although it should be avoided in patients who have hepatic or metabolic disease. The usual dose of sodium pentobarbital is 6 mg/kg (intramuscular) for the first 15 kg of body weight, followed by 5 mg for each additional kilogram up to a total dose of 200 mg. Administer the drug 35–45 min before the anticipated imaging time.

In the previous edition of this book, the safest drug for sedating children was stated to be chloral hydrate (11). Others have also reported on the safety and efficacy of chloral hydrate, especially in infants under the age of 18 months (5) and even up to age 4 years (12). However, questions have recently been raised concerning the potential mutagenicity of this drug (13). At the time of publication of this book, this question is not adequately answered. If used, chloral hydrate is administered orally in a dose of 75–100 mg/kg for the first 10 kg of body weight, then 50 mg/kg for each kg of body weight above 10 kg. If the child is still awake after 20 min, give supplementary doses up to a total dose of 2,000 mg.

After an oral, rectal, or IM sedative has been administered, move the patient and parent to a dark, quiet room. Otherwise the noise and activity of a waiting room will keep the child awake. Sleep deprivation is also helpful. If the imaging study is performed in the morning, keep the child awake several hours past normal bedtime the night preceding the exam and awaken the child earlier than usual on the morning of the exam. If the imaging is performed in the afternoon, deprive the child of his or her normal naps. Do not allow the child to fall asleep during travel to the MR facility. Finally, permit a parent to enter the scanner with the patient, if desired, to reassure the child that security is nearby. The second body will not create artifact.

IV sedation offers a number of advantages over the other routes of administration. Once intravenous access is obtained, sedation can be rapidly achieved. Moreover, supplemental doses are easily administered without disturbing the patient. Finally, the effects of many drugs (e.g., opiates) can be rapidly reversed.

The most popular drug used for IV sedation is pentobarbital (Nembutal) (2,5), which is administered intravenously in the following manner. Approximately 2.5 mg/kg is given over 30–40 sec while closely observing the patient. If the patient does not fall asleep within 60 sec, a second dose of 1.0 mg/kg is administered. If the patient remains awake, a third and fourth administration of 1.0 mg/kg can be given up to a total dose of 6 mg/kg. Repeated doses of 1–1.25 mg/kg are then administered, as needed, to maintain sedation during the exam. Small motions of the arms and legs are usually an indication that the level of sedation is diminishing.

At UCSF, our pediatric anesthesiologists have recommended that pentobarbital be used in conjunction with morphine sulfate, as the two drugs have complementary actions. Our regimen consists of an initial dose of 1–2 mg/kg pentobarbital, followed by 0.05 mg/kg morphine, followed by another dose of pentobarbital, another of morphine, and so on, until the patient is adequately sedated. Additional doses are given, as needed, if the level of sedation appears to be diminishing.

TABLE 1.1. *Some MR-compatible monitoring equipment*

Device and manufacturer	Function
Model 1040 pulse oximeter. Biochem International, Waukesha, WI	Heart rate, oxygen saturation
Omega 1400. In Vivo Research, Inc; Winter Park, FL	Blood pressure, heart rate
Omni-Trak 3100 MR vital signs monitor. In Vivo Research, Inc; Winter Park, FL	Heart rate, ECG, oxygen saturation, respiratory rate, temperature
MR fiber-optic pulse oximeter. Nonin Medical, Inc; Plymouth, MN	Oxygen saturation
Laserflow blood perfusion monitor. Vasomed, Inc; St Paul, MN	Skin blood flow
LD 5000 laser-Doppler perfusion monitor. Medpacific Corporation; Seattle, WA	Skin blood flow
Respiratory rate monitor, models 515 and 525. Biochem International; Waukesha, WI	Respiratory rate
MicroSpan capnometer 8800. Biochem International; Waukesha, WI	Respiratory rate, end-tidal carbon dioxide
Aneuroid chest bellows. Coulbourn Instruments; Allentown, PA	Respiratory rate
Fluoroptic thermometry system, model 3000. Luxtron; Mountain View, CA	Temperature
Omni-Vent, series D. Columbia Medical Marketing; Topeka, KS	Ventilator
Ventilator, models 225 and 2500. Monaghan Medical Corp. Plattsburgh, PA	Ventilator
Anesthesia ventilator. Ohio Medical; Madison, WI	Ventilator
Infant ventilator MVP-10. Bio-Med Devices, Inc; Madison, CT	Ventilator
Datex carbon dioxide monitor. Puritan-Bennett Corporation. Los Angeles, CA	Percentage of carbon dioxide
Wenger precordial stethoscope. Anesthesia Medical Supplies; Santa Fe Springs, CA	Heart sounds

Adapted from refs. 6, 41. Note that these devices may require modifications to make them MR compatible, and none of them should be positioned closer than 8 ft (240 cm) from the entrance of the bore of a 1.5-T MR imager. Also, monitors with metallic cables, leads, or probes may cause imaging artifacts if placed near the imaging area of interest. Consult manufacturers to determine compatibility with specific MR imagers.

Intravenous sedation using propofol has been successfully used instead of pentobarbital in some studies (8); however, we have no experience with that drug.

MONITORING

The American Academy of Pediatrics and the American Society of Anesthesiologists recommends that the following parameters be monitored in all sedated infants and children: heart and respiratory rates, blood pressure, and arterial oxygen saturation (10). Although monitoring a patient in a CT suite is relatively simple, a patient who is undergoing MR examination is difficult to monitor because of the distortion of the magnetic field created by electric currents and paramagnetic metals. The monitoring must be performed using equipment composed of diamagnetic metals (e.g., aluminum) and plastics. A plastic stethoscope with very long tubing may be taped to the patient's chest so that heart rate can be monitored from outside the bore of the magnet. EKG leads, if necessary, may be run under the patient and as far away as possible from the body part being imaged. A CO_2-sensitive apnea monitor connected by long, small-caliber tubing to the patient in the scanner provides visual display of respiration and audio and visual alarms during apnea episodes without affecting image quality. Disposable, pediatric-sized nasal cannulae are available. Fortunately, MR-compatible monitoring equipment is now available (Table 1.1).

As a general rule, CT is adequate for the identification of most treatable life-threatening conditions in unstable patients. Although some lower-field-strength magnets and some shielding configurations will allow life support equipment to be in close proximity to the patient, most high-field MR suites require significant modifications to achieve intense, close-in electronic monitoring. Rarely, unstable patients may require imaging with MR. Ventilators made of aluminum or plastic are available (Table 1.1); in their absence, respirator-dependent patients must be manually ventilated. If a patient is very unstable, the physician or nurse may sometimes have to crawl into the bore of the magnet and observe the child from this extremely uncomfortable position throughout the examination.

SPECIAL PROBLEMS IN THE IMAGING OF PREMATURE INFANTS

Premature infants present the special problems of small size and inability to maintain body temperature. In general, premature infants should be imaged with ultrasound in the neonatal intensive care unit. Cranial ultrasound imaging is the examination of choice in these patients because it is inexpensive and portable (exams can be performed without moving the infant from the neonatal intensive care unit). Moreover, transfontanel ultrasonography is excellent for the examination of the deep areas of the brain, the location of most central nervous system pathology in the premature infant (see Chapter 4). If MR examination is thought necessary, the infant should be wrapped in an air bag that is warmed to body temperature. Others have wrapped the neonatal bodies in prewarmed towels. A stockinet hat prevents heat loss from the head. Monitoring of the vital signs in these infants is critical.

CONTRAST AGENTS

CT scans in children should initially be performed without intravenous contrast. If review of the noncontrast scan reveals a suspected abnormality, contrast should be given. The exact type of *iodinated contrast* is not important, as long as the concentration is approximately 300 mg/ml. The recommended dose is 3 ml/kg of body weight up to a total dose of 120 ml. The child should be scanned as soon as possible after the contrast has been administered.

The administration of *paramagnetic MR contrast agents* has been shown to be efficacious in the identification and evaluation of primary and metastatic brain tumors (especially extraparenchymal tumors), infections (cerebritis and meningitis), and neoplasms of the spinal cord and spinal canal (14). No significant difference has been demonstrated among the different paramagnetic contrasts that are commercially available. All are given intravenously; the standard dose is 0.1 mmol/kg. After infusion of contrast, only short TR/TE spin echo images or three-dimensional Fourier transformed gradient echo images with gradient spoilers (i.e., "T1-weighted" images) should be obtained; long TR/TE ("T2-weighted") images are not of value in this situation. It is likely that higher doses of contrast (0.3 mmol/kg) allow a higher sensitivity of detection of enhancing lesions, particularly CSF-borne metastases from brain tumors (15). Other conditions in which higher doses are indicated have not yet been defined.

CT SCANNING TECHNIQUES

In general, techniques for scanning older children with CT are identical to those for scanning adults. Axial images parallel to the canthomeatal line are obtained using 5-mm slice thickness. As CT scanning has become more rapid, little time penalty is paid for relatively thin slice profiles, and significant additional information may be acquired, especially in the small heads of infants and young children. An image thickness of 10 mm is too large.

Because the newborn brain has a very high water content, proper *windowing* of the CT scan is essential for optimal analysis of brain abnormalities. In general, CT images of the newborn brain should be photographed with a window of 60 and level of 20. Use of normal adult brain windows will result in pathology being missed.

There is one special situation in pediatric CT imaging where standard adult techniques should be modified. This is in the scanning of patients with craniofacial anomalies or craniosynostosis. These patients should be scanned using 3-mm slice thickness. Thicker (5–10-mm) slices allow too much averaging and obscure detail. Programs that give high detail bone resolution should be used; however, a soft tissue algorithm is also mandatory to assess the underlying brain for abnormality. Software is available from most manufacturers that allows three-dimensional reformations of the bones of the face and skull; these are of great value in planning reconstructive surgery.

ROUTINE MR IMAGING SEQUENCES

Brain

A sagittal, T1-weighted sequence should be performed on all patients. This sequence allows assessment of the midline structures that are frequently abnormal in congenital brain malformations. In particular, scrutinize the corpus callosum and cerebellum. The sagittal sequence then serves as a localizer for additional axial or coronal sequences. Standard parameters for this sequence are a repetition time (TR) of 500–600 msec, echo time (TE) of 11–20 msec, 3–5-mm slice thickness (1-mm gap), a 192×256 acquisition matrix, and one excitation. Using these parameters, most of the brain will be visualized. If the option of 192 acquisitions in the phase-encoding direction is not available, 128 acquisitions (at the expense of decreased spatial resolution) or 256 acquisitions (at the expense of increased imaging time and diminished signal to noise ratio) can be used. Using a short TR (500 msec) will save imaging time while still allowing assessment of the midline structures, but a price is paid in that the signal-to-noise ratio decreases and the lateral portions of the brain are not imaged.

After the sagittal images are obtained, axial T1- and T2-weighted images should be obtained in all patients less than 18 months old. For patients older than 18 months, only T2-weighted images are necessary. Both the T1- and T2-weighted sequences are necessary in younger patients for the following reasons. From birth to 6 months of age, brain maturation is evaluated best by T1-weighted images. From 6–8 months of age until approximately 18 months of age (at which time the brain is essentially mature by MR standards), T2-weighted images are more useful for assessing brain maturity. During the process of white matter maturation, the gray matter and subcortical white matter of the brain become isoin-

tense for a variable period of time on MR images; this isointensity of the cortex to the subcortical white matter obscures structural detail (see Chapter 2). Therefore, during the first 6 months of life (while the white matter is maturing on T1-weighted images) T2-weighted images are necessary to see the details of the gyral and sulcal patterns. Similarly, as the white matter matures on T2-weighted images between 6 and 18 months of age, T1-weighted images are essential to evaluate for structural abnormalities.

The optimal imaging parameters may vary from scanner to scanner. Although inversion recovery (IR) sequences give better T1 information than any spin echo sequences, an SE 600/11-20 sequence (identical to that outlined for the sagittal images) can be routinely used for T1-weighted images on high-field scanners. Use of this imaging sequence produces excellent images; moreover, the imaging time is markedly shorter than with inversion recovery sequences, resulting in less motion artifact. New "fast" inversion recovery imaging techniques, now available from some manufacturers, allow IR studies to be obtained in relatively short times; however, T1-weighted spin echo images are still faster. Three-dimensional gradient echo (GE) techniques using gradient pulses to "spoil" residual transverse magnetization (SPGR, 3D-FLASH, CE-FEE-T1, T1-FAST) can also be used to acquire T1-weighted images. These techniques have the ability to acquire very thin (1 mm or less) contiguous images through the brain in a relatively short imaging time. These spoiled GE techniques are particularly useful in looking for small, subtle cortical anomalies, such as cortical dysplasia (see Chapter 5). Moreover, they can be reformatted in any plane (sagittal, axial, coronal, or any obliquity) on an independent console, allowing acquisition of only one T1-weighted sequence. For T2-weighted sequences, spin echo sequences with a 4–5-mm slice thickness (2–2.5-mm gap), TR of 2,500–3,000 msec, TE of 30–60 msec (first echo), and 70–120 msec (second echo), 192×256 acquisition matrix, and 0.75–1 excitation should be used. In infants less than 12 months old, heavily T2-weighted sequences are highly recommended, as the water content of the brain in young children is considerably higher than that in older children and adults (16,17). We routinely use TR = 3,000 msec and TE = 60, 120 msec (first and second echoes) for this patient group. Although fast spin echo (FSE) images are used by some groups for infants and children, we have not been satisfied with the sensitivity of commercially available FSE sequences in the analysis of cortical and white matter detail. Although missing a single small white matter lesion in an adult is relatively unimportant, the same type of abnormality may be the only clue to the correct diagnosis in a child (18). Therefore, we continue to use the standard spin echo sequences in infants with nonspecific developmental delay. However, FSE sequences are adequate for infants with focal neurologic signs or symptoms and for evaluation of congenital anomalies or tumors (19). Moreover, FSE sequences continue to improve and will likely eventually replace standard SE sequences in most instances. Typical FSE parameters include TR = 2,500–3,000 msec, effective TE = 17–100 msec, echo train length = 8.

Mid-field and low-field scanners, however, do not produce adequately T1-weighted images with this standard spin echo technique. The reasons for the poorer images are twofold. First, T1 relaxation times increase with increasing static magnetic field strength; therefore, images obtained with identical parameters will be more T1 weighted at higher field strengths than at lower field strengths. Second, lower-field-strength scanners, in general, cannot achieve echo times as short as those of high-field scanners. The combination results in unsatisfactory T1-weighted spin echo images in infants scanned on most mid- and low-field scanners. Inversion recovery or 3D GE images with gradient spoilers should be used instead.

After the sagittal and axial images have been obtained, the coronal sequence may be helpful in some patients for further elucidation of pathology. Coronal images are particularly helpful in the imaging of schizencephaly (see Chapter 5), holoprosencephaly (Chapter 5), and periventricular leukomalacia (Chapter 4). They are also very valuable in the imaging of tumors where the relationship of the mass to the surrounding brain and dura is of great importance to the surgeon.

T2*-weighted GE images are sometimes useful in pediatric imaging, particularly when looking for areas of old hemorrhage, as in suspected trauma or vascular malformations. GE T1-weighted images can be obtained by using a large angle (60° to 90°), a short TR (20–100 msec), and a short TE (10–20 msec). GE T2-weighted images are obtained using a small flip angle (5° to 20°), a short TR (50–500 msec), and a long TE (20–100 msec). The T2*-weighted GE images are particularly useful in the evaluation of vascular lesions and hemorrhage because they are quite sensitive to the magnetic susceptibility changes and local heterogeneity of magnetic fields that are caused by blood breakdown products. Images show marked signal loss in the regions of the blood products (see Chapters 4 and 11).

Spine

In imaging the spine, different techniques are used, depending upon the clinical situation. When scanning a child with suspected or confirmed spinal *dysraphism*, sagittal T1-weighted images (TR = 600, TE = 20) should be obtained initially using 3-mm slice thickness. Axial images should then be obtained through any areas of abnormality or suspected abnormality. T1-weighted images are most helpful in these axial sequences; the exact

repetition time may be determined by the length of the spinal cord that needs to be evaluated. For example, if a large area of the cord needs to be examined, a repetition time in the range of 1,200 or 1,400 msec may be necessary to allow the entire region of the spine to be scanned in one imaging sequence. A relatively T1-weighted sequence can still be obtained by the use of a very short (20 msec) echo time.

Patients with *scoliosis* present a challenge. Initially, a coronal T1- or T2-weighted image should be obtained to assess vertebral anomalies and look for a split cord malformation (Chapter 10). Oblique sagittal and oblique axial planes can then be defined to give optimal information. If a split spinal cord is seen, axial T2*-weighted GE images should be obtained through the entirety of the split to look for a fibrocartilagenous or calcified spur.

Patients who present with *myelopathy* with no suspicion of dysraphism should have 3-mm T2-weighted images through the entire spinal cord, in addition to the T1-weighted sagittal and axial images. Axial GE images can then localize any abnormal region of T2 prolongation within the cord. Infusion of intravenous paramagnetic contrast is often very helpful in the evaluation of intrinsic spinal cord pathology, particularly when neoplasia is suspected.

The use of gradient moment nulling ("flow compensation") is very important in children because their extremely pulsatile cerebral vessels cause phase dispersion in the surrounding cerebrospinal fluid, resulting in increased spatial misregistration of the signal from moving protons when compared with adults. The gradient moment nulling option is available at present on most commercial scanners and should be used routinely on the long TR images.

SPECIAL MR TECHNIQUES

Magnetic Resonance Angiography (MRA)

For studies of the intracranial vasculature, three-dimensional Fourier transformed time of flight (3D TOF) is the most useful (20,21). For 3D TOF studies, a gradient echo (GE) 50/6.9 sequence is performed with flip angle (*theta*) of 35°, partition thickness of .9 mm, 128 partitions, and one acquisition. Velocity compensation gradients are applied in the read and phase-encoding directions. After data acquisition is completed and each of the partitions is reconstructed, separate MR angiograms are created by means of the maximum-intensity projection (MIP) technique described by Laub and Kaiser (22). *The reader should remember that the process of creating the MIP generates a number of artifacts (23,24) and that therefore the individual partition images should always be scrutinized in every MRA or MRV.*

For studies of the cervical carotid and vertebral arteries, two-dimensional Fourier transform time of flight (2D TOF) images are optimal (20,25,26). 2D TOF is also useful in place of 3D TOF for studies of intracranial vessels when complicated by excessive patient motion, although it is primarily used for imaging of vessels in the neck. We perform 2D TOF studies using a GE 45/7 sequence. Fifty-five consecutive axial MR images are obtained with a section thickness of 1.5 mm, theta of 60°, and bipolar gradients for flow compensation. Walking superior saturation pulses are applied cephalad to the axial images to eliminate signal intensity from venous blood returning via the jugular veins. MIP images are reconstructed in multiple planes.

Phase contrast images are useful for imaging slow flow, analyzing flow direction, and reducing saturation effects from slow flow (20,27). In pediatric neuroimaging, multislice 2D phase contrast (PC) is most often used to determine flow direction, as it is significantly quicker than 3D PC imaging. 2D PC studies are performed using a GE 27/4.5 sequence, a 192×256 acquisition matrix, slice thickness 5 mm, theta of 20°, and 15 excitations. The image is obtained using a presaturation band technique. Encoding velocity (V_{enc}), the velocity at which a phase shift of 180° between acquisitions, is set at 80 mm/sec for arterial studies and at 30 mm/sec for venous studies.

Studies of the dural venous sinuses are best achieved using 2D TOF techniques (28). 2D TOF venograms are acquired in the coronal plane to avoid saturation effects in the transverse sinuses secondary to in-plane flow. Contiguous 1.5-mm GE 45/6.9 images are obtained using theta of 60°, 256×128 matrix, and one excitation. Walking saturation pulses are applied posteriorly for coronal acquisition.

CSF Flow Studies

Cerebrospinal fluid (CSF) flow can be visualized and quantitatively analyzed using phase contrast studies (29,30). MR studies of CSF flow are most useful when looking for interruptions of normal flow patterns. In particular, we use these studies in patients with Chiari I and II malformations (see Chapter 5) when they are being considered for foramen magnum decompressions. We use phase contrast sagittal studies centered at the foramen magnum. Our typical parameters include V_{enc} of 10 cm/sec, TR = 27 msec, TE = 11.7 msec, theta = 30°, 22 cm field of view, a 128×256 acquisition matrix, and two excitations. Peripheral gating is used.

Magnetization Transfer

The technique of *magnetization transfer contrast (MTC)* is useful in assessing myelination and demyelination (31,32). MTC imaging relies on detecting differ-

ences in relaxation properties of free and bound water (32–34). The technique is based on the fact that water protons bound to macromolecules (such as those composing myelin) have very short T1 and T2 relaxation times; thus, bound protons do not contribute to the signal obtained by MR imaging. However, a constant exchange of water molecules is occurring between the free water molecules and the bound water molecules. Those protons in water molecules that are bound to macromolecules at the time of the initial radiofrequency pulse and that separate from the macromolecule before the readout gradient is applied will have considerably shorter T1 and T2 relaxation times than the rest of the free water proton molecules. The measured relaxation times of the entire population of water protons will be shortened by this process, which is known as magnetization transfer. The amount of magnetization transfer will depend upon the quantity of macromolecular components available to bind within the free water molecules and the rate of exchange of the two pools of water molecules.

If a radiofrequency (RF) pulse is applied slightly (5–10 kHz) off the peak resonance for free water, it will saturate the bound water protons, which have a much broader absorption peak, with minimal effect upon the free water protons. Application of the off-resonance RF pulse will therefore negate any contribution of bound water protons to the overall T1 and T2 relaxation times and to the MR image. Subtraction of the image obtained with the off-resonance RF saturation pulse will show the contribution from the bound protons (i.e., the amount of magnetization transfer). The amount of magnetization transfer can be quantitated (35).

Magnetization transfer images can be obtained by acquiring two sets of gradient echo scans with gradient spoilers. Data is best acquired using a repetition time of 300 msec, echo time of 7 msec, theta of 20°, 3 mm partition thickness, 12 cm field of view, and three-dimensional Fourier transform reconstruction techniques. A radiofrequency saturation band applied to the second set at 5 kHz off the resonance frequency of free water will saturate the pool of bound protons. Subtraction of the second data set from the first results in a magnetization transfer image. The amount of magnetization transfer in the different regions of the brain, which should reflect the state of myelination, can be calculated from region of interest measurements from those regions of brain.

Perfusion Imaging

Several approaches exist for performing dynamic MR imaging after administration of a contrast agent (36,37). One method is the use of fast gradient echo sequences with inversion prepulses [FSPGR (General Electric)]. This sequence allows strongly T1-weighted sequences to be acquired in as little as 1 sec. Enhancement with paramagnetic contrast is manifested as an increase in brain signal intensity of the images. Alternatively, T2*-weighted [susceptibility-weighted, MPGR (General Electric)] pulse sequences can be used. During first pass of the paramagnetic contrast agent through the brain, the shortened T2 results in a loss of signal intensity (38). Our initial experience and that of others (37) indicate that superior contrast to noise is obtained using the T2*-weighted sequence, so we use that method to evaluate for brain ischemia.

The patients are imaged during infusion of paramagnetic contrast, given intravenously as a bolus injection. The imaging sequence is rapid gradient echo, using TR = 35 msec, TE = 25 msec, θ = 10°, 1 excitation, 10-mm slice thickness, and 256 × 64 acquisition matrix. This sequence allows acquisition of images every 2 sec, acquired over 30 sec. As the cerebral circulation time (including arterial, capillary, and venous phases) varies from 7 sec to 9 sec, 30 sec provides adequate "buffer" capacity for the timing. Data analysis can provide local blood volume, local blood flow, and perfusion delay measurements (36,37). If echo planar imaging is available, it should be used, as, with 70-msec imaging times, echo planar imaging will allow acquisition of images at six levels, from the frontal to the occipital lobes, with a single bolus administration of gadoteridol.

Spectroscopy

Proton MR spectroscopy is sometimes useful in the analysis of inborn errors of metabolism. Spectra are obtained from volumes of approximately 8 cm^3. The voxel is prescribed from MR images obtained in an imaging sequence during the same examination. A stimulated echo sequence (39,40) combined with chemical shift-selective pulses is used for localization and water suppression, yielding only a signal from the region of interest at the spatial intersection of three section selective pulses. Field homogeneity is optimized from the localized volume by shimming of the water proton signal (water line widths after shimming should be 8–10 Hz, or less). Following the shimming process, a chemical shift-selective excitation (CHESS) type sequence is used to suppress the unwanted water signal (by a factor of up to 1,000). The water suppression pulse should not distort the remainder of the observed spectra appreciably. One hundred averages (TR = 2.0 sec, TE = 20 msec, TM = 10.7 msec) are obtained to achieve adequate signal to noise. Spectra are acquired with a standard imaging quadrature head coil.

COILS FOR MR IMAGING

When very young infants (especially younger than 4–5 months of age) are being imaged, an attempt should be made to fit the patient into an extremity coil. As opposed to most surface coils that act only as receivers of radio-frequency energy pulses, extremity coils in general function as both receiving and transmitting coils. This dual function increases field homogeneity and signal-to-noise ratio. The improved signal-to-noise ratio allows the operator to use a 256 × 192 or 256 × 256 acquisition matrix with one excitation or fractional excitations, thus improving spatial resolution while reducing imaging time, and consequently, the likelihood of motion artifact. In very young infants, the extremity coil can also be used for imaging of the spine. If the extremity coil proves too small, employ the standard head coil, using a 20-cm field of view for head studies. If the child is small enough, the head coil can be used for imaging the spine as well. Once the child outgrows the head coil, standard surface coils should always be used for imaging the spine.

REFERENCES

1. Zimmerman RA, Gusnard DA, Bilaniuk LT. Pediatric craniocervical spiral CT. *Neuroradiology* 1992;34:112–116.
2. Strain JD, Campbell JB, Harvey LA, Foley LC. IV nembutal: safe sedation for children undergoing CT. *Am J Roentgenol* 1988;151:975–979.
3. Thompson JR, Schneider S, Ashwal S, Holden BS, Hinshaw DB Jr, Hasso AN. The choice of sedation for computed tomography in children: a prospective evaluation. *Radiology* 1982;143:475–479.
4. Keeter S, Benator RM, Weinberg SM, Hartenberg MA. Sedation in pediatric CT: national survey of current practice. *Radiology* 1990;175:745–752.
5. Hubbard AM, Markowitz RI, Kimmel B, Kroger M, Bartko MB. Sedation for pediatric patients undergoing CT and MRI. *J Comput Assist Tomogr* 1992;16:3–6.
6. Holshouser BA, Hinshaw DB Jr, Shellock FG. Sedation, anesthesia, and physiologic monitoring during MRI. In: Hasso AN, Stark D, eds. *Spine and body MRI: categorical course syllabus*. Boston: American Roentgen Ray Society, 1991.
7. Burckhart GJ, White TJ III, Siegle RL, Jabour JT, Ramey DR. Rectal thiopental versus an intramuscular cocktail for sedating children before computerized tomography. *Am J Hosp Pharm* 1980;37:222–224.
8. Bloomfield EL, Masaryk TJ, Caplin A, et al. Intravenous sedation for MR imaging of the brain and spine in children: pentobarbital versus Propofol. *Radiology* 1993;186:93–97.
9. Berger PE, Kuhn JP, Brusehaber J. Techniques for computed tomography in infants and children. *Radiol Clin North Am* 1981;19:399–408.
10. American Academy of Pediatrics Committee on Drugs. Guidelines for monitoring and management of pediatric patients during and after sedation for diagnostic and therapeutic procedures. *Pediatrics* 1992;89:1110–1115.
11. Barkovich AJ. Techniques and methods in pediatric imaging. In: Barkovich A, eds. *Pediatric neuroimaging*. New York: Raven, 1990:1–4.
12. Greenberg SB, Faerber EN, Aspinall CL, Adams RC. High-dose chloral hydrate sedation for children undergoing MR imaging: safety and efficacy in relation to age. *Am J Roentgenol* 1993;161:639–641.
13. Smith MT. Chloral hydrate warning [Letter]. *Science* 1990;249:359.
14. Ge HL, Hirsch WL, Wolf GL, Rubin RA, Hackett RK. Diagnostic role of gadolinium-DTPA in pediatric neuroradiology: a retrospective review of 655 cases. *Neuroradiology* 1992;34:122–125.
15. Zimmerman RA, Bilaniuk L, Harris C, Phillips P. Use of 0.3 mmol/kg Gadoteridol in the evaluation of pediatric central nervous system diseases. *Radiology* 1993;189P:222.

16. Barkovich AJ, Kjos BO, Jackson DE Jr, Norman D. Normal maturation of the neonatal and infant brain: MR imaging at 1.5 T. *Radiology* 1988;166:173–180.
17. Holland BA, Haas DK, Norman D, Brant-Zawadzki M, Newton TH. MRI of normal brain maturation. *AJNR* 1986;7:201–208.
18. Kjos BO, Umansky R, Barkovich AJ. MR of the brain in children with developmental retardation of unknown cause. *AJNR* 1990;11:1035–1040.
19. Tice HM, Jones KM, Mulkern RV, et al. Fast spin-echo imaging if intracranial neoplasms. *J Comput Assist Tomogr* 1993;17:425–431.
20. Edelman RR, Mattle HP, Atkinson DJ, Hoogewoud HM. MR angiography. *Am J Roentgenol* 1990;154:937–946.
21. Ruggieri PM, Gerhard AL, Masaryk TJ, Modic MT. Intracranial circulation: pulse-sequence considerations in three-dimensional (volume) MR angiography. *Radiology* 1989;171:785–791.
22. Laub GA, Kaiser WA. MR angiography with gradient motion refocusing. *J Comp Assist Tomogr* 1989;12:377–382.
23. Anderson CM, Saloner D, Tsuruda JS, Shapeero LG, Lee RE. Artifacts in maximum-intensity-projection display of MR angiograms. *Am J Roentgenol* 1990;154:
24. Tsuruda JS, Saloner D, Norman D. Artifacts associated with MR neuroangiography. *AJNR* 1992;13:1411–1422.
25. Heiserman JE, Drayer BP, Fram EK, et al. Carotid artery stenosis: clinical efficacy of two-dimensional time-of-flight angiography. *Radiology* 1992;182:761–768.
26. Keller PJ, Drayer BP, Fram EK, Williams KD, Dumoulin CL, Souza SP. MR angiography with two-dimensional acquisition and three-dimensional display. *Radiology* 1989;173:527–532.
27. Huston J III, Rufenacht DA, Ehman RL, Wiebers DO. Intracranial aneurysms and vascular malformations: comparison of time-of-flight and phase-contrast MR angiography. *Radiology* 1991;181:721–730.
28. Mattle HP, Wentz KU, Edelman RR, et al. Cerebral venography with MR. *Radiology* 1991;178:453–458.
29. Nitz WR, Bradley WG Jr, Watanabe AS, et al. Flow dynamics of cerebrospinal fluid: assessment with phase-contrast velocity MR imaging performed with retrospective cardiac gating. *Radiology* 1992;183:395–405.
30. Enzmann DR, Pelc NJ. Normal flow patterns of intracranial and spinal cerebrospinal fluid defined with phase-contrast cine MR imaging. *Radiology* 1991;178:467–474.
31. Chew WM, Rowley HA, Barkovich AJ. Magnetization transfer contrast imaging in pediatric patients. *Radiology* 1992;185(P):281.
32. Dousset V, Grossman RI, Ramer KN, et al. Experimental allergic encephalomyelitis and multiple sclerosis: lesion characterization with magnetization transfer imaging. *Radiology* 1992;182:483–491.
33. Wolff SD, Balaban RS. Magnetization transfer contrast (MTC) and tissue water proton relaxation *in vivo*. *Magn Reson Med* 1989;11:135–144.
34. Wolff SD, Eng J, Balaban RS. Magnetization transfer contrast: method for improving contrast in gradient-recalled-echo images. *Radiology* 1991;179:133–137.
35. Eng J, Ceckler TL, Balaban RS. Quantitative 1H magnetization transfer imaging in Vivo. *Magn Reson Med* 1991;17:304–314.
36. Zigun JR, Frank JA, Barrios FA, et al. Measurement of brain activity with bolus administration of contrast agent and gradient-echo MR imaging. *Radiology* 1993;186:353–356.
37. Warach S, Li W, Ronthal M, Edelman RR. Acute cerebral ischemia: evaluation with dynamic contrast-enhanced MR imaging and MR angiography. *Radiology* 1992;182:41–47.
38. Villringer A, Rosen RB, Belliveau JW, et al. Dynamic imaging with lanthanide chelates in normal brain: contrast due to magnetic susceptibility effects. *Magn Reson Med* 1988;6:164–174.
39. Frahm J, Merboldt K-D, Hanicke W. Localized proton spectroscopy using stimulated echoes. *J Magn Reson* 1987;72:502–508.
40. Kimmich R, Hoepfel D. Volume-selective multipulse spin-echo spectroscopy. *J Magn Reson* 1987;72:379–384.
41. Kanal E, Shellock FG. Patient monitoring during clinical MR imaging. *Radiology* 1992;185:623–629.

CHAPTER 2

Normal Development of the Neonatal and Infant Brain, Skull, and Spine

The brain matures in an organized, predetermined pattern that correlates with the functions the newborn or infant performs at various stages of development. The myelination of white matter is an important component of brain maturation because it facilitates the transmission of neural impulses through the central nervous system. Before the development of x-ray computed tomography (CT) and magnetic resonance imaging (MR), it was impossible to analyze normal brain maturation *in vivo*. Only autopsy studies had been performed, and they suffered from skewing of the sample population by the various causes of infant demise. Both CT and MR show gross morphologic changes in the maturing brain; however, only the high-contrast resolution of MR permits highly sensitive assessment of gray and white matter changes. Imaging correlations of the changes that occur during normal brain maturation will be described in this chapter.

NORMAL PRENATAL BRAIN DEVELOPMENT

Embryology

The bilateral cerebral vesicles that will form the cerebral hemispheres first appear at about 35 days of gesta-

tion as out-pouchings of the telencephalon from the regions of the foramina of Monro. At this time, the walls of the vesicles are uniformly thin and are connected in the midline by the lamina terminalis. The lamina terminalis does not grow; however, the cerebral vesicles exhibit marked expansion laterally, rostrally, ventrally, and caudally. As the vesicles expand, cellular layers develop within their walls, forming the germinal matrices from which the cells that form the cerebrum will eventually develop. Vascular areas develop on the dorsal medial aspect of each vesicle, marking the primordia of the choroid plexuses of the lateral ventricles. Details of the development of the hemispheres are described in more detail in Chapter 5. For the purposes of the discussion to follow, it is sufficient to understand that the occipital pole begins to develop at about the 43rd gestational day and the temporal pole at approximately the 50th gestational day. During the early weeks of gestation, the surfaces of the cerebral hemispheres are smooth. The fetal sulci appear in an orderly sequence; the phylogenetically older sulci appear first, and the more recently acquired sulci appear later. The principal sulci and gyri form the characteristic pattern of the human cortex that can be identified in the full-term infant. The primitive Sylvian fissure, the earliest fetal sulcus, first appears during the

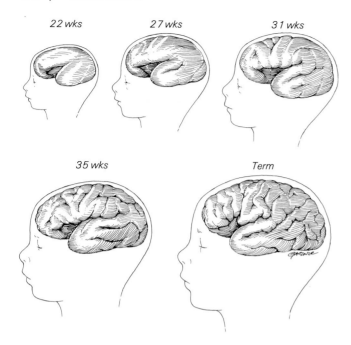

22 wks   27 wks   31 wks

35 wks   Term

FIG. 2.1. Schematic demonstrating normal development of the fetal brain. During the early weeks of gestation, the cerebral hemispheres are smooth. The earliest fetal sulcus is the Sylvian fissure, which first appears during the fifth gestational month. By about 27 weeks, the rolandic, interparietal, and superior temporal sulci have appeared. Secondary and tertiary sulci develop during the last 2 months of gestation. Because of the different appearance of the brain in premature infants as compared with term infants, it is important to know the gestational age of a child at the time of delivery before assessing the structure of the brain.

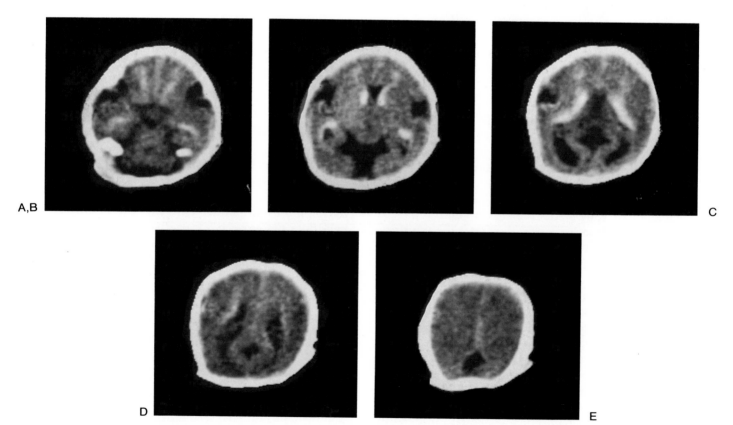

A,B

C

D

E

FIG. 2.2. CT of normal 24-week premature infant. **A:** Axial image through the level of the fourth ventricle shows a large subarachnoid space around the cerebellum and wide Sylvian fissures. The fourth ventricle is visible, an unusual finding at this age. **B:** The germinal matrix adjacent to the frontal horns and the atria of the lateral ventricles is quite prominent because this is a post mortem CT. The interhemispheric fissure is prominent posteriorly. **C:** The germinal matrix has an extremely high attenuation along the bodies of the lateral ventricles. The occipital horns are dilated, a normal finding at this age. **D:** At this level, the normally dilated occipital horns of the lateral ventricles are well visualized. **E:** Near the vertex, the posterior interhemispheric fissure remains prominent. This is probably the result of incomplete development of the occipital lobes and remains a feature of the normal brain through term and for several months postnatally. (These images are courtesy of Dr. C. Fitz.)

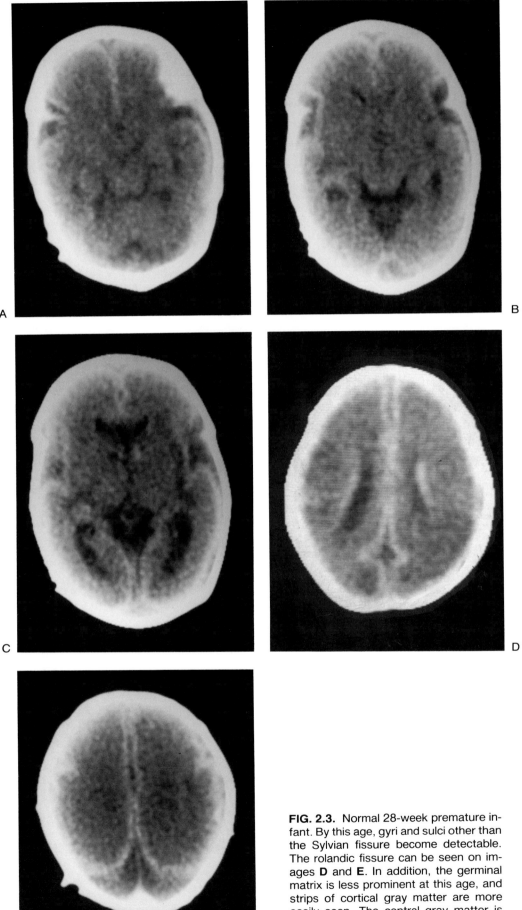

FIG. 2.3. Normal 28-week premature infant. By this age, gyri and sulci other than the Sylvian fissure become detectable. The rolandic fissure can be seen on images **D** and **E**. In addition, the germinal matrix is less prominent at this age, and strips of cortical gray matter are more easily seen. The central gray matter is more easily visible at this age.

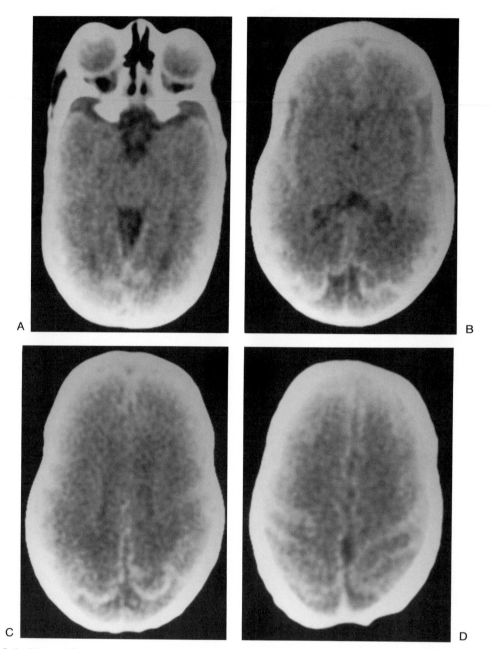

FIG. 2.4. Normal 31-week premature infant. The cortex is somewhat thicker and therefore more easily seen on CT **(A–D)**. Moreover, there is more sulcal formation by this age. This is most apparent in the areas around the rolandic fissure and in the parieto-occipital region. The gray matter of the basal ganglia and thalami has higher attenuation at this age, resulting in an appearance of very-low-density white matter in the frontal, temporo-occipital, and parietal regions. The occipital horns remain prominent.

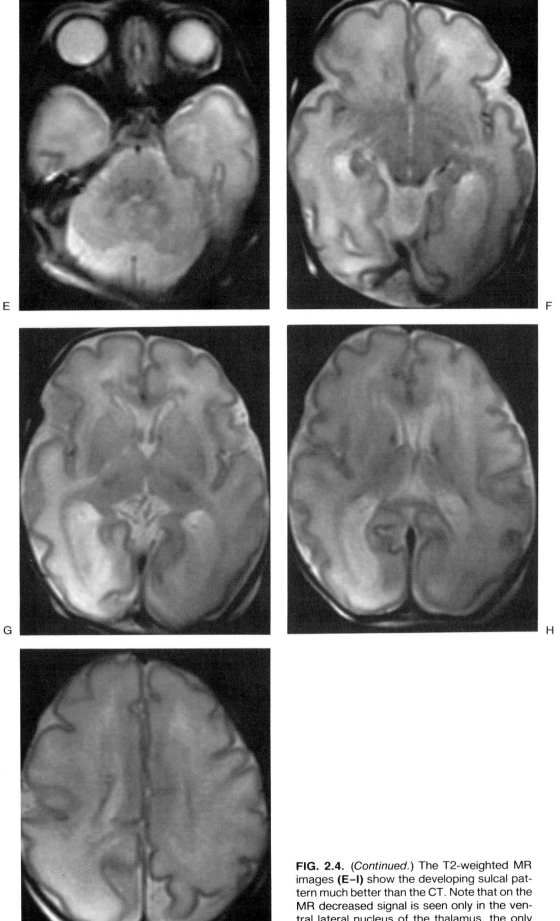

FIG. 2.4. (*Continued.*) The T2-weighted MR images **(E–I)** show the developing sulcal pattern much better than the CT. Note that on the MR decreased signal is seen only in the ventral lateral nucleus of the thalamus, the only myelinated supratentorial structure at this age.

E

F

G

H

I

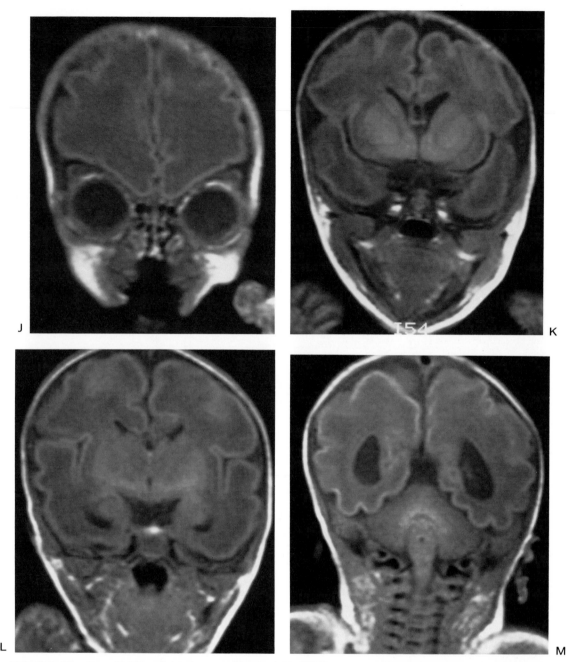

FIG. 2.4. (*Continued.*) T1-weighted coronal images **(J–M)** show some high signal in the cerebellar peduncles, indicating myelination in those structures.

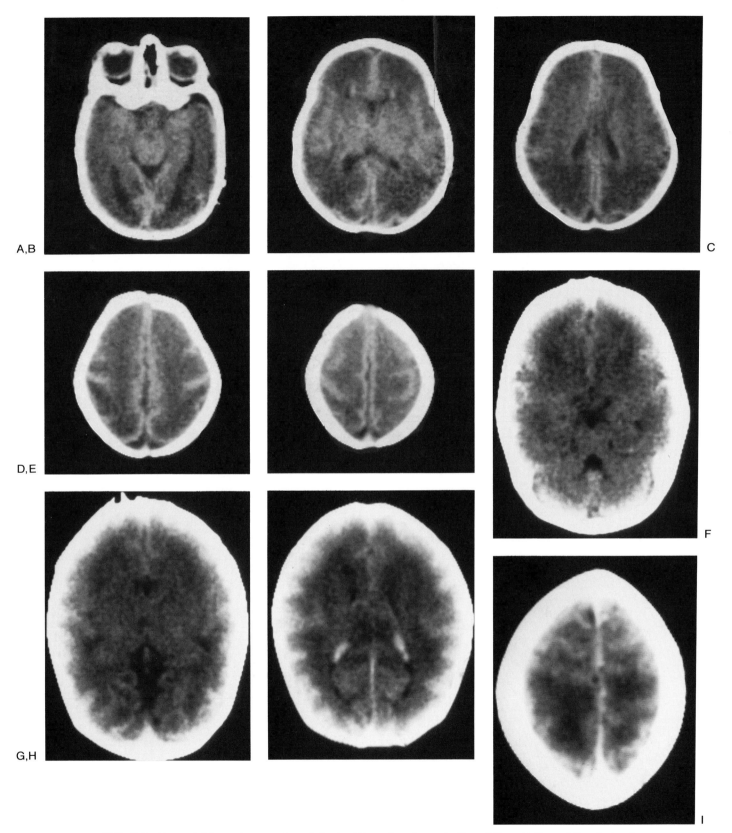

FIG. 2.5. Normal 34-week premature infants. There has been further differentiation of the thalamic-basal ganglia region on CT. Moreover, gray matter is now visible in the inferior operculum. More sulci are forming, as can be seen along the interhemispheric fissure, as well as over the convexities. The Sylvian fissures have markedly diminished in prominence. The frontal lobes still remain essentially agyric. There is significant variation in development at this age. The patient illustrated in figures **A–E** shows less gyral development and lower signal intensity of the white matter than the infant shown in **F–J** (see **J** on next page).

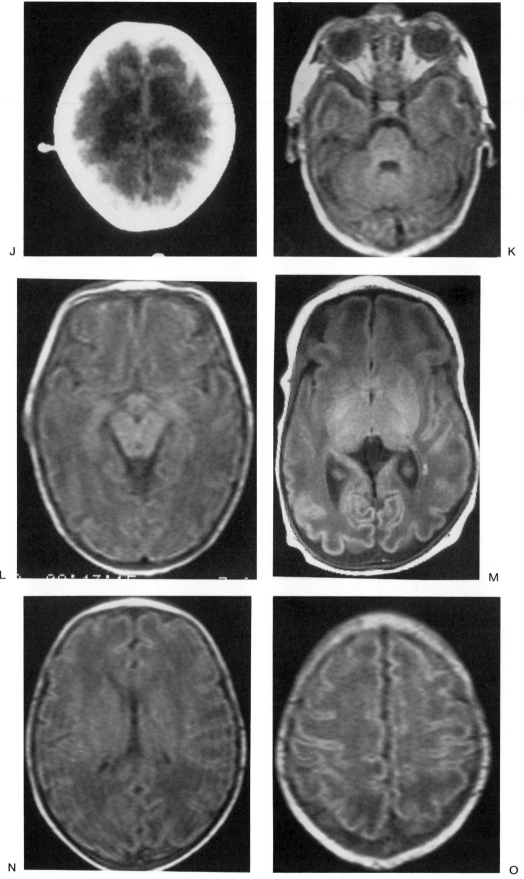

FIG. 2.5. (*Continued.*)Notice on the axial T1-weighted MR **(K–O)** how dorsal brain stem and lentiform nuclei have increased in intensity.

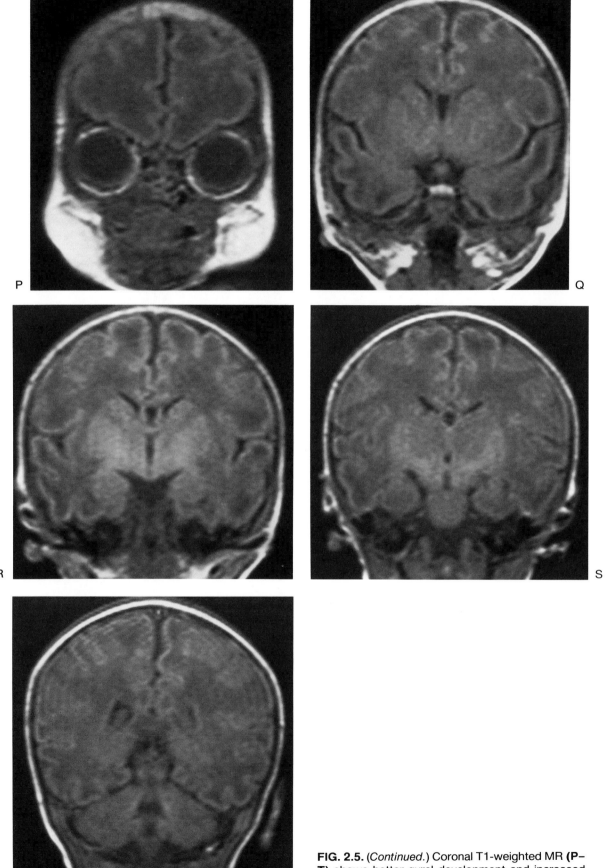

FIG. 2.5. (*Continued.*) Coronal T1-weighted MR (**P–T**) shows better gyral development and increased signal in the inferior corticospinal tracts.

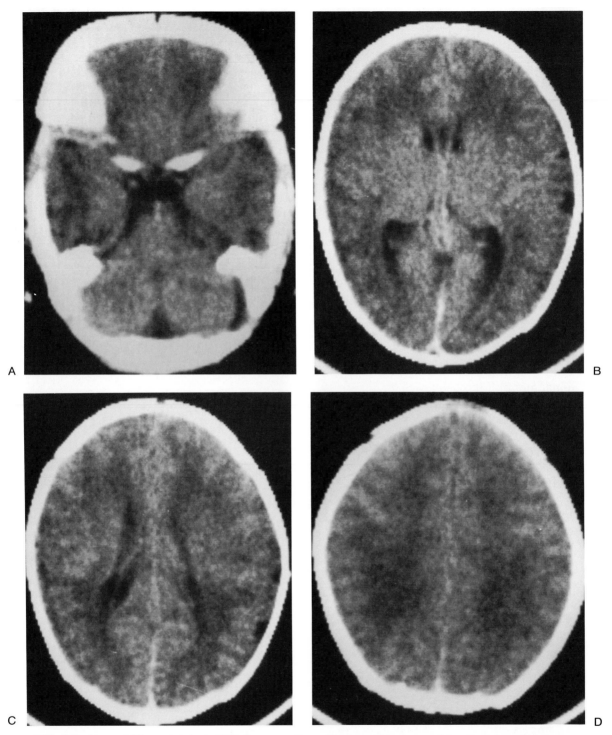

FIG. 2.6. Normal 38-week infant. With the exception of increased lucency of the frontal and temporo-parieto-occipital white matter, the CT scan of this infant resembles any normal infant during the first year of life. The cavum septi pellucidi is always prominent at this age. The MR scan **(E)** shows that the cortical sulcal pattern is not as well developed as in the 42-week term infant (Fig 2.7).

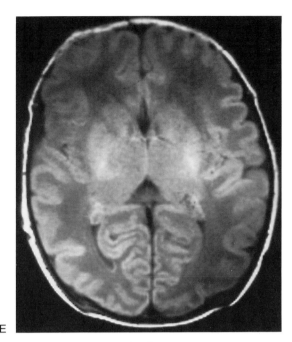

E

FIG. 2.6. *Continued.*

fifth gestational month. This is followed by the rolandic (central), interparietal, and superior temporal sulci, which appear toward the end of the sixth and beginning of the seventh gestational months (1) (Fig. 2.1). Because sulcal formation occurs so late in gestation, CT and MR studies of premature infants show sulci that are shallow and few in number. *It is therefore important to know the gestational age of a child at the time of delivery before assessing the sulcal pattern.* Otherwise a false diagnosis of lissencephaly may be made.

CT and MR of the Premature Brain

Before 28 weeks of gestation, the brain viewed by CT or MR is essentially agyric, with the exception of the wide, vertically oriented Sylvian fissures. The cerebral cortex is extremely thin, and the sections adjacent to the calvarium are barely visible on CT. The thin, cortical stripe is more easily identified in the insular and interhemispheric regions as a tissue of relatively high attenuation in comparison to white matter (Fig. 2.2). On MR, short TR/TE images show the cortex to be very hyperintense with respect to the underlying white matter. Before 28 weeks, the germinal matrix has not yet involuted and is visible on CT as an area of high density (significantly higher than gray or white matter) along the lateral surface of the lateral ventricles. The germinal matrix is thickest at the region of the caudate heads (the last portion of the matrix to involute, also called the *ganglionic eminence*) and should not be mistaken for a germinal matrix hemorrhage at this location. For unknown reasons, germinal matrix is poorly seen on MR (2). The lat-

eral ventricles and the cisterns around the brain stem and cerebellum are visible and more prominent at this age than in the mature infant. The third and fourth ventricles are often not visualized on routine imaging studies at this age because the size of the brain is so small (2,3).

By *28 to 30 weeks,* gyri and sulci other than the Sylvian fissure became detectable. The rolandic and the parieto-occipital fissures may be seen as infoldings of the cortex in the lateral and posteromedial aspects of the hemispheres (Fig. 2.3). The Sylvian fissures retain their immature appearance. The germinal matrix has involuted to some degree, but some high attenuation remains along the lateral walls of the lateral ventricles on CT, most prominently seen in the region of the caudate heads (Fig. 2.3). The cisterns around the brain stem and cerebellum remain large at this age and the CSF spaces in the occipital region and in the interhemispheric fissure remain prominent. The cavum septi pellucidi and cavum Vergae are prominent and will remain so throughout the first 40 postconceptual weeks (2,3).

At *32–33 weeks* of gestation, a large number of cortical sulci become visible. The cerebral cortex thickens and the gyral pattern becomes more pronounced, permitting improved visualization of the cortex on CT (Fig. 2.4). The CSF spaces remain prominent in the Sylvian and occipital regions, but the interhemispheric fissure and posterior fossa cisterns are considerably smaller at this age. The germinal matrix continues to involute but can still be seen on CT in the region of the caudate heads as an area of increased attenuation. The thalami and basal ganglia are well defined and easily identified for the first time. On T1-weighted MR, they are of high intensity compared to the hemispheric white matter but cannot be distinguished from the internal capsule at this age (2,3) (Fig. 2.4). T2-weighted MR shows hypointensity in the ventrolateral thalamic nucleus.

At *35 or 36 weeks,* the cerebral cortex has further thickened, and more gyri have developed. The density of the basal ganglia and thalami increase on CT, accentuating the relative lucency of the hemispheric white matter, which is most pronounced in the frontal and parieto-occipital regions (Fig. 2.5). On T1-weighted MR, the internal capsule is iso- to slightly hyperintense as compared to the lentiform nucleus. By this age, the germinal matrix has usually completely involuted. The Sylvian fissures and, to a lesser extent, the CSF spaces near the occipital pole, remain prominent. The fourth ventricle is routinely identified on posterior fossa images. Considerable variation in brain maturity can be seen at this age, with some infants having a gyral pattern that resembles a term infant and others still appearing quite immature (2,3).

By *38–40 weeks,* the brain has a nearly normal adult sulcal pattern (Fig. 2.6); the sulci are formed but are not as deep as they will become in the next several weeks. On T1-weighted MR studies, the dorsal brainstem, internal capsule (posterior limb), and central portion of the corona radiata are hyperintense compared to the rest of the brain. There are few differences between the CT images of a newborn term infant and those of older infants. The frontal white matter and parieto-occipital white matter remain relatively low in attenuation compared to the gray matter (Fig. 2.7). This probably results from the known high water content of the newborn brain and the lack of myelination. The MR appearance of the newborn brain, on the other hand, is considerably different from that in older children, as discussed in the following section. The Sylvian fissures may remain prominent in the immediate newborn period; the occipital CSF spaces may also remain somewhat large for several months. A cavum vergae and cavum septi pellucidi are usually present at birth; they disappear rapidly after birth as the septal leaves fuse.

The cisterna magna and basilar cisterns are relatively large throughout infancy. This enlargement is quite apparent on MR scans but less so on CT, where only the axial plane is available and beam-hardening artifact frequently obscures details in the basilar cistern area.

NORMAL POSTNATAL BRAIN DEVELOPMENT

Embryology

From the imaging perspective, postnatal brain development consists primarily of changes in signal intensity secondary to the process of myelination. Pathologically, myelination of the brain begins during the fifth fetal month with the myelination of the cranial nerves and continues throughout life. In general, the myelination progresses from caudal to cephalad, and from dorsal to ventral. The brain stem therefore myelinates prior to the cerebellum and basal ganglia. Similarly, the cerebellum and basal ganglia myelinate prior to the cerebral hemispheres. Another generalization is that, within any particular portion of the brain, the posterior region tends to myelinate first. Therefore, the dorsal brain stem, containing the medial lemniscus and medial longitudinal fasciculus, myelinates prior to the ventral brain stem, which contains the corticospinal tracts. Likewise, the occipital lobes of the cerebral hemispheres myelinate early, whereas the frontal lobes myelinate late.

Another general trend in the maturation of the brain is that myelination of fiber systems mediating sensory input to the thalamus and the cerebral cortex precedes myelination of those fiber systems carrying cortical impulses relating to movement. Therefore, in the brain stem the medial longitudinal fasciculus, lateral and medial lemnisci, and inferior and superior cerebellar peduncles, which transmit vestibular, acoustic, tactile, and proprioceptive sense, are myelinated at birth, whereas the middle cerebellar peduncles, which transmit motor im-

pulses into the cerebellum, acquire myelin later and more slowly. Similarly, in the cerebrum, the geniculate and calcarine (optic), postcentral (somesthetic), and precentral (propriokinesthetic) regions acquire myelin early, whereas the posterior parietal, temporal, and frontal areas, which integrate the sensory experience, acquire myelin later (4–7). Yakovlev and Lecours (7), staining the brain with the Weigert stain for myelin, showed that myelination proceeds rapidly within the brain up to about two years of age. The process slows markedly after 2 years, although fibers to and from the association of areas of the brain continue to myelinate well into the third and fourth decades of life.

MR of Postnatal Brain Development

In general, changes in white matter maturation are seen best on T1-weighted images during the first 6–8 months of life and on the second echo of T2-weighted images between the ages of 6 and 18 months. Maturation of both the brain stem and cerebellum seems to be more sensitively assessed on T2-weighted images (8,9). We obtain both T1- and T2-weighted axial sequences for imaging patients in these age groups, using conventional spin echo sequences. Our parameters are a maximum TR of 600 msec and a maximum TE of 20 msec for T1-weighted images and a TR of 3,000 msec and TEs of 60 (first echo) and 120 msec (second echo) for T2-weighted images. Other imaging sequences that give heavily T1-weighted and T2-weighted sequences will work as well. The rationale for obtaining both sequences and some suggested alternate sequences were explained in Chapter 1.

T1-Weighted Images

Brain maturation occurs at different rates and at different times on the T1-weighted images than on the T2-weighted images. On short TR/TE images, the appearance of the newborn brain is similar to that of long TR/TE images in adults in that white matter is of lower signal intensity than gray matter. With maturation, the intensity of white matter increases relative to gray matter.

Neonatal posterior fossa structures that exhibit high signal intensity at birth include the dorsal brain stem and the inferior and superior cerebellar peduncles (Fig. 2.7). An increase in signal intensity of the deep cerebellar white matter appears near the end of the first month of life and steadily increases, with high signal intensity developing in the subcortical white matter of the cerebellar folia by the third month. At 3 months of age, the cerebellum has an appearance similar to that seen in the adult on both axial and sagittal images. Signal intensity in the

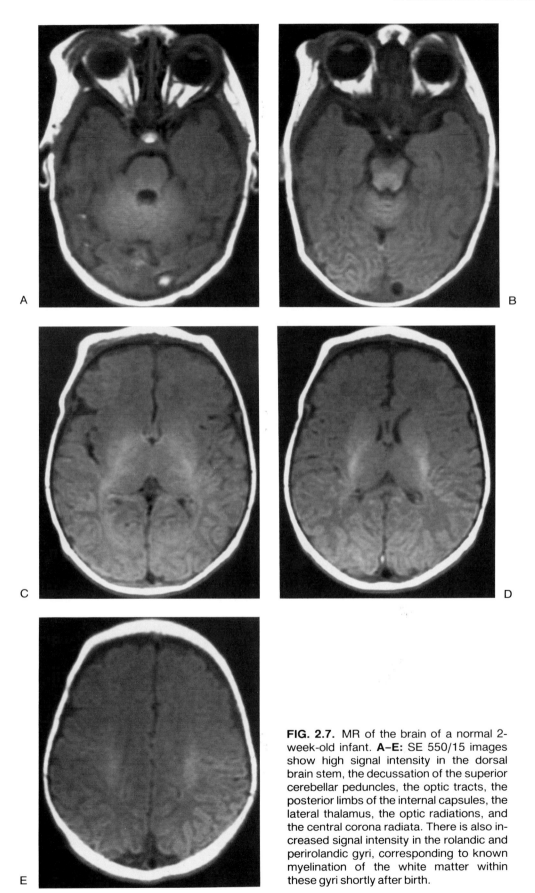

FIG. 2.7. MR of the brain of a normal 2-week-old infant. **A–E:** SE 550/15 images show high signal intensity in the dorsal brain stem, the decussation of the superior cerebellar peduncles, the optic tracts, the posterior limbs of the internal capsules, the lateral thalamus, the optic radiations, and the central corona radiata. There is also increased signal intensity in the rolandic and perirolandic gyri, corresponding to known myelination of the white matter within these gyri shortly after birth.

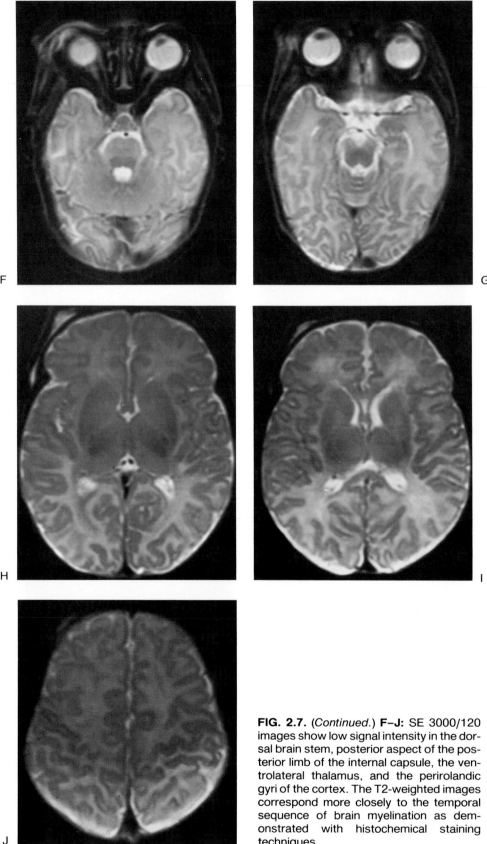

FIG. 2.7. (*Continued.*) **F–J:** SE 3000/120 images show low signal intensity in the dorsal brain stem, posterior aspect of the posterior limb of the internal capsule, the ventrolateral thalamus, and the perirolandic gyri of the cortex. The T2-weighted images correspond more closely to the temporal sequence of brain myelination as demonstrated with histochemical staining techniques.

basis pontis (ventral pons) increases less rapidly, occurring during the third through the sixth months.

In the supratentorial region, the decussation of the superior cerebellar peduncles, the ventral lateral region of the thalamus, the dorsal putamen, and the posterior limb of the internal capsule exhibit high signal intensity at birth (Fig. 2.7). The development of high signal intensity proceeds rostrally from the pons along the corticospinal tracts into the cerebral peduncles, the posterior limb of the internal capsule, and the central portion of the centrum semiovale. The white matter of the pre- and postcentral gyri are of high signal intensity compared with surrounding cortex by about 1 month of age (Fig. 2.7). The change to high signal intensity in the subcortical motor tracts is essentially complete by age 3 months. In infants less than 1 month old, high signal intensity is present in the optic nerve, optic tracts, and optic radiations; by age 3 months, the occipital white matter surrounding the calcarine fissure is of high signal intensity. The posterior limb of the internal capsule is of high signal intensity at birth; high signal intensity does not develop in the anterior limb until 2–3 months of age. The splenium of the corpus callosum shows high signal intensity in all infants by 4 months (Fig. 2.8). The increase in signal intensity proceeds rostrally; the genu is always of high signal intensity by age 6 months (Fig. 2.9). Typically, at 4–5 months of age the splenium is high in signal intensity, and the genu is low in signal intensity. Maturation of the subcortical white matter, other than the visual and motor regions, begins at 3 months. The deep white matter matures in a posterior-to-anterior direction, with the deep occipital white matter maturing first and the frontal and temporal white matter last. Peripheral extension and increasing complexity of arborization of the subcortical white matter continues until approximately age 7 months in the occipital white matter and 8–11 months in the frontal and temporal white matter (Fig. 2.10). Only minimal changes are seen on the T1-weighted images after 8 months, consisting of increasing signal intensity in the most peripheral regions of the frontal, temporal, and parietal white matter (4).

T2-Weighted Images

The overall appearance of the newborn brain on T2-weighted images is similar to that of adult T1-weighted images in that the white matter has a higher signal intensity than the gray matter. On T2-weighted sequences, white matter maturation is seen as a reduction in signal intensity. As stated earlier, T2-weighted images are probably superior to T1-weighted images for assessment of maturation of the cerebellum (10) and brain stem (8).

At birth, the inferior and superior cerebellar peduncles and the dorsal brain stem are of low signal intensity (Fig. 2.7). The middle cerebellar peduncles begin to decrease

in signal intensity during the second to third months of life. Arborization (low signal intensity developing in the subcortical white matter of the cerebellar folia) begins to develop within the cerebellum at approximately the eighth month, and the cerebellum reaches an adult appearance at approximately 18 months.

Supratentorial structures that show low signal intensity at birth include the decussation of the superior cerebellar peduncles, the ventral lateral region of the thalamus, small patches of the posterior portion of the posterior limb of the internal capsule, and, to a limited extent, the posterior putamen. By less than 1 month of age, the cortex in the pre- and postcentral gyri has lower intensity than the surrounding cortex (Fig. 2.7). By age 2 months, patches of low signal intensity are seen in the central centrum semiovale, but the paracentral gyri are harder to distinguish from the surrounding gyri because the adjacent gyri and subjacent white matter are diminished in intensity. By age 4 months, the intensity of the paracentral gyri is indistinguishable from that of adjacent gyri (Fig. 2.8). Low signal intensity is seen in the optic tracts at age 1 month; the decrease in signal intensity extends posteriorly along the optic radiations during the subsequent 2 months; by 4 months of age, the calcarine fissure shows some low signal intensity.

Most deep white matter tracts of the cerebrum decrease in signal intensity between 6 and 12 months of age (Figs. 2.9–2.12). The internal capsule matures in a posterior to anterior fashion. The more anterior portion of the posterior limb contains a thin strip of hypointensity by approximately 7 months; progressive thickening of the hypointense area continues up to 10 months of age. The anterior limb of the internal capsule is completely hypointense by 11 months in all patients; hypointensity can be detected as early as 7 months in some patients but is always preceded by detectability of low signal intensity in the posterior limb. The corpus callosum matures from posterior to anterior; the splenium shows low signal intensity by age 6 months and the genu by age 8 months (Figs. 2.9, 2.10). The basal ganglia begin to diminish in signal intensity relative to the subcortical white matter at 7 months of age. This appearance gradually fades as the surrounding brain decreases in signal intensity as a result of myelination. The basal ganglia appear essentially isointense with the subcortical white matter by the age of approximately 10 months (Fig. 2.11). The globus pallidus will become hypointense with respect to white matter again around the end of the first decade of life; this decrease in intensity results from iron deposition and will be described later in this chapter.

The subcortical white matter (other than the calcarine and rolandic areas) matures last, proceeding from the occipital region anteriorly to the frontal and temporal lobes. This process begins at 9–12 months of age in the occipital lobe and at 11–14 months frontally (Figs. 2.12, 2.13); temporal lobe white matter matures last. Periph-

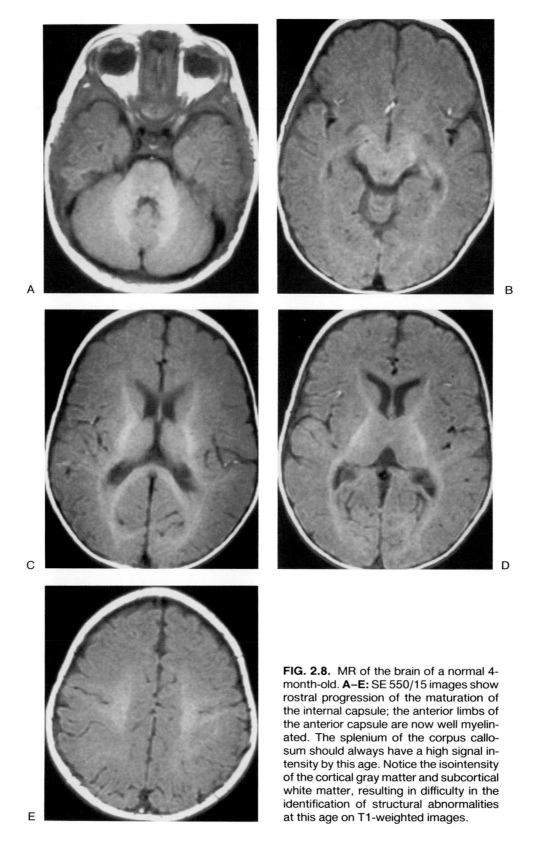

FIG. 2.8. MR of the brain of a normal 4-month-old. **A–E:** SE 550/15 images show rostral progression of the maturation of the internal capsule; the anterior limbs of the anterior capsule are now well myelinated. The splenium of the corpus callosum should always have a high signal intensity by this age. Notice the isointensity of the cortical gray matter and subcortical white matter, resulting in difficulty in the identification of structural abnormalities at this age on T1-weighted images.

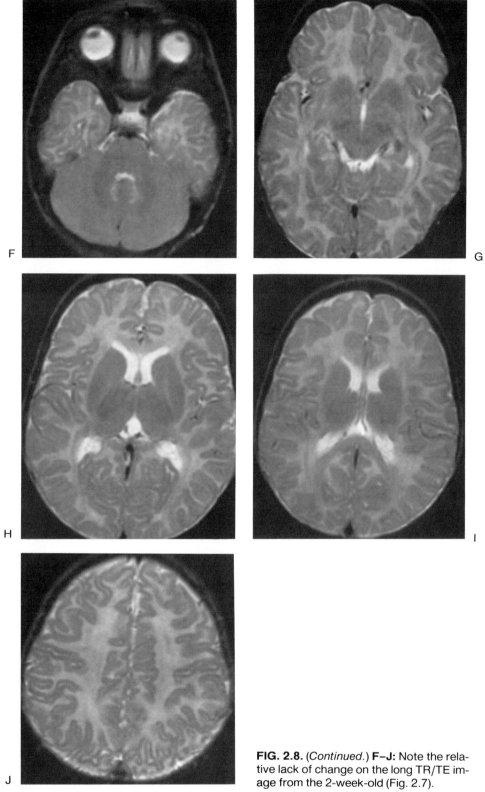

FIG. 2.8. (*Continued.*) **F–J**: Note the relative lack of change on the long TR/TE image from the 2-week-old (Fig. 2.7).

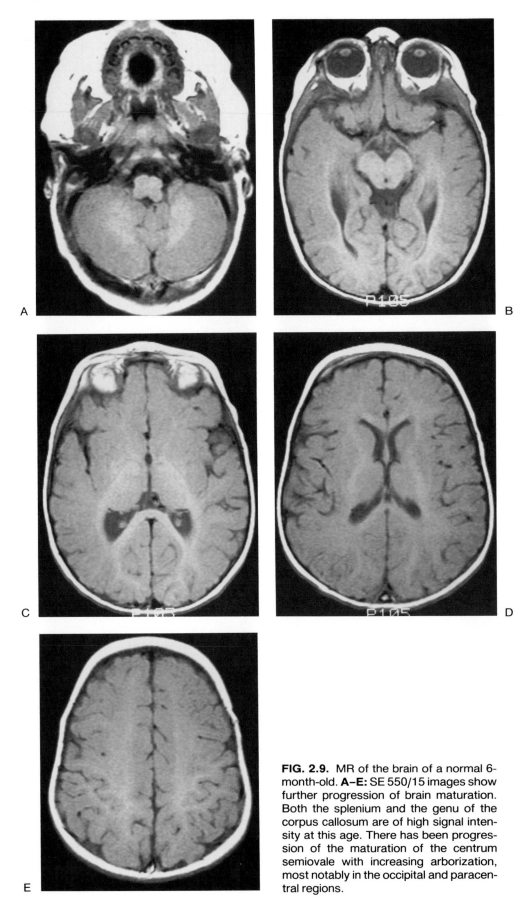

FIG. 2.9. MR of the brain of a normal 6-month-old. **A–E:** SE 550/15 images show further progression of brain maturation. Both the splenium and the genu of the corpus callosum are of high signal intensity at this age. There has been progression of the maturation of the centrum semiovale with increasing arborization, most notably in the occipital and paracentral regions.

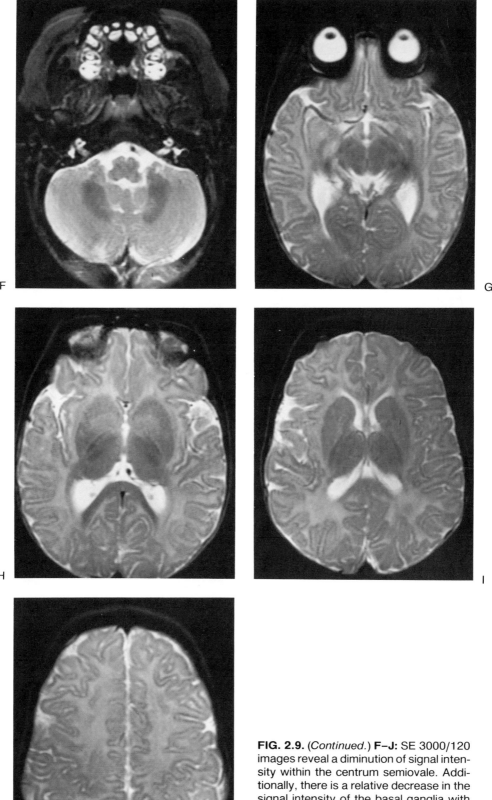

FIG. 2.9. (*Continued.*) **F–J:** SE 3000/120 images reveal a diminution of signal intensity within the centrum semiovale. Additionally, there is a relative decrease in the signal intensity of the basal ganglia with respect to the surrounding brain. The splenium of the corpus callosum is of low signal intensity at this age, and there are patches of low signal intensity within the callosal genu.

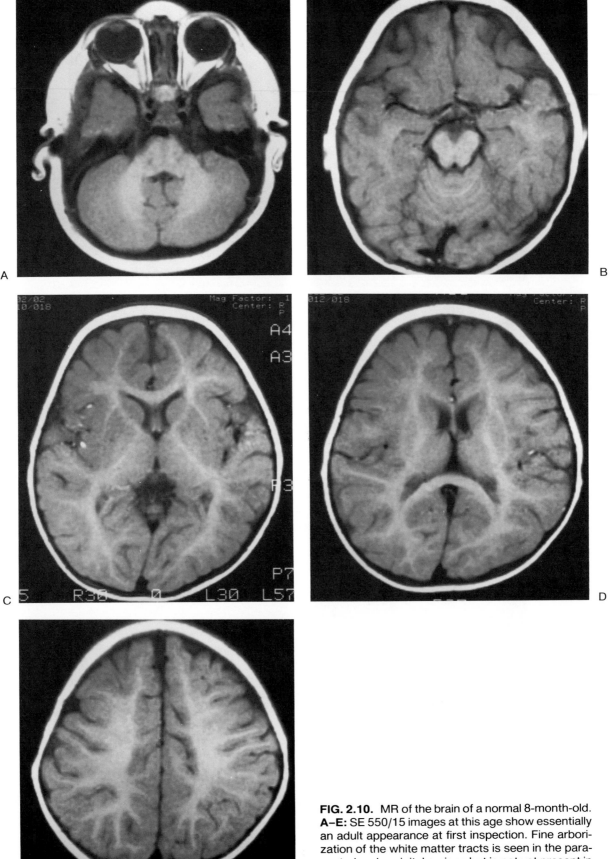

FIG. 2.10. MR of the brain of a normal 8-month-old. **A–E:** SE 550/15 images at this age show essentially an adult appearance at first inspection. Fine arborization of the white matter tracts is seen in the paracentral and occipital regions but is not yet present in the frontal or parietal regions.

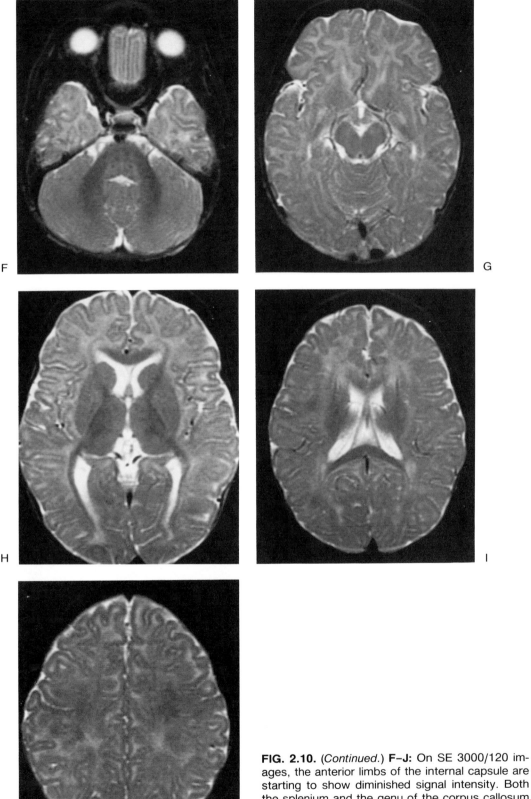

FIG. 2.10. (*Continued.*) **F–J:** On SE 3000/120 images, the anterior limbs of the internal capsule are starting to show diminished signal intensity. Both the splenium and the genu of the corpus callosum are of low signal intensity at this age. The white matter in the occipital and paracentral regions is now isointense with the overlying cortex.

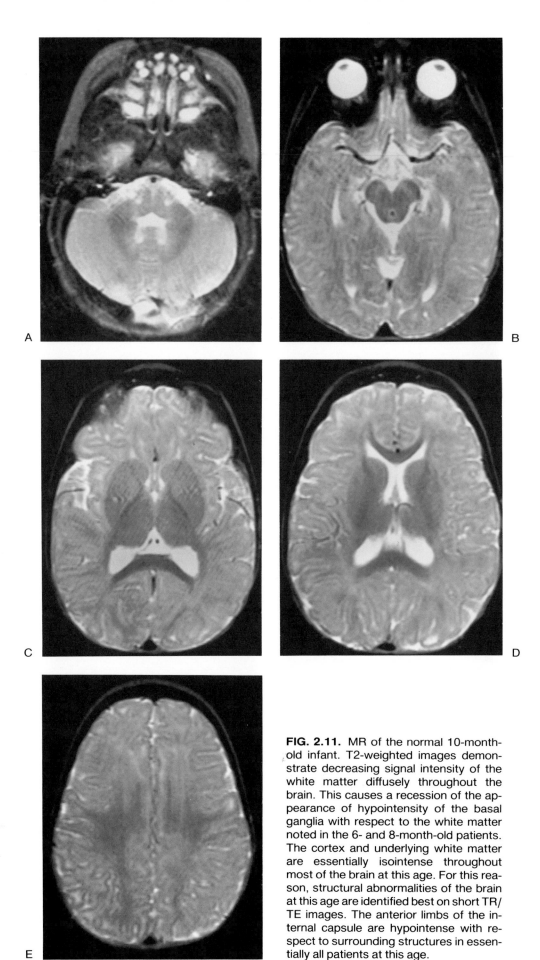

FIG. 2.11. MR of the normal 10-month-old infant. T2-weighted images demonstrate decreasing signal intensity of the white matter diffusely throughout the brain. This causes a recession of the appearance of hypointensity of the basal ganglia with respect to the white matter noted in the 6- and 8-month-old patients. The cortex and underlying white matter are essentially isointense throughout most of the brain at this age. For this reason, structural abnormalities of the brain at this age are identified best on short TR/TE images. The anterior limbs of the internal capsule are hypointense with respect to surrounding structures in essentially all patients at this age.

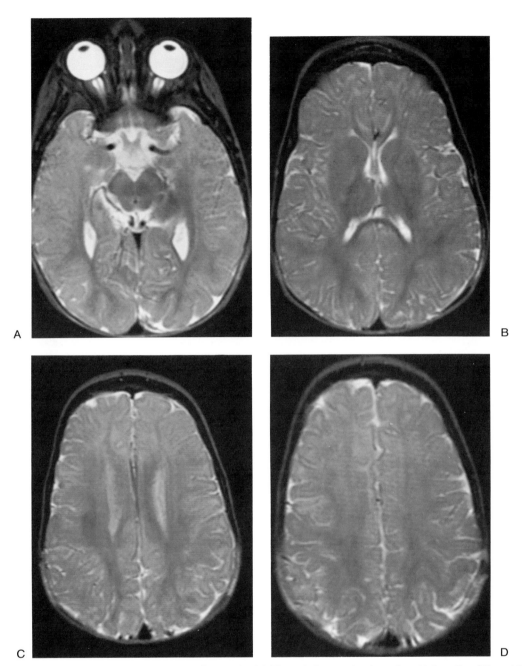

FIG. 2.12. MR of the brain of a normal 12-month-old. There is increasing low signal intensity of the white matter in the paracentral and occipital regions. The images are otherwise very similar to those of the 10-month-old infant.

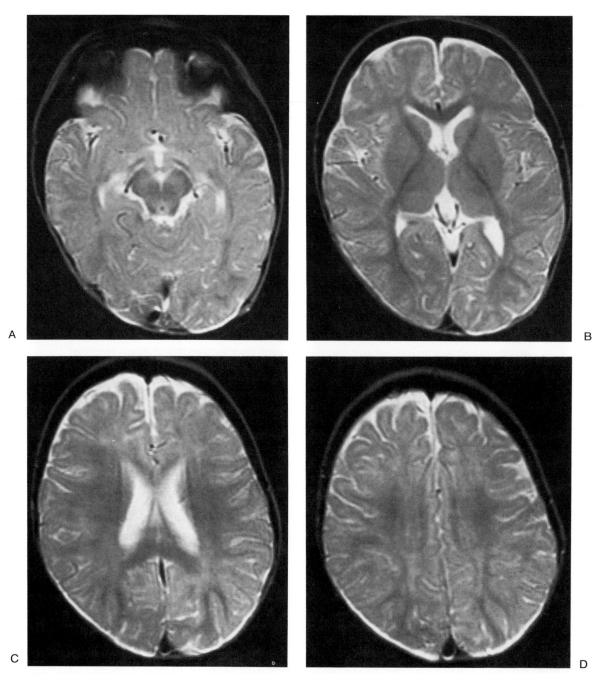

FIG. 2.13. MR of the brain of a normal 15-month-old. The maturation of the deep white matter has progressed significantly since the 12-month-old stage. Although somewhat patchy, the supratentorial white matter now shows a great deal of arborization throughout the hemispheres. The arborization and maturation of the white matter is slowest in the frontal regions.

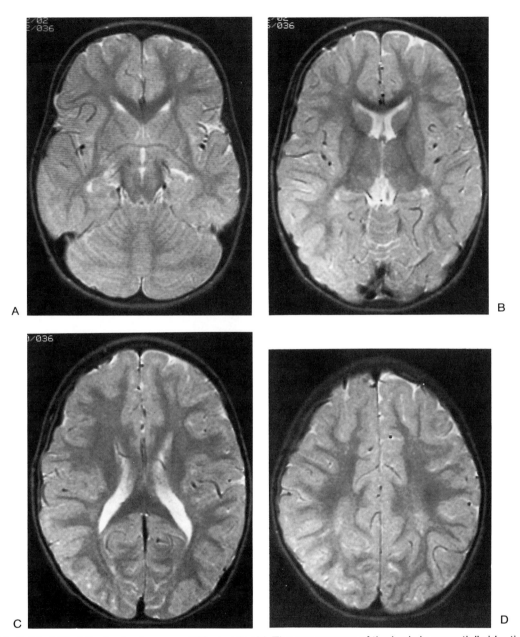

FIG. 2.14. MR of the brain of a normal 22-month-old. The appearance of the brain is essentially identical to that of an adult. Notice, however, that there is still some patchy high-signal intensity parallel to the lateral ventricles. This is most prominent dorsal to the bodies and trigones of the lateral ventricles.

eral extension of the low signal intensity into the subcortical white matter begins at about 1 year and is essentially complete by 22–24 months (Fig. 2.14). Thus, with the exception of the so-called terminal zones (see the next section), white matter maturation, as assessed by MR, is complete by the end of the second year of life. During the progress of the peripheral extension of the low signal intensity within the white matter, the mantle of gray matter gives the appearance of progressive thinning, and the subcortical white matter often has a heterogeneous appearance.

Terminal Zones

As maturation in the centrum semiovale progresses, nearly all subjects have persistent areas of high signal intensity in the white matter dorsal and superior to the ventricular trigones on long TR/TE images (Fig. 2.15). The margins of these areas are indistinct, and they may extend anteriorly lateral to the bodies of the lateral ventricles. The areas are most often homogeneous, although in some patients they may be patchy. They are more difficult to identify on the first echo of the long TR se-

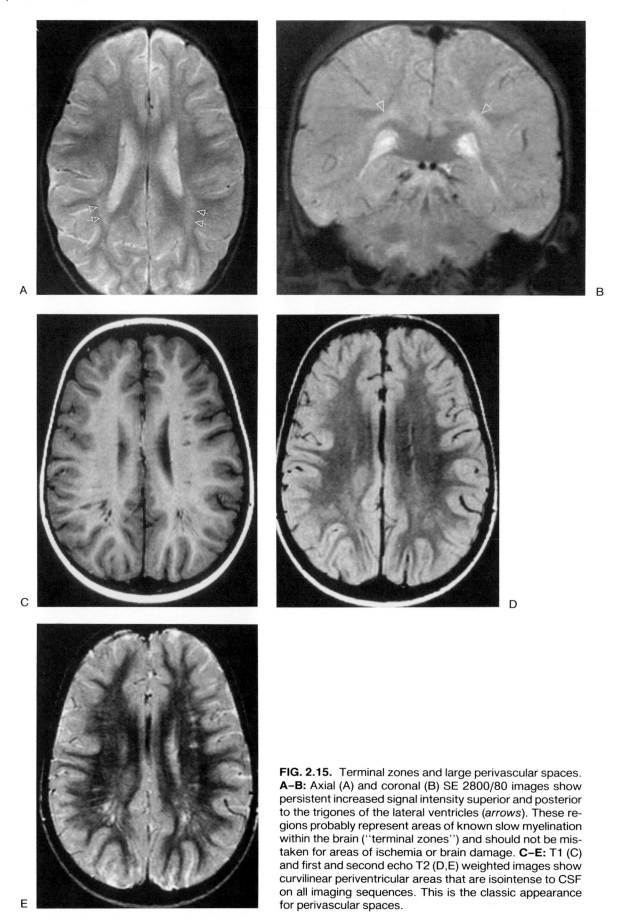

FIG. 2.15. Terminal zones and large perivascular spaces. **A–B:** Axial (A) and coronal (B) SE 2800/80 images show persistent increased signal intensity superior and posterior to the trigones of the lateral ventricles (*arrows*). These regions probably represent areas of known slow myelination within the brain ("terminal zones") and should not be mistaken for areas of ischemia or brain damage. **C–E:** T1 (C) and first and second echo T2 (D,E) weighted images show curvilinear periventricular areas that are isointense to CSF on all imaging sequences. This is the classic appearance for perivascular spaces.

quence than on the second. The cause of this high signal intensity is probably the known delayed myelination of the fiber tracts involving the association areas of the posterior and inferior parietal and posterior temporal cortex. Yakovlev and Lecours have called these regions the "terminal zones" because some of the axons in these regions do not stain for myelin until the fourth decade (7). These areas of persistent high signal intensity are seen throughout the first decade and, in some patients, into the second decade of life.

It is important to differentiate the terminal zones from periventricular leukomalacia (see Chapter 4), which also is associated with areas of prolonged T2 relaxation in the peritrigonal region. In general, the periventricular leukomalacia lesions are more sharply defined. They are situated more inferiorly, lateral to the trigones and near the optic radiations. They are of very high intensity and are easily detected on the first echo of the long TR sequence. Moreover, periventricular leukomalacia is associated with loss of periventricular brain tissue typically resulting in irregularity of the ventricular wall, abnormally deep cortical sulci that may extend down to the ventricular surface, and thinning of the posterior body of the corpus callosum (see examples of periventricular leukomalacia in Chapter 4). Baker and colleagues (11) have suggested that the differentiation between these normal peritrigonal areas of high signal intensity and periventricular leukomalacia is very difficult. They noted, however, that a layer of myelinated white matter is present between the trigone of the ventricle and the terminal zones in normal patients (Fig. 2.15). When the peritrigonal high signal is due to periventricular leukomalacia, this layer of normally myelinated white matter is absent.

Another feature that can mimic both the terminal zones and periventricular leukomalacia on MR is dilated perivascular spaces, which are most commonly seen in the peritrigonal region (Fig. 2.15C–E). Although most patients with dilated perivascular spaces are normal, evidence has been presented that affected patients have a higher incidence of neuropsychiatric disorders than the general pediatric population (12).

Milestones

Barkovich and colleagues (4) charted the ages at which the changes of myelination appeared on T1- and T2-weighted images, as well as normal MR imaging milestones for myelination of brain (Table 2.1). During the first 6 months of life, T1-weighted images are most useful for assessing normal brain maturation. On these short TR/TE images, high signal intensity should appear in the anterior limbs of the internal capsules and should extend distally from deep cerebellar white matter into the cerebellar folia by 3 months of age. The splenium of the cor-

TABLE 2.1. *Ages when changes of myelination appear*

Anatomic region	Age when changes of myelination appear	
	T1-weighted images	T2-weighted images
Middle cerebellar peduncle	Birth	Birth to 2 mo
Cerebral white matter	Birth to 4 mo	3–5 mo
Posterior limb internal capsule		
Anterior portion	Birth	4–7 mo
Posterior portion	Birth	Birth to 2 mo
Anterior limb internal capsule	2–3 mo	7–11 mo
Genu corpus callosum	4–6 mo	5–8 mo
Splenium corpus callosum	3–4 mo	4–6 mo
Occipital white matter		
Central	3–5 mo	9–14 mo
Peripheral	4–7 mo	11–15 mo
Frontal white matter		
Central	3–6 mo	11–16 mo
Peripheral	7–11 mo	14–18 mo
Centrum semiovale	2–6 mo	7–11 mo

pus callosum should be of moderately high signal intensity by the fourth month, and the genu of the corpus callosum should be of high signal intensity by age 6 months. An essentially adult pattern is seen by approximately 8 months of age, with the exception that some of the most peripheral white matter fibers have not acquired high signal intensity. After age 6 months, T2-weighted images are more useful in the assessment of normal brain maturation. On these long TR/TE images, the splenium of the corpus callosum should be of low signal intensity by 6 months of age, the genu of the corpus callosum by 8 months of age, and the anterior limb of the internal capsule by 11 months of age. The deep frontal white matter should be of low signal intensity by age 14 months, and the entire brain should have an adult appearance (except for the most peripheral fibers) by 18 months.

Postulated Causes of T1 and T2 Shortening Associated with Myelination

It is interesting to note that brain maturation occurs at different rates and times on T1-weighted SE images, T2-weighted SE images, and inversion recovery images with short inversion time (STIR) (4,13). The exact reasons for these differences have not been entirely worked out. However, it is known that the T1 shortening correlates temporally with the increase in cholesterol and glycolipids that accompany the formation of myelin from oligodendrocytes (4,14). Furthermore, the T2 shortening correlates temporally with the tightening of the spiral of myelin around the axon (which is associated with conformational changes of myelin proteins and the saturation of polyunsaturated fatty acids within the myelin membranes [i.e., the maturation of the myelin sheath (4,15–17)]). Portions of the proteins, cholesterol, and glycolipids that compose myelin are hydrophilic; that is, they hydrogen-bond strongly with water molecules (18,19). Therefore, it is likely that the initial T1 shortening seen by MR results from an increase in the amount of bound water in the brain (and consequent decrease in the amount of free water) secondary to hydrogen bonding of free water to the accumulating building blocks of myelin. Koenig and colleagues (20) postulate that the T1 shortening is accentuated by a thermally activated transmembrane diffusion of water and, hence, more rapid mixing of free axonal water and bound myelin water molecules. The decrease in signal intensity on the T2-weighted images probably reflects changes in water distribution and, most likely, magnetization transfer resulting from myelin maturation (and the consequent tightening of the spiral of myelin around the axon).

Other Approaches to Brain Maturation by MR

Many different approaches have been used in assessing the changes in T1 and T2 relaxation times of the newborn brain by MR imaging. Some authors (13,21–23) have been largely descriptive. Others (2,4) have tried to quantitate myelination and create milestones of normal myelination by which delayed myelination can be identified. Dietrich and colleagues (24) approached the subject of normal brain maturation by dividing the appearance of the brain on T2-weighted spin echo images into three patterns: (1) infantile (birth to 6 months); (2) isointense (8–12 months); and (3) early adult (10 months onward). In the infantile pattern, the cerebral white matter is hyperintense relative to gray matter, whereas the adult pattern shows hypointense white matter. The appearance of the isointense and early adult patterns is delayed in patients with developmental delay. Bird and colleagues (25) determined that the gray and white matter should be isointense by age 4 months on T1-weighted images and by 9–10 months on T2-weighted images. They considered the age at which gray and white matter are isointense as a critical factor in evaluating patients for developmental delay. Finally, some authors have analyzed the images in terms of patterns and attempted to assess degree of, and delay in, maturation on the basis of the pattern (8,9,26,27). We choose to assess maturation through the use of the normal milestones described earlier. However, any of the methods can be used reliably.

A number of studies (28,29) have postulated the existence of a window of time during which delayed myelination can be detected by MR. This window seems to be between the ages of 4 months and 2 years. Delayed myelination can be detected in patients older than 24 months only when it is very severe.

NORMAL POSTNATAL MR DEVELOPMENT OF THE CORPUS CALLOSUM

The corpus callosum forms between 8 and 20 weeks of gestation. The embryological development is discussed in Chapter 5. Briefly, the corpus callosum develops primarily from anterior to posterior, with the exception of the rostrum. Axons forming the posterior portion of the genu develop first, followed by axons of the body, the splenium, the anterior genu, and, lastly, the rostrum (30). The bed for ingrowth of the callosal fibers forms between approximately 8 and 16 weeks of gestation. Callosal fibers of the genu first cross at approximately 12 weeks; the fibers of the rostrum are the last to cross the midline, doing so at 18–20 weeks of gestation. Although all the components of the corpus callosum are present by 20 weeks, growth of the structure is far from complete. From 20 weeks to term, the length increases 25%; the thickness of the body increases by 30%; and the genu grows by 270% (30). As all the callosal axons are present at the time of birth, the postnatal callosal growth presumably directly reflects the myelination of the axons. Because the corpus callosum is easily evaluated by magnetic resonance imaging, an understanding of the normal postnatal development of the corpus has become important.

The appearance of corpus callosum is quite different in the neonate when compared to the adult; an adult appearance evolves slowly over the first 8–10 months of life. In the neonate, the corpus callosum is thin and flat; the bulbous enlargements seen at the adult genu and splenium are not present (31) (Fig. 2.16A). The first postnatal change is a substantial, albeit variable in time, thickening of the genu, which frequently occurs as early as the second and third months of life. DeLacoste and colleagues (32) have demonstrated that the fibers crossing through the genu come from the inferior frontal and anterior, inferior parietal regions. The enlargement of the genu, therefore, presumably relates to the myelination of the interhemispheric connections of the inferior portions of the precentral and postcentral gyri; these areas, which are involved with basic motor and sensory function, develop early in life.

At birth, the splenium is intermediate in size between the body and the genu of the corpus callosum. It enlarges slowly until the fourth or fifth postnatal month and then rapidly increases in size (Fig. 2.16B, C). By the end of the seventh month, the splenium is equal in size to the genu; it then gradually enlarges in proportion with the genu and the rest of the brain through the remainder of the first year (31) (Fig 2.16C, D). By about 9 months, the

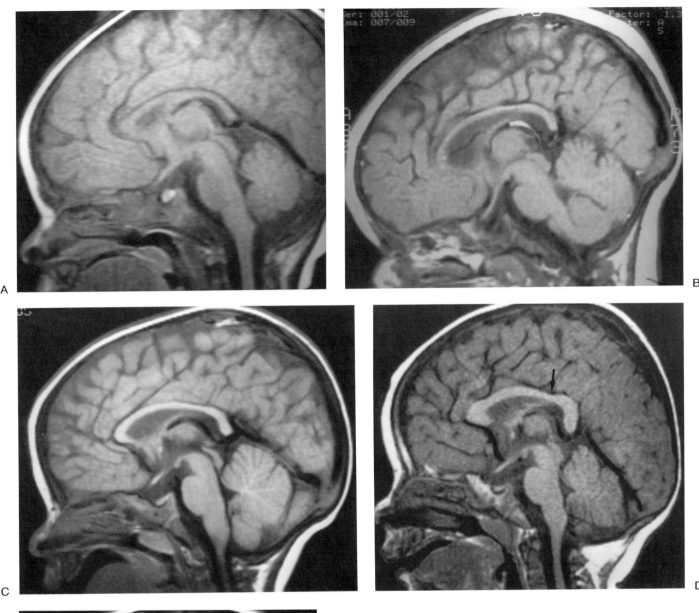

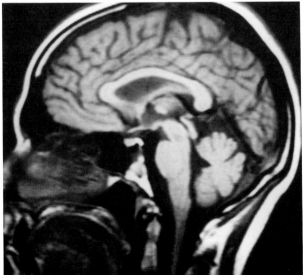

FIG. 2.16. Normal corpus callosum development. **A:** Normal 1-month-old. On this SE 600/20 image, the corpus callosum is isointense with the rest of the brain. The corpus callosum is uniformly thin at this age without the normal bulbous enlargement of the genu and splenium; the genu, body, and splenium are all of the same thickness. **B:** Normal 4-month-old. By 3–4 months of age, the splenium of the corpus callosum increases in size and begins to show an increased signal intensity as compared to the rest of the brain on SE 600/20 images. These changes probably result from the process of myelination in the visual association fibers. **C:** Normal 7-month-old. By 6–7 months of age, the corpus callosum is of a uniformly high signal intensity as compared with surrounding brain. The genu and splenium of the corpus are now large, compared to the body. The corpus is still relatively thin. **D:** Normal 10-month-old. By 8–9 months, the corpus callosum begins to thicken in the genu and splenium, taking on more of an adult appearance. The thinning of the corpus at the junction of the posterior body and splenium (*arrow*) is a normal variant and does not connote pathology. **E:** Normal mature corpus callosum in a 15-year-old.

appearance of the corpus callosum becomes similar to that in the adult (Fig. 2.16E). The fibers in the splenium arise from the visual and visual association areas of the cortex (32). Not surprisingly, the rapid development of the splenium corresponds temporally with increasing visual awareness at 4–6 months of age. It is during this period that the infant develops binocular vision and visual accommodation and begins to identify objects (33). Both binocular vision and object identification are dependent on interhemispheric connection. Thus, the enlargement of the splenium presumably relates to the myelination of connections between the visual cortex and the association areas of the brain in the increasingly visually aware child.

The body of the corpus callosum steadily enlarges throughout childhood without any detectable growth spurts. The size of the body is relatively uniform, except that a focal thinning is frequently seen at the junction of the body and splenium (Fig. 2.16D). This focal thinning is seen in adults as well. McLeod and colleagues (34) found narrowing at this location in 22% of 450 randomly selected patients. The narrowing is almost unquestionably a normal variant.

The absence of significant enlargement of the body compared with the genu and splenium probably represents the anatomic origin of these fibers and the phylogenetic development of the brain. Sensory and visual function are important early in life for all animals. It is therefore unsurprising that the areas of the brain serving these functions myelinate first and that the association tracts related to these functions, which run through the corpus callosum, develop early as well. The more gradual growth of the body of the corpus callosum probably reflects the lesser importance of association areas in the temporal and parietal lobes (from which these fibers originate) in early life and in lower orders of animal life. The fact that the fibers from the association areas myelinate later as well (as seen by the late myelination of the temporal lobes and the persistent areas of prolonged T2 relaxation superior and dorsal to the trigones) further supports this hypothesis.

The length of the corpus callosum changes slowly and erratically during the first year of life. Callosal length seems to vary more with respect to head size and shape than with respect to age (31), probably because normal infants vary more in head size and shape than in head enlargement during the first year of life. This hypothesis is supported by the fact that the ratio of callosal length to AP brain diameter is quite constant in infants throughout the first year of life (31). Because of the insensitivity of callosal length as a marker of normal growth, the changes in callosal shape and signal intensity (see the section on normal myelination) are the preferred means of judging normal maturation of the corpus callosum and, thereby, normal brain development.

NORMAL MR DEVELOPMENT OF THE PITUITARY GLAND

In neonates, the pituitary gland is convex with a shorter T1 than the remainder of the brain (Fig. 2.17A) (35,36). The signal intensity and size slowly diminish until approximately age 2 months of age (Fig. 2.17B), the

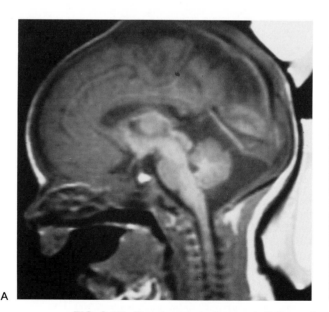
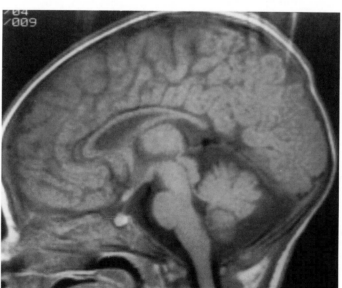

A   B

FIG. 2.17. Development of normal pituitary gland. **A:** Normal newborn pituitary. The gland is upwardly convex and is uniformly bright on T1-weighted images. **B:** Normal infant pituitary gland. By age 2–3 months the adenohypophysis (anterior pituitary) loses its high signal on T1-weighted images, allowing the bright neurohypophysis (posterior pituitary) to be identified as a separate structure.

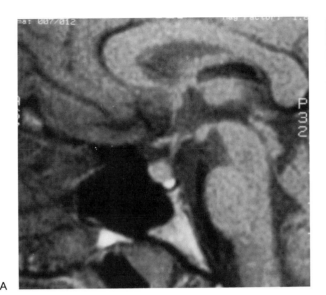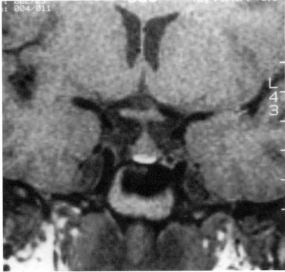

A   B

FIG. 2.18. Menarchal pituitary gland. Children entering puberty have enlarged pituitaries, typically larger in girls than in boys.

time at which the pituitary gradually assumes the appearance of an older child's, with a flat superior margin and a signal intensity of normal gray matter on T1-weighted spin echo images (37,38). During childhood, the pituitary gland slowly grows in all dimensions, maintaining a flat or mildly concave upper surface, with a height of 2–6 mm in the sagittal plane. The size of the pituitary stalk is difficult to measure. The size of the stalk relative to the size of the brain never changes, and it should never be as large as the basilar artery on axial images (39).

With the arrival of puberty, the pituitary gland increases dramatically in size and (in girls, but not boys) demonstrates a marked upward convexity (Fig. 2.18). The height of the gland may reach 10 mm in girls and 7–8 mm in boys (40,41). The appearance then slowly evolves into that of the adult gland over the subsequent 5–8 years.

NORMAL MR DEVELOPMENT OF THE SKULL AND PARANASAL SINUSES

The Skull

At birth, the signal intensity of the bone marrow in the clivus and in the diploic space of the calvarium is of low signal intensity with respect to brain and to the spheno-occipital synchondrosis (Fig. 2.19A). The low signal intensity is believed to result from the presence of red (actively hematopoietic) marrow. By the end of the second year of life, the marrow in the crista galli and the nasal processes of the frontal bone develop high signal intensity on T1-weighted images (Fig. 2.19B). During the third year of life, patchy areas of increased signal inten-

sity begin to appear in the clivus on T1-weighted images (Fig. 2.19C). These foci of T1 shortening may initially appear in the basi-occiput or the basi-sphenoid. Slowly, over the next 3–4 years, these foci of short T1 relaxation time enlarge and coalesce (Fig. 2.19C–E). By 10 years of age, the marrow in almost all children is almost entirely of high signal intensity on the short TR/TE images (Fig. 2.19F). A few small foci of low signal intensity may remain well into the second decade.

After intravenous administration of paramagnetic contrast, the immature skull and skull base show variable enhancement in infants and young children (42). Most likely, the enhancement is the result of the vascularity of the hematopoietic marrow in the calvarial diploë and, particularly, the skull base of infants. The amount of enhancement is age related, as the immature homogeneous marrow of younger children enhances more and to a greater degree than the heterogeneous marrow of older children (42). The amount of enhancement seen in older children after fat suppression pulses have been applied is unknown. The normal enhancement of bone marrow in infants can be problematic in patients with such diseases as leukemia and neuroblastoma; differentiation of normal hematopoietic marrow from metastatic neuroblastoma may not be possible by MR alone unless the bone is expanded or periosteum is lifted from the surface of the bone. Correlation with CT and radionuclide studies is essential.

Before pneumatization of the sphenoid sinus, an area of markedly increased signal intensity appears in the presphenoid portion of the sphenoid bone (Fig. 2.19C). This high signal, believed to represent fatty change, appears between 7 months and 2 years of age; then it regresses as pneumatization of the sphenoid sinus occurs after the

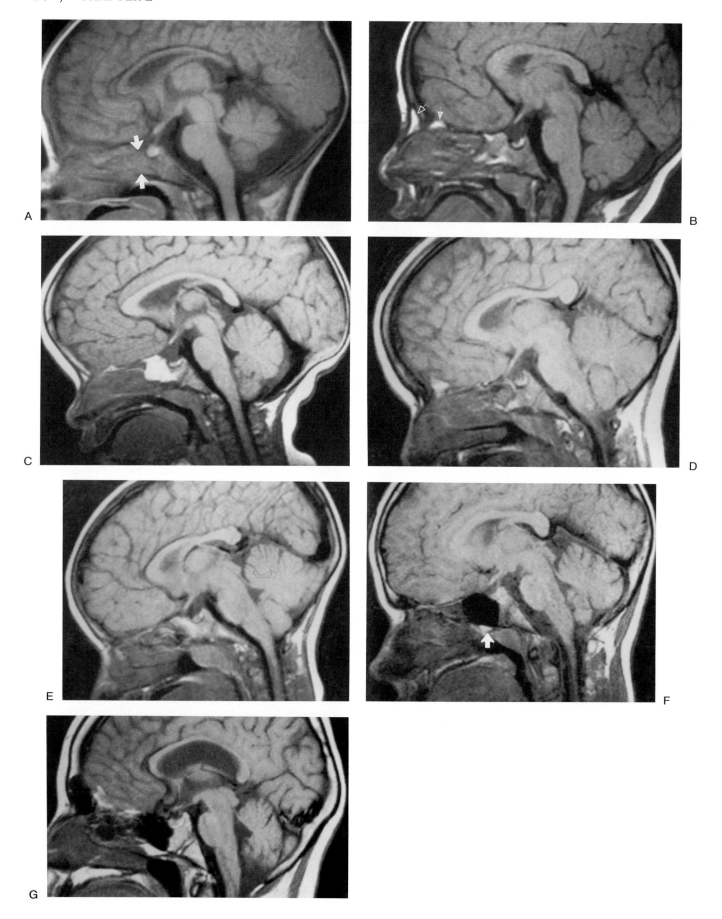

age of 2 years (Fig. 2.19D–G). Some of the high signal may persist into the second decade (43).

The maturation of the diploic space of the calvarium occurs at almost the identical time as the clivus. Foci of high signal intensity on short TR/TE images begin to appear within the diploic space at approximately 3 years of age. More and more areas of high signal intensity develop over the next 4 years, until, at about 7 years of age, the diploic space is of nearly uniform high signal intensity (44). Enhancement of the diploic space parallels that of the clivus.

The spheno-occipital synchondrosis remains prominent throughout childhood and can be seen well into the third decade of life.

The importance of understanding the normal temporal sequence of skull maturation lies in the evaluation of the patient with systemic disease. For example, several disease entities will cause reactivation of erythropoiesis within the bone marrow. In particular, states of chronic anemia, such as sickle cell disease and thalassemia, will cause a reversion of bone marrow to the immature low signal intensity. Other disease processes, such as leukemia, can infiltrate the bone marrow; such infiltration will also cause a lengthening of the T1 relaxation time resulting from replacement of fat by a proliferative marrow. If low signal intensity is seen diffusely throughout the clivus beyond the age of 4 years, some underlying condition, such as an anemia or a systemic, infiltrative disease, should be sought.

The Paranasal Sinuses

The *maxillary sinus* is the first of the paranasal sinuses to develop. The sinuses are rudimentary at birth, lying entirely medial to the orbit. They are commonly partially or completely opacified. The sinuses grow rapidly through childhood, with a growth rate of 2 mm/year in the vertical dimension and 3 mm/year in the anteropos-

terior dimension (45). Growth continues until the end of puberty, when facial growth ceases. The following milestones are useful: (1) Lateral margin of the sinus projects under the medial orbital wall by the end of the first year; (2) sinus extends laterally past the infraorbital canal by age 4 years; (3) sinus reaches maxillary bone and plane of hard palate by age 9 years (46).

At birth, the *ethmoid sinuses* are developed more anteriorly than posteriorly. Lack of aeration of the posterior ethmoid sinuses is considered normal until the age of approximately 6 years (45). Pneumatization progresses posteriorly, with resultant enlargement of the posterior air cells. By the late phases of pneumatization, the posterior cells are larger and fewer than the anterior cells. The last phase of ethmoid pneumatization involves development of the extramural air cells, the agger nasi, Hallers cells, and concha bullosa, which lie in the anterior ethmoidal region (46).

The fetal *sphenoid sinuses* consist of small cavities (conchal sinuses) within the developing sphenoid bones. Soon after birth, the conchal sinuses fuse to the sphenoid bone and begin to pneumatize (45). High-resolution CT may show pneumatization of the sphenoid sinuses as early as age 2 years. Pneumatization proceeds inferiorly, posteriorly, and laterally, with the presphenoid portion developing first, followed by the basi-sphenoid and, in some patients, greater sphenoid wings and pterygoid processes. As noted in the previous section, care must be taken not to mistake the normal fatty changes that occur prior to pneumatization (43) for hemorrhage, proteinaceous fluid, or inclusion tumor.

The *frontal sinuses* are the last of the paranasal sinuses to develop. They originate as extensions of the anterior ethmoidal air cells (45). At birth, they are normal bone containing red marrow. They follow the same prepneumatization transition as the sphenoid sinuses, in that yellow, fatty marrow develops prior to pneumatization (46). Earliest pneumatization is seen around the age of 2 years

FIG. 2.19. Development of normal bone marrow in the clivus. **A:** Normal clivus of a 3-month-old. The marrow within the basi-occiput and basi-sphenoid is of uniform low signal intensity as compared to the spheno-occipital synchondrosis. The presphenoid region of the sphenoid bone is isointense to the basi-sphenoid. **B:** Normal 12-month-old infant. During the second year of life, the crista galli (*closed arrow*) and the nasal process of the frontal bone (*open arrow*) develop high signal intensity within their marrow. **C:** Normal 18-month-old infant. Between the ages of 6 months and 2 years, fatty change occurs within the presphenoid portion of the sphenoid bone. The basi-sphenoid and basi-occiput remain of uniform low intensity. **D:** Normal 4-year-old child. The fatty change in the presphenoid region has begun to recede as pneumatization occurs. There are patches of high signal intensity within the basi-sphenoid and basi-occiput as normal yellow marrow begins to appear. **E:** Normal 5-year-old child. The regions of high signal intensity within the basi-sphenoid and basi-occiput are becoming more apparent and beginning to coalesce. **F:** Normal 10-year-old. The sphenoid sinus is nearly completely pneumatized at this age. Only a small amount of fatty change remains in the inferior-most portion of the presphenoid (*arrow*). The basi-sphenoid and basi-occiput are now composed of mainly yellow marrow; the clivus therefore shows mainly a high signal intensity compared to the synchondrosis with a few patchy areas of low signal intensity persisting. **G:** Mature clivus in a normal 16-year-old. The basi-occiput and basi-sphenoid are now of uniform high signal intensity.

in the orbital processes of the frontal bone. By age 4 years, pneumatization reaches the nasion, advancing to the level of the orbital roof by age 8 years and into the vertical portion of the frontal bone by age 10 years. Growth continues until the end of puberty. The extent of frontal sinus development is extremely variable (46).

NORMAL MR DEVELOPMENT OF BRAIN IRON

In the adult, certain regions of the brain show a marked diminution in signal intensity on long TR, long TE images, particularly at high field strength. This diminished T2 relaxation time has been suggested to result from the presence of relatively high quantities of iron in those locations (47), although the cause and effect relationship is disputed (48). The most prominent areas in which these phenomena occur are the basal ganglia, particularly the globus pallidus, the substantia nigra (mostly in the medial pars reticularis), the red nuclei, and the dentate nuclei of the cerebellum.

At birth, this accentuated T2 shortening is not seen anywhere in the brain (49) (Fig. 2.20). The basal ganglia begin to manifest low intensity with respect to the cerebral cortex on long TR/TE images at approximately age 6 months. However, the globus pallidus and putamen at this age are isointense to one another and hypointense with respect to the internal capsule. This initial decrease in signal intensity on T2-weighted images is therefore believed to be secondary to myelination of the axons within the lentiform nuclei. Indeed, as the cerebral white matter begins to myelinate, the basal ganglia become hyperintense with respect to the surrounding white matter on T2-weighted images. A second phase of T2 shortening in the globus pallidus, substantia nigra, and red nuclei becomes noticeable at 9 or 10 years of age (49) (Fig. 2.21). At this age, the intensity of these areas becomes equal to, and then less than, that of the surrounding white matter. The globus pallidus will be of lower signal intensity than surrounding brain in 90% of patients by age 15 years (49) (Fig. 2.22). The signal intensity continues to diminish on long TR/long TE images throughout the second decade and may continue at a slower rate throughout life.

The dentate nuclei of the cerebellum begin to show lower signal intensity at a slightly later age, with noticeable changes beginning to occur at about age 15 years (Fig. 2.21). This low signal intensity also progresses slowly throughout life; however, there is less accumulation of iron in the dentate nucleus than in the other iron-containing regions of the brain. The dentate nucleus will be of lower signal intensity than surrounding cerebellum in only 30% of patients at age 25 years (49).

NORMAL MR DEVELOPING OF THE SPINE

Embryology

At the end of the second gestational week, the normal human embryo is a bilaminar structure comprised of a flat sheet of cells adjacent to the amnion, termed the *epiblast*, and a second layer adjacent to the yolk sac, known as the *hypoblast*. The hypoblast will eventually be replaced by the *endoderm*, which is believed to be a derivative of the epiblast. Soon after, cells in the caudal midline of the embryo proliferate to form a *primitive knot* (also known as Hensen's node) and the *primitive streak* caudal to it. By about embryonic day 16, the primitive streak begins to regress and cells at the rostral lip of the primitive knot migrate between the epiblast and hypoblast, forming the *notochordal process.* The notochordal process elongates as cells from the primitive knot are added to it at its caudal end; after canalization, the more caudal portion will be known as the *notochord*. The notochord induces surrounding mesoderm (the paraxial mesoderm, derived from the primitive streak) to condense into paired blocks of somites and, eventually, into *myotomes*, which will form the paraspinous muscles and overlying skin, and *sclerotomes*, which will form the cartilage, bones, and ligaments of the vertebral column (50,51).

During the fourth or fifth gestational week, resegmentation of the sclerotomes occurs, with eventual development of the vertebral bodies. In this resegmentation, the cells within the caudal half of each sclerotome separate from the cranial half (of the same sclerotome) at the sclerotomal cleft and then fuse with the cranial half of the inferior sclerotome (Fig. 2.23) to form a new, primitive vertebral body (50,51). As a result, the intersegmental arteries become trapped in the centers of the new vertebral bodies. At the same time, the segments of notochord within the newly formed vertebrae disintegrate and the notochordal segments in the intervertebral regions proliferate and convert into nucleus pulposis. The mesenchymal vertebrae then undergo chondrification, starting at specific chondrification centers within the vertebrae, between days 40 and 60. Finally, ossification begins in four ossification centers (two in the vertebral body and one in each side of the vertebral arch), a process that continues into postnatal life (50,51).

The newborn vertebral body has a membranous central component, with ossification centers and end-plates of hyaline cartilage that lie superior and inferior to the central component. The end-plates are each about one-half the size of the central vertebral component (52). Both the vertebral body and cartilaginous end-plates of the newborn have a more substantial vascular supply than those of adults. The vertebral bodies contain hematopoietic marrow, with large vascular pools and sinusoi-

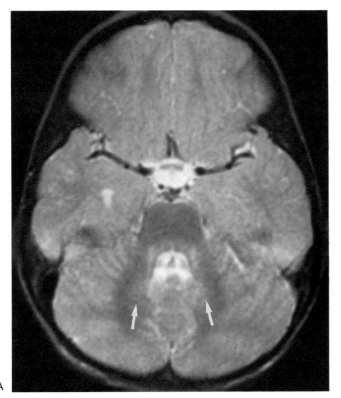

A

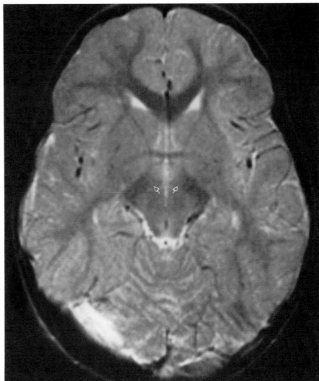

B

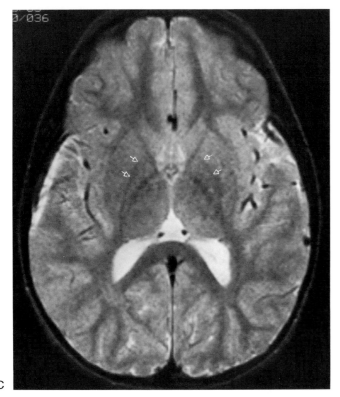

C

FIG. 2.20. Immature pattern of brain iron. **A–C:** In this normal 4-year-old, we see that the globus pallidus, red nucleus, pars reticularis of the substantia nigra, and dentate nuclei of the cerebellum are all hyperintense as compared to normal white matter of the brain (*arrows*). This appearance usually changes to isointensity with white matter before the age of 10 in the globus pallidus, substantia nigra, and red nucleus. The changes in the dentate nucleus occur later and less consistently.

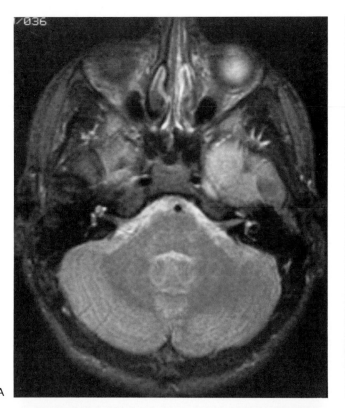

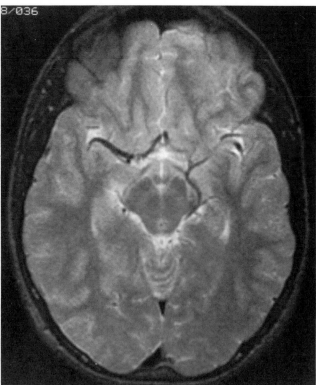

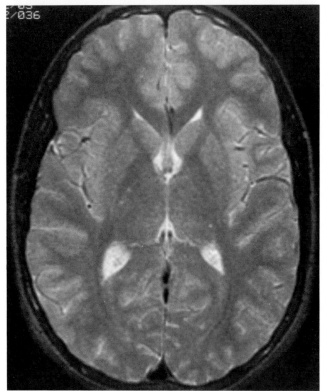

FIG. 2.21. Intermediate stage of maturation of brain iron. **A–C:** In this normal 13-year-old, the iron-concentrating regions of the brain are now isointense with white matter. Iron accumulates more rapidly in the globus pallidus than in the other areas of the brain, and the globus pallidus will be of lower signal intensity than surrounding brain in 90% of patients by age 15. The substantia nigra and red nuclei are hypointense with respect to white matter in 50% of normal patients by age 20.

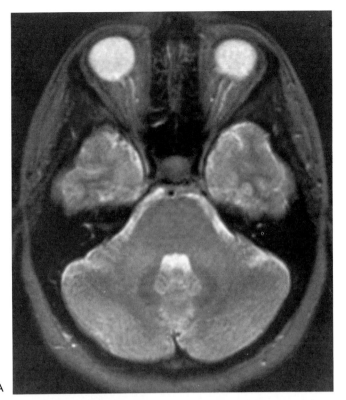

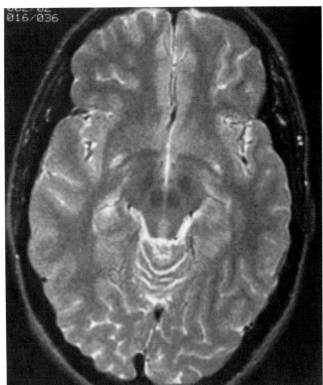

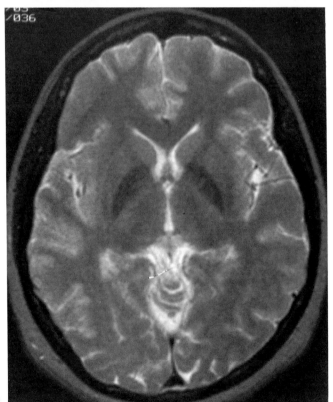

FIG. 2.22. Brain iron in normal young adult. **A–C:** By the age of 25, the globus pallidus, substantia nigra, and red nuclei will be hypointense with respect to white matter in 80% of normals. However, only 30% of normal 25-year-old people will show hypointensity of the dentate nuclei, which accumulate iron more slowly and less consistently than the other areas.

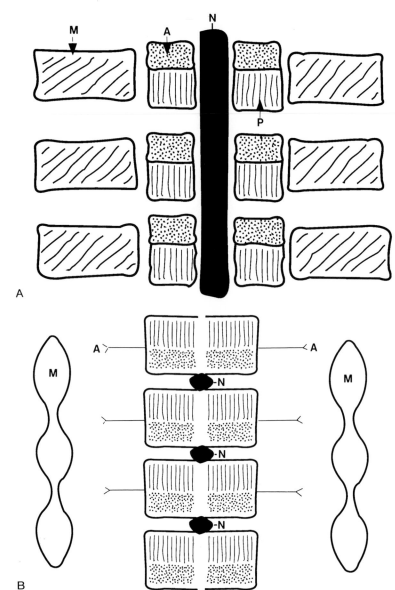

FIG. 2.23. Formation of vertebral bodies. **A:** Each sclerotome consists of a cranial mass of loosely packed cells (anterior sclerotome, A, *dotted areas*) and a caudal mass of densely packed cells (posterior sclerotome, P, *vertical lines*). The sclerotomes are closely related to the notochord (N) and the myotomes (M, *cross-hatched areas*). **B:** The caudal, dense cell mass of one sclerotome unites with the cranial loose cell mass of the adjacent caudal sclerotome to form a structure (the centrum of the vertebral body) that contains equal parts of adjacent sclerotomes. The notochord has regressed; its remnants (N) will become nuclei pulposi. Myotomes are evolving into paraspinous muscles (M). Note the relationship of intersegmental arteries (A) to the vertebrae and sclerotomal segments.

dal channels that lack blood-brain barrier and contain large extracellular spaces. The cartilaginous end-plates are perfused by vessels from the margins of the vertebral bodies and by vessels branching from the lumbar arteries (53,54).

MR of Spine Development

The MR appearance of the infant spinal column has been described as evolving through three stages (55). *Stage I*, occurring from birth through the first month of life, is characterized by biconvex vertebral bodies that are markedly hypointense, compared to muscle, on short TR images. A horizontal band of high intensity is located within the center of the vertebral body, probably repre-

senting the basivertebral venous plexus. The cartilaginous end-plates of the vertebral bodies, which are about one-half the size of the osseous body at this age, are mildly hyperintense compared with muscle, but markedly hyperintense compared with the central osseous portion (Fig. 2.24). T2-weighted images show the ossification centers to be markedly hypointense and the endplates mildly hyperintense compared with muscle. Administration of paramagnetic contrast at this age will result in mild to marked enhancement of both the vertebral body and the cartilaginous end-plates. The intervertebral disc does not change significantly during childhood. It appears hypointense on T1-weighted images and hyperintense on T2-weighted images, and shows minimal to no enhancement (55,56).

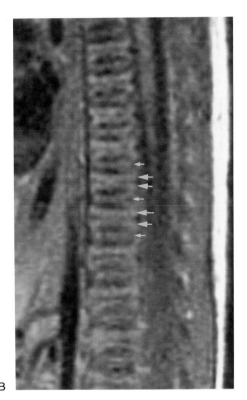
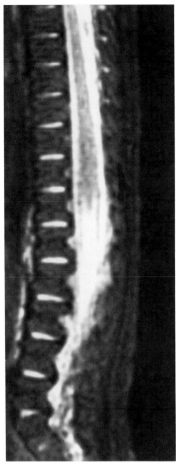

A,B

FIG. 2.24. Neonatal spine, stage I. A: T1-weighted image shows horizontal bands of high intensity (*small white arrows*) located within the centers of the vertebral bodies, probably representing the basivertebral venous plexuses. The cartilaginous end-plates of the vertebral bodies (*larger white arrows*), which are about one-half the size of the osseous body at this age, are mildly hyperintense compared with muscle, but markedly hyperintense compared with the central osseous portion. B: T2-weighted image shows the ossification centers to be markedly hypointense and the end-plates mildly hyperintense compared with muscle. The intervertebral discs are markedly hyperintense.

Stage II (Fig. 2.25), taking place from approximately 1–6 months, is characterized by T1 shortening in the vertebral bodies that starts at the superior and inferior borders of the body and moves centrally, eventually affecting the entire vertebral body. T2-weighted images also show increasing intensity in the superior and inferior portions of the vertebrae; the vertebral body slowly becomes isointense with the end-plates by about age 3 months. The enhancement pattern of the vertebral body and end-plate at stage II is not significantly different from that at stage I (55,56).

Stage III (Fig. 2.25) takes place from about age 7 months onward. At this stage, the vertebral bodies are hyperintense with respect to the cartilaginous end-plates and surrounding muscle on T1-weighted images. The cartilaginous end-plates gradually become ossified and incorporated into the vertebral body, which becomes rectangular in shape by about age 2 years. T2-weighted images show the vertebral bodies to be homogeneous, isointense with the cartilaginous end-plates, and mildly hyperintense compared with surrounding muscle. Uniform contrast enhancement of variable intensity is seen in the end-plates and vertebral bodies in most children up to the age of 9 or 10 years, during which time the hematopoietic marrow is being slowly replaced (55,56).

EVALUATION OF BRAIN DEVELOPMENT USING NEW MR TECHNIQUES

MR Spectroscopy

The evaluation of the developing brain with MR spectroscopy is at a very early stage of development. Let us first discuss the different peaks seen on proton (^{1}H) MR spectra (Fig. 2.26), the origin of their signals, and their significance. After understanding the origin of the signals, the changes that occur during development will be discussed.

N-acetylaspartate (NAA) is the most obvious peak on ^{1}H MRS and is the peak (at 2.01 ppm) that is used as a reference for chemical shift determination (57,58). The peak actually includes contributions from NAA, *N*-acetylaspartylglutamate, glycoproteins, and amino-acid residues in peptides (57,58). Therefore, the peak is perhaps more appropriately termed *N-acetyl groups*. NAA

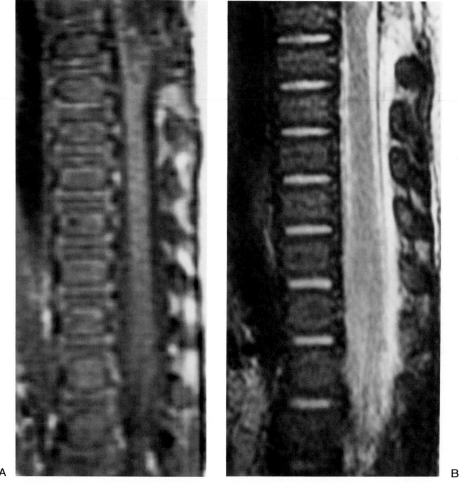

A   B

FIG. 2.25. Spine at age 4 months (stage II) and 14 months (stage III). **A:** Sagittal SE 500/11 image at age 4 months. T1 shortening has occurred at the superior and inferior borders of the vertebral body and is moving centrally. **B:** T2-weighted image shows increasing intensity in the superior and inferior portions of the vertebral bodies, which have slowly become isointense with the end-plates.

has been postulated to have at least two functions in the adult brain: (1) It is a precursor of brain lipids and (2) it is involved in coenzyme A interactions (59). Others have suggested that NAA is metabolically inert and functions only to balance the "anion deficit" of neural tissues, that it is a neurotransmitter/neuromodulator precursor, and that it functions as a free storage form for aspartate (60,61). In adult brains, NAA concentrations are higher in the cortex than in the white matter (62), as most NAA is located in neurons and their branches; an absolute or relative (to Cr) decrease of this peak is an indicator of neuronal and/or axonal damage (9,63–66). In the infant, concentrations of NAA in the gray and white matter are similar. The relatively high NAA concentrations of immature white matter have been attributed to very active lipid synthesis (59). Recent work in the immature brain has shown that oligodendroglia precursors contain twice as much NAA as immature neurons (67). As a conse-

quence, NAA levels have potential as an indicator of normal oligodendroglial development.

The *choline* peak at 3.21 ppm is composed of contributions of the trimethylammonium ($-N[CH_3]_3^+$) protons in choline, betaine, and carnitine plus the H_5 proton of *myo*-inositol and taurine (57,58). The "choline" contribution is a sum signal from several choline-containing compounds (i.e., phosphocholine, glycerophosphocholine, and free choline) in conjunction with the choline that is present as a polar head group in membrane lipids. It reflects the structural components of cell membranes, especially myelin sheaths (57,58).

The *creatine* peak at 3.03 ppm is from methyl (CH_3) protons of creatine and phosphocreatine plus minor contributions from γ-amino butyrate, lysine, and glutathione (57,58). Phosphocreatine appears to be a crucial molecule in maintenance of energy-dependent systems in all brain cells (68). Its concentration is highest in the

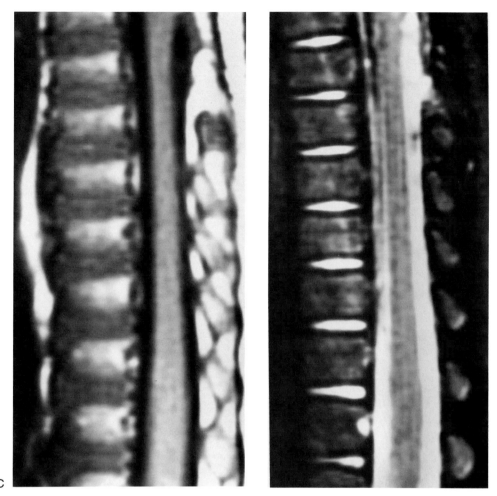

C   D

FIG. 2.25. *(Continued.)* **C:** Sagittal SE 500/16 image shows that the vertebral bodies are now hyperintense with respect to the cartilaginous end-plates and surrounding muscle. The cartilaginous end-plates are gradually becoming ossified and incorporated into the vertebral bodies, which are more rectangular. They will look completely rectangular at about age 24 months. **D:** T2-weighted image shows the vertebral bodies to be homogeneous, isointense with the cartilaginous end-plates, and mildly hyperintense compared with surrounding muscle.

cerebellum, followed by the gray matter and white matter (69).

Myo-inositol, which absorbs at 3.56 and at 4.06 (two peaks), is thought to be the storage pool for membrane phosphoinositides, which play a role in synapse transmission (70,71). Other possible roles include osmoregulation, cell nutrition, and detoxification (70,71). *Taurine*, with a small peak at 3.35 ppm, is present in high concentration within the synaptosomes at the time of synaptogenesis, and may facilitate synaptic contacts (72). *Scyllo-inositol* is a nonmetabolized isomer of *myo*-inositol that may inhibit the transport and incorporation of *myo*-inositol into phospholipids (73,74). Most experts now believe that the singlet peak at 3.35 ppm is from the six equivalent methine protons of the cyclic alcohol of scyllo-inositol, not from taurine, based upon the exact

chemical shift, the singlet nature of the resonance, agreement with biochemical concentration levels, a link to *myo*-inositol levels, and exclusion of other metabolites in ¹H MR spectra of mammalian brain *in vivo* and *in vitro* (69,74). Cerebral *glucose* may be detected on short TE ¹H MR spectra by a singlet at 3.43 ppm. The area under the singlet may be used as a gross measurement of glucose concentration in the brain (75).

Lactate, detected by a characteristic doublet seen at 1.4 ppm on ¹H MRS, is an abnormal finding in term neonates (see Chapter 3). However, lactate is a normal finding on ¹H MRS in premature infants, diminishing in amount as the infant reaches the age of 40 postconceptual weeks.

Presently, the progressive decrease of *phosphomonoester* (PME) and the complementary increase of *phos-*

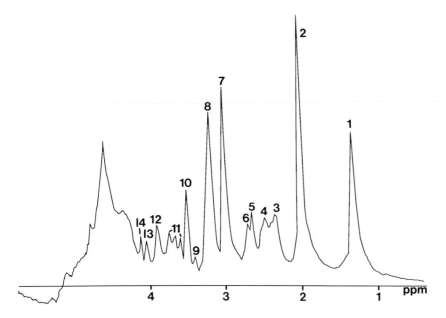

FIG. 2.26. ^{1}H spectral peak identification. (1) CH_3 of lactate; (2) CH_3 of NAA and *N*-acetylaspartylglutamate, C-2 CH_2 of glutamate and glutamine, C-3 CH_2 of gamma aminobutyric acid (GABA); (3) C-4 CH_2 of glutamate and C-2 CH_2 of GABA; (4) C-4 CH_2 of glutamine and C-3 CH_2 of NAA; (5,6) C-3 CH_2s of NAA; (7) CH_3 of creatine and C-4 CH_2 of GABA; (8) CH_3 of cholines; (9) C-1 CH_2 of taurine; (10) C-1 and C-3 CH of inositol and C-2 CH_2 of glycine; (11) C-2 CH of glutamate and glutamine, C-4 and C-6 CH of inositol; (12) C-2 CH_2 of creatine; (13) CH_2's of cholines; (14) C-2 CH of lactate.

phodiester (PDE), caused by lipid metabolism, seem to be the best indicators of brain development on ^{31}P MRS (76). Additionally, the correlation of ^{31}P MRS and neurologic exam (examination of reflexes, motor, and sensory functions) in newborn dogs demonstrated that exponential increases in phosphocreatine, inorganic phosphate, and PDE, with maintenance of the phosphocreatine/inorganic phosphate ratio, preceded maturational changes in the neurologic examination (77). The spectroscopic evolution is postulated to result from increasing ATP turnover in the maturing mitochondria.

Changes in *in vivo* MR spectra with brain maturation vary with technique. Spectra acquired with short echo times have a different appearance from those acquired with long echo times because T2 relaxation and J-coupling cause broadening and decreased amplitude of peaks (70). The maximum information is obtained by using short echo times. Changes in MRS that reflect brain maturation include a relative decrease in the size of the phosphomonoester peak and relative increases in the size of the phosphocreatine and phosphodiester peaks on ^{31}P spectra and increase in the size of the large *N*-acetylaspartate peak [at chemical shift 2.01 parts per million (ppm)] relative to the choline (at 3.21 ppm) and the creatine-phosphocreatine peaks (at 3.03 ppm) on ^{1}H spectra (Fig. 2.27) (70,78). In addition, the large *myo*-inositol peak present at 3.56 ppm in the spectra of newborns (Fig. 2.27) diminishes substantially during the first year of life (71). The taurine [scyllo-inositol (74)] peak is highest in newborns (71,79).

Absolute concentrations of metabolites are very

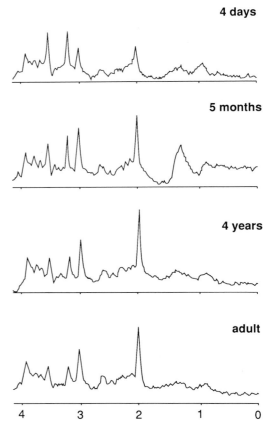

FIG. 2.27. Changes in ^{1}H spectra with maturation. *myo*-Inositol is the dominant peak in neonates. Choline is the dominant peak in older infants. Creatine and *N*-acetyl groups are the dominant peaks in older children and adults. (Reprinted with permission from ref. 68.)

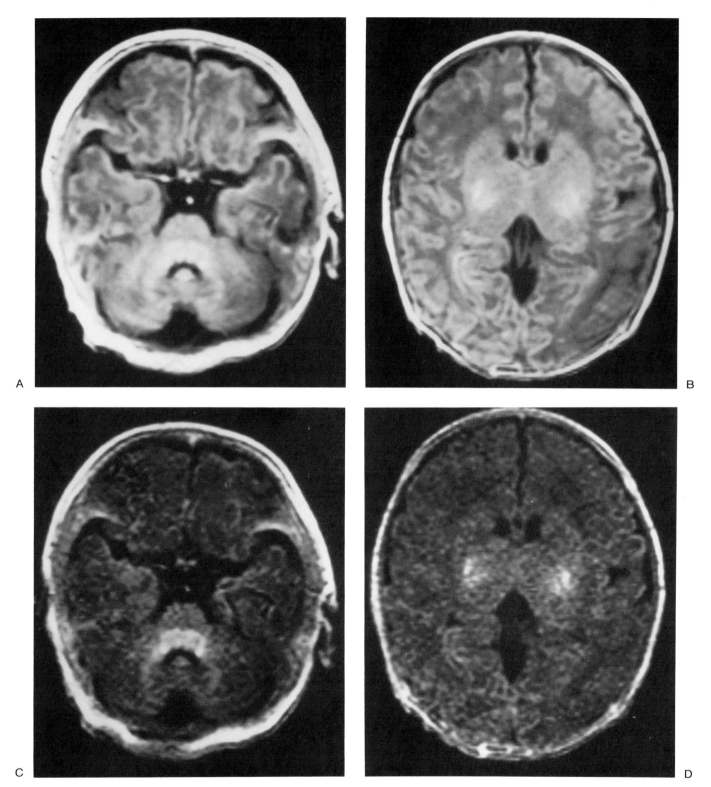

FIG. 2.28. Magnetization transfer images in a neonate. **A,B:** SE 550/15 images show T1 shortening in the dorsal brain stem and the posterior limb of the internal capsule/lateral thalamus. **C,D:** Magnetization transfer images show considerable magnetization transfer in the areas of T1 shortening on the T1-weighted images, but nowhere else.

difficult to determine by *in vivo* MR spectroscopy (80,81). Therefore, the time course of most metabolites has been expressed most exactly by comparing the spectral peaks with each other and calculating ratios (60,64,71). Compared to Cr, for example, a decrease of choline (the Ch/Cr ratio) and *myo*-inositol (*myo*-Ins/ Cr ratio) develops as maturation progresses (64); the choline/*myo*-inositol ratio is stable (60,71). In addition, the temporal evolution of the peaks differs in gray matter as compared to white matter. Whereas the Cr/Ch ratio stays nearly constant in white matter, the ratio increases in gray matter during the first 2 years of life (64).

The reader should be aware that new methods for absolute quantification of peak areas have been developed and, because they are more reproducible and reliable, may soon become the standard way of analyzing spectra (68,70,82). Using absolute measurements, *myo*-inositol was found to be the dominant peak in neonates, with a concentration of 10–12 mmol/kg (70). Choline, with a concentration of 2.5 mmol/kg, is the dominant peak in older infants (70). Creatine and *N*-acetyl groups, which have concentrations of 6 mmol/kg and 5 mmol/kg, respectively, in the neonate, increase in concentration to 7 mmol/kg and 9 mmol/kg, respectively, in the adult. Thus, they become the dominant peaks in the adult proton spectrum. *myo*-Inositol, conversely, decreases to a concentration of 6 mmol/kg in the adult, resulting in its decreasing prominence in the spectrum of the older child and adult (70).

Diffusion Imaging

Using special techniques that were initially developed in the 1960s (83,84), MR can be used to measure the rate of *diffusion* of water in the brain (65,85). MR of the newborn brain demonstrates isotropic diffusion of water molecules; that is, water diffuses at equal rates in all directions (65,86). As the brain matures, diffusion becomes anisotropic, more rapid parallel to the longitudinal axes of major axonal bundles of the cerebral white matter than perpendicular to them (65). Although it has been suggested that anisotropy develops as a result of the development of myelin sheaths, the initial development of anisotropy seems to precede that of myelination (87). Additionally, diffusion anisotropy occurs in unmyelinated nerve bundles (87,88). Thus, diffusion-weighted imaging (DWI) has potential in the assessment of cerebral maturation, although the cause(s) of anisotropy are yet to be determined.

Magnetization Transfer Imaging

Another technique that may be useful in the analysis of brain development is *magnetization transfer*. As discussed in Chapter 1, almost all magnetization transfer in the brain seems to result from the interaction of the free water in the brain with components of myelin, in particular the hydroxyl and amine moieties of cholesterol and glycocerebrosides on the myelin surface (89,90). Destruction of myelin results in decreased magnetization transfer (91). Moreover, the onset of T1 shortening seen during the early phases of myelination on T1-weighted images corresponds temporally and topographically to the onset of magnetization transfer (Fig. 2.28) (92). Thus, it appears that the T1 shortening on spin echo images results from a magnetization transfer interaction of glycocerebrosides and cholesterol on the surface of the myelin molecule with free water in the brain. Increases in magnetization transfer can therefore be used to evaluate brain maturation.

REFERENCES

1. Lemire RJ, Loeser JD, Leech RW, Alvord EC. *Normal and abnormal development of the human nervous system.* New York: Harper & Row, 1975.
2. McArdle CB, Richardson CJ, Nicholas DA, Mirfakhraee M, Hayden CK, Amparo EG. Developmental features of the neonatal brain: MR imaging. Part I. Gray–white matter differentiation and myelination. *Radiology* 1987;162:223–229.
3. Fitz CR. Developmental anomalies of the brain. In: Heinz ER, ed. *Neuroradiology.* In: Rosenberg R, ed. *The clinical neurosciences.* New York: Churchill Livingstone, 1984:215–224.
4. Barkovich AJ, Kjos BO, Jackson DE Jr, Norman D. Normal maturation of the neonatal and infant brain: MR imaging at 1.5 T. *Radiology* 1988;166:173–180.
5. Brody BA, Kinney HC, Kloman AS, Gilles FH. Sequence of central nervous system myelination in human infancy. I. An autopsy study of myelination. *J Neuropathol Exp Neurol* 1987;46:283–301.
6. Kinney HC, Brody BA, Kloman AS, Gilles FH. Sequence of central nervous system myelination in human infancy. II. Patterns of myelination in autopsied infants. *J Neuropathol Exp Neurol* 1988;47:217–234.
7. Yakovlev PI, Lecours AR. The myelogenetic cycles of regional maturation of the brain. In: Minkowski A, ed. *Regional development of the brain in early life.* Oxford: Blackwell, 1967:3–70.
8. Martin E, Krassnitzer S, Kaelin P, Boesch C. MR imaging of the brainstem: normal postnatal development. *Neuroradiology* 1991; 33:391–395.
9. Van der Knaap MS, Valk J. MR imaging of the various stages of normal myelination during the first year of life. *Neuroradiology* 1990;31:459–470.
10. Van der Knaap MS, Valk J, de Neeling N, Nauta JJP. Pattern recognition in MRI of white matter disorders in children and young adults. *Neuroradiology* 1991;33:478–493.
11. Baker LL, Stevenson DK, Enzmann DR. End stage periventricular leukomalacia: MR imaging evaluation. *Radiology* 1988;168:809–815.
12. Rollins NK, Deline C, Morriss MC. Prevalence and clinical significance of dilated Virchow-Robin spaces in childhood. *Radiology* 1993;189:53–57.
13. Hittmair K, Wimberger D, Rand T, et al. Spin echo (SE) sequences and short inversion time inversion recovery (STIR) sequences in the assessment of brain myelination, *Am J Neuroradiol* (in press).
14. Poduslo SE, Jang Y. Myelin development in infant brain. *Biochem Res* 1984;9:1615–1626.
15. Barkovich AJ. Brain development: normal and abnormal. In: Atlas SW, ed. *Magnetic resonance imaging of the brain and spine.* New York: Raven, 1991:129–175.
16. Husted C, Montez B, Le C, Moscarello MA, Oldfield E. Carbon-13 "magic-angle" sample-spinning nuclear magnetic resonance

studies of human myelin, and model membrane systems. *Magn Reson Med* 1993;29:168–178.

17. Husted C. *Carbon-13 magic angle spinning NMR studies of myelin membranes.* (Ph.D. Thesis) University of Illinois at Urbana–Champaign, 1991.

18. Kosaras B, Kirschner DA. Radial component of CNS myelin: junctional subunit structure and supramolecular assembly. *J Neurocytol* 1990;19:187–199.

19. Braun PE. Molecular organization of myelin. In: Morell P, ed. *Myelin*, 2nd ed. New York: Plenum, 1984:97–116.

20. Koenig SH, Brown RD III, Spiller M, Lundbom N. Relaxometry of the brain: why white matter appears bright on MRI. *Magn Reson Med* 1990;14:482–495.

21. Johnson MA, Peccock JM, Bydder GM, et al. Clinical NMR of the brain in children: normal and neurologic disease. *AJR* 1983;141:1005–1018.

22. Holland BA, Haas DK, Norman D, Brant-Zawadzki M, Newton TH. MRI of normal brain maturation. *Am J Neuroradiol* 1986;7:201–208.

23. Christophe C, Muller MF, Baleriaux D, et al. Mapping of normal brain maturation on phase-sensitive inversion-recovery images. *Neuroradiology* 1990;32:173.

24. Dietrich RB, Bradley WG, Zagaroza EJ, et al. MR evaluation of early myelination patterns in normal and developmentally delayed infants. *Am J Neuroradiol* 1988;9:69–76.

25. Bird C, Hedberg M, Drayer BP, et al. MR assessment of myelination in infants and children: usefulness of marker sites. *Am J Neuroradiol* 1989;10:731–740.

26. Van der Knaap MS. *Myelination and myelin disorders: a magnetic resonance study in infants, children and young adults.* (Ph.D. Thesis) Free University of Amsterdam and University of Utrecht, Netherlands, 1991.

27. Martin E, Boesch C, Zuerrer M, et al. MR imaging of brain maturation in normal and developmentally handicapped children. *J Comput Assist Tomogr* 1990;14:685–692.

28. Kjos BO, Umansky R, Barkovich AJ. MR of the brain in children with developmental retardation of unknown cause. *Am J Neuroradiol* 1990;11:1035–1040.

29. Barkovich AJ, Truwit CL. MR of perinatal asphyxia: correlation of gestational age with pattern of damage. *Am J Neuroradiol* 1990;11:

30. Rakic P, Yakovlev PI. Development of the corpus callosum and cavum septae in man. *J Comp Neurol* 1968;132:45–72.

31. Barkovich AJ, Kjos BO. Normal postnatal development of the corpus callosum as demonstrated by MR imaging. *Am J Neuroradiol* 1988;9:487–491.

32. DeLacoste MC, Kirkpatrick JB, Ross ED. Topography of the corpus callosum. *J Neuropathol Exp Neurol* 1985;44:578–591.

33. Liebman SD, Gellis SS. *The pediatrician's ophthalmology.* St Louis: CV Mosby, 1966.

34. McLeod NA, Williams JP, Machen B, Lum GB. Normal and abnormal morphology of the corpus callosum. *Neurology* 1987;37:1240–1242.

35. Wolpert XM, Osborne M, Anderson M, Runge VM. Bright pituitary gland: a normal MR appearance in infancy. *Am J Neuroradiol* 1988;9:1–3.

36. Cox TD, Elster AD. Normal pituitary gland: changes in shape, size, and signal intensity during the first year of life at MR imaging. *Radiology* 1991;179:721–724.

37. Konishi Y, Kuriyama M, Sudo M, Hayakawa K, Konishi K, Nakamura K. Growth patterns of the normal pituitary gland and in pituitary adenoma. *Dev Med Child Neurol* 1990;32:69–73.

38. Hayakawa K, Konishi Y, Matsuda T, et al. Development and aging of brain midline structures: assessment with MR imaging. *Radiology* 1989;172:171–177.

39. Peyster RG, Hoover ED, Adler LP. CT of the normal pituitary stalk. *Am J Neuroradiol* 1984;5:45–47.

40. Peyster RG, Hoover ED, Viscarello RR, et al. CT appearance of the adolescent and preadolescent pituitary gland. *Am J Neuroradiol* 1983;4:411–414.

41. Elster AK, Chen MYM, Williams DW III, Key LL. Pituitary gland: MR imaging of physiologic hypertrophy in adolescence. *Radiology* 1990;174:681–685.

42. Applegate GR, Hirsch WL, Applegate LJ, Curtin HD. Variability

43. Aoki S, Dillon WP, Barkovich AJ, Norman D. Marrow conversion prior to pneumatization of the sphenoid sinus: assessment with MR imaging. *Radiology* 1989;172:373–375.

44. Okada Y, Aoki S, Barkovich AJ, et al. Cranial bone marrow in children: assessment of normal development with MR imaging. *Radiology* 1989;171:161–164.

45. Hasso AN, Vignaud J. Normal anatomy of the paranasal sinuses, nasal cavity and facial bones. In: Newton TH, Hasso AN, Dillon WP, eds. *Computed tomography of the head and neck.* In: Newton TH, ed. *Modern neuroradiology.* New York: Raven, 1988:6.1–6.18.

46. Scuderi A, Harnsberger HR, Boyer RS. Pneumatization of the paranasal sinuses: normal features of importance to the accurate interpretation of CT scans and MR images. *Am J Roentgenol* 1993;160:1101–1104.

47. Bizzi A, Brooks RA, Brunetti A, et al. Role of iron and ferritin in MR imaging of the brain: a study in primates at different field strengths. *Radiology* 1990;177:59–65.

48. Chen JC, Hardy PA, Kucharczyk W, et al. MR of human postmortem brain tissue: correlative study between T2 and assays of iron and ferritin in Parkinson and Huntington disease. *Am J Neuroradiol* 1993;14:275–281.

49. Aoki S, Okada Y, Nishimura K, et al. Normal deposition of brain iron in childhood and adolescence: MR imaging at 1.5 T. *Radiology* 1989;172:381–385.

50. Sarwar M, Kier EL, Varapongse C. Development of the spine and spinal cord. In: Newton TH, Potts DG, eds. *Computed tomography of the spine and spinal cord.* In: Newton T, Potts D, eds. *Modern neuroradiology.* San Anselmo: Clavedel, 1983:15–30.

51. Naidich T, McLone D. Growth and development. In: Kricun M, ed. *Imaging modalities in spinal disorders.* Philadelphia: WB Saunders, 1988:1–19.

52. Ho PSP, Yu S, Sether LA, Wagner M, Ho KC, Haughton VM. Progressive and regressive changes in the nucleus pulposus. I. The neonate. *Radiology* 1988;169:87–91.

53. Guida G, Cigala F, Riccio V. The vascularization of the vertebral body in the human fetus at term. *Clin Orthop* 1969;65:229–234.

54. Ferguson W. Some observations on the circulation on foetal and infant spines. *J Bone Joint Surg (Am)* 1950;32:640–648.

55. Sze G, Baierl P, Bravo S. Evolution of the infant spinal column: evaluation with MR imaging. *Radiology* 1991;181:819–827.

56. Sze G, Bravo S, Baierl P, Shimkin PM. Developing spinal column: gadolinium-enhanced MR imaging. *Radiology* 1991;180:497–502.

57. Kreis R, Ross BD, Farrow NA, Ackerman Z. Metabolic disorders of the brain in chronic hepatic encephalopathy detected with H-1 MR spectroscopy. *Radiology* 1992;182:19–27.

58. Kreis R, Ross BD. Cerebral metabolic disturbances in patients with subacute and chronic diabetes mellitus: detection with proton MR spectroscopy. *Radiology* 1992;184:123–130.

59. Burri R, Steffen C, Herschkowitz N. N-acetyl-L-aspartate is a major source of acetyl groups for lipid synthesis during rat brain development. *Dev Neurosci* 1991;13:403.

60. Hueppi PS, Boesch C, Fusch C, et al. Concentrations of cerebral metabolites in the developing human brain: comparison of autopsy data (HPLC) and *in vivo* 1H-MRS data. Society of Magnetic Resonance in Medicine, Eleventh Annual Scientific Meeting, August 8–14, Berlin, Germany 1992;1:231.

61. Yakovlev PI, Wadsworth RC. Schizencephalies. A study of the congenital clefts in the cerebral mantle. 2. Clefts with hydrocephalus and lips separated. *J Neuropathol Exp Neurol* 1946;5:169–206.

62. Miyake M, Kakimoto Y. Developmental changes of N-acetyl-L-aspartic acid, N-acetyl-L-aspartylglutamic acid, and beta-cityrl-L-glutamic acid in different brain regions and spinal cords of rat and guinea pig. *J Neurochem* 1981;37:1064–1067.

63. Krägeloh-Mann I, Grodd W, Niemann G, Haas G, Ruitenbeek W. Assessment and therapy monitoring of Leigh disease by MRI and proton spectroscopy. *Pediatr Neurol* 1992;8:60.

64. Bruhn H, Kruse B, Korenke GC, et al. Proton NMR spectroscopy of cerebral metabolic alterations in infantile peroxisomal disorders. *16* 1992;3:335.

65. Sakuma H, Nomura Y, Takeda K, et al. Adult and neonatal hu-

man brain: diffusional anisotropy and myelination with diffusion-weighted MR imaging. *Radiology* 1991;180:229–233.

66. Moseley ME, Cohen Y, Kucharczyk J, et al. Diffusion-weighted MR imaging of anisotropic water diffusion in cat central nervous system. *Radiology* 1990;176:439–445.

67. Urenjak J, Williams SR, Gadian DG, Noble M. Specific expression of *N*-acetylaspartate in neurons, oligodendrocyte-type-2 astrocyte progenitors, and immature oligodendrocytes in vitro. *J Neurochem* 1992;59:55.

68. Kreis R, Ernst T, Ross BD. Development of the human brain: *in vivo* quantification of metabolite and water content with proton magnetic resonance spectroscopy. *Magn Reson Med* 1993;30:424–437.

69. Michaelis T, Merboldt K-D, Bruhn H, Hänicke W, Frahm J. Absolute concentrations of metabolites in the adult human brain *in vivo*: quantification of localized proton MR spectra. *Radiology* 1993;187:219–227.

70. Kreis R, Ernst T, Ross BD. Absolute quantitation of water and metabolites in the human brain. II. Metabolite concentrations. *J Magn Reson* 1993;102:9–15.

71. Hueppi PS, Posse S, Lazeyras F, et al. Developmental changes im 1H spectroscopy in human brain. In: Lafeber HN, ed. *Fetal and neonatal physiological measurements*. New York: Elsevier, 1991:33.

72. Lleu PL, Croswell S, Huxtable RJ. Synaptosomes of the developing rat brain. *Adv Exp Med Biol* 1992;315:221.

73. Weisinger H. *myo*-Inositol transport in mouse astroglia-rich primary cultures. *J Neurochem* 1991;56:1698–1709.

74. Michaelis T, Helms KD, Merboldt W, Haenicke W, Bruhn H, Frahm J. First observation of scyllo-inositol in proton NMR spectra of human brain *in vitro* and *in vivo*. Presented at Society of Magnetic Resonance in Medicine, Berlin 1992:541.

75. Gruetter R, Rothman DL, Novotny EJ, Shulman GI, Prichard JW, Shulman RG. Detection and assignment of the glucose signal in H-1 NMR difference spectra of the human brain. *Magn Reson Med* 1992;27:183–188.

76. Pettegrew JW, Panchalingam S, Withers G, McKeag D, Strychor S. Changes in brain energy and phospholipid metabolism during development and aging in the Fischer 344 rat. *J Neuropathol Exp Neurol* 1990;49:237.

77. Nioka S, Zaman A, Yoshioka H, et al. 31P magnetic resonance spectroscopy study of cerebral metabolism in developing dog brain and its relationship to neuronal function. *Dev Neurosci* 1991;13:61.

78. Van der Knaap MS, van der Grond J, van Rijen PC, Faber JAJ, Valk J, Willemse K. Age-dependent changes in localized proton and phosphorus MR spectroscopy of the brain. *Radiology* 1990;176:509–515.

79. Hida K. In vivo 1H and 31P NMR spectroscopy of the developing rat brain. *Hokkaido J Med Sci* 1992;67:272.

80. Hennig J, Pfister H, Ernst T, Ott D. Direct absolute quantification of metabolites in the human brain with in vivo localized proton spectroscopy. *NMR Biomed* 1992;5:193–199.

81. Hüppi PS, Posse S, Lazeyras F, Burri R, Bossi E, Herschkowitz N. Magnetic resonance in preterm and term newborns: 1-H spectroscopy in developing human brain. *Pediatr Res* 1991;30:574–578.

82. Ernst T, Kreis R, Ross BD. Absolute quantitation of water and metabolites in the human brain. I. Compartments and water. *J Magn Reson* 1993;102:1–8.

83. Stejskal EO, Tanner JE. Spin diffusion measurements: spin echoes in the presence of a time-dependent field gradient. *J Chem Phys* 1965;42:288–292.

84. Stejskal EO. Use of spin echo in pulsed magnetic-field gradient to study anisotropic, restricted diffusion and flow. *J Chem Phys* 1965;43:3597–3603.

85. Chenevert TL, Brunberg JA, Pipe JG. Anisotropic diffusion in human white matter: demonstration with MR techniques in vivo. *Radiology* 1990;177:401–405.

86. Rutherford MA, Cowan FM, Manzur AY, et al. MR imaging of anisotropically restricted diffusion in the brain of neonates and infants. *J Comput Assist Tomogr* 1991;15:188–198.

87. Wimberger D, Roberts TP, Kucharczyk J, Barkovich AJ, Kozniewska E, Prayer LM. *Diffusion-weighted imaging at 4.7T in the assessment of brain maturation in albino rats*. Presented at Society of Magnetic Resonance Imaging, San Francisco 1993:62.

88. Beaulieu C, Allen PS. *Diffusional anisotropy of water in nerve cords without myelination*. Presented at Society of Magnetic Resonance in Medicine, Berlin 1992:1728.

89. Ceckler TL, Wolff SD, Yip V, Simon SA, Balaban RS. Dynamic and chemical factors affecting water proton relaxation by macromolecules. *J Magn Reson* 1992;98:637–645.

90. Fralix TA, Ceckler TL, Wolff SD, Simon SA, Balaban RS. Lipid bilayer and water proton magnetization transfer: effect of cholesterol. *Magn Reson Med* 1991;18:214–223.

91. Dousset V, Grossman RI, Ramer KN, et al. Experimental allergic encephalomyelitis and multiple sclerosis: lesion characterization with magnetization transfer imaging. *Radiology* 1992;182:483–491.

92. Chew WM, Rowley HA, Barkovich AJ. Magnetization transfer contrast imaging in pediatric patients. *Radiology* 1992;185(P):281.

CHAPTER 3

Toxic and Metabolic Brain Disorders

Inborn errors of metabolism form a very diverse group of brain disorders. The disorders are generally caused by a biochemical alteration involving one or more metabolic pathways. Clinical symptoms are the result of either lack of production of a normal biochemical or accumulation of an abnormal biochemical that may be toxic to the brain. As both endogenous (caused by inborn metabolic errors) and exogenous (ingested or inhaled) toxins may cause similar patterns of brain damage, both are included in this chapter. Autoimmune diseases involving the brain can have similar patterns of brain injury and are, therefore, included as well.

The diagnosis of the disorders discussed in this chapter is a challenge for both the clinician and the radiologist. The presenting symptoms are usually nonspecific (e.g., seizures, spasticity, or delay in achieving developmental milestones), and the imaging study typically shows nonspecific patterns. Even the classification of these disorders is challenging. Some clinicians classify them by the clinical syndrome; others classify them according to results of laboratory studies. The latter classifications may involve the staining characteristics of tissue, specific biochemical assays, the cellular organelle in which the abnormal biochemical process takes place, or the genomic location of the genetic defect.

Some method of organizing the diseases from an imaging perspective is helpful to both the radiologist and the clinician, as narrowing the differential diagnosis facilitates the clinical work-up. Even in the future, when inborn errors of metabolism will be diagnosed, classified, and treated according to the underlying genetic anomaly, narrowing of the differential diagnosis by imaging will shorten the time and expense of the biochemical and genetic work-ups. In this chapter, metabolic disorders will be classified by the initial pattern of brain involvement. By proper analysis of the early pattern of brain involvement, many disorders can be excluded. It is important to recognize that most metabolic brain disorders have a similar imaging appearance in the late stages of the disease. Therefore, if an imaging study is to have a role in the diagnosis of inborn metabolic errors, the study should be performed early in the course of the disease.

The first part of this chapter is a listing of many metabolic disorders based solely upon their imaging characteristics; this section should be useful for those who merely want a list of differential diagnoses for a particular pattern of brain involvement. The second part of the chapter is a more extensive discussion of the same disorders, including some biochemical and clinical information, as well as references for those interested in pursuing more information about the diseases.

A PATTERN APPROACH TO METABOLIC DISEASE

Metabolic brain diseases can be very confusing to the radiologist. The white matter, which nearly always seems abnormal, may be involved primarily or secondarily. Both the ventricles and sulci are often big. Involvement of the basal nuclei (the thalami and basal ganglia) may be the result of gray matter or white matter injury (about

TABLE 3.1. *Disorders involving gray matter only*

A. Cortical gray matter
   1. Ceroid lipofuscinoses
   2. GM$_1$ gangliosidoses
   3. Mucolipidoses
B. Deep gray matter
   1. Prolonged T2 in striatum
      a. Leigh's disease
      b. Juvenile Huntington's disease
      c. MELAS
      d. Hypoxic–ischemic injury
      e. Hypoglycemic injury
   2. Short T2 in pallidum—Hallervorden-Spatz disease
   3. Long T2 in pallidum
      a. Methylmalonic acidemia
      b. Propionic acidemia
      c. Carbon monoxide poisoning
      d. Kernicterus

TABLE 3.3. *Disorders involving gray matter and white matter*

A. Cortical gray matter only
   1. Normal bones
      a. Cortical dysplasia
         i. Generalized peroxisomal disorder
         ii. Congenital cytomegalovirus infection
         iii. Fukuyama's congenital muscular dystrophy
         iv. Walker-Warburg syndrome
      b. No cortical dysplasia
         i. Alper's disease
         ii. Menkes' disease
   2. Abnormal bones
      a. Mucopolysaccharidoses
      b. Lipid storage disorders
B. Deep gray matter involvement
   1. Primary thalamic involvement
      a. Krabbe's disease
      b. GM$_2$ gangliosidoses
      c. Profound neonatal asphyxia
   2. Primary globus pallidus involvement
      a. Canavan's disease
      b. Kearns-Sayre syndrome
      c. Methylmalonic/propionic acidemia
      d. Carbon monoxide poisoning
      e. Maple syrup urine disease
   3. Primary striatal involvement
      a. Leigh's disease
      b. MELAS
      c. Wilson's disease
      d. Toxins (i.e., cyanide)
      e. Asphyxia in child
      f. Cockayne's disease

half of the basal nuclei is composed of white matter). This section presents a systematic approach to the analysis of these disorders based upon the pattern of brain involvement (Tables 3.1–3.3). Please recognize that this approach is a simplification because many of the metabolic disorders will have a different appearance on imaging studies when imaged at different stages of the disease. This approach is, therefore, most useful in the early stages of the disease. In the end stage, most of these diseases have very similar appearances, with diffuse loss of brain tissue and increased water in the remaining tissue. Another potential source of error is that the disorders can

TABLE 3.2. *Disorders involving white matter only*

A. Peripheral white matter early
   1. Large head
      a. Large NAA peak on MRS—Canavan's disease
      b. Frontal involvement, small NAA peak on MRS—Alexander's disease
   2. Normal head size—galactosemia
B. Deep white matter early
   1. Abnormal thalami—Krabbe's disease
   2. Normal thalami
      a. Specific brain stem trace involvement—peroxisomal disorders
      b. No specific brain stem tracts involved
         i. Metachromatic leukodystrophy
         ii. Phenylketonuria
         iii. Maple syrup urine disease (+ cerebellum and cerebral peduncles)
         iv. Lowe's disease
         v. Radiation/chemotherapy
C. Lack of myelination
   1. Pelizaeus–Merzbacher disease
   2. Trichothiodystrophy
D. Nonspecific white matter pattern (diffuse, unilateral or bilateral, asymmetric)
   1. Nonketotic hyperglycinemia
   2. Urea cycle disorders
   3. Collagen vascular diseases
   4. Demyelinating diseases
   5. End stage of any white matter disease

(for unknown reasons) have atypical patterns. Finally, classification of many diseases is likely to change as we gain knowledge and experience. Nonetheless, this systematic approach will allow the user to get close to the diagnosis much of the time.

White Matter Versus Gray Matter

The first important decision is whether the disease involves primarily gray matter, primarily white matter, or both. In general, disorders that primarily affect cortical gray matter will show prominent cortical sulci. Those disorders primarily affecting deep gray matter will show low attenuation (CT) or prolonged T1 and T2 relaxation times (MR) in the involved structures acutely and may show short T2 relaxation times in a more chronic stage, especially in the cerebral cortex. The cerebral *white* matter will often have an abnormal appearance in disorders of *gray* matter, as Wallerian degeneration of axons causes diminished white matter volume and decreased white matter attenuation (CT) or mildly to moderately prolonged white matter T2 (MR). This white matter appearance can often be differentiated from that of primary white matter disorders. Disorders primarily affecting white matter cause marked hypoattenuation (CT) or T1 and T2 prolongation (MR) before any volume loss is apparent. The white matter disorders sometimes have an inflammatory component in the early stages that causes edema, with accompanying mass effect upon adjacent sulci. Moreover, many white matter disorders (e.g., adrenoleukodystrophy and Alexander's disease) start locally and advance to involve adjacent areas. White matter diseases can result in devastation of the involved areas, with necrosis and cavitation of the affected brain and marked *ex vacuo* dilatation of the ventricles, whereas the abnormal white matter in gray matter disorders appears less severely damaged. Finally, the clinical presentation of patients with cortical gray matter disorders (seizures, dementia in early stages) differs from that of deep gray matter disorders (chorea, athetosis, dystonia), and both differ from the presentation of white matter disorders (spasticity, hyperreflexia, ataxia). *Clinical information is often very useful to get started on the right track.*

Gray Matter Disorders

Once a disorder is identified as being primarily of gray matter, the next step is to determine whether it is cortical or deep gray matter that is primarily involved. This is most easily determined by examining the deep gray nuclei to look for abnormal attenuation (CT) or abnormal T2 relaxation (MR). For confirmation of cortical involvement, a specific search for sulcal enlargement, cortical thinning, and abnormal signal intensity of the cortex may be helpful.

If the pattern of the imaging study indicates that it is primarily one of cortical involvement (cortical thinning with enlarged cortical sulci), consideration should be given to such disorders as the ceroid lipofuscinoses, the mucolipidoses, glycogen storage diseases, or GM$_1$ gangliosidosis.

If only deep gray matter is involved the signal intensity and location of the affected structures is crucial. Involvement of the *striatum* (caudate and putamen) is seen in mitochondrial disorders (primarily Leigh's disease, MELAS, and the glutaric acidurias), Wilson's disease, juvenile Huntington's disease, asphyxia, and hypoglycemia. Many of these disorders may occur in conjunction with white matter injury. If involvement is restricted to the *globus pallidus* and consists of T2 shortening or T2 shortening with central T2 prolongation, the diagnosis of Hallervorden-Spatz disease can be made with some confidence. If isolated globus pallidus involvement shows T2 prolongation, then methylmalonic acidemia, propionic acidemia, carbon monoxide poisoning, or kernicterus (see Chapter 4) should be considered.

White Matter Disorders

If the imaging abnormality is limited to the white matter, the *subcortical white matter* should be carefully analyzed to see if the subcortical U fibers are involved. If

so, an attempt should be made to find out whether the patient has macrocephaly. Bilateral, symmetrical, frontal white matter involvement in which the U fibers are affected in a macrocephalic patient is quite specific for Alexander's disease. Diffuse subcortical involvement with T2 prolongation extending into the internal and external capsules suggests Canavan's disease, which can be confirmed by a very large NAA peak on proton spectroscopy. Bilateral, symmetric, peripheral white matter involvement without macrocephaly should raise suspicion for galactosemia.

If early involvement is restricted to primarily *deep white matter,* the thalami should be specifically analyzed. High attenuation (CT) or short T2 (MR) bilaterally in the thalami strongly suggest Krabbe's disease. If the thalami are normal, the brain stem should be evaluated for involvement of specific tracts, particularly the corticospinal tracts. If specific tracts (the corticospinal tracts, in particular) are affected, a peroxisomal disorder is suggested. If not, consideration should be given to metachromatic leukodystrophy, phenylketonuria, Lowe's disease (oculocerebrorenal syndrome), and, in the proper clinical setting, damage from radiation or chemotherapy. If the internal capsules, cerebral peduncles, and cerebellar white matter are affected in a newborn, maple syrup urine disease should be considered.

The pattern of a *lack of myelination,* as opposed to damaged or destroyed myelination, is seen in Pelizaeus-Merzbacher disease and trichothiodystrophy. Occasionally, some amino and organic acidopathies will have a similar appearance.

Nonspecific white matter patterns include those with involvement of both superficial and deep white matter, those with unilateral involvement, those with diffuse involvement, and those with bilateral asymmetric involvement of white matter. Included under this heading are the urea cycle disorders (which are asymmetric and can at times affect overlying cortex); collagen vascular diseases, such as systemic lupus erythematosus (which tend to involve the white matter bilaterally and asymmetrically); and demyelinating diseases, such as multiple sclerosis and acute disseminated encephalomyelitis (which affect the white matter bilaterally and asymmetrically and may affect deep cerebral nuclei). End-stage white matter disease of any cause results in diffuse (superficial and deep), bilateral white matter damage that is completely nonspecific.

Disorders Affecting Gray and White Matter

Disorders involving both gray and white matter can be divided into those involving only the cerebral cortex and those involving deep gray matter (with or without cortical involvement). Those disorders affecting *only cortical gray matter* can be subdivided, depending on whether the patient has normal long bones and spinal column. If the *bones are normal,* the cortex should be analyzed for areas of cortical dysplasia (polymicrogyria). If cortical dysplasia is present in addition to a lack of myelination, the differential diagnosis includes the generalized peroxisomal disorders, such as Zellweger's syndrome, congenital cytomegalovirus disease (see Chapter 11), Fukuyama's congenital muscular dystrophy (see Chapter 5), and the Walker-Warburg syndrome (see Chapter 5). If no cortical dysplasia is present, differential considerations include Alper's disease and Menkes' disease, both of which cause considerable brain destruction. If the *bones are abnormal*, the differential includes primarily storage diseases, such as the mucopolysaccharidoses and lipid storage disorders.

If *deep gray matter is involved*, differential diagnosis is dependent upon which nuclei are primarily involved. If the *thalami* are primarily involved, differential considerations include Krabbe's disease and the GM$_2$ gangliosidoses (both of which have high attenuation on CT and short T2 on MR) and neonatal profound asphyxia (in which posterior putaminal involvement is almost always present). Primary *globus pallidus* involvement suggests a differential diagnosis of Canavan's disease, Kearns-Sayre syndrome, methylmalonic or propionic acidemia, maple syrup urine disease, or carbon monoxide poisoning. Kearns-Sayre and Canavan's diseases always have peripheral white matter involvement superimposed upon the deep gray matter involvement. Maple syrup urine disease typically affects the internal capsules, cerebral peduncles, dorsal pons, and cerebellar white matter. Primary *striatal* (*putamen and caudate*) involvement suggests Leigh's disease, MELAS, Wilson's disease, toxic exposure, or childhood asphyxia or hypoglycemia. Cockayne' s disease will show calcification of the striatum, as well as characteristic facies and other aspects of the syndrome.

GRAY MATTER DISEASES AND WHITE MATTER DISEASES

The simplest way to organize inborn metabolic errors is to separate those disorders that primarily involve gray matter, known as poliodystrophies, from those restricted to white matter, known as leukodystrophies. Patients with gray matter disorders classically present with seizures, dementia, and visual loss, whereas those with white matter disorders present with motor dysfunction, particularly spasticity, hyperreflexia, and ataxia. The separation of these disorders based on clinical criteria needs to be established early in the course of the disease, as the symptoms and signs become nearly identical in the late stages.

Diseases Primarily Affecting White Matter

White matter diseases of children are traditionally divided into the categories of dysmyelinating and myelin-oclastic diseases. *Dysmyelinating* diseases result from an inherited enzymatic deficiency that causes abnormal formation or increased breakdown of the components of myelin. Areas of abnormal myelination in dysmyelinating diseases are relatively symmetrical, are central (sparing subcortical U fibers in early stages), affect both cerebral and cerebellar white matter, and are poorly marginated (1). *Myelinoclastic* disorders involve destruction of intrinsically normal myelin. Their causes include infection, chemotherapy, radiation, and autoimmune disorders, such as multiple sclerosis. Myelinoclastic injury is characteristically sharply defined, is asymmetric, spares the cerebellar white matter, and involves the subcortical U fibers early in the course of the disease (1). Unfortunately, these patterns are not absolute and many exceptions are found. In the following sections, the disorders of white matter are organized by the pattern of initial white matter involvement.

White Matter Diseases Initially Affecting Central White Matter

In many sources, disorders of white matter are classified by the intracellular organelle in which the malfunctioning enzyme is located (1–3). The disorder is then classified by the organelle (e.g., as a lysosomal disorder or a peroxisomal disorder). However, the phenotypic appearance of the brain (e.g., white matter involvement versus gray matter involvement) depends more upon the specific enzyme involved than the organelle the enzyme is in; therefore, classification by organelle is impractical from the imaging perspective. Nonetheless, some understanding of the organelle approach to classification is necessary if one is to read and understand the literature. Therefore, one should know that *lysosomes* are intracellular organelles that contain lysosymes, hydrolytic enzymes that aid in the phagocytosis of undesirable molecules and particles. Dysfunction of specific lysosomal enzymes results in a variety of disorders that affect the brain. Those that affect oligodendrocytes result in white matter diseases (2). One should also know that *peroxisomes* are small organelles measuring 0.2–1.0 μm. They are limited by a single membrane and contain a minimum of one oxidase, to form hydrogen peroxide, and one catalase to decompose it (1). Although peroxisomes can contain many enzymes, their most important function from the perspective of this chapter is to break down very-long-chain (more than 26 carbon atoms) fatty acids. When very-long-chain fatty acids are incorporated into myelin, they form unstable myelin that is more easily broken down by normal metabolic processes of the body (2,3).

Metachromatic Leukodystrophy

Metachromatic leukodystrophy causes diffusely abnormal myelination of the cerebral hemispheres; it can become manifest in a variety of forms. All forms of this disorder are caused by decreased activity of arylsulfatase-A. The result is a failure of myelin to be broken down and reutilized in the central and peripheral nervous systems and the accumulation of ceramide sulfatide within macrophages and Schwann cells. The most common form of metachromatic leukodystrophy is the *late infantile variant*, which typically presents with a gait disorder and strabismus early in the second year of life. Impairment of speech, spasticity, and intellectual deterioration appear gradually. Progression is steady, with death occurring usually within 4 years of the onset of symptoms (4). The *juvenile form* is slightly rarer; neurologic symptoms become evident between 5 and 7 years of age and progress slowly (4,5). In the uncommon *adult form*, patients develop an organic mental syndrome and progressive corticospinal, corticobulbar, cerebellar, or extrapyramidal signs (6).

The imaging findings in metachromatic leukodystrophy are nonspecific. CT scans show progressive atrophy and diffuse low attenuation in the central cerebral white matter. No enhancement occurs after contrast administration (6,7). MR scans show progressive symmetrical areas of prolonged T1 and T2 relaxation times in the deep cerebral white matter (Fig. 3.1); the peripheral white matter is spared until late in the course of the disease (2,7). The low signal intensity on the short TR/TE images can easily be differentiated from normal white matter, and the high signal intensity on long TR/TE images clearly represents increased water from tissue injury distinct from a lack of myelination (as seen in Pelizaeus-Merzbacher disease). Regions of normal myelination are present in metachromatic leukodystrophy (Fig. 3.1). A progressive loss of hemispheric brain tissue is seen with progression of the disease.

Globoid Cell Leukodystrophy (Krabbe's Disease)

Krabbe's disease, also known as globoid cell leukodystrophy, begins acutely between 3 and 6 months of age with restlessness, irritability, intermittent fever, feeding problems, and delayed development. Optic atrophy and hyperacusis often develop. Terminally, the infants are flaccid and develop bulbar signs; they die within the first few years of life (4,5). The basic defect in this condition is a deficiency of galactosylceramide beta-galactosidase. For reasons that are not entirely clear, absence of this enzyme results in the destruction of oligodendrocytes. A contributing factor may be an accumulation of psychosine within affected cells (4).

Although diagnosis in these patients is based upon the assay of beta-galactosidase from white blood cells or skin

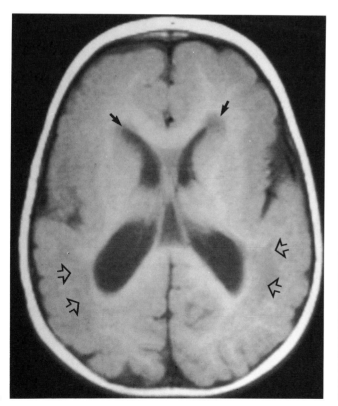

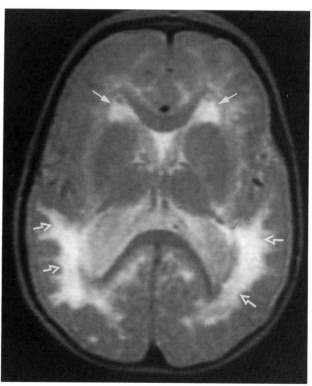

A B

FIG. 3.1. Metachromatic leukodystrophy. **A:** Axial SE 600/20 image shows decreased intensity of the periventricular white matter around the frontal horns (*solid arrows*) and trigones (*open arrows*) of the lateral ventricles. **B:** Axial SE 2800/70 image at the same level shows abnormal T2 prolongation in the same regions (*arrows*). Note that the abnormal regions have a much higher signal intensity than the surrounding unmyelinated white matter.

fibroblasts, the CT features can occasionally be very helpful. Early in the disease, high signal intensity is seen bilaterally in the thalami (Fig. 3.2), caudate nuclei, and corona radiata before and in conjunction with the development of decreased attenuation in the white matter (8). With progression of the disease, diffuse white matter atrophy ensues; at this stage, the CT appearance of Krabbe's disease resembles that of the end stage of all other dysmyelinating diseases (8,9). The MR appearance of Krabbe's disease is that of nonspecific T1 and T2 prolongation in the deep cerebral and cerebellar white matter; the cerebrum is particularly affected in the parietal lobes (Fig. 3.2) (10,11). The peripheral white matter is spared early in the course of the disease (12). The thalami may be normal or show decreased T1 or T2 relaxation times (7). They are involved rather late in the course of the disease (13).

Classic X-Linked Adrenal Leukodystrophy/ Peroxisomal Disorders with Single Enzyme Deficits

Classic X-linked adrenal leukodystrophy, seen exclusively in males, usually presents between ages 5 and 10 years with a gradual disturbance in gait and slight intellectual impairment. Abnormal skin pigmentation or other signs and symptoms of adrenal insufficiency sometimes precede neurologic abnormalities; in other cases, adrenal symptoms never become present. Progression of the disease is usually fairly rapid. Hypotonia, seizures, visual complaints, and difficulty in swallowing appear with time. Spinal cord and peripheral nerve involvement may occur without central symptoms; rarely, adrenal insufficiency may occur without neurologic involvement (14–16).

Some patients present in adolescence or adulthood; when it occurs after the age of 12 years, this disorder is called adrenomyeloneuropathy (17). Adrenomyeloneuropathy and X-linked adrenoleukodystrophy, therefore, are the same disease presenting at different ages (18,19).

The diagnosis of adrenal leukodystrophy, and of all other peroxisomal disorders, is made by assay of plasma, red cells, or cultured skin fibroblasts for the presence of increased amounts of very-long-chain fatty acids (14–16).

Imaging studies show a characteristic pattern in most patients. In classic X-linked adrenoleukodystrophy, CT reveals low attenuation in the central occipital white matter extending into the splenium of the corpus callosum. The anterior edge of this low attenuation region often shows contrast enhancement, believed to be secondary to an inflammatory leading edge of active demyelination (Fig 3.3). MR scans demonstrate marked prolongation of T1 and T2 relaxation times in the affected area (Fig. 3.3) with enhancement of the inflammatory leading edge of demyelination if paramagnetic contrast is administered. In the early phases of the disease, the peripheral white matter is spared (2,3). The corticopontine and corticospinal tracts in the brain stem often show T2 prolongation (Fig. 3.3D) (3) and enhancement. The splenium of the corpus callosum is typically involved. It appears atrophic and of low signal intensity on the midline sagittal, T1 weighted image (20). Adrenomyeloneuropathy more commonly involves the cerebellar white matter and brain stem corticospinal tract than the classic childhood form of adrenoleukodystrophy (17).

Less common patterns have been described (3,21,22). Calcification can be seen in the parieto-occipital region. Patients have also been described in which the white matter involvement was predominantly frontal (Fig. 3.4), predominantly unilateral involving the entire hemisphere, and both frontal and occipital. However, well over two-thirds of the patients will present with the classical bilateral occipital distribution. Proton MRS shows decreased NAA, increased choline, glutamine, and glutamate, decreased *myo*-inositol, and increased aliphatic hydrocarbon resonances (23,24). MRS shows abnormalities before the MR imaging study becomes abnormal in some patients (23).

Imaging findings in a number of other peroxisomal disorders have been described, including *Refsum's disease, infantile Refsum's disease*, and *rhizomelic chondrodysplasia calcificans punctata*. All these disorders show T1 and T2 prolongation in deep white matter and in white matter tracts in the brain stem. No other distinctive features have been described (7,25), other than bilateral lesions in the cerebellar dentate nuclei in infantile Refsum's disease (26).

Infantile Adrenal Leukodystrophy/Generalized Peroxisomal Disorders

The generalized peroxisomal disorders include the *Zellweger cerebro-hepato-renal syndrome, neonatal adrenal leukodystrophy, and hyperpipecolic acidemia* (14–16,27). These disorders are associated with severe psychomotor retardation, dysmorphic facial features, hypotonia, seizures, and impaired liver function. They differ from X-linked adrenal leukodystrophy, Refsum's disease, and rhizomelic chondrodysplasia calcificans punctata in many respects; in particular, severe abnormalities are present at birth and involve nearly every organ. Very-long-chain fatty acid oxidation is impaired in the generalized peroxisomal disorders, as it is in X-linked adrenal leukodystrophy, Refsum's disease, and rhizomelic chondrodysplasia calcificans punctata, but in the former this impairment is only part of a spectrum of enzyme defects that result from a defect in peroxisome structure, whereas in the latter it is thought that the primary defect involves only a single enzyme (15). A number of researchers are presently investigating these disor-

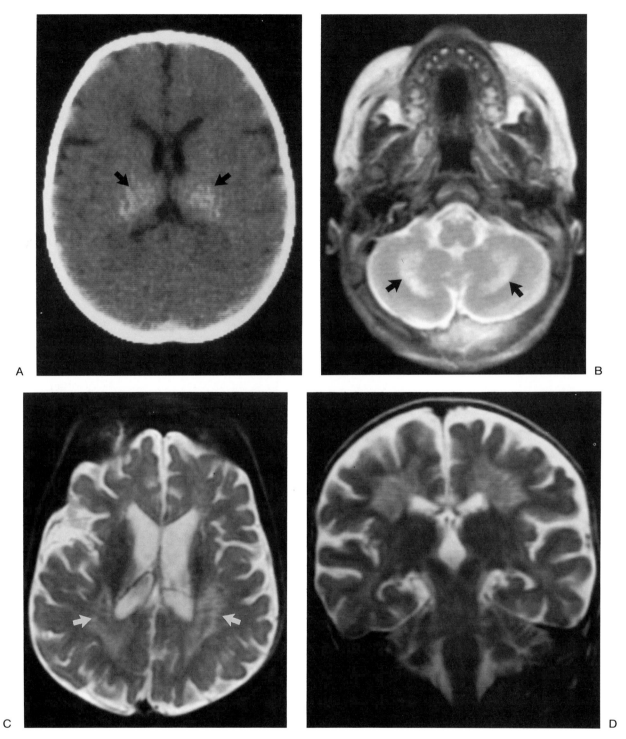

FIG. 3.2. Krabbe's disease. **A:** Axial CT image shows calcification (*arrows*) in the thalami. **B:** Axial SE 2500/70 image shows abnormal high intensity (*arrows*) in the cerebellar white matter. **C:** Axial SE 2500/ 70 image shows high intensity (*arrows*) in the parietal white matter. **D:** Coronal SE 2500/70 image shows the periventricular location of the high signal intensity with sparing of the subcortical white matter.

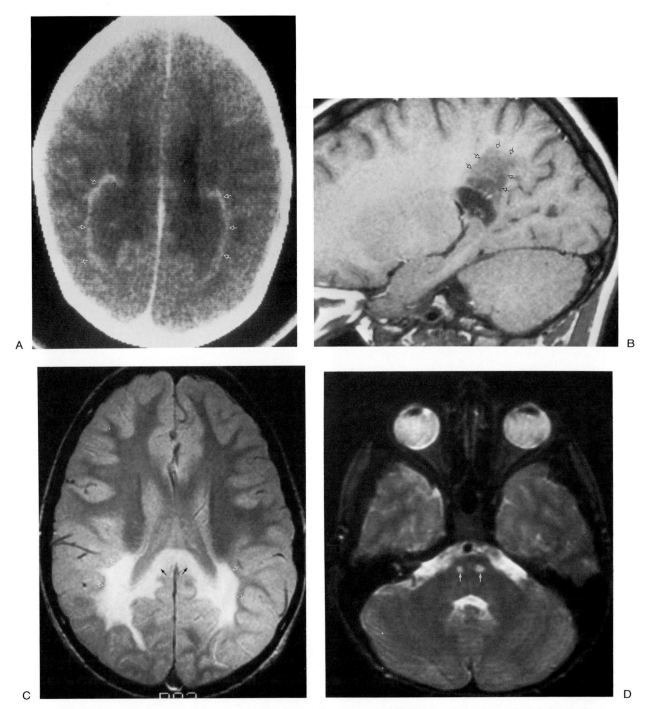

FIG. 3.3. X-linked adrenal leukodystrophy. **A:** Axial postcontrast CT image shows low attenuation in the parieto-occipital white matter with a leading edge (*arrows*) of enhancement. **B:** Parasagittal SE 600/20 image shows low intensity (*arrows*) in the parietal white matter. **C:** Axial SE 2500/30 image shows high signal intensity (*open white arrows*) in the occipital white matter. The splenium (*black arrows*) is involved. The peripheral white matter is spared. **D:** Axial SE 2500/70 image shows high signal intensity (*arrows*) in the corticospinal tracts.

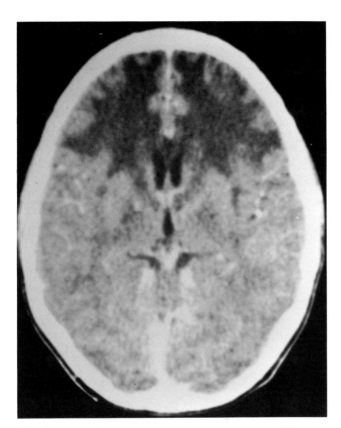

FIG. 3.4. Atypical adrenoleukodystrophy. Axial CT image shows predominant involvement of the frontal white matter. The cause of this atypical pattern is unknown.

ders; therefore, our concepts of them may change considerably in the near future.

Neonatal adrenal leukodystrophy differs fundamentally from X-linked adrenal leukodystrophy both radiologically and clinically. A nearly complete absence of myelin is present in the cerebral white matter throughout the hemispheres, causing severe loss of white matter volume (3). Subtle polymicrogyria may be present (1). The head size is small and the corpus callosum extremely atrophic as a result of the white matter atrophy. *Zellweger's syndrome* is the most severe of the peroxisomal disorders, the patients exhibiting dysmorphic facies, hepatosplenomegaly, and congenital ocular dysplasias (14,15). Imaging findings include profound hypomyelination, prominent cortical dysplasia, gray matter heterotopia, and subependymal cysts (Fig. 3.5).

Pelizaeus-Merzbacher Disease

Pelizaeus-Merzbacher disease is a rare, X-linked leukodystrophy that usually manifests itself in the neonatal period. The name Pelizaeus-Merzbacher disease has been used to describe five different types of sudanophilic leukodystrophies, all of which present similar clinical signs and anatomic anomalies but differ from each other

by age of onset, rate of progression, and genetic transmission (28,29). Other authors limit the term *Pelizaeus-Merzbacher disease* to the classical X-linked recessive form that presents in infancy and leads to death in adolescence or early adulthood (30,31). All forms of the disease seem to result from a deficiency of proteolipid protein, one of the primary components of myelin (32–34). Patients with all forms of Pelizaeus-Merzbacher disease present with clinical signs of abnormal eye movement, often bizarre pendular nystagmus coexisting with head shaking, cerebellar ataxia, and slow psychomotor development. The early infantile (connatal) form of the disease is more rapidly progressive than the other forms. The symptoms are progressive in all forms of the disease (1,35).

On CT scans Pelizaeus-Merzbacher disease appears as low signal intensity in the white matter with progressive white matter atrophy; it is therefore indistinguishable from most other white matter diseases (36). The MR appearance of this disorder is that of a lack of myelination, without frank evidence of white matter destruction (2,31). The brain may retain the appearance of a newborn, with high signal intensity only appearing in the internal capsule, optic radiations, and proximal corona radiata on T1-weighted images and a near complete absence of low signal intensity in the supratentorial region on the T2-weighted images (Fig. 3.6). The amount of myelination slowly diminishes over time (31). In late or very severe cases, a total absence of myelin may be seen (31). The cortical sulci show slowly progressive enlargement (37,38).

Trichothiodystrophy

Trichothiodystrophy, also known as sulfur-deficient brittle hair disease, is a rare autosomal recessive disorder (39,40). Clinical features vary widely in both nature and severity, ranging from patients with only a hair defect (the single common feature in all patients) to those with intellectual impairment, short stature, ichthyosis, photosensitivity, nail dystrophy, cataracts, decreased fertility, neurologic deficits, and immunodeficiency. The underlying biochemical abnormalities are probably altered synthesis of high sulfur-containing proteins and defects in excision repair of chromosomal damage (41).

Imaging findings in trichothiodystrophy are of diffuse lack of myelination (Fig. 3.7), similar to the pattern seen in Pelizaeus-Merzbacher disease (42). Ventriculomegaly has been present in one patient we have examined.

Phenylketonuria

Phenylketonuria is an autosomal recessive disorder that is usually the result of phenylalanine hydroxylase deficiency, although other biochemical defects can cause

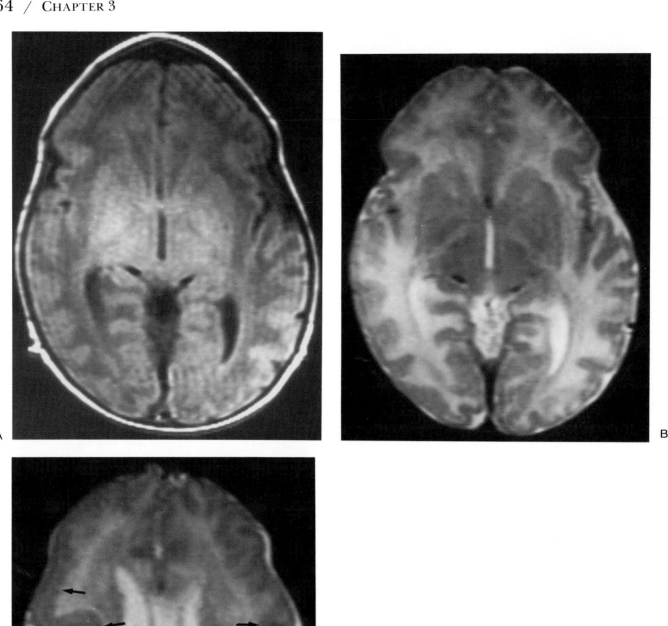

FIG. 3.5. Zellweger's syndrome. **A:** Axial SE 600/20 image shows a nearly complete lack of myelination. Note that the posterior limbs of the internal capsules are hypointense compared to the adjacent thalami and putamina. **B:** Axial SE 3000/120 image shows that the normal focus of hypointensity is absent in the posterior limb of the internal capsule. **C:** Axial SE 600/20 image shows thickened cortex (*arrows*) with a simplified gyral pattern in both hemispheres.

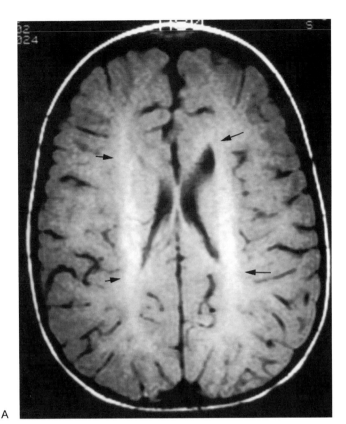

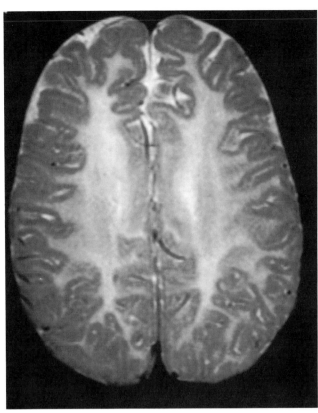

FIG. 3.6. Pelizaeus–Merzbacher disease in a 5-year-old child. **A:** Axial SE 600/16 image shows high signal of myelination (*arrows*) only in the central coronal radiata. **B:** Axial SE 2500/70 at a higher level shows no evidence of the low signal of myelination.

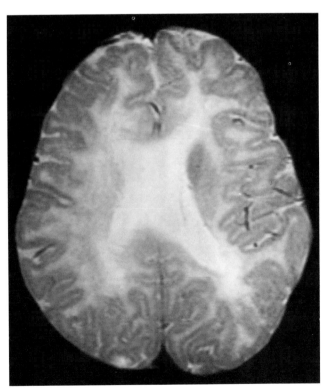

FIG. 3.7. Trichothiodystrophy in a 7-year-old child. Axial SE 2500/70 image shows no evidence of myelination.

the disease (43). The deficiency results in the production of compounds (phenylpyruvic and phenylacetic acids and phenylacetylglutamine) that are toxic to the developing brain (7,43). Untreated patients are characterized by growth retardation and global developmental delay, eczematous dermatitis, hypopigmentation, and a peculiar musty odor of the urine, skin, and hair. Treatment is by dietary control and, occasionally, dietary supplements (43,44).

Imaging studies show primarily abnormal signal in the white matter that corresponds to delayed and defective myelination. In older patients, ventriculomegaly is found as a result of white matter degeneration (45). MR shows T2 prolongation that is initially found in the periventricular white matter of the cerebral hemispheres (7,46). The peripheral white matter is initially spared. Contrast enhancement has not been reported.

Maple Syrup Urine Disease

Maple syrup urine disease is an autosomal recessive disorder, caused by abnormal oxidative decarboxylation of the branched chain amino acids leucine, isoleucine, and valine. Onset of clinical signs and symptoms occurs during the first week of life when poor feeding, vomiting, dystonia, opisthotonic posturing, and seizures become manifest (43). If the disease is not recognized and treated, infants develop signs of increased intracranial pressure, become comatose, and may die in a few weeks (43,47).

Imaging findings are normal in the first few days of life. Starting with the onset of symptoms, the CT and MR findings are quite characteristic, revealing profound localized edema (low density on CT, long T1, T2 on MR) in the deep cerebellar white matter, dorsal brain stem, cerebral peduncles, posterior limb of the internal capsule, and sometimes globi palladi (Figs. 3.8, 3.9) (7,47). The regions involved correspond to those that are myelinated or myelinating at the time of birth. Generalized edema of the cerebral hemispheres may be superimposed on the localized abnormalities (47). After the acute phase of the disease has resolved, the patients are left with a variable degree of brain damage, dependent upon how quickly treatment was initiated (43,47).

Oculocerebrorenal Syndrome (Lowe's Syndrome)

Lowe's syndrome (oculocerebrorenal syndrome) is an X-linked recessive disorder, the etiology of which has yet to be determined. Primary clinical manifestations include congenital ocular abnormalities, mental retardation, renal tubular dysfunction (Fanconi syndrome), and metabolic bone disease leading to arthropathy (48,49). CT shows nonspecific hypodensity in the cerebral white matter. MR shows two distinct lesions: (1) multiple small spherical foci in deep and subcortical white matter that parallel CSF intensity; (2) confluent regions of long T1 and T2 that spare the subcortical U fibers in the early course of the disease (48,50,51).

White Matter Injury from Radiation and Chemotherapy

With a few exceptions, the clinical and imaging manifestations of white matter injury secondary to radiation or chemotherapy in children are not significantly different from those in adults. Radiation injury to the brain is most commonly divided into three major groups: (1) acute reactions (1–6 weeks after treatment); (2) early delayed reactions (3 weeks to several months after treatment); and (3) late delayed reaction (several months to years following treatment).

Acute and *early delayed* reactions are mild, often asymptomatic, and self-limiting, consisting of mild localized edema or perhaps transient myelin injury. They are seen on imaging studies as subtle low density (CT) or T1 and T2 prolongation (MR) without significant mass effect or change in contrast enhancement (52,53).

Late delayed injury is believed to result from damage to blood vessels. Breakdown of the capillary endothelium leads to blood-brain barrier breakdown and exudation of fibrin from the blood vessel lumen. Eventually, endothelium becomes hyalinized and proliferates, compromising the lumen of the vessel and decreasing local blood flow, with subsequent white matter infarction (54). Pathologically, the white matter exhibits areas of necrosis, with rarefaction and fragmentation of myelin, and cellular disruption. Patients may develop localized neurologic deficits or obtundation.

Imaging studies show variable patterns of injury, ranging from single, focal lesions to diffuse white matter abnormality. Signal abnormalities reflect the edema and loss of myelin, as CT shows low attenuation and MR shows T1 and T2 prolongation (Fig. 3.10) (52,53). Contrast enhancement is common, but not invariable, and may be transitory. Significant mass effect can be present. Central necrosis within the lesions is uncommon in children (53). Petechial hemorrhage may be present, appearing as multifocal areas of short T1 and T2 superimposed upon the edema. Knowledge of the ports for radiotherapy can be extremely useful in making the proper diagnosis as the injury is limited to the irradiated field (Fig. 3.11).

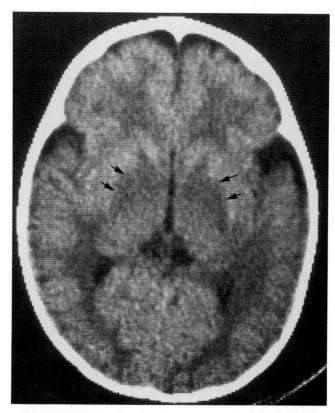

FIG. 3.8. Maple syrup urine disease. Axial CT image shows low attenuation (*arrows*) in the globi palladi and posterior limbs of the internal capsules.

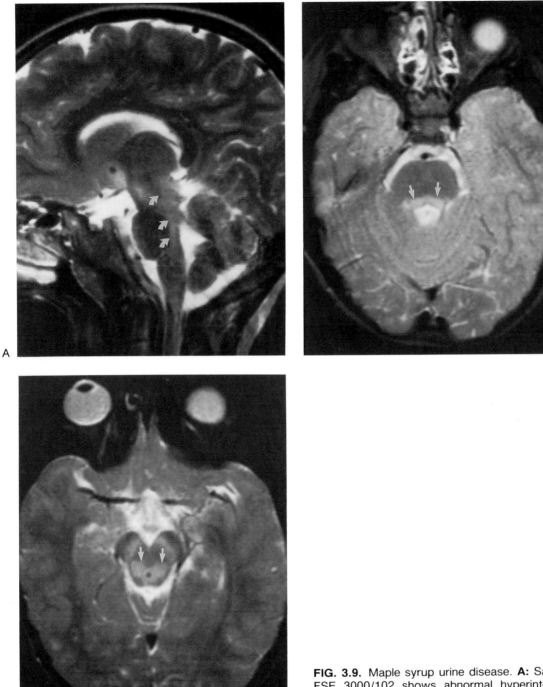

FIG. 3.9. Maple syrup urine disease. **A:** Sagittal FSE 3000/102 shows abnormal hyperintensity (*curved arrows*) in the dorsal brain stem. **B, C:** Axial SE 2500/70 images show abnormal hyperintensity (*arrows*) in the dorsal mesencephalon and pons.

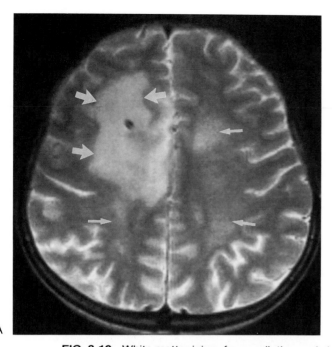
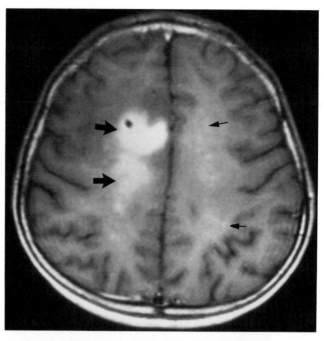

FIG. 3.10. White matter injury from radiation and chemotherapy. This patient was treated with intrathecal methotrexate and radiation to the right frontal lobe. **A:** Axial SE 2500/70 image shows mild hyperintensity diffusely in the periventricular white matter [presumably from the chemotherapy (*small arrows*)] with more pronounced hyperintensity [presumably from the radiation (*large arrows*)] in the right frontal lobe. **B:** Postcontrast axial SE 600/20 image shows enhancement (*arrows*) in many of the areas that showed hyperintensity in A.

Hemorrhagic lesions may be seen in white matter of children who have been irradiated (55). The exact cause of these lesions has not been ascertained; the imaging and surgical appearance is that of occult vascular malformations, or cavernomas (see Chapter 12). Affected children may present with headaches, seizures, or focal neurologic signs and symptoms, or they may be asymptomatic (55). Currently, the lesions are only resected if they are symptomatic or have caused symptomatic hemorrhage.

Young children are more susceptible than adults to radiation injury of the large vessels of the circle of Willis. Children at greatest risk are those younger than 4 years old who receive large doses of radiation to the sellar/suprasellar/parasellar region for suprasellar tumors (56,57). Patients develop progressive narrowing of the supraclinoid carotid artery (Fig. 3.12) and the proximal anterior and middle cerebral arteries, and may evolve into a moyamoya vascular pattern (see Chapter 12). Clinically, this condition is manifest as recurrent TIAs, frank infarction, or developmental delay secondary to chronic cerebral ischemia.

Abnormalities of the cerebral white matter can also result from treatment with *chemotherapeutic agents* (58). The drugs that most commonly cause leukoencephalopathy are methotrexate, cisplatin, arabinosylcytosine,

carmustine, and thiotepa (58,59). The white matter abnormalities seen on imaging studies may be transient or permanent and may be present with or without associated clinical abnormalities (59–61). In contradistinction to the focal white matter abnormalities seen in radiation-induced leukoencephalopathy, T1 and T2 prolongation secondary to chemotherapy tends to be symmetric, widespread, and often diffuse (Fig. 3.10). The T2 prolongation is seen primarily in the central and periventricular white matter, with *relative sparing of the subcortical U fibers* (44,53,59–61). The corpus callosum, anterior commissure, and hippocampal commissure are most often spared (52,53). When enhancement occurs after contrast administration, it tends to be multifocal, usually deep within the centrum semiovale (53).

When patients who have received radiation and chemotherapy begin to rapidly deteriorate clinically in conjunction with diffuse white matter injury, the condition is called *diffuse necrotizing leukoencephalopathy* (62). This form of leukoencephalopathy is pathologically differentiated from other forms by the presence of more extensive areas of white matter necrosis. If the patient survives, the necrotic areas shrink and the volume of white matter diminishes (53). The appearance of the white matter on imaging studies does not correlate well with the severity of the clinical syndrome.

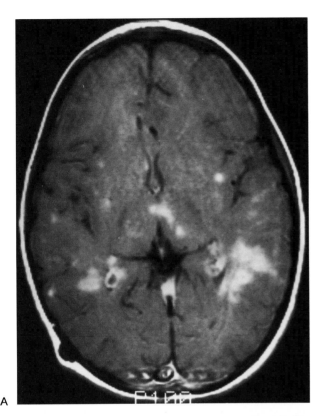

A

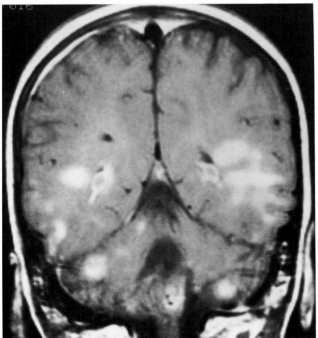

B

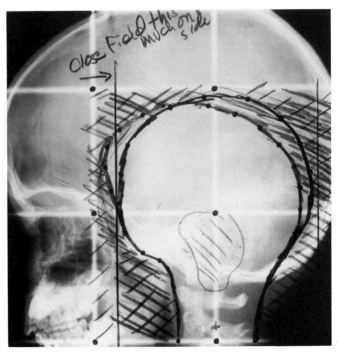

C

FIG. 3.11. Radiation injury in patient treated for brain stem glioma. **A:** Postcontrast axial SE 600/20 image shows enhancement in the middle of the brain with sparing of the anterior frontal and occipital lobes. **B:** Postcontrast coronal SE 600/20 image shows sparing of the superior half of the cerebrum. **C:** Diagram of radiation ports. When lesions are so localized, radiation ports should be examined.

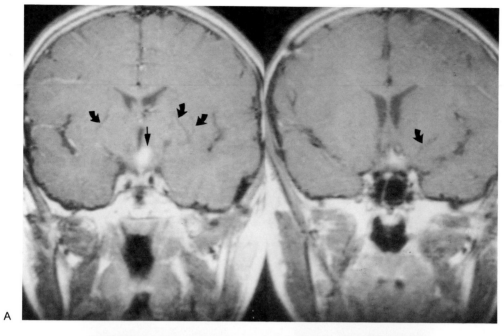

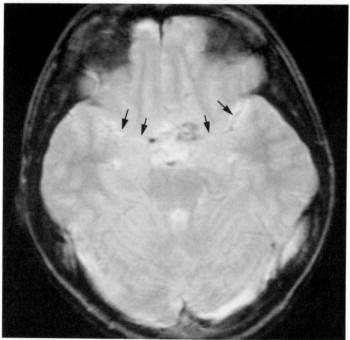

FIG. 3.12. Radiation-induced vasculopathy. **A, B:** Postcontrast SE 600/20 images show dilated lenticulostriate arteries (*curved arrows*) in the basal ganglia. Straight arrow points to residual craniopharyngioma. **C:** Axial SE 2500/70 image shows threadlike middle cerebral arteries (*arrows*).

White Matter Disorders Initially Affecting Peripheral White Matter

Canavan's Disease (Spongiform Leukodystrophy)

Canavan's disease is an autosomal recessive disorder, most common in Ashkenazi Jews, that is caused by a deficiency of aspartoacylase; the biochemical disorder results in N-acetyl aspartic aciduria (63). In the first few weeks of life, affected infants may show marked hypotonia, macrocephaly, and seizures. With further progression of the disease, spasticity, intellectual failure, failure to attain motor milestones, and optic atrophy develop. Death usually occurs in the second year of life (35).

CT and MR in these affected patients reveal diffuse, symmetric abnormalities of the cerebral white matter without any focal predominance. CT shows a diffuse low density in the cerebral and cerebellar white matter. MR reveals prolongation of T1 and T2 relaxation times, resulting in low signal intensity on T1-weighted images and high signal intensity on T2-weighted images (Fig. 3.13) (64). The peripheral white matter is preferentially affected early in the course of the disease (distinguishing this disorder from Krabbe's disease and metachromatic leukodystrophy) and may appear swollen (1,2). Contrast enhancement is not reported. Specific involvement of the globus pallidus can be present, with sparing of the adjacent putamen (1,44). As the disease progresses, diffuse atrophy of the white matter and, subsequently, cerebral cortex is seen (7). Proton spectroscopy (Fig. 3.13F) shows significant enlargement of the N-acetyl aspartate peak (65), a finding that appears specific for this disorder.

Alexander's Disease

Patients with Alexander's disease, also known as fibrinoid leukodystrophy, typically present during the first year of life, sometimes as early as the first few weeks of life. The most frequent initial manifestations are macrocephaly and failure to attain developmental milestones. Progressive psychomotor retardation may become prominent; death usually ensues in infancy or early childhood (5,35). The cause is unknown. Diagnosis is made by the combination of macrocephaly, early onset of clinical findings, and the result of imaging studies.

CT shows low density in the frontal white matter that gradually extends posteriorly into the parietal region and internal capsule. Contrast enhancement is often seen near the tips of the frontal horns early in the disease (66,67) (Fig 3.14). The MR findings are those of prolonged T1 and T2 relaxation times beginning in the frontal white matter and progressing posteriorly to the parietal white matter and the internal and external capsules (Fig. 3.14). Peripheral white matter is affected early in

the course of the disease. In the late stages of the disease, cysts may develop in affected regions of the brain.

Cockayne Syndrome

Cockayne syndrome is an autosomal recessive disorder that is characterized by cutaneous photosensitivity, dwarfism, optic atrophy, cataracts, and progressive neurologic dysfunction. Affected patients typically present with psychomotor retardation between the ages of 6 and 12 months. Both development and growth fall farther and farther from the norm (68,69). Patients are further characterized by accentuated thoracic kyphosis, lumbar lordosis, and characteristic facies (44,68).

CT in Cockayne syndrome reveals brain calcification, most commonly in the basal ganglia and cerebellar dentate nuclei, and cerebral and cerebellar atrophy (44,70). MR shows atrophy and T2 prolongation, initially in the periventricular white matter, basal ganglia, and cerebellar dentate nuclei (71,72). The subcortical U fibers can be involved early in the disease but are more commonly affected only in later stages (1). Gradient echo, and sometimes spin echo, images will show hypodensity of the calcified deep cerebral and cerebellar nuclei (Fig. 3.15) (71).

Other Disorders with Cerebral Calcifications and Abnormal Myelination

Other disorders have radiologic findings similar to those in Cockayne syndrome but without the characteristic clinical findings. Basal ganglia calcification occurs in pediatric AIDS, which will be discussed in Chapter 11. References for the other disorders are provided for interested readers (73–76).

Galactosemia

Galactosemia is an autosomal recessive disorder that is most commonly the result of galactose-1-phosphate-uridyl transferase deficiency, although other causes have been reported (77). Affected patients present as newborns and young infants with signs of increased intracranial pressure and vomiting. If untreated, patients develop severe liver disease, profound mental retardation, epilepsy, and choreoathetosis (78). Treatment is dietary restriction of galactose; however, even compliant patients show some neurologic and neuropsychologic abnormalities (79).

CT scans of patients with galactosemia are nonspecific, showing extensive low attenuation in the cerebral white matter (7). MR studies seem somewhat more specific, showing delayed myelination (persistent high signal) in the subcortical white matter on T2-weighted images, although the same white matter seems to mature

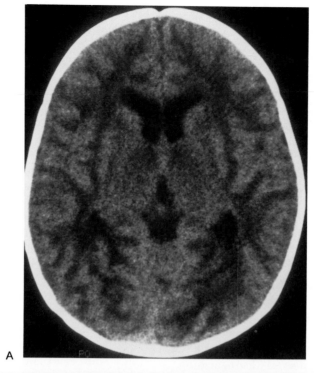

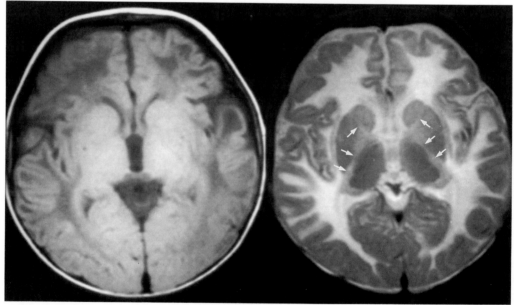

FIG. 3.13. Canavan's disease. **A:** Axial CT image shows diffuse white matter hypodensity. **B–E:** Axial T1- and T2-weighted spin echo images show diffuse T1 and T2 prolongation of the white matter with involvement of the internal (*arrows*) and external capsules and the subcortical U fibers. **F:** ¹H MRS shows an enlarged NAA peak.

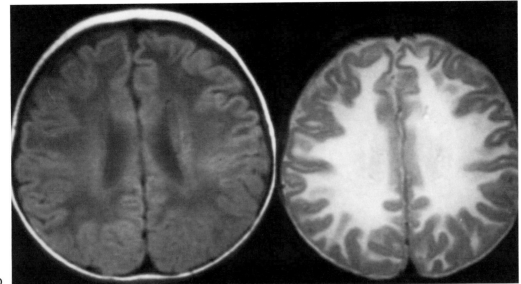

D   E

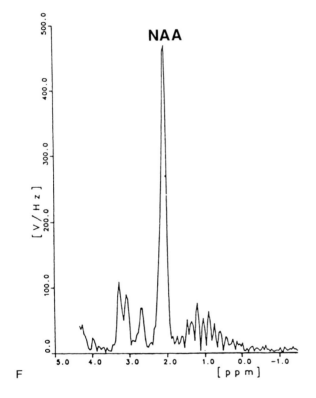

F   **FIG. 3.13.** *(Continued.)*

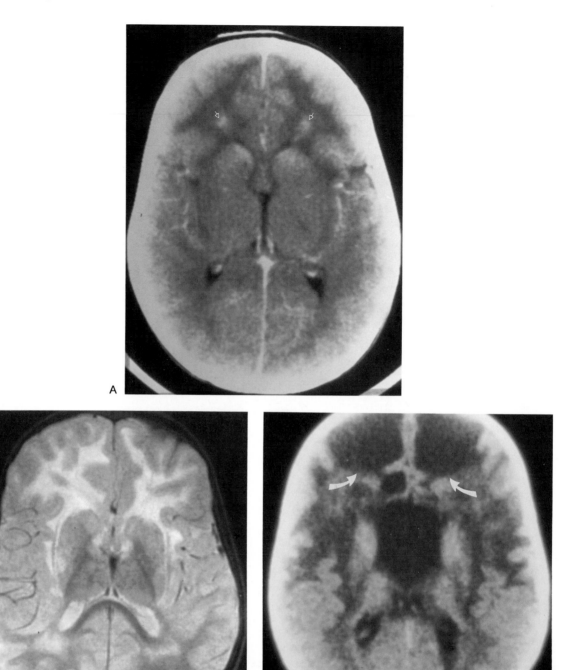

FIG. 3.14. Alexander's disease. **A:** Postcontrast axial CT image shows low attenuation in the frontal white matter bilaterally. Enhancement (*arrows*) is present around the tips of the frontal horns of the lateral ventricles. **B:** Axial SE 2500/70 image shows high signal intensity in the frontal white matter, involving the subcortical U fibers and extending posteriorly into the external capsules. **C:** Axial CT scan 1 year after that in A shows that the white matter injury has extended posteriorly into the parieto-occipital regions. Cysts (*arrows*) have formed in the frontal lobes.

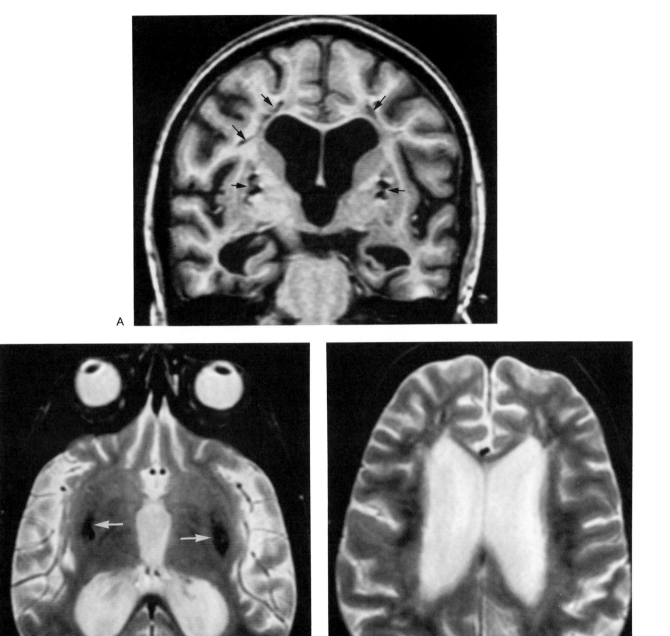

FIG. 3.15. Cockayne syndrome. **A:** Coronal spoiled gradient echo image shows susceptibility artifact (*arrows*) from multiple foci of calcification in the basal ganglia and white matter. **B:** Axial SE 2500/70 image shows low intensity (*arrows*) secondary to calcification in the basal ganglia and prominent CSF spaces. **C:** Axial SE 2500/70 image at a higher level shows diminished quantity of white matter, prominent CSF spaces, and abnormally high intensity in the white matter, the latter presumably secondary to loss of myelin.

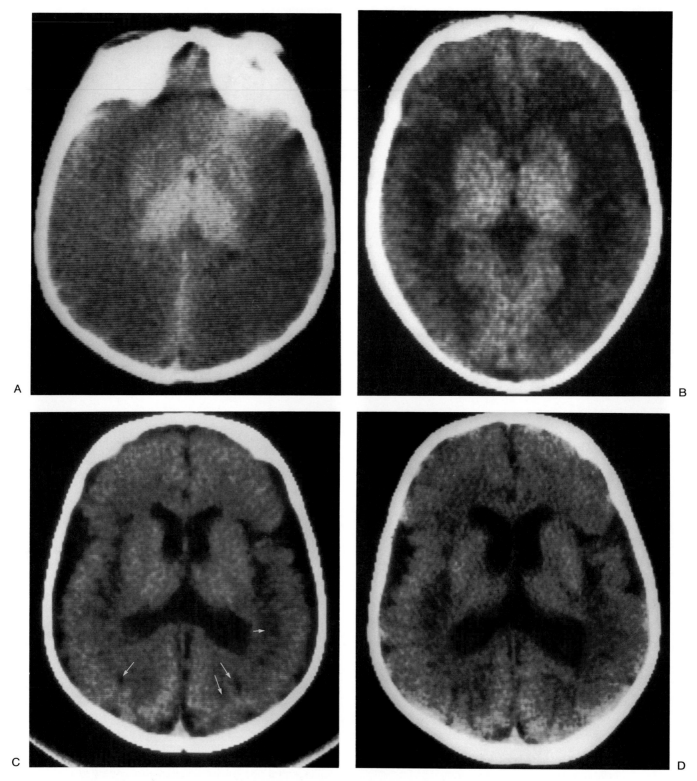

FIG. 3.16. Citrullinemia. **A:** Axial CT image at age 2 days shows diffuse cerebral edema involving the cerebral cortex, cerebral white matter, and basal ganglia. **B:** At age 2 weeks, after treatment, the edema is resolving in the basal ganglia and parts of the cerebral cortex. **C:** At age 6 months, the CSF spaces are slightly large and foci of low attenuation (*arrows*) are scattered in the white matter. **D:** At age 3 years, white matter atrophy has progressed with consequent enlargement of the ventricles.

normally on T1-weighted images (80). Cerebral and cerebellar atrophy are seen in older patients. Focal white matter lesions are occasionally seen and are of uncertain significance (80).

Mitochondrial Disorders

Although mitochondrial encephalopathies can cause demyelination, gray matter is almost always involved. Therefore, mitochondrial disorders are included in the section "Metabolic Disorders Affecting Both Gray and White Matter."

White Matter Diseases with Nonspecific Patterns

Nonketotic Hyperglycinemia

Nonketotic hyperglycinemia is a hereditary disorder of amino acid metabolism in which large quantities of glycine accumulate in plasma, urine, and CSF. It is caused by a disturbance in the breakdown of glycine. Onset of clinical symptoms is most often in early infancy with seizures, dystonia, and pronounced developmental delay (43).

CT studies have revealed cerebral and cerebellar volume loss with hypoattenuation of the periventricular white matter (81). MR shows a nonspecific pattern of decreased volume and prolonged T2 relaxation time of the cerebral hemispheric white matter, with consequent thinning of the corpus callosum, which is abnormally thin (82).

^{1}H MRS studies show an abnormal peak at 3.56 ppm, believed to represent glycine, in patients with nonketotic hyperglycinemia (83). Abnormal spectra are reported in patients with normal MR imaging studies. Moreover, the clinical course of the patients seems to correlate more closely to the glycine level, as detected by MRS, than to plasma or CSF concentrations of glycine (83). To separate the glycine peak from that of *myo*-inositol, which has a similar chemical shift, the spectra should be obtained with a long echo time. The *myo*-inositol peak, which has a short T2 relaxation time, disappears on the long TE spectra. Properly performed, MRS may become the method of choice for following patients with nonketotic hyperglycinemia.

Disorders of the Urea Cycle and Ammonia

Disorders of the urea cycle include *ornithine carbamyl transferase deficiency, carbamyl phosphate synthetase deficiency, argininosuccinic aciduria, citrullinemia,* and *hyperargininemia.* All result in hyperammonemia that may be worsened by high protein intake or illness. The timing of onset of these disorders depends upon the nature of the molecular defect and the degree to which the patient sustains some capacity for elimination of nitrogen waste products (84). Affected patients typically have intermittent neurologic dysfunction that may present as movement disorders, seizures, ataxia, or confusion.

The CT and MR patterns in these disorders are nonspecific. Patients may initially present with a pattern of diffuse edema (Fig. 3.16). Images later in the course of the disease may show both focal and diffuse areas of hypodensity on CT and prolongation of T1 and T2 relaxation times on MR (Figs. 3.16, 3.17). Moreover, the cerebral cortex may be affected in the acute stage. In advanced cases, atrophy is often severe. Two characteristics of brain involvement are noteworthy: (1) The subcortical U fibers are *not* spared; and (2) cerebral involvement is most often asymmetric.

Autoimmune and Infectious Disorders Affecting White Matter

Multiple Sclerosis

Although usually considered an adult disease, multiple sclerosis (MS) can begin to be manifest during

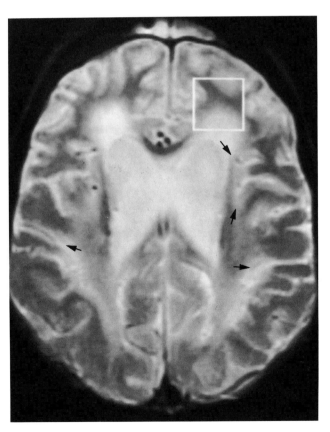

FIG. 3.17. Citrullinemia. Axial SE 2500/70 image shows abnormal high signal intensity in the white matter. Note the involvement of the subcortical U fibers (*arrows*) in several locations. The box shows the location in which a ^{1}H MRS (not shown) was obtained.

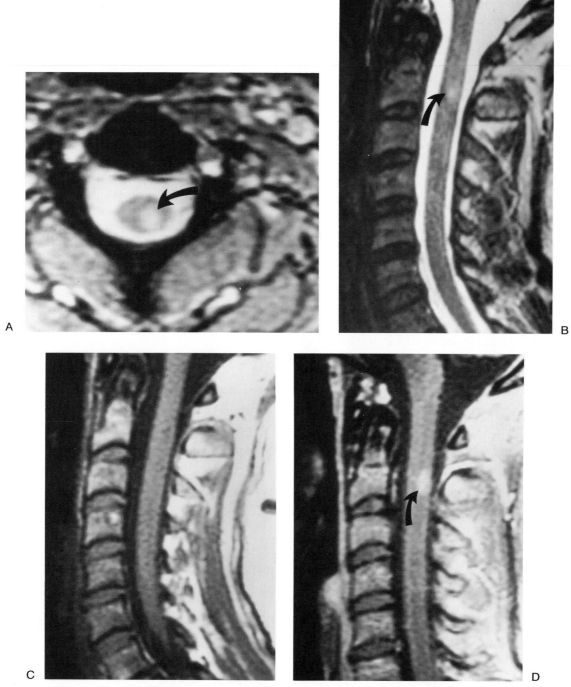

FIG. 3.18. Childhood multiple sclerosis resembling the disease in adults. **A, B:** Axial GE 600/20 and sagittal FSE 3000/102 images show a focus of hyperintensity (*arrows*) in the spinal cord at the C2 level. **C, D:** Precontrast (C) and postcontrast (D) SE 600/20 images show that the lesion (*arrow*) enhances.

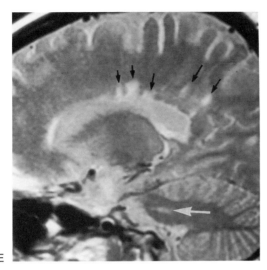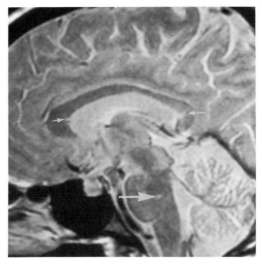

E F

FIG. 3.18. (*Continued.*) **E, F:** Sagittal FSE 3000/102 images show foci of hyperintensity in the corpus callosum (*small white arrows*), posterior fossa (*large white arrows*), and periventricular white matter of the cerebrum (*black arrows*).

childhood. It has been estimated that between 0.3% and 2% of all patients with MS present during childhood (85,86). However, a number of reports describing patients presenting with multiple sclerosis before the age of 5 years have appeared in the recent medical literature (see the listing in ref. 87), suggesting that the number of cases in childhood may have been underreported. The clinical presentation of the disease in early childhood can range from school problems and paresthesias to dra-

matic presentations suggesting diffuse encephalopathy with cerebral edema, meningismus, and impaired consciousness (87).

Imaging findings in children with multiple sclerosis are not significantly different from those in adults (Fig. 3.18), although the incidence of tumefactive plaques (Figs. 3.19, 3.20) (88) and posterior fossa plaques (Fig. 3.19) (89) may be somewhat higher. Tumefactive plaques can sometimes be differentiated from tumors by the pres-

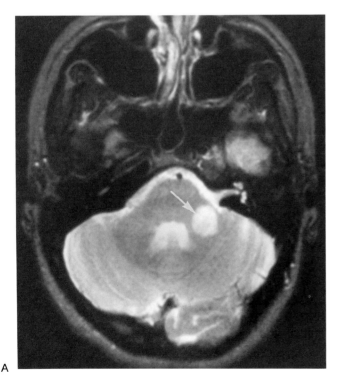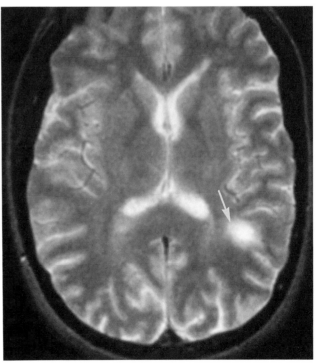

A B

FIG. 3.19. Tumefactive multiple sclerosis in a child. Axial SE 2500/70 images show large, tumefactive plaques of demyelination (*arrows*). Tumefactive plaques seem to be more common in childhood multiple sclerosis.

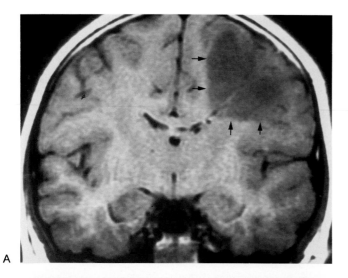

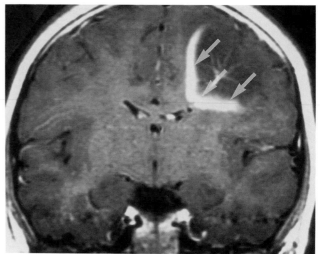

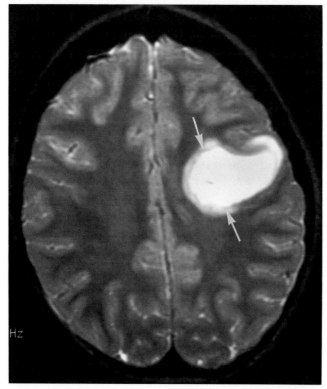

FIG. 3.20. Tumefactive multiple sclerosis. **A, B:** Coronal SE 600/16 and axial SE 2500/70 images shows an area (*arrows*) with prolonged T1 and T2 relaxation times in the left frontal lobe. The lesion abuts the left lateral ventricle and has essentially no mass effect. **C:** Postcontrast coronal SE 600/16 image shows enhancement (*arrows*) on only one side of the lesion, suggesting that it is not a tumor.

ence of other, more typical plaques, lack of mass effect, location adjacent to the ventricular surface, and enhancement limited to only one side of the lesion (in contradistinction to a complete ring, Fig. 3.20). Readers interested in further information concerning imaging findings in multiple sclerosis are referred to any standard adult neurology or neuroradiology text.

Localized proton spectroscopy from white matter plaques of children with MS shows a decrease in NAA and creatines and an increase in cholines and *myo*-inositol relative to age-matched controls (24). Adjacent white matter is normal, but adjacent cortical gray matter shows reduced NAA.

Preliminary work shows that magnetization transfer techniques may be useful in differentiating the inflammation associated with MS from actual demyelination (90).

Acute Disseminated Encephalomyelitis (ADEM)

Children may develop acute encephalitis late in the course of a viral illness or after a vaccination; less commonly, encephalitis may occur after a bacterial infection (particularly mycoplasma) or drug ingestion (91,92). This disorder is called acute disseminated encephalomyelitis (ADEM) or parainfectious encephalomyelitis. The most common clinical presentation is the onset of seizures and focal neurologic signs 4–7 days after the clinical onset of the viral infection. Less fulminant cases present with headache, fever, irritability, drowsiness, or vomiting; nuchal rigidity is often present. The neurologic findings resolve over a period of weeks. Most patients make a complete recovery with no neurologic sequelae; 10% to 20% will have some permanent neurologic damage (93,94). Measles, mumps, chickenpox, rubella, and pertussis are the best-described viruses that cause this disease; however, many cases seem to occur "spontaneously," or follow nonspecific infections (93,94).

ADEM is likely caused by an autoimmune response; it is postulated that the precipitating illness induces a host-antibody response against a central nervous system antigen. This postulate is supported by the fact that the gross pathologic and histologic manifestations of acute disseminated encephalomyelitis closely resemble those of experimental allergic encephalitis, an experimentally induced autoimmune disease caused by antibodies to myelin. Pathologically, a diffuse perivenous inflammatory process causes confluent areas of demyelination. Cortical and deep gray matter are involved, but to a lesser extent than white matter.

On imaging studies, moderate to large areas of demyelination (low density on CT, prolonged T1 and T2 on MR) are seen in the subcortical white matter of one or both hemispheres, usually asymmetrically (Fig. 3.21)

(95,96). MR reveals abnormalities of the deep cerebral nuclei (Fig. 3.22) in approximately 50% of affected pediatric patients (97,98) (Fig. 3.22). The brain stem, spinal cord, and cerebellar white matter can also be affected, although less commonly than the supratentorial structures (97). In the subacute phase, the lesions will show various patterns of enhancement after infusion of contrast (98,99).

Acute Hemorrhagic Encephalomyelitis

Acute hemorrhagic encephalomyelitis is a variant of acute disseminated encephalomyelitis in which the involved regions of brain undergo hemorrhagic necrosis. Patients often progress rapidly into delirium and coma, and most die within the first few days to a week of onset (93). The few survivors have serious neurologic sequelae. Imaging findings are similar to those in ADEM except that the lesions are hemorrhagic and have more associated edema and mass effect (44,100).

Progressive Multifocal Leukoencephalitis

Progressive multifocal leukoencephalitis is a rare demyelinating disease caused by a papovavirus. It causes a combination of isolated and confluent areas of T2 prolongation, primarily in the white matter. Mass effect and

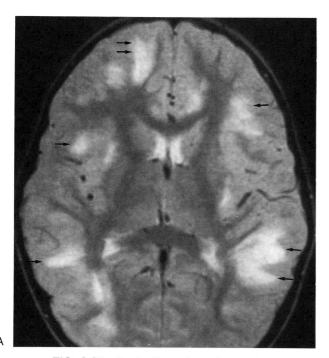
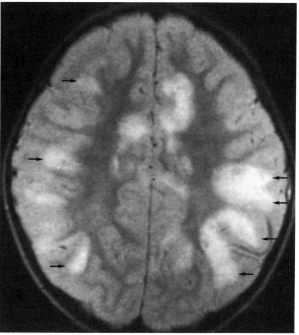

FIG. 3.21. Acute disseminated encephalomyelitis. Axial SE 2500/70 images show multiple foci of T2 prolongation (*arrows*) located bilaterally and asymmetrically at the gray matter–white matter junction.

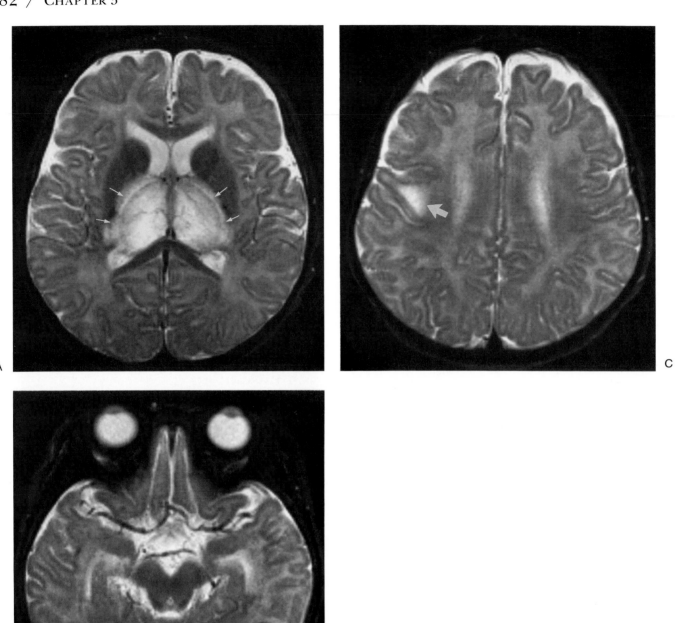

A

C

B

FIG. 3.22. Acute disseminated encephalomyelitis. **A:** Axial SE 2500/70 image shows abnormal hyperintensity in the thalami (*arrows*). **B, C:** Subcortical foci of demyelination (*arrows*) are seen at the gray matter—white matter junction of the right hemisphere.

contrast enhancement are minimal, if present at all. This disease is more fully discussed in Chapter 11.

Subacute Sclerosing Panencephalitis

Subacute sclerosing panencephalitis is a slow virus infection of the CNS that occurs secondary to measles infection. Imaging studies show a nonspecific pattern of increased water in white matter with localized cortical lesions in some cases. This disease is discussed more fully in Chapter 11.

Collagen Vascular Diseases

Collagen vascular diseases are immunologically mediated syndromes in which antigen-antibody complexes are found in various body tissues, resulting in multiorgan dysfunction. The most common of these disorders presenting with neurologic signs and symptoms in children and adolescents is systemic lupus erythematosus (SLE). Affected patients may present with seizures, acute focal neurologic deficits, intracranial hypertension, dementia, psychiatric disorders, chorea, visual disturbances, paresthesias, aseptic meningitis, or a host of other signs or symptoms (101–103). Although neurologic events commonly occur in SLE, they are frequently difficult to assess, because they may be related to therapy, infection, complications, or functional problems related to the underlying disorder (101,102). A variety of pathologic abnormalities have been identified in SLE, including cerebral atrophy, cerebral infarcts due to emboli, vasculitis, petechial hemorrhages, and areas of demyelination. These are all believed to result from the action of cytotoxic antibodies that vary in their composition and antigenicity and thus attack various vulnerable parts of the central nervous system (101–103).

Imaging studies in SLE are nonspecific. Most commonly, the appearance is of small or large areas of low attenuation (CT) or long T1 and T2 (MR) in the white matter of the cerebrum, cerebellum, brain stem, or spinal cord. Some peripheral enhancement may be present in the subacute phase. These areas tend to spare the overlying cortex (Fig. 3.23) and may revert to normal on subsequent scans. When symptoms are the result of vasculitis, both superficial and deep gray matter may be involved. Infarcted tissue will, obviously, not return to a normal appearance.

Toxins

Several exogenous toxins can cause demyelination. Most of these intoxications result in a spongiform leukoencephalopathy that initially affects the peripheral white matter, including the subcortical U fibers. Among

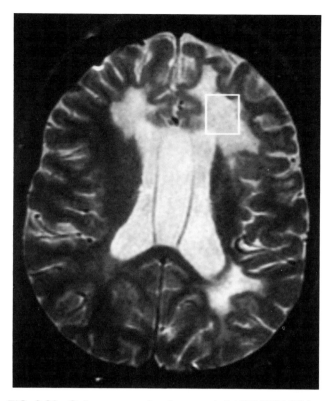

FIG. 3.23. Collagen vascular disease. Axial SE 2500/70 image shows multiple foci of abnormal hyperintensity in the cerebral white matter with sparing of the overlying cortex. These regions may revert to normal on subsequent scans. The box in the left frontal lobe was a site for MRS.

the toxic substances that cause demyelination are triethyl tin, hexachlorophene, cuprizone, actinomycin D, and isoniazid (44, 104–106). All these disorders cause bilateral symmetric white matter injury that involves the subcortical U fibers early in the course of the clinical illness.

Special mention must be made of *lead encephalopathy*. The typical clinical presentation of lead intoxication is abdominal cramping, nausea, and vomiting. Neurologic signs and symptoms vary from mild behavioral change to frank obtundation, with occasional ataxia, aphasia, or psychological disturbance (104,107). Rarely, lead intoxication may lead to localized edema in the cerebellum causing hydrocephalus and presentation as a posterior fossa mass (107,108). CT and MR (Fig. 3.24) show localized cerebellar edema with mass effect and mild enhancement after intravenous contrast infusion (107,108). The appearance is identical to that of acute cerebellitis from viral illnesses (see Chapter 11 and Fig. 11.26).

Metabolic Disorders Primarily Affecting Gray Matter

A large number of conditions affecting the pediatric central nervous system affect the gray matter, including

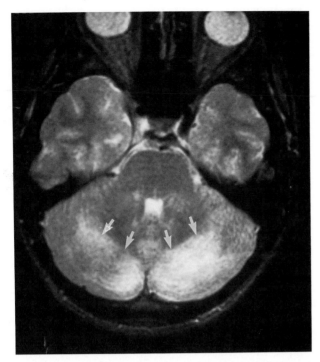

FIG. 3.24. Lead encephalopathy. Axial SE 2500/70 image shows edema in the cerebellar white matter. A similar pattern of cerebellar edema can be seen in viral and parainfectious cerebellitis (see Chapter 11 and Fig. 11.26).

infections, malformations, and injuries, in addition to inborn errors of metabolism. The imaging findings in many gray matter disorders are nonspecific. In some disorders, such as the mucolipidoses, Gaucher's disease, and some forms of Niemann-Pick disease, the brain appears normal. In others, such as the ceroid lipofuscinoses, the cerebral cortex is thin and the cerebral white matter is diminished in volume and has low attenuation (CT) and prolonged T1 and T2 relaxation times (MR), compared to those of normal white matter, particularly in the periventricular regions (Fig. 3.25) (109–111). However, the T2 prolongation is not as marked as in the leukodystrophies (see Figs. 3.1–3.3, for example), presumably because the white matter abnormality results from Wallerian degeneration of the axons and is not associated with an inflammatory response or with an active destructive process. In this section, only those disorders are discussed that have distinctive abnormalities on imaging studies.

Hallervorden-Spatz Disease

Hallervorden-Spatz disease is a rare metabolic disorder that is characterized clinically by progressive gait impairment, gradually increasing rigidity of all limbs, slowing of voluntary movements, choreo-athetotic movement disorder, dysarthria, and mental deterioration. Although the age of onset varies considerably, most

patients begin to show some neurologic deterioration during the second decade of life. Iron is concentrated in the basal ganglia, resulting in the hyperpigmentation and symmetrical destruction of the globus pallidus and substantia nigra that is seen pathologically (112).

Imaging studies reflect the underlying pathology. CT scans may show low- or high-density foci in the globus pallidus. Although the cause of this variability has not been proven pathologically, it is likely that the low-density lesions reflect tissue destruction, whereas the high-density foci are a result of subsequent dystrophic calcification. MR will initially show hypodensity in the globus pallidus on T2-weighted images (more pronounced hypodensity than is normally seen in the second decade; see Chapter 2), resulting from iron deposition (113–115). Foci of prolonged T2 develop within the globus pallidus soon thereafter and subsequently enlarge; these foci presumably represent pallidal destruction and gliosis (Fig. 3.26) (114). *Of the many disorders that affect the basal ganglia in children (Tables 3.4–3.6) thus far, only Hallervorden-Spatz disease has shown T2 shortening.*

Juvenile Huntington's Disease

Huntington's disease is a chronic, degenerative disease characterized by choreiform movements, mental deterioration, and an autosomal dominant transmission. About 5% of patients present prior to the age of 14 years (5). The clinical presentation in children is one of hypokinesia, rigidity, seizures, and mental deterioration

TABLE 3.4. *Childhood diseases involving the basal ganglia*

Acute
  Hypoxia
  Hypoglycemia
  Carbon monoxide poisoning
  Hemolytic–uremic syndrome
  Osmotic myelinolysis
  Encephalitis
  Parainfectious encephalomyelitis
Chronic
  Inborn errors of metabolism
    Mitochondrial disorders
    Glutaric aciduria types I and II
    Methylmalonic acidemia
    Propionic acidemia
    Maple syrup urine disease
    Wilson's disease
    Canavan's disease
    Hallervorden-Spatz disease
Degenerative diseases
  Juvenile Huntington disease
  Sequelae of acute insults
  Basal ganglia calcification syndromes (i.e., Cockayne's)
Other diseases
  Neurofibromatosis type I

TABLE 3.5. *Disorders resulting in basal ganglia calcification*

Endocrine
    Hypoparathyroidism
    Pseudohypoparathyroidism
    Pseudopseudohypoparathyroidism
    Hyperparathyroidism
    Hypothyroidism
Metabolic
    Mitochondrial disorders
    Fahr disease (familial cerebrovascular ferrocalcinosis)
    Hallervorden-Spatz disease
Congenital or developmental
    Familial idiopathic symmetric basal ganglia calcification
    Hastings–James syndrome
    Cockayne syndrome
    Lipoid proteinosis (hyalinosis cutis)
    Neurofibromatosis
    Tuberous sclerosis
    Oculocraniosomatic disease
    Methemoglobinopathy
    Down's syndrome
Inflammatory
    Toxoplasmosis
    Congenital rubella
    Cytomegalovirus
    Measles
    Chicken pox
    Pertussis
    Coxsackie B virus
    Cysticercosis
    Systemic lupus erythematosus
    Acquired immunodeficiency syndrome
Toxic
    Hypoxia
    Cardiovascular event
    Carbon monoxide intoxication
    Lead intoxication
    Radiation therapy
    Methotrexate therapy
    Nephrotic syndrome

(116). Imaging studies are normal early in the course of the disease. However, the striatum develops T2 prolongation and atrophies as the disease progresses; atrophy of the caudate heads result in a characteristic enlargement of the frontal horns of the lateral ventricles, which become convex laterally (Fig. 3.27). Atrophy in the putamen, seen better by MR than by CT, is equal to or more severe than that in the caudate (117). Cortical atrophy is most prominent in the frontal lobes. F^{18}-fluorodeoxyglucose PET scanning is sensitive to decreased glucose uptake in the striatum before CT scans become positive (118). Comparisons of the sensitivity of PET to that of MR have not been published.

Neuroaxonal Dystrophy

Patients with the infantile form of neuroaxonal dystrophy usually present during the end of the first year or the second year of life. Affected patients develop a lack of spontaneous movement, followed by nystagmus and progressive deterioration of posture, gait, speech (if developed), and visual acuity. Deep dementia, blindness, and complete lack of motor function eventually ensue. Choreoathetosis and epilepsy develop in some patients.

Pathology shows atrophy of the cerebellar and cerebral cortices. MR shows prominent sulci, diminished cerebral white matter, and marked T2 prolongation of the cerebellar cortex (Fig. 3.28).

TABLE 3.6. *Anatomic distribution of diseases affecting basal ganglia*

Diagnosis	Globus pallidus	Caudate	Putamen	White matter
Acute				
Hypoxia	+	+	+	+
Hypoglycemia	+	+	+	+
Carbon monoxide intoxication	++	+	+	+
Hemolytic–uremic syndrome	+	+	+	+
Osmotic myelinolysis	+	+	+	++pons
Encephalitis	+	+	+	+
Chronic				
Mitochondrial disorders	+	+	++	+
Wilson's disease	++	+	++	+
Glutaric aciduria type I		+	+	
Glutaric aciduria type II			+	+
Juvenile Huntington's Dz		++	++	
Methylmalonic acidemia	+			+
Propionic acidemia	+			+
Huntington disease	+	++	++	+
Hallervorden-Spatz disease	++			

Note: Common involvement indicated by ++.

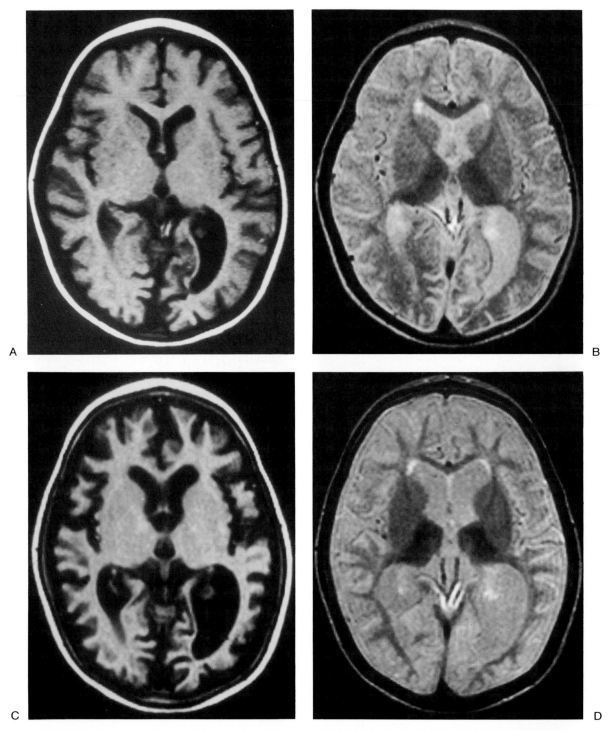

FIG. 3.25. Neuronal ceroid lipofuscinosis, a gray matter disease. **A:** Axial SE 500/25 image at age 3 years shows prominent CSF spaces without focal abnormalities. **B:** Axial SE 2200/80 image shows that the hemispheric white matter has higher signal intensity than in a normal 3-year-old. However, the signal is not as high as in a typical leukodystrophy (compare with Figs. 3.1–3.3). **C:** Axial SE 500/25 1 year after the study shown in (A) and (B). Progressive gray matter atrophy has resulted in more pronounced cortical thinning with resultant enlargement of cortical sulci. The ventricles have probably enlarged secondary to Wallerian degeneration of the white matter tracts. **D:** Axial SE 2200/40 image from the same study as (C) shows that the deep gray matter nuclei are more hypointense than the hemispheric white matter. This phenomenon may be the result of iron deposition in these structures.

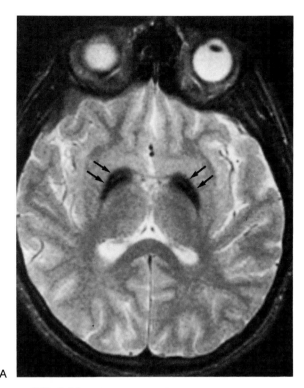 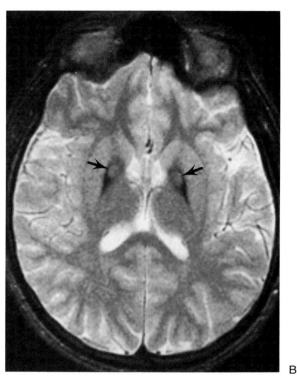

A   B

FIG. 3.26. Hallervorden-Spatz disease in a 14-year-old child. **A:** Axial SE 2800/70 image shows markedly hypointense signal (*arrows*) in the inferior globus pallidus. This region is much more hypointense than is seen in the normal 14-year-old child. **B:** Image 7.5 mm superior to (A) shows an area of higher signal intensity (*arrows*), possibly due to tissue destruction, within the hypointense globus pallidus.

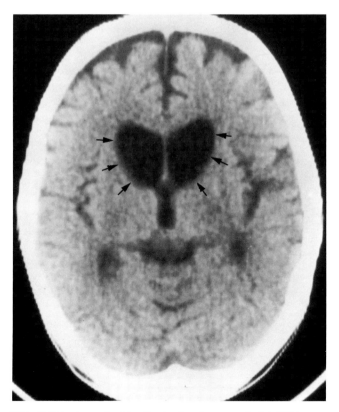

FIG. 3.27. Juvenile Huntington's disease. Axial CT image shows enlarged frontal horns (*arrows*) secondary to atrophy of the heads of the caudate nuclei and putamina.

Metabolic Disorders Affecting Both Gray and White Matter

Mucopolysaccharidoses

The mucopolysaccharidoses are lysosomal storage disorders that result from deficiency of specific lysosomal enzymes involved in the degradation of mucopolysaccharides (glycosaminoglycans). Mucopolysaccharide deposits in the lysosomes interfere with the degradation of other macromolecules, resulting in the intralysosomal accumulation of other materials in addition to mucopolysaccharides. Incompletely degraded mucopolysaccharides accumulate in the tissues and are excreted in the urine as dermatan sulfate, heparan sulfate, and keratan sulfate. Diagnosis is made by combining the clinical picture with characteristic urinary mucopolysaccharides (119,120).

Table 3.7 summarizes the main genetic and biochemical aspects of the various mucopolysaccharidoses. The clinical manifestations of these disorders vary. Most patients with mucopolysaccharidoses have macrocephaly. Developmental retardation is a prominent feature of mucopolysaccharidoses I, II, III, and VII, probably resulting from neuronal damage by the intralysosomal mucopolysaccharides. Skeletal involvement dominates the clinical picture in mucopolysaccharidoses IV and VI,

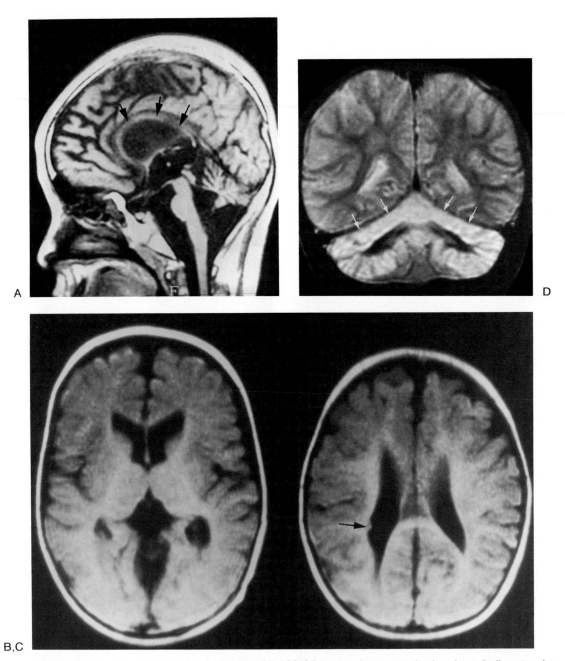

FIG. 3.28. Neuroaxonal dystrophy. **A:** Sagittal SE 500/25 image shows cerebral and cerebellar atrophy and a very thin corpus callosum (*arrows*). **B, C:** Axial SE 500/25 images show diminished cerebral white matter and deficient myelination. A subependymal heterotopion (*arrow*) is incidentally noted. **D:** Coronal SE 2000/80 image shows abnormal hyperintensity (*arrows*) of the cerebellar cortex.

TABLE 3.7. *Mucopolysaccharidoses*

Type	Eponym	Inheritance	Enzyme deficiency	Urinary glycosaminoglycan	Neurologic signs
IH	Hurler	Autosomal recessive	α-L-Iduronidase	Dermatan sulfate	Marked
II	Hunter	X-Linked recessive	Iduronate sulfatase	Dermatan or heparan sulfate	Mild to moderate
III	Sanfillipo A–D	Autosomal recessive	Heparan sulfate sulfatase	Heparan sulfate	Mental deterioration
			N-Acetyl-α-D-glucosaminidase α-Glucosamine-N-acetyltransferase N-Acetylglucosamine-6-sulfate sulfatase		
IV	Morquio A–D (B is milder form)	Autosomal recessive	N-Acetylgalactosamine-6-sulfate sulfatase β-Galactosidase	Keratan sulfate	None
IS (V)	Scheie	Autosomal recessive	α-L-Iduronidase	Heparan sulfate	None
VI	Maroteaux-Lamy	Autosomal recessive	Arylsulfatase B	Dermatan sulfate	None
VII	Sly	Autosomal recessive	β-Glucuronidase	Dermatan sulfate Heparan sulfate	Variable

mainly as a result of vertebral subluxation, which occurs most frequently at the atlanto-axial joint (119,120).

Imaging studies of the brain in the mucopolysaccharidoses are usually ordered when hydrocephalus or spinal cord compression is suspected. CT and MR usually reveal delayed myelination, atrophy, varying degrees of hydrocephalus, and white matter changes (121–123). The white matter abnormalities are manifested as diffuse low attenuation within the cerebral hemispheric white matter on CT and as focal and diffuse areas of prolonged T1 and T2 relaxation times on MR studies (Figs. 3.29, 3.30). The sharply defined foci are commonly present in the corpus callosum and basal ganglia, as well as the cerebral white matter (7). They are isointense with CSF on all imaging sequences (Fig. 3.30) and are probably mucopolysaccharide-filled perivascular spaces, as are described in pathology texts (124). With progression of the disease, the lesions become larger and more diffuse, reflecting the development of infarcts and demyelination. Diffuse white matter haziness is seen on T2-weighted images in mucopolysaccharidoses types IH, II, and III, resulting in diminished contrast between cortex and underlying white matter (122). The atrophy and white matter changes occur earlier in types I, II, III, and VII, usually becoming apparent within the first few years of life. In mucopolysaccharidoses types IV and VI, the white matter changes and atrophy may not become apparent until the second decade of life (119,121–123). Affected patients are commonly macrocephalic, probably resulting from a combination of hydrocephalus and mucopolysaccharide deposition within the brain, meninges, and skull.

The spine abnormalities in the mucopolysaccharidoses consist of characteristic vertebral body changes that are well described in pediatric radiology texts. These children are usually imaged to determine the site and cause of cord compression, which occurs frequently in

mucopolysaccharidoses types IV and VI (7,119,120, 125). The most common location for the cord compression is at the atlanto-axial (C1–C2) joint. Atlanto-axial subluxation may occur in these patients as a result of laxity of the transverse ligament or because of hypoplasia or absence of the odontoid (Fig. 3.31). Flexion/extension views are often necessary to demonstrate the laxity of the transverse odontoid ligament. Ligamentous hypertrophy (Fig. 3.31) may develop in response to chronic subluxation at the C1–C2 level, causing additional compression on the upper cervical spinal cord. Another cause of cord compression at the C1–C2 level is dural thickening resulting from intradural deposition of collagen and mucopolysaccharidoses. This is seen as a thickening of the soft tissues posterior to the dens, resulting in a narrowing the subarachnoid space at that level. One final cause of cord compression in these patients is gibbous formation in the thoracic spine. This results from the vertebral deformities (Fig. 3.32) and is most common in Morquio's disease (mucopolysaccharidosis type IV) (7,119,120, 125). Meningeal thickening may result in cyst formation in MPS types 1H and II (7).

Proton MR spectroscopy results have been reported in a few of the mucopolysaccharidoses (126). A patient with Sanfilippo (type IIIa) syndrome showed a decreased NAA/choline ratio and elevated glutamate, glutamine, and inositol. A patient with Hurler's syndrome had decreased NAA/choline and larger-than-normal peaks in the inositol and glutamate/glutamine regions.

Wilson's Disease

Wilson's disease, also known as hepatolenticular degeneration, results from an inborn error of copper metabolism that is transmitted in an autosomal recessive manner. When the disease manifests itself in children,

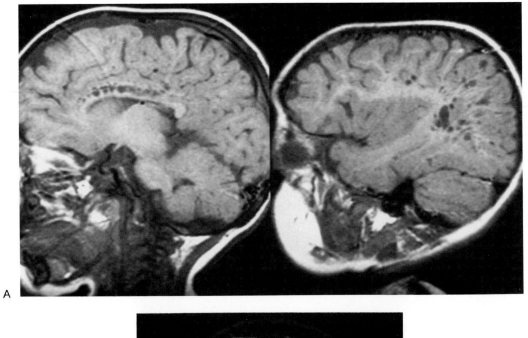

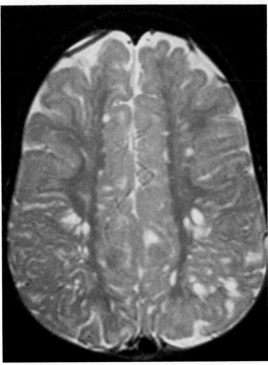

FIG. 3.29. Mucopolysaccharidosis 1H (Hurler). **A, B:** Sagittal SE 600/16 images show multiple well-defined focal areas of hypointensity, probably mucopolysaccharide-filled perivascular spaces, in the cerebral white matter and corpus callosum. **B:** Axial SE 2800/70 image shows well-marginated foci of hyperintensity superimposed upon some subtle, diffuse hyperintensity in the centrum semiovale.

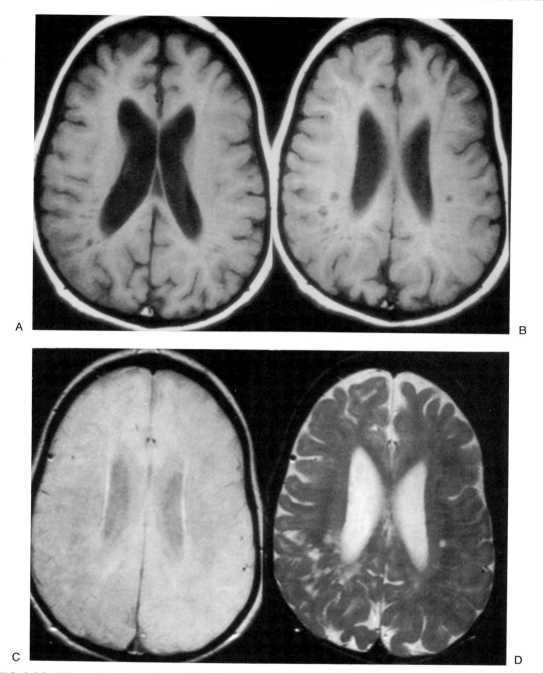

FIG. 3.30. Mucopolysaccharidosis II (Hunter). **A, B:** Axial SE 600/20 images show large lateral ventricles and well-marginated foci of hypointensity in the cerebral white matter. **C, D:** First and second echoes of a T2-weighted sequence show that the well-marginated foci are isointense to CSF on all sequences.

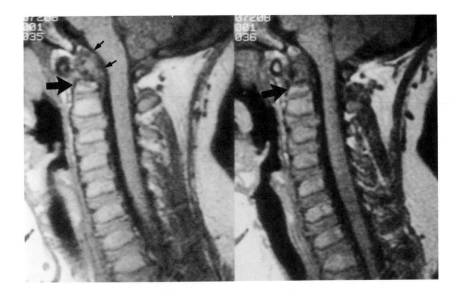

FIG. 3.31. Mucopolysaccharidosis IV (Morquio). Sagittal SE 550/15 images show characteristic vertebral anomalies with thickened intervertebral discs. The odontoid (*large arrow*) is hypoplastic. Ligamentous hypertrophy results in a pseudomass (*small arrows*) of the odontoid, which compresses the upper cervical spinal cord.

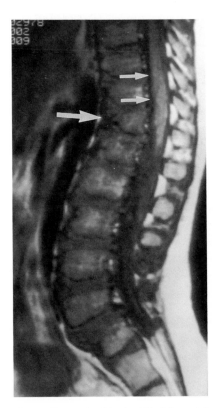

FIG. 3.32. Mucopolysaccharidosis IV (Morquio). Anterior narrowing of the L1 vertebral body (*large arrow*) results in a mild gibbous deformity with resultant impending cord compression (*small arrows*).

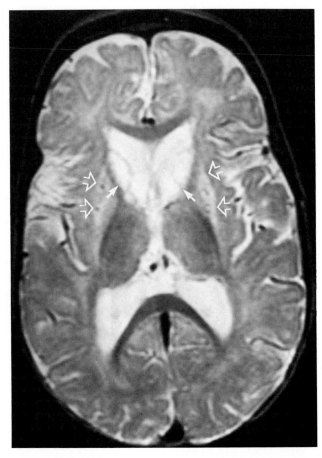

FIG. 3.33. Wilson's disease. Axial SE 2000/56 image shows abnormal hyperintensity of the putamina (*open arrows*) and caudates (*closed arrows*). The cerebral white matter is hyperintense.

initial symptoms result from liver failure (jaundice or portal hypertension). When neurologic symptoms predominate, the appearance of the illness is delayed until the age of 10 or 20 years, and progression is slower than in the hepatic form (5). The most common presenting symptoms are indistinct speech and difficulty in swallowing. Intellectual impairment or emotional disturbances may also be observed. The diagnosis is usually made from the presence of Kayser-Fleischer rings, rings of green pigmentation in the cornea. However, when Wilson's disease presents with hepatic symptoms, Kayser-Fleischer rings may not yet be present.

CT findings of Wilson's disease consist of low density in the basal ganglia and variable cerebral white matter atrophy (127). MR findings consist of prolongation of T1 and T2 relaxation times in the basal ganglia and, less commonly, the thalamus (Fig. 3.33). Patients with hepatic failure will usually have bilateral, symmetric T1 shortening (high intensity on T1-weighted images) in the globus pallidus and dorsal midbrain, secondary to the hepatic failure (128). White matter atrophy is frequently present and, occasionally, focal areas of prolonged T1 and T2 relaxation time are seen in the cerebral hemispheric white matter, primarily frontally and temporally (129,130). Although cerebral involvement is most commonly bilateral and symmetrical, asymmetric or unilateral involvement can occur (131).

Mitochondrial Disorders

The mitochondrial disorders (Table 3.8) are a group of diseases characterized by disorders of mitochondrial function that result in impaired adenosine triphosphate (ATP) production in affected cells (132–136). Single or multiple organs can be involved, with the striated muscles and brain most commonly affected (132–136).

Certain clinical features are characteristic of many of the mitochondrial disorders, including seizures, short stature, mental deterioration, muscle weakness, exercise intolerance, and neurosensory hearing loss (133–135,137). When these symptoms occur in patients who have the classic symptom complex of a specific mitochondrial disorder, a specific diagnosis is rather straightforward. However, patients often have signs and symptoms that are less classic, and diagnosis of a specific mitochondrial "syndrome" becomes difficult. This blurring of symptom complexes has created controversy concerning the classification of mitochondrial disorders. Some groups (133,136,138) believe that certain clinical features are adequately clustered in some patients to allow the identification of syndromes that are useful in patient management. Others believe that the overlap of features among the "syndromes" is too great to make the clinical classifications useful; they await a biochemical/ molecular genetic classification (134,135,139,140). Although I will discuss the various mitochondrial "syndromes," the reader should be aware that the syndromes are often not clearly distinct from one another. Moreover, the imaging findings are not entirely distinctive. *The important point to remember about mitochondrial disorders is that they should be considered in any infant or child who has abnormalities of the deep gray matter, in particular if white matter disease is present as well.* Certain mitochondrial disorders, such as MERRF (myoclonus, epilepsy, ragged red fibers) and Leber's hereditary optic neuropathy are seen primarily in adults and therefore are not included in this chapter.

Mitochondrial Encephalomyopathy with Lactic Acidosis and Stroke (MELAS)

MELAS refers to a group of disorders that present with episodes of nausea, vomiting, and strokelike events (hemianopsia and hemiparesis) in conjunction with some of the signs and symptoms of generalized mitochondrial disease (133,141–146). The strokelike events, probably the result of a proliferation of dysfunctional mitochondria in the smooth muscle cells of small arteries (147,148), may give rise to permanent or reversible deficits. Patients can present at any age, most commonly in the second decade (146). Serum and CSF lactate are usually elevated.

Imaging studies show increased water in the affected areas of the brain, primarily the parietal and occipital lobes (Fig. 3.34) (145,149) and in the basal ganglia (Fig. 3.35) (150). Sequential scans may show resolution and subsequent reappearance of the abnormal areas (145,149,151). The lesions are not restricted to a specific vascular distribution. MR spectroscopy shows high lactate in affected areas of brain (150,152,153). However, as infarcts of any cause seem to result in local increases in lactate (154), the presence of lactate in a patient with acute onset of neurologic deficit is certainly not specific for MELAS.

Kearns-Sayre Syndrome

To establish the diagnosis of Kearns-Sayre syndrome, patients must have, as a minimum, external ophthalmoplegia, retinitis pigmentosa, and onset of neurologic or muscular dysfunction before the age of 20 years (133,136,143,144,155). Some authors require, in addition, elevated CSF protein (156) or heart block (7,155) for clinical diagnosis. Patients may also have ataxia, dementia, short stature, sensorineural hearing loss, endocrine dysfunction, elevated serum and CSF lactate, and muscle weakness (133,136,156,157).

CT scans show cortical and white matter atrophy, hypodensity of cerebral and cerebellar white matter, and

TABLE 3.8. *Mitochondrial disorders*

1. Exclusive or predominant muscle involvement
   a. Fatal infantile myopathy
   b. Benign infantile myopathy
2. Predominant brain involvement
   a. Subacute necrotizing encephalomyelopathy (Leigh's disease)
   b. Alper's syndrome
   c. Myoclonic epilepsy with ragged-red fibers (MERRF)
   d. Trichopoliodystrophy (Menke's disease)
   e. Mitochondrial encephalopathy with lactic acidosis and strokelike episodes (MELAS)
   f. Glutaric acidurias types I and II
3. Other
   a. Progressive external ophthalmoplegia
      1. Isolated
      2. With retinitis pigmentosa and other organ involvement (Kearns–Sayre syndrome)
      3. Encephalomyopathy in adults
      4. *Myo*-neuro-gastrointestinal encephalopathy

variable hypodensity or calcification of the deep cerebral and cerebellar nuclei (7,158). It is not clear whether the calcification is the result of the primary disorder or the associated hypoparathyroidism that often accompanies the syndrome (159). MR scans (Fig. 3.36) show T2 prolongation in the deep gray matter nuclei, particularly the thalami and the globi palladi, and patchy white matter involvement (7,150,160). The white matter involvement is predominantly peripheral, with early involvement of the subcortical U fibers and sparing of periventricular fibers.

Subacute Necrotizing Encephalomyelopathy (Leigh's Disease)

Leigh's disease refers to a symptom complex with characteristic, but variable, clinical and pathologic manifestations (77,161). Affected infants and children typically present toward the end of the first year of life with hypotonia and psychomotor deterioration. Ataxia, ophthalmoplegia, ptosis, dystonia, and swallowing difficulties almost inevitably ensue. Characteristic pathologic abnormalities include microcystic cavitation, vascular proliferation, neuronal loss, and demyelination in the midbrain, basal ganglia, cerebellar dentate nuclei, and, occasionally, cerebral white matter (77,162–164). Several biochemical and genetic abnormalities, including pyruvate dehydrogenase deficiency (165), pyruvate carboxylase deficiency (166), and cytochrome c oxidase deficiency (167), have been identified in patients with a clinical phenotype identical to Leigh's disease. Thus, many experts separate Leigh's disease [with the classical pathologic findings initially described by Dr. Leigh (161)] from Leigh's syndrome (the characteristic combination of clinical features). Both disorders are considered

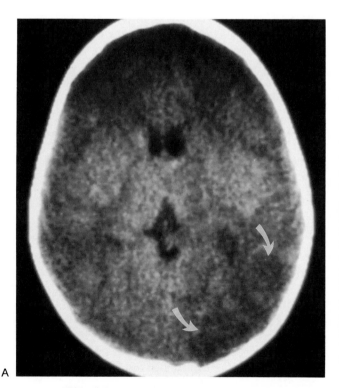
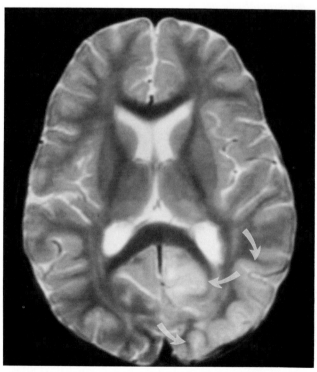

A   B

FIG. 3.34. Mitochondrial encephalopathy with lactic acidosis and strokelike episodes (MELAS). Axial CT (**A**) and MR (**B**) images show increased free water [low attenuation on CT, long T2 on MR (*arrows*)] in the left parieto-occipital region. The abnormality involves both middle cerebral artery and posterior cerebral artery distributions.

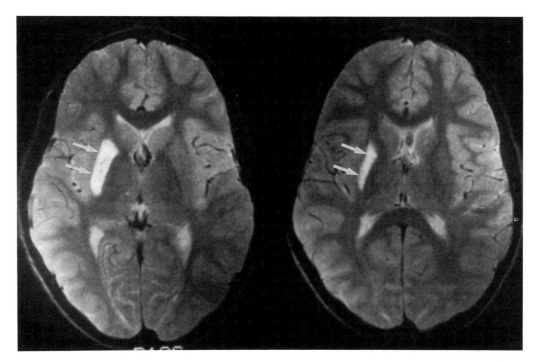

FIG. 3.35. Mitochondrial encephalopathy with lactic acidosis and strokelike episodes (MELAS). Axial SE 2800/70 images show hyperintensity (*arrows*) involving the right putamen. (Reprinted from ref. 150 with permission.)

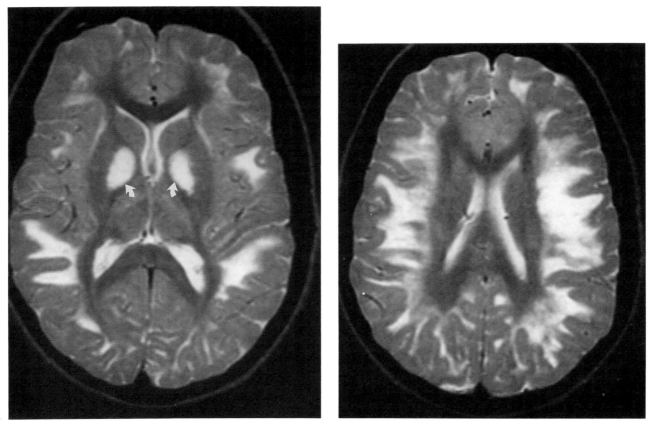

A

B

FIG. 3.36. Kearns–Sayre syndrome. **A:** Axial SE 2800/70 image shows abnormal high signal intensity in the globi palladi (*arrows*) and the peripheral cerebral white matter. **B:** At a higher level, the involvement of the peripheral white matter, including the subcortical U fibers, with sparing of the periventricular white matter is clearly shown. (Reprinted from ref. 150 with permission.)

to be the end result of a number of different defects affecting many aspects of mitochondrial function (77,133,157,162,163).

The imaging findings in Leigh's disease include areas of hypoattenuation (CT) and prolonged T1 and T2 relaxation (MR) in the putamina, globi pallidi, caudate nuclei, periaqueductal region, and cerebral peduncles, with occasional involvement of the cortical gray matter, subthalamic nuclei, restiform bodies, decussation of the superior cerebellar peduncles, and cerebral white matter (Figs. 3.37, 3.38) (168–173). The dorsal pons seems to be affected in those patients with cytochrome c oxidase deficiency (173). Significant demyelination may be present (Fig. 3.39) but is very uncommon (150).

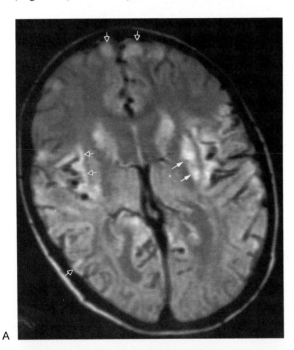

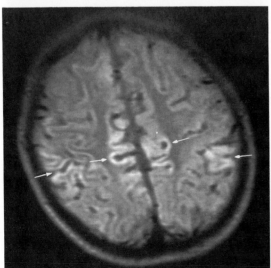

FIG. 3.37. Leigh's syndrome. Axial SE 2000/35 images show abnormal high signal intensity in the left putamen (*closed arrows*) and in multiple cortical foci (*open arrows*).

MR spectroscopy has shown decreased NAA and elevated lactate, with the lactate elevation most pronounced in those areas most severely affected on the imaging studies (Fig. 3.38) (150,152,153). Because most other nonmitochondrial disorders involving the basal ganglia (Wilson's disease, other causes of lactic acidemia, chronic infarction, maple syrup urine disease) do not have elevated basal ganglia lactate detected by proton spectroscopy (174), spectroscopy may be useful in confirming the diagnosis of Leigh's disease. Response to therapy has been monitored by a combination of MRI and MRS (175).

Progressive Cerebral Poliodystrophy (Alper's Disease)

Alper's disease is a rare multisystem disorder characterized by predominant involvement of the cerebral gray matter and the liver (137,164,176–178). Patients typically present with intractable seizures, particularly myoclonic jerks, following some early developmental delay or failure to thrive (137,164,178,179). Onset is usually in the first few years of life and may be as early as the first few weeks. Overt evidence of hepatic disease is variable, but abnormalities of hepatic chemistry may be detected early (178,180). Pathologically, the brain shows spongiform cortical atrophy, which is most pronounced in the occipital region, and atrophy of the basal nuclei, particularly the thalami and globi palladi (7,164,178).

Imaging analyses of patients with Alper's disease are few. Reported CT findings include focal hypodensities of both gray and white matter, followed by diffuse atrophy (7,137). Others note diminished white matter, delayed myelination, and cortical thinning that is most severe in the frontal, posterior temporal, and occipital lobes (150,178). No reports of MRS in Alper's disease have been published.

Trichopoliodystrophy (Menkes' Disease)

Trichopoliodystrophy (181) is an X-linked recessive mitochondrial disorder that results from impaired intestinal absorption of copper with consequent impairment of cytochrome oxidase activity in the mitochondria [cytochrome c contains two copper atoms (164)]. Patients typically present in infancy with hypotonia, hypothermia, failure to thrive, and seizures (164,181). Head circumference at birth may be normal or decreased; a reduction with respect to the normal growth curve soon becomes evident. Patients have coarse, stiff, sparse hair with broken, nodular, frayed ends (164,181); hence, the disease is referred to as "kinky hair disease." Most patients die before the second year of life. Pathologic examination shows diffuse atrophy of cerebral and cerebellar hemispheres with thin-walled, tortuous cerebral arteries (164). Microscopic examination shows widespread spongiform degeneration of the gray matter, sometimes ex-

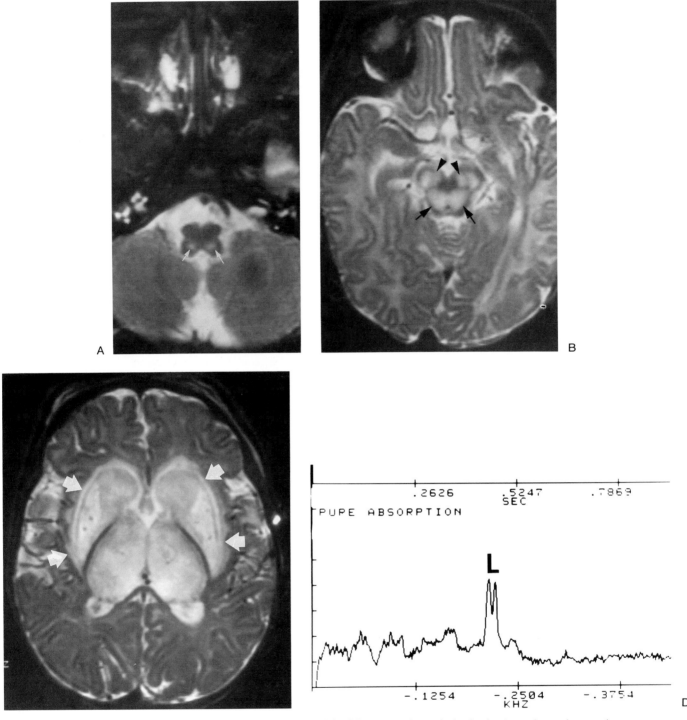

FIG. 3.38. Leigh's syndrome. **A, B:** Axial SE 3000/120 images through the brain stem show abnormal high signal intensity in the dorsal medulla (*white arrows*), dorsal midbrain (*black arrows*), and cerebral peduncles (*black arrowheads*). **C:** Axial SE 3000/120 image shows swelling and abnormal high signal intensity (*arrows*) in the basal ganglia and thalami bilaterally. **D:** ¹H MRS from the basal ganglia shows a large lactate doublet (L) 2 kHz downfield from water. No normal peaks can be identified. (Reprinted from ref. 150 with permission.)

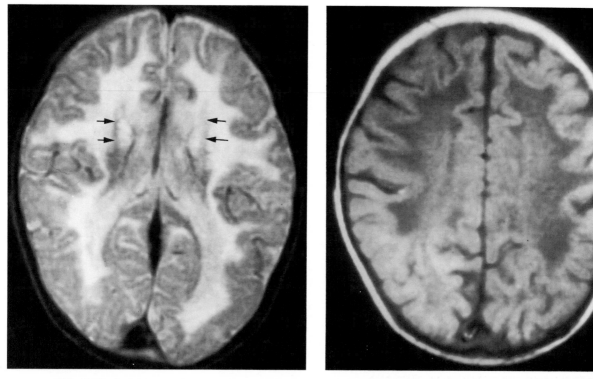

FIG. 3.39. Leigh's syndrome with demyelination in an 11-month-old child. **A:** Axial SE 2500/70 image shows abnormal high signal intensity in the putamina (*arrows*) and cerebral white matter. **B:** Axial SE 600/20 image shows a complete lack of myelin in the cerebral white matter. (Reprinted from ref. 150 with permission.)

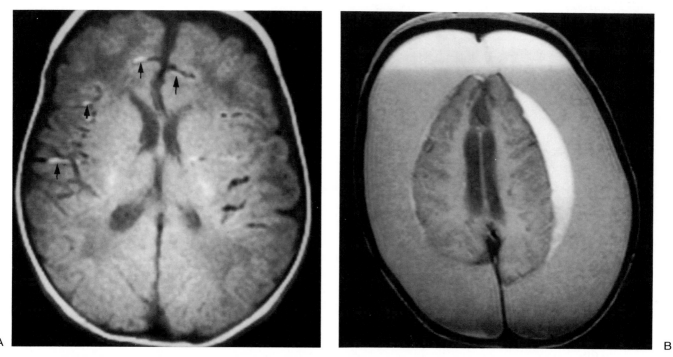

FIG. 3.40. Trichopoliodystrophy (Menkes' kinky hair disease). **A:** Axial SE 600/20 image at age 1 month shows abnormal high signal (*arrows*) in several areas of cerebral cortex. **B:** Follow-up SE 600/20 image at age 5 months shows profound atrophy with enormous bilateral subdural hematomas. (Reprinted from ref. 150 with permission.)

hibiting frank cavitation. The volume of white matter is reduced, and the white matter is hypomyelinated (164).

Radiologic studies of Menkes' disease show cerebral atrophy, large subdural collections, and tortuosity of cerebral blood vessels (182–185). More recently, the rapid progression of the atrophy and T1 and T2 shortening in the cerebral cortex have been observed (Fig. 3.40) (150,185–187). *An important point in this respect is that rapid brain atrophy in the presence of large bilateral subdural hematomas and apparent cortical blood is not necessarily a manifestation of asphyxic or physical trauma.*

Glutaric Aciduria Type I

Glutaric aciduria type I is an autosomal recessive disorder caused by deficiency of glutaryl-CoA dehydrogenase, an enzyme located in mitochondria. Patients may present with an acute encephalopathy or with gradual neurologic deterioration, including hypotonia, progressive dystonia, and tetraplegia. Pathology shows defective myelination and degeneration of the basal ganglia (44,143).

Imaging studies show retarded myelination, degeneration of the basal ganglia (low attenuation on CT, long T1, T2 on MR), and frontotemporal atrophy, manifest as widening of the Sylvian fissures (7,188).

Glutaric Aciduria Type II

Glutaric aciduria type II, also known as multiple acyl CoA dehydrogenase deficiency, results from a defect of the mitochondrial electron transport chain at coenzyme Q. Affected patients may present as neonates or infants, usually with hypoglycemia, hypotonia, and acidosis. Those presenting in infancy rarely survive beyond a few weeks. Those presenting later in infancy are managed by dietary means (143). Rare reports of adolescent or adult presentation are published (189); these older patients are reported to have movement disorders (190). Imaging studies show basal ganglia involvement (143,190). We have seen one patient with proven glutaric aciduria type II in whom a brain MR showed T2 prolongation in the caudate head, putamen, and cerebral hemispheric white matter (Fig. 3.41).

Nonspecific Mitochondrial Disorders

As discussed in the opening paragraph of this section, some brain disorders that are associated with mitochondrial dysfunction do not fit into any of the syndromes that have been described. These nonspecific mitochondrial disorders can present in patients of any age, from the neonates (191) to senior citizens (192). Presenting signs and symptoms are variable, as in all mitochondrial disorders (133,150), with seizures, short stature, mental deterioration, muscle weakness, exercise intolerance, and neurosensory hearing loss being the most common (133–135,137).

Imaging findings are nonspecific with increased water (low attenuation on CT, long T1 and T2 on MR) in the basal ganglia and cerebral white matter (Fig. 3.42).

Methylmalonic and Propionic Acidemias

Both methylmalonic and propionic acidemia are autosomal recessive disorders that result in deficiency of CoA carboxylases, with subsequent ketoacidosis and excretion of the respective acids in the urine. Both diseases present early in life with vomiting, tachypnea, and seizures, often leading to coma and death. Survivors suffer from quadriparesis and psychomotor retardation with episodic vomiting, ketosis, and coma (143). CT and MR reveal increased water (low attenuation and long T1, T2, respectively) in the basal ganglia, primarily the globi palladi, which sometimes resolves after therapy (7,193–195). Low attenuation has also been described in the cerebral white matter on CT (7,194).

GM₂ Gangliosidoses

GM_2 gangliosidoses are autosomal recessive disorders of sphingolipid storage caused by a deficiency of hexosaminidase enzymes; the two most common forms are Tay-Sachs disease and Sandhoff disease. Clinical and imaging findings are similar in the two diseases, which are separated biochemically. Patients present with psychomotor retardation followed by neurologic deterioration during the second half of the first year of life. Progressive motor weakness, spasticity, blindness, macrocephaly, and seizures ensue (44,143). CT studies show high attenuation in the thalami (Fig. 3.43A) and low attenuation in the white matter in early stages, with cerebral and cerebellar atrophy in later stages (196). MR shows diffuse, mild T2 prolongation in the white matter (Fig. 3.43) and sometimes low signal intensity in the thalami (7).

AMINO AND ORGANIC ACIDOPATHIES

The amino and organic acidopathies form a large and diverse group of disorders that can affect both gray matter and white matter. As amino and organic acids are present in all cellular organelles and exhibit various patterns of brain damage, they are listed in this chapter

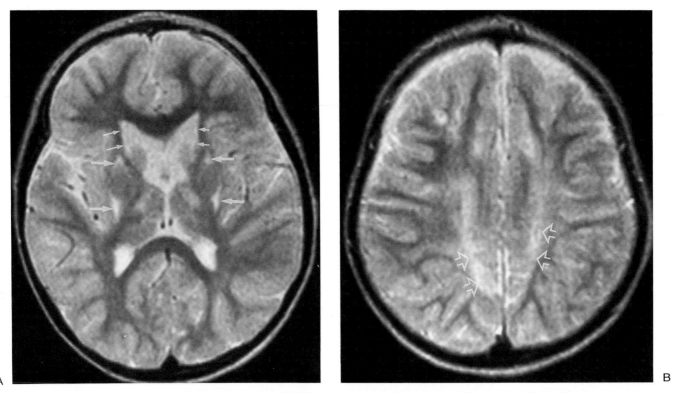

A B

FIG. 3.41. Glutaric aciduria type II. Axial SE 2500/80 images show abnormal hyperintensity in the caudate heads (*small closed arrows*), putamina (*large closed arrows*), and cerebral white matter (*open arrows*).

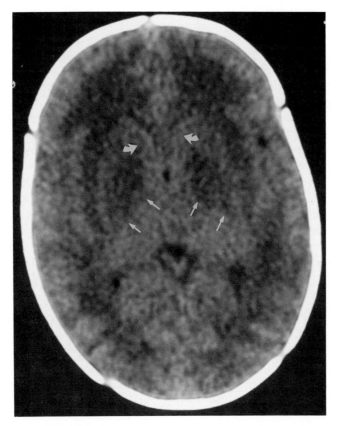

FIG. 3.42. Nonspecific mitochondrial disorder. Axial CT image shows low attenuation in the lentiform nuclei (*straight arrows*), caudate heads (*curved arrows*), and cerebral white matter.

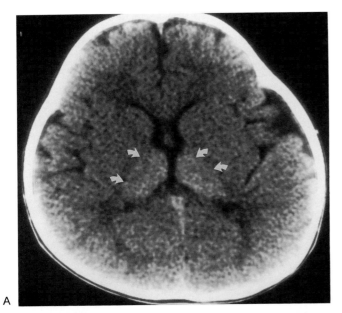

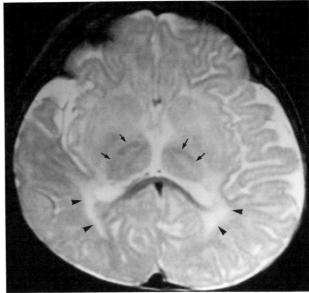

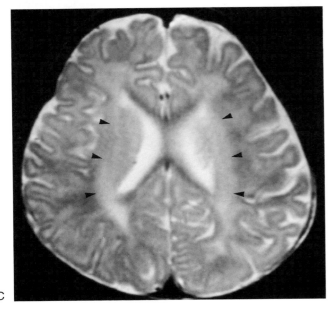

FIG. 3.43. GM$_2$ gangliosidosis (Sandhoff's disease). A: Axial CT image shows abnormal high attenuation of the thalami (*arrows*). B, C: Axial SE 2500/70 images show slight hypointensity of the thalami (*arrows*) compared to the basal ganglia and hyperintensity (*arrowheads*) of the periventricular white matter.

according to the pattern of brain abnormality. For example, glutaric aciduria types I and II are reported under "Disorders Affecting Gray and White Matter," phenylketonuria is discussed under "White Matter Diseases Initially Affecting Central White Matter," and citrullinemia and ornithine transcarbamylase deficiency are discussed under "White Matter Diseases with Nonspecific Patterns." Many disorders in this category remain unclassified at the present time. A full discussion of the biochemistry and clinical manifestations of these disorders is beyond the scope of this book. Readers are referred to any good pediatric neurology text for details. Because some texts classify these diseases as "disorders of organic acids" and "disorders of amino acids," selected amino and organic acidopathies are listed in Table 3.9.

TABLE 3.9. *Amino and organic acidopathies*

Phenylketonuria
Hyperphenylalaninemia
Tyrosinemia
Maple syrup urine disease
Argininosuccinic aciduria
Citrullinemia
Ornithine transcarbamylase deficiency
Hyperargininemia
Homocystinuria
Cystathioninuria
Hypermethioninemia
Propionic acidemia
Methylmalonic acidemia
Nonketotic hyperglycinemia
Hyperprolinemia
Glutaric acidurias types I and II

REFERENCES

1. Becker LE. Lysosomes, peroxisomes and mitochondria: function and disorder. *Am J Neuroradiol* 1992;13:609–620.
2. Van der Knaap MS. *Myelination and myelin disorders: a magnetic resonance study in infants, children and young adults.* (Ph.D. Thesis) Free University of Amsterdam and University of Utrecht, Netherlands, 1991.
3. Van der Knaap MS, Valk J. The MR spectrum of peroxisomal disorders. *Neuroradiology* 1991;33:30–37.
4. Brady RO. Disorders of lipid metabolism. In: Berg BO, ed. *Neurologic aspects of pediatrics.* Boston: Butterworth-Heinemann, 1992:145–165.
5. Menkes JH. *Textbook of child neurology,* 3rd ed. Philadelphia: Lea & Febiger, 1985.
6. Alves D, Pires MM, Guimaraes A, Miranda MD. Four cases of late onset metachromatic leukodystrophy in a family: clinical, biochemical, and neuropathological studies. *J Neurol Neurosurg Psychiatr* 1986;49:1417–1422.
7. Kendall BE. Disorders of lysosomes, peroxisomes, and mitochondria. *Am J Neuroradiol* 1992;13:621–653.
8. Kwan E, Drace J, Enzmann D. Specific CT findings in Krabbe disease. *AJR* 1984;143:665–670.
9. Ieshima A, Eda I, Matsui A, Yoshino K, Takashima S, Takeshita K. CT in Krabbe's disease: comparison with neuropathology. *Neuroradiology* 1983;25:323–327.
10. Lyon G, Hagberg B, Evrard P, Allaire C, Pavone L, Vanier M. Symptomology of late onset Krabbe's leukodystrophy: the European experience. *Dev Neurosci* 1992;13:240–244.
11. Demaerel P, Wilms G, Verdru P, Carton H, Baert AL. MR findings in globoid leukodystrophy. *Neuroradiology* 1990;32:520–522.
12. Sasaki M, Sakuragawa N, Takashima S, Hanaoka S, Arima M. MRI and CT findings in Krabbe disease. *Pediatr Neurol* 1991;7:283–288.
13. Farley TJ, Ketonen LM, Bodensteiner JB, Wang DD. Serial MRI and CT findings in infantile Krabbe disease. *Pediatr Neurol* 1992;8:455–458.
14. Naidu S, Moser AE, Moser HW. Phenotypic and genotypic variability of generalized peroxisomal disorders. *Pediatr Neurol* 1988;4:5–12.
15. Moser HW, Mihalik SJ, Watkins PA. Adrenoleukodystrophy and other peroxisomal disorders that affect the nervous system, including new observations on L-pipecolic acid oxidase in primates. *Brain Dev* 1989;11:80–90.
16. Moser HW. Adrenoleukodystrophy: from bedside to molecular biology. *J Child Neurol* 1987;2:140–150.
17. Moser H, Moser A, Naidu S, et al. Clinical aspects of adrenoleukodystrophy and adrenomyeloneuropathy. *Dev Neurosci* 1991;13:254–261.
18. Snyder RD, King JN, Keck GM, Orrison WW. MR imaging of the spinal cord in 23 subjects with ALD–AMN complex. *AJNR* 1991;12:1095–1098.
19. Aubourg P, Adamsbaum C, Lavallard-Rousseau MC, et al. Brain MRI and electrophysiologic abnormalities in preclinical and clinical adrenomyeloneuropathy. *Neurology* 1992;42:85–91.
20. Kumar AJ, Rosenbaum AE, Naidu S, et al. Adrenoleukodystrophy: correlating MR imaging with CT. *Radiology* 1987;165:497–504.
21. Aubourg P, Diebler C. Adrenoleukodystrophy—its diverse CT appearances and an evolutive or phenotypic variant. *Neuroradiology* 1982;24:33–42.
22. Hong-Magno ET, Muraki AS, Huttenlocher PR. Atypical CT scans in adrenoleukodystrophy. *J Comput Assist Tomogr* 1987;11:333–336.
23. Tzika A, Ball W Jr, Vigneron D, Dunn RS, Nelson SJ, Kirks D. Childhood adrenoleukodystrophy: assessment with proton MR spectroscopy. *Radiology* 1993;189:467–480.
24. Bruhn H, Kruse B, Korenke GC, et al. Proton NMR spectroscopy of cerebral metabolic alterations in infantile peroxisomal disorders. *J Comput Assist Tomogr* 1992;16:335–344.
25. Williams DW III, Elster AD, Cox TD. Cranial MR imaging in rhizomelic chondrodysplasia punctata. *Am J Neuroradiol* 1991;12:363–365.
26. Dubois J, Sebag G, Argyropoulou M, Brunelle F. MR findings in infantile Refsum disease: case report of two family members. *Am J Neuroradiol* 1991;12:1159–1161.
27. Goldfischer S, Collins J, Rapin I, Calthoff-Schiller B. Peroxisomal defects in neonatal-onset and X-linked adrenoleukodystrophies. *Science* 1985;227:67–70.
28. Scheffer IE, Baraitser M, Harding B, Kendall B, Brett EM. Pelizaeus-Merzbacher disease: classical or connatal? *Neuropediatrics* 1991;22:71–78.
29. Renier WD, Gabreels FJM, Justinx TW, et al. Connatal Pelizaeus-Merzbacher disease with congenital stridor in two maternal cousins. *Acta Neuropathol* 1981;54:11–24.
30. Seitelberger F. Pelizaeus-Merzbacher disease. In: Vinken P, Bruyn G, eds. *Handbook of clinical neurology.* Amsterdam: Elsevier-North Holland, 1970:150–202.
31. Van der Knaap MS, Valk J. The reflection of histology in MR imaging of Pelizaeus-Merzbacher disease. *Am J Neuroradiol* 1989;10:99–103.
32. Pham Dinh D, Popot JL, Boespflug Tanguy O, et al. Pelizaeus-Merzbacher disease: a valine to phenylalanine point mutation in a putative extracellular loop of myelin proteolipid. *Proc Natl Acad Sci USA* 1991;88:7562–7566.
33. Mattei MG, Alliel PM, Dautigny A, et al. The gene encoding for the major brain proteolipid (PLP) maps on the q-22 band of the human X chromosome. *Hum Genet* 1986;72:352–353.
34. Koeppen AH, Ronca NA, Greenfield E, Hans MB. Defective biosynthesis of proteolipid protein in Pelizaeus-Merzbacher disease. *Ann Neurol* 1987;21:159–170.
35. Volpe JJ. *Neurology of the newborn,* 2nd ed. Philadelphia: WB Saunders, 1987.
36. Barnes DM, Enzmann D. The evolution of white matter diseases as seen on computed tomography. *Radiology* 1981;138:379–383.
37. Journel H, Roussey M, Gandon Y, Allaire C, Carsin M, le Marec B. MR imaging in Pelizaeus-Merzbacher disease. *Neuroradiology* 1987;29:403–405.
38. Penner MW, Li KC, Gebarski SS, Allen RJ. MR imaging of Pelizaeus-Merzbacher disease. *J Comput Assist Tomogr* 1987;11:591–593.
39. Price VH, Odom RR, Ward WH, Jones FT. Trichothiodystrophy. *Arch Dermatol* 1980;116:1375–1384.
40. Price VH. Trichothiodystrophy: update. *Pediatr Dermatol* 1992;9:369–370.
41. Gillespie JM, Marshall RC, Rogers M. Trichothiodystrophy—biochemical and clinical studies. *Aust J Dermatol* 1988;29:85–93.
42. Peserico A, Battistella PA, Bertoli P. MRI of a very rare hereditary ectodermal dysplasia: PIBI(D)S. *Neuroradiology* 1992;24:316–317.
43. Sweetman L, Haas RH. Abnormalities of amino acid metabolism. In: Berg BO, ed. *Neurologic aspects of pediatrics.* Boston: Butterworth-Heinemann, 1992:3–32.
44. Valk J, van der Knaap MS. *Magnetic resonance of myelin, myelination, and myelination disorders.* Berlin: Springer-Verlag, 1989.
45. Pearsen KD, Gean-Marton AD, Levy HL, Davis KR. Phenylketonuria: MRI of the brain with clinical correlation. *Radiology* 1990;177:437–440.
46. Shaw DW, Maravilla KR, Weinberger E, Garretson J, Trahms CM, Scott CR. MR imaging of phenylketonuria. *AJNR* 1991;12:403–406.
47. Brismar J, Aqueel A, Brismar G, et al. Maple syrup urine disease. *Am J Neuroradiol* 1990;11:1219–1228.
48. Charnas L, Bernar J, Pezeshkpour GH, Kalakas M, Harper GS, Gahl WA. MRI findings and peripheral neuropathy in Lowe's syndrome. *Neuropediatrics* 1988;19:7–9.
49. Lowe CU, Terrey M, MacLachlan EA. Organic-aciduria, decreased renal ammonia production, hydrophthalmos, and mental retardation: a clinical entity. *Am J Dis Child* 1952;83:164–184.
50. O'Tauma DA, Lasker DW. Oculocerebrorenal syndrome: case report with CT and MR correlates. *AJNR* 1987;8:555–557.
51. Carroll WJ, Woodruff WW, Cadman TE. MR findings in oculocerebrorenal syndrome. *Am J Neuroradiol* 1993;14:449–451.
52. Valk PE, Dillon WP. Radiation injury of the brain. *Am J Neuroradiol* 1991;12:45–62.
53. Ball WS Jr, Prenger EC, Ballard ET. Neurotoxicity of radio/che-

motherapy in children: pathologic and MR correlation. *AJNR* 1992;13:761–776.

54. Burger PC, Boyko OB. The pathology of central nervous system radiation injury. In: Gutin PH, Liebel SA, Sheline GF, eds. *Radiation injury to the nervous system.* New York: Raven, 1991: 191–208.

55. Young-Poussaint T, Barnes P, Burrows P, Goumnerova L, Tarbell N. Hemorrhagic radiation vasculopathy of the central nervous system in childhood: diagnosis and follow-up. *Radiology* 1993;189(P):194.

56. Wright TL, Bresnan MJ. Radiation induced cerebrovascular disease in children. *Neurology* 1976;26:540–543.

57. Painter MJ, Chutorian AM, Hilal SK. Cerebrovasculopathy following irradiation in childhood. *Neurology* 1975;25:189–194.

58. Glass JP, Lee YY, Bruner J, Fields WS. Treatment-related leukoencephalopathy. *Medicine* 1986;65:154–162.

59. Lien HH, Blomlie V, Saeter G, Solheim O, Fossa SD. Osteogenic sarcoma: MR signal abnormalities of the brain in asymptomatic patients treated with high dose methotrexate. *Radiology* 1991;179:547–550.

60. Ebner F, Ranner G, Slavc I, et al. MR findings in methotrexate-induced CNS abnormalities. *Am J Neuroradiol* 1989;10:959–964.

61. Wilson CA, Nitschke R, Bowman ME, Chaffin MJ, Sexauer CL, Prince JR. Transient white matter changes on MR images in children undergoing chemotherapy for acute lymphocytic leukemia: correlation with neuropsychologic deficiencies. *Radiology* 1991;180:205–209.

62. Kay HEM, Knapton PJ, O'Sullivan JP, et al. Encephalopathy in acute leukemia associated with methotrexate therapy. *Arch Dis Child* 1972;47:344–354.

63. Matalon R, Michals K, Sebesta D, et al. Aspartoacylase deficiency and *N*-acetylaspartic aciduria in patients with Canavan disease. *Am J Med Genet* 1988;29:463–471.

64. Brismar J, Brismar G, Gascon G, Ozand P. Canavan disease: CT and MR imaging of the brain. *Am J Neuroradiol* 1990;11:805–810.

65. Grodd W, Krageloh-Mann I, Petersen D, Trefz FK, Harzer K. In vivo assessment of *N*-acetylaspartate in brain in spongy degeneration (Canavan's disease) by proton spectroscopy (letter). *Lancet* 1990;2:437–438.

66. Farrell K, Chuang S, Becker LE. Computed tomography in Alexander's disease. *Ann Neurol* 1984;15:605–609.

67. Trommer BL, Naidich TP, Del Cento MC, et al. Noninvasive CT diagnosis of infantile Alexander disease: pathologic correlation. *J Comput Assist Tomogr* 1983;7:509–512.

68. Guzzetta F. Cockayne-Neill-Dingwall syndrome. In: Vinken PJ, Bruyn GW, eds. *Handbook of clinical neurology.* Amsterdam: North-Holland, 1972:431–440.

69. Brumback RA. Cockayne's syndrome diagnosis. *Neurology* 1984;34:842–843.

70. Demaerel P, Kendall BE, Kingsley D. Cranial CT and MRI in diseases with DNA repair defects. *Neuroradiology* 1992;34:117–121.

71. Demaerel P, Wilms G, Verdru P, Carton H, Baert AL. MRI in the diagnosis of Cockayne's syndrome. One case. *J Neuroradiol* 1990;17:157–60.

72. Boltshauser E, Yalcinkaya C, Wichmann W, Reutter A, Prader A, Valvanis A. MRI in Cockayne syndrome type I. *Neuroradiology* 1989;31:276–277.

73. Billard G, Dulac O, Bouloche J, et al. Encephalopathy with calcifications of the basal ganglia in children. *Neuropediatrics* 1989;20:12–19.

74. Boltshauser E, Steinlin M, Boesch CH, Martin E, Schubiger G. MRI in infantile encephalopathy with cerebral calcification and leukodystrophy. *Neuropediatrics* 1991;22:33–35.

75. Aicardi J, Goutieres F. A progressive familial encephalopathy in infancy with calcifications of the basal ganglia and chronic cerebrospinal fluid lymphocytosis. *Ann Neurol* 1984;15:49–54.

76. Razavi-Encha FJ, Larroche J-C, Gaillard D. Infantile familial encephalopathy with cerebral calcifications and leukodystrophy. *Neuropediatrics* 1988;19:72–79.

77. Snodgrass SR. Abnormalities of carbohydrate metabolism. In: Berg B, ed. *Neurologic aspects of pediatrics.* Boston: Butterworth-Heinemann, 1992:93–124.

78. Donnell GN, Collado M, Koch R. Growth and development of children with galactosemia. *J Pediatr* 1961;58:836–839.

79. Lo W, Packman S, Nash S, et al. Curious neurologic sequelae in galactosemia. *Pediatrics* 1964;73:309–312.

80. Nelson MD Jr, Wolff JA, Cross CA, Donnell GN, Kaufman FR. Galactosemia: evaluation with MR imaging. *Radiology* 1992;184:255–261.

81. Valvanis A, Schubiger O, Hayek J. Computed tomography in nonketotic hyperglycinemia. *Comput Radiol* 1981;5:265–270.

82. Press GA, Barshop BA, Haas RH, Nyhan WL, Glass RF, Hesselink JR. Abnormalities of the brain in nonketotic hyperglycinemia: MR manifestations. *Am J Neuroradiol* 1989;10:315–321.

83. Heindel W, Kugel H, Roth B. Noninvasive detection of increased glycine content by proton MR spectroscopy in the brains of two infants with nonketotic hyperglycinemia. *Am J Neurorad* 1993;14:629–635.

84. Bartholomew DW, Brusilow SW. Abnormalities of urea cycle and ammonium. In: Berg B, ed. *Neurologic aspects of pediatrics.* Boston: Butterworth-Heinemann, 1992:33–46.

85. Lowis GW. The social epidemiology of multiple sclerosis. *Sci Total Environ* 1990;90:163–190.

86. Duquette P, Murray TJ, Pleines J, et al. Multiple sclerosis in childhood: clinical profile in 125 patients. *J Pediatr* 1987;111: 359–363.

87. Hanefeld F, Bauer HJ, Christen H-J, Lrise.B, Bruhn H, Frahm J. Multiple sclerosis in childhood: report of 15 cases. *Brain Dev* 1991;13:410–416.

88. Ebner F, Millner MM, Justich E. Multiple sclerosis in children: value of serial MR studies to monitor patients. *Am J Neuroradiol* 1990;11:1023–1027.

89. Osborn AG, Harnsberger HR, Smoker WR, Boyer RS. Multiple sclerosis in adolescents: CT and MR findings. *Am J Neuroradiol* 1990;11:489–494.

90. Dousset V, Grossman RI, Ramer KN, et al. Experimental allergic encephalomyelitis and multiple sclerosis: lewion characterization with magnetization transfer imaging. *Radiology* 1992;182:483–491.

91. Johnson RT, Griffin DE, Gendelman HE. Postinfectious encephalomyelitis. *Semin Neurol* 1985;5:180–190.

92. Nasralla CAW, Pay N, Goodpasture HC, Lin JJ, Svoboda WB. Postinfectious encephalopathy in a child following *Campylobacter jejuni* enteritis. *AJNR* 1993;14:444–448.

93. DiMario FJ, Younkin D. Disorders of the respiratory system. In: Berg B, ed. *Neurologic aspects of pediatrics.* Boston: Butterworth-Heinemann, 1992:339–356.

94. Sriram S, Steinman L. Postinfectious and postvaccinial encephalomyelitis. *Neurol Clin* 1984;2:341–353.

95. Okuno T, Fuseya Y, Ito M, et al. Reversible multiple hypodense areas in white matter diagnosed as acute disseminated encephalomyelitis. *J Comput Assist Tomogr* 1981;5:119–121.

96. Atlas SW, Grossman RI, Goldberg HI, Hackney DB, Bilaniuk LT, Zimmerman RA. MR diagnosis of acute disseminated encephalomyelitis. *J Comput Assist Tomogr* 1986;10:798–801.

97. Baum P, Barkovich AJ, Koch T. MR of acute disseminated encephalomyelitis: a high incidence of basal nuclei involvement. *Am J Neuroradiol* (in press).

98. Ohtaki E, Murakami Y, Komori H, Yamashita Y, Matsuishi T. Acute disseminated encephalomyelitis after Japanese B encephalitis vaccination. *Pediatr Neurol* 1992;8:137–139.

99. Caldmeyer KS, Harris TM, Smith RR, Edwards MK. Gadolinium enhancement in acute disseminated encephalomyelitis. *J Comput Assist Tomogr* 1991;15:673–675.

100. Reich H, Lin SR, Goldblatt D. Computerized tomography in acute hemorrhagic leukoencephalopathy: case report. *Neurology* 1979;29:255–258.

101. Szer IS. The diagnosis and management of systemic lupus erythematosus in childhood. *Pediatr Ann* 1986;15:596–604.

102. Kaell AT, Shetty M, Lee BCP, et al. The diversity of neurologic events in systemic lupus erythematosus: prospective clinical and computed tomographic classification of 82 events in 71 patients. *Arch Neurol* 1986;43:273–276.

103. Spiro AJ, Pack DR. Disorders of immunologic dysfunction. In: Berg B, ed. *Neurologic aspects of pediatrics.* Boston: Butterworth-Heinemann, 1992:501–527.

104. Vinken PJ, Bruyn GW. *Intoxications of the central nervous system*, ed. Amsterdam: North-Holland, 1979.
105. Valk J, van der Knaap MS. Toxic encephalopathy. *Am J Neuroradiol* 1992;13:747–760.
106. Lorenzo AV, Jolesz FA, Wallman JK, Ruenzel PW. Proton magnetic resonance studies of triethyltin-induced edema during perinatal brain development in rabbits. *J Neurosurg* 1989;70:432–440.
107. Pappas CL, Quisling RG, Ballinger WE, Love LC. Lead encephalopathy: symptoms of a cerebellar mass lesion and obstructive hydrocephalus. *Surg Neurol* 1986;26:391–394.
108. Harrington JF, Mapstone TB, Selman WR, Galloway P, Bundschuh C. Lead encephalopathy presenting as a posterior fossa mass. *J Neurosurg* 1986;65:713–715.
109. Wisniewski K, Kida E, Connell F, Elleder M, Eviatar L, Konkol R. New subform of the late infantile form of neuronal ceroid lipofuscinosis. *Neuropediatrics* 1993;24:155–163.
110. Machen BC, Williams JP, Lum GB, et al. Magnetic resonance imaging in neuronal ceroid lipofuscinosis. *J Comput Assist Tomogr* 1987;11:160–166.
111. Autti T, Raininko R, Launes J, Nuutila A, Santavuori P. Jansky-Bielschowsky variant disease: CT, MRI, and SPECT findings. *Pediatr Neurol* 1992;8:121–126.
112. Wigboldus JM, Bruyn GW. Hallervorden-Spatz disease. In: Vinken PJ, Bruyn GW, eds. *Handbook of clinical neurology: diseases of basal ganglia*. Amsterdam: North-Holland, 1968:604–631.
113. Rutledge JN, Hilal SK, Silver AJ, Defendini R, Fahn S. Study of movement disorders and brain iron by MR. *AJNR* 1987;8:397–411.
114. Savoiardo M, Halliday WC, Nardocci N, et al. Hallervorden-Spatz disease: MR and pathologic findings. *Am J Neuroradiol* 1993;14:155–162.
115. Schaffert DA, Johnsen SD, Johnson PC, Drayer BP. Magnetic resonance imaging in pathologically proven Hallervorden-Spatz disease. *Neurology* 1989;39:440–442.
116. Jervis GA. Huntington's chorea in childhood. *Arch Neurol* 1963;9:244–251.
117. Harris GJ, Pearlson GD, Peyser CE, et al. Putamen volume reduction on magnetic resonance imaging exceeds caudate changes in mild Huntington's disease. *Ann Neurol* 1992;31:69–73.
118. Kuhl DE. Cerebral metabolism and atrophy in Huntington's disease determined by 18FDG and CT scan. *Ann Neurol* 1982;12:425–431.
119. McKusick VA, Neufeld EF. The mucopolysaccharide storage diseases. In: Stanbury JB, eds. *The metabolic basis of inherited disease*. New York: McGraw-Hill, 1983:751–823.
120. Butler IJ. Disorders of connective tissue and bone. In: Berg BO, ed. *Neurologic aspects of pediatrics*. Boston: Butterworth-Heinemann, 1992:468–483.
121. Lee C, Dineen TE, Brack M, Kirsch JE, Runge VM. Mucopolysaccharidoses: characterization by cranial MR imaging. *Am J Neuroradiol* 1993;14:1285–1292.
122. Murata R, Nakajima S, Tanaka A, et al. MR imaging of the brain in patients with mucopolysaccharidosis. *AJNR* 1989;10:1165–1170.
123. Watts RWE, Spellacy E, Kendall BE, du Boulay G, Gibbs DA. CT studies on patients with mucopolysaccharidoses. *Neuroradiology* 1981;21:9–23.
124. Becker LE, Yates A. Inherited metabolic disease. In: Davis R, Robertson D, eds. *Textbook of neuropathology*, 2nd ed. Baltimore: Williams and Wilkins, 1990:331–427.
125. Kulkarni MV, Williams JC, Yeakley JW. MR in the diagnosis of the cranio-cervical manifestations of the mucopolysaccharidoses. *Magn Reson Imag* 1987;5:317–323.
126. Tzika AA, Ball WS Jr, Vigneron D, Dunn RS, Kirks D. Clinical proton MR spectroscopy of neurodegenerative disease in childhood. *Am J Neuroradiol* 1993;14:1267–1281.
127. Kvicala V, Vymazal J, Nevsimalova S. CT of Wilson's disease. *Am J Neuroradiol* 1983;4:429–430.
128. Kim I, Yeon K, Kim W, Seo J, Han M. MR imaging of the brain in Wilson disease of childhood. *Radiology* 1993;189(P):195.
129. Aisen AM, Martel W, Gabrielsen TO, et al. CT of Wilson's disease. *AJNR* 1985;4:429–430.
130. Starosta-Rubenstein S, Young AB, Kluin K, et al. Clinical assessment of 31 patients with Wilson's disease: correlations with structural changes on magnetic resonance imaging. *Arch Neurol* 1987;44:365–370.
131. Prayer L, Wimberger D, Kramer J, Grimm G, Oder W. Cranial MRI in Wilson's disease. *Neuroradiology* 1990;32:211–212.
132. DiMauro S, Bonilla E, Zeviani M, Nakagawa M, DeVivo D. Mitochondrial myopathies. *Ann Neurol* 1985;17:521–538.
133. DiMauro S, Bonilla E, Lombes A, Shanske S, Minetti C, Moraes CT. Mitochondrial encephalomyopathies. *Neurol Clin* 1990;8:483–506.
134. Petty RKH, Harding AE, Morgan-Hughes JA. The clinical features of mitochondrial myopathy. *Brain* 1986;109:915–923.
135. Holt IJ, Harding AE, Cooper JM, et al. Mitochondrial myopathies: clinical and biochemical features of 30 patients with major deletions of muscle mitochondrial DNA. *Ann Neurol* 1989;26:699–708.
136. Wallace DC. Mitochondrial genetics: a paradigm for aging and degenerative diseases? *Science* 1992;256:628–632.
137. Tulinius MH, Holme E, Kristiansson B, Larsson NG, Oldfors A. Mitochondrial encephalomyopathies in childhood. II. Clinical manifestations and syndromes. *J Pediatr* 1991;119:251–259.
138. Berenberg RA, Pellock JM, DiMauro S, et al. Lumping or splitting? "Ophthalmoplegia-plus" or Kearns-Sayre syndrome? *Ann Neurol* 1977;1:37–54.
139. Morgan-Hughes JA. The mitochondrial myopathies. In: Engel AG, Banker BQ, eds. *Myology*. New York: McGraw-Hill, 1986:1709–1743.
140. Truong DD, Harding AE, Scaravilli F, Smith SJM, Morgan-Hughes JA, Marsden CD. Movement disorders in mitochondrial myopathies. A study of nine cases with two autopsy studies. *Movement Disorders* 1990;5:109–117.
141. Pavlakis SG, Phillips PC, DiMauro S, et al. Mitochondrial myopathy, encephalopathy, lactic acidosis, and stroke-like episodes: a distinctive clinical syndrome. *Ann Neurol* 1984;16:481–488.
142. Rowland LP, Blake DM, Hirano M, et al. Clinical syndromes associated with ragged red fibers. *Rev Neurol* 1991;147:467–473.
143. Haas RH, Nyhan WL. Disorders of organic acids. In: Berg BO, ed. *Neurologic aspects of pediatrics*. Boston: Butterworth-Heinemann, 1992:47–91.
144. DiMauro S, Moraes CT, Shanske S, et al. Mitochondrial encephalomyopathies: biochemical approach. *Rev Neurol* 1991;147:443–449.
145. Allard JC, Tilak S, Carter AP. CT and MR of MELAS syndrome. *AJNR* 1988;9:1234–1238.
146. Van Hellenberg Hubar JLM, Gabreels FJM, Ruitenbeek W, et al. MELAS syndrome: report of two patients, and comparison with data of 24 patients derived from the literature. *Neuropediatrics* 1991;22:10–14.
147. Sakuta R, Nonaka I. Vascular involvement in mitochondrial myopathy. *Ann Neurol* 1989;25:594–601.
148. Ohama E, Ohara S, Ikuta F, Tanaka K, Nishizawa M, Miyatake T. Mitochondrial angiopathy in cerebral blood vessels of mitochondrial encephalomyopathy. *Acta Neuropathol (Berl)* 1987;74:226–33.
149. Rosen L, Phillips S, Enzmann D. Magnetic resonance imaging in MELAS syndrome. *Neuroradiol* 1990;32:168–171.
150. Barkovich AJ, Good W, Koch TK, Berg BO. Mitochondrial disorders: analysis of their clinical and imaging characteristics. *Am J Neuroradiol* 1993;14:1119–1137.
151. Abe K, Invi T, Hirono N, et al. Fluctuating MR images with mitochondrial encephalomyopathy, lactic acidosis, stroke-like syndrome (MELAS). *Neuroradiol* 1990;32:77.
152. Detre JA, Wang Z, Bogdan AR, et al. Regional variation in brain lactate in Leigh syndrome by localized 1-H magnetic resonance spectroscopy. *Ann Neurol* 1991;29:218–221.
153. Grodd W, Krageloh-Mann I, Klose U, Sauter R. Metabolic and destructive brain disorders in children: findings with localized proton MR spectroscopy. *Radiology* 1991;181:173–181.
154. Dujin JH, Matson GB, Maudsley AA, Hugg JW, Weiner MW. Human brain infarction: proton MR spectroscopy. *Radiology* 1992;183:711–718.
155. Kearns T, Sayre GP. Retinitis pigmentosa, external ophthalmoplegia, and complete heart block. *Arch Ophthalmol* 1958;60:280–289.

156. Guggenheim MA, Becker LE, Jagadha V. CPC: muscle weakness in an adolescent male. *Pediatr Neurosci* 1985–1986;12:320–325.

157. DiMauro S, Lombes A, Nakase H, et al. Cytochrome c oxidase deficiency. *Pediatr Res* 1990;28:536–541.

158. Seigel RS, Seeger JF, Gabrielsen TO, Allen RJ. Computed tomography in oculocraniosomatic disease (Kearns-Sayre syndrome). *Radiology* 1979;130:159–164.

159. Pellock JM, Behrens M, Lewis L, Holub D, Carter S, Rowland LP. Kearns-Sayre syndrome and hypoparathyroidism. *Ann Neurol* 1978;3:455–458.

160. Demange P, Gia HP, Kalifa G, Sellier N. MR of Kearns-Sayre Syndrome. *Am J Neuroradiol* 1989;10:S91.

161. Leigh D. Subacute necrotizing encephalomyelopathy in an infant. *J Neurol Neurosurg Psychiatry* 1951;14:216–221.

162. Walter GF, Brucher JM, Martin JJ, Ceuterick C, Pilz P, Freund M. Leigh's disease: several nosological entities with an identical histopathological complex? *Neuropathol Appl Neurobiol* 1986;12:95–107.

163. Robinson J, Norman MG. CPC: feeding problems and lactic acidosis in a 10-week-old boy. *Pediatr Neurosci* 1989;15:28–35.

164. Friede RL. *Developmental neuropathology*, 2nd ed. Berlin: Springer-Verlag, 1989.

165. DeVivo DC, Haymond MW, Obert KA, et al. Defective activation of the pyruvate dehydrogenase complex in subacute necrotizing encephalomyelopathy. *Ann Neurol* 1979;6:483–494.

166. Van Biervliet JP, Duran M, Wadman SK, et al. Leigh's disease with decreased activities of pyruvate carboxylase and pyruvate decarboxylase. *J Inherited Metab Dis* 1980;2:15–18.

167. Willems JL, Monnens LAH, Trijbels JMF, et al. Leigh's encephalomyelopathy in a patient with cytochrome c oxidase deficiency in muscle tissue. *Pediatrics* 1977;60:850–857.

168. Koch TK, Yee M, Hutchinson H, Berg BO. Magnetic resonance imaging in subacute necrotizing encephalomyelopathy (Leigh's disease). *Ann Neurol* 1986;19:605–607.

169. Paltiel HJ, O'Gorman PM, Meagher-Villemure K, Rosenblatt B, Silver K, Watters GV. Subacute necrotizing encephalomyelopathy (Leigh disease): CT study. *Radiology* 1987;162:115–118.

170. Medina L, Chi TL, DeVivo DC, Hilal SK. MR findings in patients with subacute necrotizing encephalomyelopathy (Leigh syndrome): correlation with biochemical defect. *AJNR* 1990;11:379–384.

171. Greenberg SB, Faerber EN, Riviello JJ, de Leon G, Capitanio MA. Subacute necrotizing encephalopathy (Leigh disease): CT and MRI appearances. *Pediatr Radiol* 1990;21:5–8.

172. Geyer CA, Sartor KJ, Prensky AJ, Abramson CL, Hodges FJ, Gado MH. Leigh disease (subacute necrotizing encephalomyelopathy): CT and MR in five cases. *J Comput Assist Tomogr* 1988;12:40–44.

173. Savoiardo M, Uziel G, Strada L, Visciani A, Grisoli M, Wang G. MRI findings in Leigh's disease with cytochrome-c-oxidase deficiency. *Neuroradiology* 1991;33(suppl):507–508.

174. Krägeloh-Mann I, Grodd W, Schöning M, Marquard K, Nägele T, Ruitenbeek W. Proton spectroscopy in five patients with Leigh's disease and mitochondrial enzyme deficiency. *Dev Med Child Neurol* 1993;35:769–776.

175. Krägeloh-Mann I, Grodd W, Niemann G, Haas G, Ruitenbeek W. Assessment and therapy monitoring of Leigh disease by MRI and proton spectroscopy. *Pediatr Neurol* 1992;8:60–64.

176. Alpers BJ. Progressive cerebral degeneration in infancy. *J Nerv Ment Dis* 1960;130:442–448.

177. Alpers BJ. Diffuse progressive degeneration of the grey matter of the cerebrum. *Arch Neurol Psychiatr* 1931;25:469–505.

178. Harding BN. Progressive neuronal degeneration of childhood with liver disease (Alpers-Huttenlocher syndrome): a personal review. *J Child Neurol* 1990;5:273–287.

179. Menkes JH. Genetic disorders of mitochondrial function. *J Pediatr* 1987;110:255–259.

180. Egger J, Harding BN, Boyd SG, et al. Progressive neuronal degeneration of childhood (PNDC) with lever disease. *Brain* 1987;26:167–173.

181. Menkes JH, Alter M, Steigleder GK, Weakley DR, Sung JH. A sex-linked recessive disorder with retardation of growth, peculiar hair, and focal cerebral and cerebellar degeneration. *Pediatrics* 1962;29:764–779.

182. Wesenberg RL, Gwinn JL, Barnes GR Jr. Radiological findings in the kinky hair syndrome. *Radiology* 1969;92:500–506.

183. Seay AR, Bray PE, Wing SD, Tompson JA, Bale JF, Williams DM. CT scan in Menkes disease. *Neurology* 1979;29:304–312.

184. Faerber EN, Grover WD, DeFilipp GJ, Capitanio MA, Liu TH, Swartz JD. Cerebral MR of Menkes kinky-hair disease. *Am J Neuroradiol* 1989;10:190–192.

185. Blaser SI, Berns DH, Ross JS, Lanska MJ, Weissman BM. Serial MR studies in Menkes disease. *J Comput Assist Tomogr* 1989;13:113–115.

186. Ichihashi K, Yano S, Kobayashi S, Miyao M, Yanagisawa M. Serial imaging of Menkes disease. *Neuroradiol* 1990;32:56–59.

187. Johnsen DE, Coleman L, Poe L. MR of progressive neurodegenerative change in treated Menkes' kinky hair disease. *Neuroradiology* 1991;33:181–182.

188. Altman NR, Rovira MJ, Bauer M. Glutaric aciduria type I: MR findings in two cases. *AJNR* 1991;12:966–968.

189. Dusheiko G, Kew MC, Joffe BI, et al. Recurrent hypoglycemia associated with glutaric aciduria type II in an adult. *N Engl J Med* 1979;301:1405–1409.

190. Goodman SI, Frerman FE, Loehr JP. Recent progress in understanding glutaric acidemias. *Enzyme* 1987;38:76–79.

191. Blaser S, Feigenbaum A, Becker L, Robinson B, Whyte H, Harwood-Nash D. *Lethal neonatal mitochondrial disease: a radiographic mimic of perinatal asphyxia*. Presented at American Society of Neuroradiology 31st Annual Meeting. Forbes G, ed. Vancouver, BC: ASNR; 1993:121.

192. Sandhu J, Dillon WP. MR in mitochondrial encephalomyelopathy. *Am J Neuroradiol* 1991;12:375–379.

193. Surtees RAH, Matthews EE, Leonard JV. Neurologic outcome of propionic acidemia. *Pediatr Neurol* 1992;8:333–337.

194. Gebarski SS, Gabrielsen TO, Knake JE, Latack JT. Cerebral CT findings in methylmalonic and propionic acidemias. *Am J Neuroradiol* 1983;4:955–957.

195. Andreula CF, De Blasi R, Carella A. CT and MR studies of methylmalonic acidemia. *AJNR* 1991;12:410–412.

196. Stalker HP, Han BK. Thalamic hyperdensity: a previously unreported sign of Sandhoff disease. *AJNR* 1989;10:S82.

CHAPTER 4

Destructive Brain Disorders of Childhood

This chapter discusses destructive lesions of the brain. In a strict sense, it is difficult to separate the brain injuries discussed in this chapter from many of those discussed in Chapter 3, as many of the inborn errors of metabolism and demyelinating disorders are, in fact, destroying myelin. However, inborn metabolic, toxic, and idiopathic (autoimmune) disorders are discussed in the previous chapter, and those resulting from physical and hypoxic–ischemic–hypoglycemic–hyperbilirubinemic trauma are described in this chapter.

PATTERNS OF BRAIN DESTRUCTION

Before considering specific patterns of brain injury from specific causes, it is useful to consider the imaging appearances that result from diffuse brain injury in the neonate and infant. Diffuse insults to the brain, causing widespread destruction, result in different radiologic and pathologic appearances, depending upon the maturity of the brain at the time of insult and on the severity of the insult. Porencephalies, multicystic encephalomalacia, and hydranencephaly are terms used to describe specific patterns of tissue reaction to injury. An understanding of these terms will be useful in further discussions in this, and subsequent, chapters.

Porencephaly

The term *porencephaly* has many definitions. Pathologists use it to describe focal cavities with smooth walls and minimal surrounding glial reaction (1,2). Those cav-

ities resulting from focal brain destruction prior to approximately the 26th gestational week are often lined by dysplastic gray matter and accompanied by anomalies of the overlying cortex, usually polymicrogyria (1). Used in this sense, porencephaly is essentially synonymous with schizencephaly, an anomaly that results from destruction of a portion of the germinal matrix and surrounding brain before the hemispheres are fully formed (see Chapter 5). Other authors have designated lesions developing late in the second trimester as *encephaloclastic porencephalies*, to differentiate them from *agenetic porencephalies (schizencephalies)* and from *encephalomalacia* (see the following discussion), a condition characterized by shaggy-walled cavities with considerable glial reaction and resulting from late gestational, perinatal, or postnatal injuries (2–4). The differentiation of an encephaloclastic porencephaly from encephalomalacia can be made because the fetal brain reacts to injuries differently from the more mature, postnatal brain. In the fetal brain there is limited capacity for astrocytic reaction; therefore, necrotic tissue is completely reabsorbed (liquefaction necrosis). The result is a smooth-walled, fluid-filled cavity (a porencephalic cyst). The mature brain, on the other hand, reacts to injury by significant astrocytic proliferation; the resulting cavity contains septations and an irregular wall composed primarily of reactive astrocytes. The ability to mount an astrocytic response to injury seems to begin sometime during the late second or early third trimester (2,5). On imaging studies (encephaloclastic) porencephalies appear as smooth walled cavities that are isointense to cerebrospinal fluid on all sequences (Figs. 4.1, 4.2). The

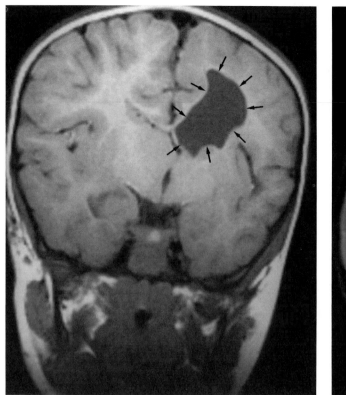

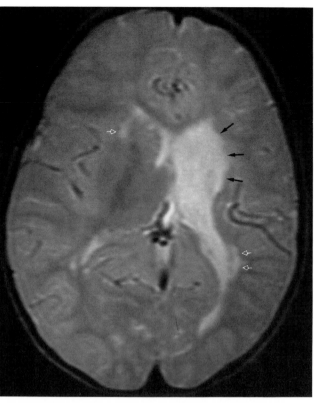

A   B

FIG. 4.1. Porencephaly. **A:** Coronal SE 600/20 image through the frontal horns shows a large, smooth-walled cystic cavity (*arrows*) adjacent to, and including, the left frontal horn. No glial septae are present within the cavity. **B:** Axial SE 2500/70 image shows that the porencephalic cavity (*arrows*) remains isointense with CSF. Multiple other nonspecific areas of increased signal (*open arrows*) are present in the white matter, indicating more extensive cerebral damage.

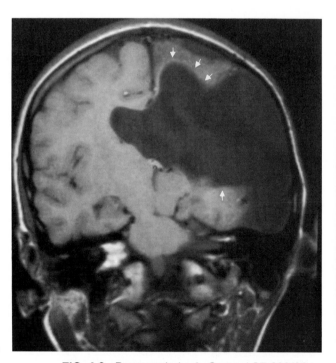

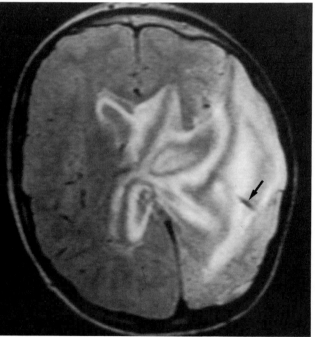

A   B

FIG. 4.2. Porencephaly. **A:** Coronal SE 600/20 image shows a large cavity (*arrows*) extending from the left lateral ventricle to the subarachnoid space. No internal structure is seen within the cavity. The cavity is lined by white matter of the cerebral hemisphere, not gray matter, differentiating it from schizencephaly (see Chapter 5). **B:** Axial SE 2500/70 image shows multiple wave patterns within the cavity, proving free communication and an absence of internal structure. The arrow points to a ventriculostomy that was used to treat this patient's hydrocephalus.

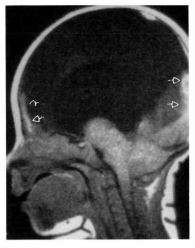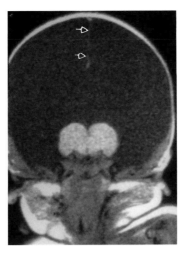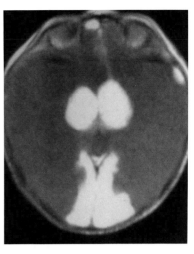

A,B
C

FIG. 4.3. Hydranencephaly. A: Axial SE 600/20 image shows absence of most of the cerebrum. Portions of the anteroinferior frontal lobe and the occipital lobe (*arrows*) are present. B: Coronal SE 600/20 image shows complete absence of the cerebral hemispheres with the exception of the thalami. The falx cerebri (*arrows*) is present. C: Axial SE 600/20 image shows preservation of the thalami and the medial temporo-occipital cortex.

cavities have no internal structure and the surrounding brain is of normal signal intensity.

Hydranencephaly

Hydranencephaly is a condition in which most of the brain mantle (cortical plate and hemispheric white matter) has been destroyed and resorbed (6). The cerebral hemispheres are largely replaced by thin-walled sacs containing CSF (1,2). The membranes of the sacs are composed of an outer layer of leptomeningeal connective tissue and an inner layer of remnants of the cortex and white matter. Although some people consider hydranencephaly a congenital anomaly, it is included in the chapter on destructive disorders because the remnants of hemispheric tissue clearly imply a destructive process. The causal injury is not entirely clear. A similar condition has been induced in laboratory animals by the occlusion of both carotid arteries *in utero*. Therefore, a vascular etiology is highly likely in some cases. However, toxoplasmosis and cytomegalovirus infections have been demonstrated to be factors in at least some cases (7). In all likelihood, any of a number of insults to the developing brain, at a time when the brain reacts by liquefaction necrosis, can result in hydranencephaly (2,7). Clinically, affected patients may be microcephalic, normocephalic, or macrocephalic, depending upon the presence and degree of associated hydrocephalus (8,9). Because of the nearly complete lack of cortical tissue, the children are developmentally delayed from an extremely early age (8,9).

On imaging studies, the cerebral hemispheres appear nearly completely replaced by CSF (2,10). The thalami are usually preserved. Often the inferior medial aspects of the frontal lobes and the inferior medial aspects of the

temporal lobes are also preserved (Fig. 4.3). The brain stem is usually atrophic; the cerebellum almost always has a normal appearance.

It is sometimes a diagnostic problem to differentiate hydranencephaly from severe hydrocephalus. This distinction is considered significant because children with hydrocephalus, even when extremely severe, typically respond well to CSF diversion procedures and can have

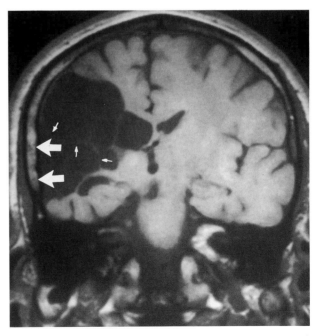

FIG. 4.4. Multicystic encephalomalacia secondary to infarction. Coronal SE 600/20 image shows a sharply defined area of hypointensity in the right cerebral hemisphere. Thin septae (*small arrows*) are present within the cavity. The overlying calvarium (*large arrows*) is thickened.

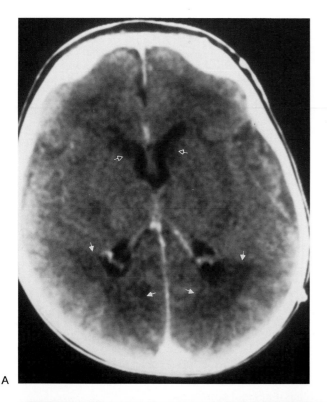

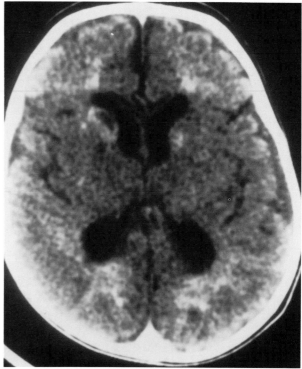

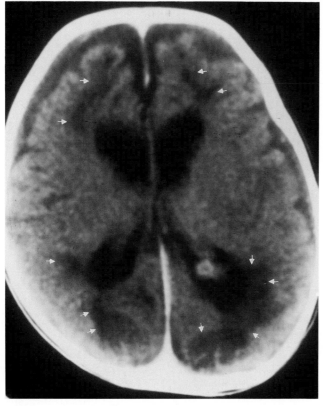

FIG. 4.5. Encephalomalacia secondary to partial asphyxia. **A:** Contrast-enhanced CT image in the acute phase shows low attenuation in the frontal and temporo-occipital (*solid arrows*) white matter and the caudate heads (*open arrows*). **B:** In the sub-acute phase (1 week after injury), the injured regions show contrast enhancement. **C:** In the chronic phase (2 months after injury), the cerebral cortex is shrunken away from the calvarium, resulting in an increased amount of extraparenchymal fluid. The ventricles have enlarged secondary to atrophy of white matter and the caudate heads. Abnormal lucency (*arrows*) representing encephalomalacia is present in the frontal and temporo-occipital white matter.

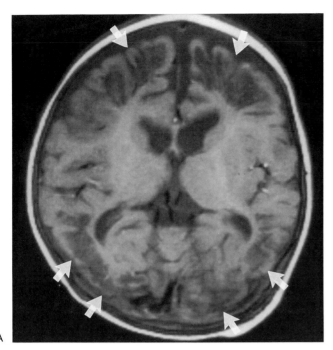
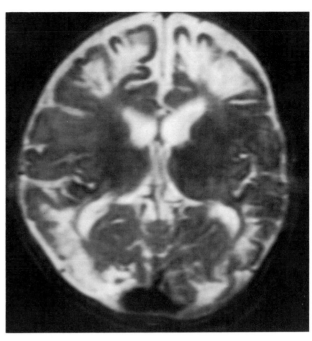

A   B

FIG. 4.6. Multicystic encephalomalacia secondary to partial asphyxia. **A:** Axial SE 600/20 image shows cortical thinning (*arrows*) in the frontal and temporo-occipital regions. The underlying white matter is hypointense, with strands of hyperintensity (glial septae). **B:** Axial SE 3000/120 image shows cortical thinning and heterogeneous hyperintensity in the affected regions.

normal intelligence and a normal life if the shunting is performed at an early age. Children with hydranencephaly, on the other hand, will not improve intellectually after shunting. On imaging studies, the diagnosis of hydrocephalus is established by identification of a thin rim of dilated white matter and cortex around the dilated ventricles. This rim of tissue may be impossible to identify on a CT scan because of artifact generated by the overlying calvarium. MR, which is not subject to the beam-hardening artifact, is useful in the detection of this thin cortical rim. In practice, this distinction may be purely academic because CSF diversion is dictated by an abnormally enlarging head in infants with either entity. Although CSF diversion will not improve intellectual development in infants with hydranencephaly, it will prevent the development of the grotesquely enlarged head size that would otherwise result from the increased intracranial pressure. In the absence of an abnormally enlarging head size, CSF shunting is not indicated and the differentiation between the two disease processes becomes equally unimportant.

Encephalomalacia

Encephalomalacia, in contradistinction to porencephalies and hydranencephaly, is characterized pathologically by astrocytic proliferation and, often, glial septations within the area of damaged brain. MR shows the reactive astrocytosis and tissue injury as areas of prolonged T1 and T2 relaxation (10). Because it has inherently poorer contrast resolution, CT will not allow

confident differentiation of porencephalies from encephalomalacia. Ultrasound is the most sensitive modality in the detection of glial septa but is less useful in the overall evaluation of the brain.

Multicystic encephalomalacia results from a diffuse insult to the brain late in gestation, during birth, or after birth (1,2). Multiple cystic cavities of variable size form in the necrotic area, separated from one another by glial septations (Fig. 4.4)(1). The location of the lesions varies with the nature of the insult. If caused by thrombotic or embolic infarction (Fig. 4.4), the affected area will be in the distribution of a branch of a major cerebral artery. In contrast, injury resulting from partial asphyxia (Figs. 4.5, 4.6) will tend to be located in the cortex and peripheral white matter, primarily in the intervascular boundary zones ("watershed areas"). When very severe, only the immediate periventricular white matter may be spared (Figs. 4.6, 4.7). When injury is the result of an infection, the site of the encephalomalacia is nonspecific; it will vary with the region of the brain that was injured by the infection. In either case, the CT appearance is that of hypodense tissue containing cysts of various sizes; septations are often seen within the damaged region (Fig. 4.7), and calcification may be present (2). On MR, the affected area appears as an ill-defined area of prolonged T1 and T2 relaxation containing loculations of fluid (Figs. 4.4, 4.6)(10). Some heterogeneity is often present, as a result of the combination of variably sized glial septae and CSF within the lesion. The heterogeneity is often most apparent on the first echo of the T2-weighted sequence, in which the glial strands are quite hyperintense and the

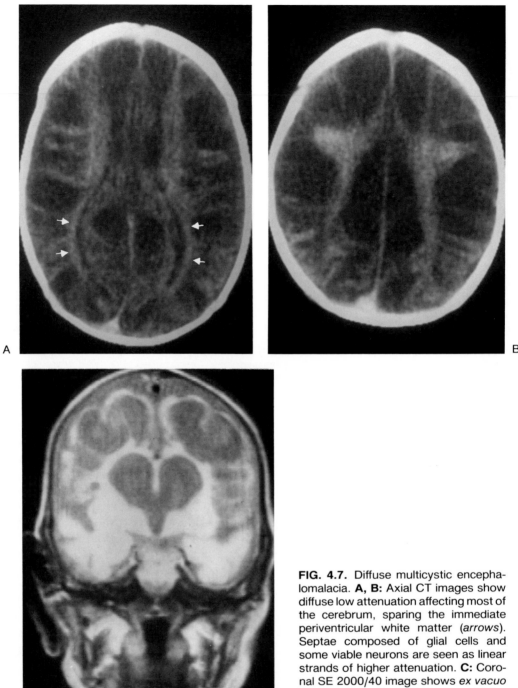

FIG. 4.7. Diffuse multicystic encephalomalacia. **A, B:** Axial CT images show diffuse low attenuation affecting most of the cerebrum, sparing the immediate periventricular white matter (*arrows*). Septae composed of glial cells and some viable neurons are seen as linear strands of higher attenuation. **C:** Coronal SE 2000/40 image shows *ex vacuo* enlargement of the lateral ventricles with multicystic encephalomalacia involving the hemispheric white matter. The overlying cerebral cortex is thinned.

CSF spaces mimic that of the ventricular CSF. The septae are better seen by MR than by CT.

HYPOXIC–ISCHEMIC BRAIN INJURY

Localized Infarctions

Causes of Infarctions in Children

Focal ischemic infarction has a variable presentation in the pediatric age group, with the presenting signs and symptoms dependent upon the region of brain affected and the age of the patient at the time of the infarct (11,12). Stroke in the neonatal period typically presents with neonatal seizures, hypotonia, or lethargy, whereas stroke presenting in infancy more commonly presents as an early hand preference. (Infants do not usually show hand preference prior to the age of 1 year.) Older infants and children present in a manner similar to adults, with an abrupt onset of neurologic deficit (11,12). Because the clinical presentation of stroke in neonates and infants can be quite subtle, imaging is often the most important component of the diagnostic work-up.

A large number of conditions can cause ischemic brain damage in infants. When infarction is focal and in the distribution of the middle cerebral artery, an embolic source is the most likely cause. In neonates, the most common cause of *embolic cerebral infarction* is congenital cyanotic heart disease. In cyanotic heart disease, emboli from the peripheral venous system are shunted through abnormal connections from the right to the left heart chambers, bypassing the filtering effect of the capillary beds within the lungs (11). In older children, causes of cerebral embolism include cardiomyopathies, carotid dissection, and mitral valve prolapse (13). *Thrombosis* of intracranial vessels can result from polycythemia (sometimes caused by congenital heart disease), direct and indirect trauma to the head and neck leading to intimal dissection, viral infection (14,15), meningitis (especially Hemophilus influenzae, tuberculous, and gram-negative meningitides) with extension of the inflammatory process into the perivascular spaces, coagulopathies [especially partial deficiencies of factors, such as proteins C and S, which are being discovered more and more frequently as a cause of neonatal stroke (16)], maternal drug use [especially cocaine (17,18)], and vasculopathies (i.e., those associated with moyamoya neurofibromatosis, Kawasaki's disease, fibromuscular disease, and sickle cell disease) that cause thickening of the intima and an obliterative arteritis. Migraine can cause ischemic infarction in children, probably secondary to vasospasm (19). *Metabolic disorders*—such as homocystinuria, progeria (20), congenital disorders of cholesterol and triglyceride metabolism (21), and MELAS (see Chapter 3)—can cause localized thrombosis and infarction. Infarcts can also result from *vascular malformations* and from congenital *CNS tumors,* which can compress and occlude vessels (11,22).

Imaging Appearances of Infarctions in Children

On cranial ultrasound, cerebral infarction most commonly appears as an ill-defined region of hyperechogenicity (Fig. 4.8) that slowly develops several days after the event. Differentiation of hemorrhagic from bland infarction is difficult; however, focal areas of marked hyperechogenicity within the echogenic zone should suggest hemorrhage.

Cerebral infarction in the neonate has a similar appearance to that in the older child or adult on CT. When the infarction involves the cerebral cortex, CT shows a well-defined, often wedge-shaped, region of hypoattenuation that affects both the cortex and the underlying white matter (Fig. 4.9). Areas of hemorrhage are unequivocally detected as regions that are hyperdense compared to normal parenchyma on noncontrast scans. The administration of iodinated contrast will result in enhancement of the infarcted region of cortex starting about 5 days after the injury; enhancement will slowly disappear starting 4–6 weeks after the injury. The appearance of the infarct is independent of the cause of the infarct.

In contrast to CT, the MR appearance of focal bland (nonhemorrhagic) infarction in a neonate is very different from that in older children and can be quite subtle (Figs. 4.8, 4.9). In newborns, the infarcted cortex becomes edematous and therefore becomes isointense with the underlying unmyelinated white matter. I look for infarcts by trying to see the entire circumference of the cerebral cortex. If a segment of the cortex appears to be "missing," especially on T2-weighted images, it probably represents focal infarction. Regions of infarction with petechial hemorrhage will show high signal on T1-weighted images and low signal on T2-weighted images (Figs. 4.9, 4.11). In older infants, the earliest sign of infarction is the appearance of a stripe of T2 prolongation near the cortical–white matter junction that corresponds to blurring of the gray matter–white matter junction on the T1-weighted images (Fig. 4.10). The exact pathologic correlation of this stripe is uncertain, although it may represent cortical laminar necrosis. The MR appearance of infarctions in older children and the MR appearance of hemorrhagic infarcts in children of any age are identical to the appearance of similar injuries in adults. Administration of intravenous paramagnetic contrast (Fig. 4.11) results in an enhancement pattern similar to that described in the preceding paragraph on CT.

Infarction of the deep gray matter nuclei in neonates and young infants can be very subtle on CT, particularly if the infarction is bilateral and associated with cerebral edema. This appearance is discussed and illustrated in the section on "profound asphyxia." The point to be stressed is that basal ganglia infarcts may be overlooked

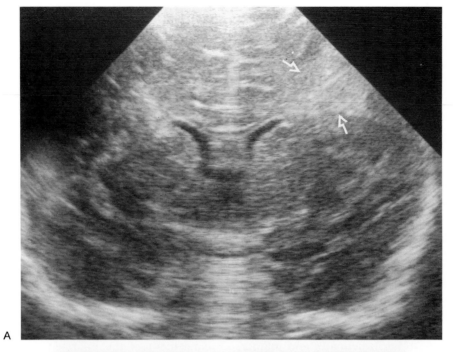

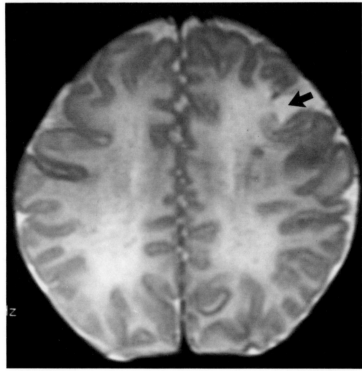

FIG. 4.8. Cerebral infarction. **A:** Sonogram in the coronal plane shows mild hyperechogenicity (*arrows*) in the white matter adjacent to the left frontal horn of the lateral ventricle. **B:** Axial SE 3000/120 MR image shows the infarct as a focus of cerebral cortex (*arrow*) that is isointense with underlying white matter.

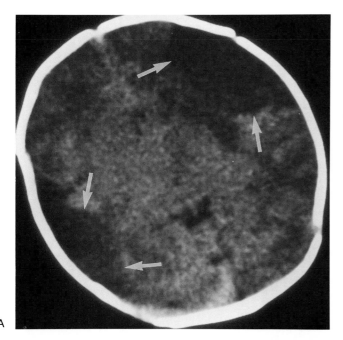

A

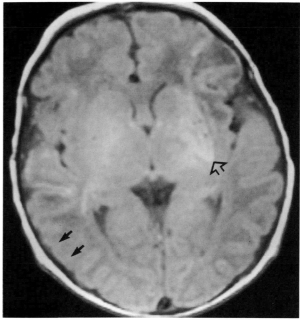

B

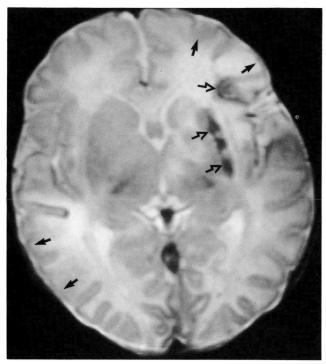

C

FIG. 4.9. Multiple infarctions in a neonate. A: Axial CT image shows wedge-shaped areas of low attenuation (*arrows*) in the left frontal lobe and lentiform nucleus, and the right temporal lobe. B: Axial SE 600/15 image shows blurring of the cerebral cortex (*solid arrows*) and underlying white matter in parts of the affected areas. Other affected areas of gray matter (*open arrows*) are hyperintense, probably secondary to petechial hemorrhage. C: Axial SE 3000/120 image shows edematous gray matter (*solid arrows*) as isointense with underlying white matter, whereas hemorrhagic gray matter (*open arrows*) is hypointense.

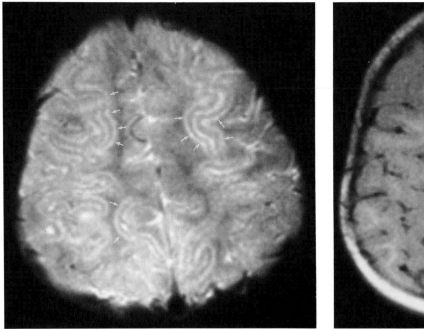
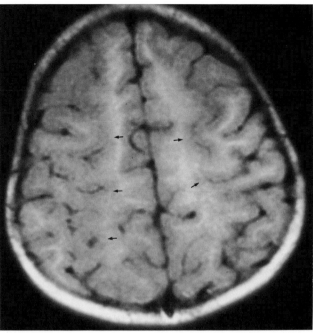

FIG. 4.10. Infarction in a 1-year-old. At this age, the first sign of infarction is a curvilinear region of hyperintensity at the cortex–white matter junction (*arrows in* **A**) on T2-weighted images and blurring of the gray matter–white matter junction (*arrows in* **B**) on T1-weighted images.

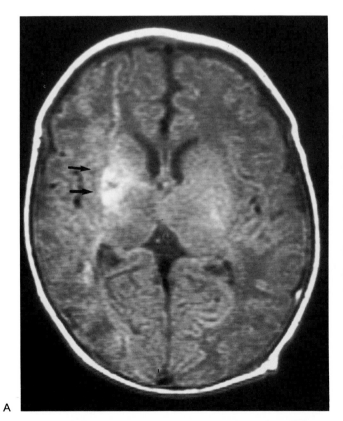
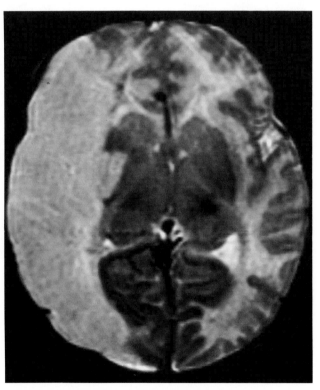

FIG. 4.11. Middle cerebral artery infarction secondary to embolus. **A:** Axial SE 600/12 image shows hyperintensity in the right lentiform nucleus (*arrows*) and poor differentiation of the cerebral cortex from the underlying white matter in the right middle cerebral artery distribution. **B:** Axial SE 3000/120 image shows hyperintensity of the cortex and underlying white matter in the right middle cerebral artery distribution.

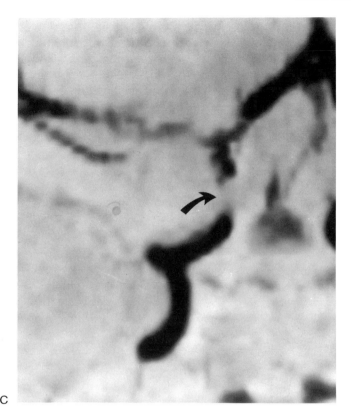

C

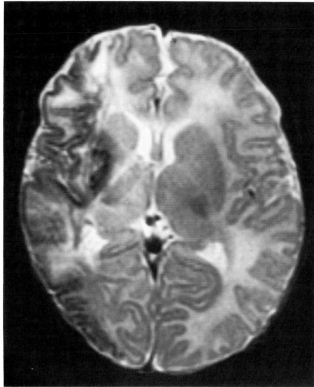

D

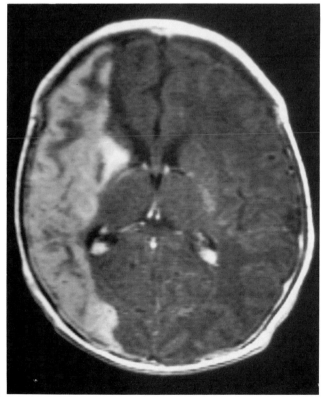

E

FIG. 4.11. (*Continued.*) **C:** MR angiogram shows an embolus (*arrow*) in the supraclinoid segment of the right internal carotid artery. **D:** Axial 3000/120 image shows abnormal hypointensity in the right lentiform nucleus and cerebral cortex in the middle cerebral artery distribution. **E:** Post-contrast SE 600/12 image from follow-up scan performed 1 week after event. Marked enhancement is seen in the injured regions of brain. (This case courtesy Dr. Chip Truwit, Minneapolis, MN.)

on CT of neonates unless the radiologist specifically looks at the basal ganglia to assess their appearance.

The MR appearance of infarcted basal ganglia is variable, depending on the amount of hemorrhage present. In the absence of hemorrhage, the basal ganglia will be nearly isointense with surrounding white matter. More often, however, some hemorrhage or myelin degradation will be present in the infarcted nuclei, resulting in a heterogeneous signal on both T1- and T2-weighted images (Figs. 4.9, 4.11).

When examining an MR scan of an infant or child who has suffered a cerebral infarction, close scrutiny of the cerebral blood vessels is essential. On routine imaging studies, the blood vessels should appear as discrete circular or ovoid regions of flow void. To avoid effects of volume averaging, the vessels are optimally viewed in the plane perpendicular to their direction of flow. Therefore, the supraclinoid carotid arteries are best viewed in the axial plane, the intracavernous carotid arteries are best evaluated in the coronal plane, and the horizontal portions of the middle and anterior cerebral arteries are best viewed in the parasagittal plane. As children have essentially no atherosclerosis, the wall of a normal cerebral blood vessel should not be seen on imaging studies. If the vessel wall is seen, it is likely to be abnormal, and either a condition of premature aging, such as progeria, or an arterial dissection (Fig. 4.12) should be suspected.

All children who suffer cerebral infarction should undergo cerebral angiography unless the patient has a known disease that predisposes to stroke and is already under treatment. In some instances, especially when the vascular disease primarily involves the arteries of the neck, skull base, or circle of Willis, MR angiography may be adequate (Fig. 4.11) (23–27). T1-weighted MR imaging may be helpful in the diagnosis of arterial dissections, as a crescent of (hyperintense) methemoglobin in the wall of the vessel is strongly suggestive of the diagnosis. However, to rule out subtle occlusions of branch vessels or vasculitis of middle-sized arteries, catheter angiography remains essential.

Diffuse Ischemic Brain Injury

A number of terms are used to describe diffuse hypoxic–ischemic brain injury in the neonate, including perinatal asphyxia, hypoxic–ischemic encephalopathy, and asphyxia neonatorum. The physiology of brain injury resulting from asphyxia is rather complex and not completely understood. Asphyxia results in a diminished oxygen content in the blood (hypoxia), elevation of the amount of carbon dioxide in the blood (hypercarbia), acidosis, and a decreased systemic blood pressure. The hypercarbia and hypoxia cause a loss of the normal vascular autoregulation in the brain (28), resulting in so-called pressure-passive flow. (In the normal situation, blood

vessels of the brain constrict when blood pressure increases and dilate when blood pressure decreases. This process, known as *autoregulation*, maintains constant cerebral blood flow.) The combination of decreased blood pressure and loss of vascular autoregulation results in decreased perfusion of the brain (9,29). Thus, almost all asphyxic brain injury is caused by hypoperfusion; the newborn brain is quite resistant to hypoxia. Hypoxia, however, has the additional effect of altering capillary permeability. Reperfusion of the weakened capillaries [particularly those within the germinal matrices, which are structurally weaker than the capillaries in the remainder of the premature brain (30)] can cause rupture of cerebral blood vessels and result in intracranial or intraventricular hemorrhage (5).

The combination of hypotension and loss of autoregulation does not explain all the patterns of brain injury seen in asphyxiated neonates, however (31–37). Many asphyxiated newborns show damage primarily to the basal ganglia or brain stem, without significant cortical or white matter damage (31–34,37–39). Two major theories have been proposed to explain these locations of brain damage. The first theory uses the fact that hypoxic–ischemic brain damage is believed to be caused by excessive release of excitatory amino acids (EAAs), primarily glutamate, into the synaptic cleft (40). If the postsynaptic neuron has proper cell surface molecules ("receptors," most commonly N-methyl-D-aspartate), the EAAs (known as *excitotoxins*) start a chain of chemical reactions in the postsynaptic neuron that result in neuronal cell death. The abundance and location of the receptor molecules within the brain varies with the stage of brain development (40,41). Thus, differing patterns of brain injury may reflect different distributions of N-methyl-D-aspartate receptors in the developing brain. The other main theory involves the status of myelination at the time of the injury (34). It is well known that neurons contributing axons to tracts that are myelinated or myelinating have much higher energy requirements than unmyelinated ones (42,43). PET studies of glucose uptake in the developing brain (44), which reflect metabolic activity, show excellent topologic correlation with the onset of myelination (45). Moreover, the pattern of brain injury detected on MR studies of profoundly asphyxiated term newborns corresponds quite closely to the pattern of myelination in the newborn (34), indicating that myelination is an important factor in determining location of brain injury in asphyxiated newborns. Still another possibility involves the fact that myelin formation inhibits axonal sprouting (personal communication, K. Mollgard). This finding raises the possibility that the entire brain is injured in profound asphyxia but that only the unmyelinated regions recover completely. In all likelihood, a combination of the preceding factors affects the ultimate pattern of brain injury as detected by imaging studies.

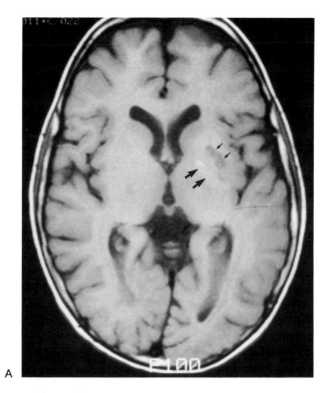

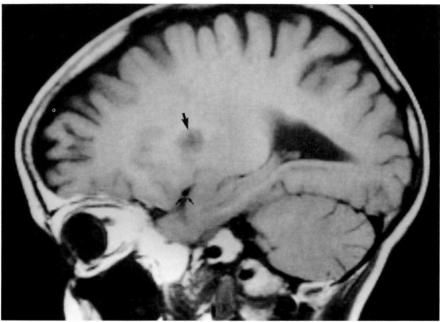

FIG. 4.12. Basal ganglia infarct secondary to intracranial dissection. **A:** Axial SE 600/20 image shows heterogeneous abnormal signal in the left lentiform nucleus. The rim of hyperintensity (*large arrows*) likely represents petechial hemorrhage. The central hypointensity (*small arrows*) is probably necrotic tissue. **B:** Sagittal SE 600/20 image shows the infarct (*large arrows*). Note that the wall (*small arrows*) of the middle cerebral artery can be seen. This is abnormal in a child. In this case, it was the result of a dissection.

Injury in the Premature Infant

Hypoxia/Ischemia in Premature Infants

Preterm infants and full-term infants experience ischemia in different regions of the brain. Classically, this has been considered to result from the changing location of the intervascular boundary zones ("watershed regions"), although this explanation is disputed (46,47). Van den Bergh (48), Takashima and Tanaka (49), and deReuck (50) postulated that the ventriculofugal blood vessels in the brain (those coursing outward into the cerebrum from the intraventricular and periventricular regions) are poorly developed during the first two trimesters of gestation. Almost all the blood supply to the cerebral white matter and cortex, therefore, comes from the ventriculopetal blood vessels coursing inward from the surface of the brain (Fig. 4.13). Moreover, Volpe and colleagues (51) have shown markedly reduced perfusion to the deep white matter in asphyxiated premature infants. Thus, it appears that, as a result of immaturity of the brain or its vascular supply, the periventricular areas are the regions at highest risk when autoregulation is compromised in premature infants. Periventricular white matter damage (periventricular leukomalacia) is there-

fore a common finding on imaging studies of stressed premature infants; it is particularly common in those with hyaline membrane disease, antepartum placental abruptions, hypocapnia, twin pregnancy, septicemia, or ischemia during delivery (32,33,35,52,53).

Other factors contribute to an increased susceptibility of premature infants to hypoxic–ischemic damage, particularly in the periventricular region. For example, the immaturity of the premature lung results in poor oxygen exchange and contributes some degree of hypoxemia and hypercarbia. In addition, the premature infant has a relatively limited vasodilatory capacity of the cerebral vessels, resulting in an inability of the body to deliver excess blood to the brain. Moreover, cerebral white matter responds to oxygen deprivation by the process of anaerobic glycolysis, an inefficient mechanism of glycogen metabolism that results in a depletion of high-energy phosphates and in localized acidosis. Both the depletion of the phosphates and the acidosis result in increased tissue destruction. Finally, the fact that the periventricular white matter is actively myelinating (and therefore has higher metabolic demands) makes the periventricular region more susceptible to injury. All the preceding factors contribute to the significant incidence of periventricular leukomalacia in premature infants with immature lungs (9,29,54).

As stated earlier, when ischemic tissue is reperfused, the weakened blood vessels often rupture, resulting in parenchymal hemorrhage. This type of hemorrhage is most frequently seen in the germinal matrix, the area within the ventricular wall in which the cells that compose the brain are generated (55,56). Cell generation is a very active metabolic process that requires a large blood supply; the germinal matrix is, therefore, extremely vascular. The germinal zones are most active between approximately 8 and 28 weeks of gestation; neurons are the primary cells produced in early stages, whereas glial cells are produced in later stages of germinal zone activity (57). Toward the end of the second trimester the germinal zones diminish in activity and begin to involute. The last area of the germinal matrix to involute is the region near the caudate heads, known as the ganglionic eminence. The incidence of subependymal hemorrhage decreases with the increasing gestational age of the infant because of the progressive involution of the germinal matrix. The ganglionic eminence, because it remains metabolically active the longest, hemorrhages most frequently. Germinal matrix hemorrhage is unusual after 34 weeks of gestation (5,9,54). The choroid plexus also frequently bleeds in premature infants, often in association with germinal matrix bleeds.

Germinal matrix hemorrhage has been divided into four grades, depending upon its severity (9). *Grade I* has been defined as germinal matrix hemorrhage with no or minimal intraventricular hemorrhage. *Grade II* is defined as extension of the subependymal hemorrhage into

VENTRICLE

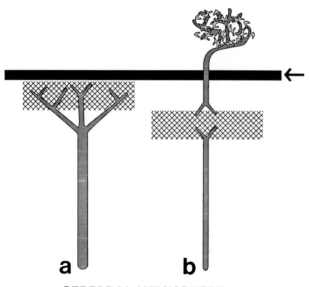

CEREBRAL HEMISPHERE

FIG. 4.13. Schematic showing postulated change in supply of blood to the cerebrum during the third trimester. **A:** The immature pattern in which the periventricular area is perfused by penetrating arteries that extend inward from the surface of the brain. The periventricular region (*hatched rectangular region*) therefore is the boundary zone. **B:** The mature pattern in which vessels extend into the brain from the lateral ventricles, moving the boundary zones peripherally. The arrow points to the ventricular wall.

the ventricles (which remain normal in size). *Grade III* bleeds (Figs. 4.14–4.16) are defined as intraventricular extension of subependymal hemorrhage with ventricular enlargement resulting from hydrocephalus. In *Grade IV* bleeds (Fig. 4.17), hemorrhage involves the cerebral hemispheres, most likely secondary to venous infarction (58). The presence of ventricular enlargement is related to the severity of the intraventricular hemorrhage and is an excellent prognosticator of the short- and long-term neurologic outcome of the patient. Only 26% of patients with grade III/IV hemorrhages survived in one large study of 484 infants, whereas 67% of infants with grade I/II hemorrhage survived (59). Patients with mild hemorrhage and normal ventricular size have approximately a 10% incidence of long-term neurologic sequelae. Patients with persistent ventriculomegaly after intraventricular hemorrhage have approximately a 50% incidence of neurologic sequelae. Those with an intraparenchymal component of hemorrhage have a 90% incidence of serious neurologic sequelae (9,59).

Even premature infants (33 weeks of gestation) with normal neurologic exams have a high incidence of cognitive impairment when examined at age 8 years (60). Mild cognitive impairment is identified in nearly 50% of preterm children with no sonographic abnormalities, although the incidence of significant impairment is less than 5% (60). The incidence of severe cognitive impairment increases significantly if hydrocephalus or loss of cerebral parenchyma can be detected by sonography (60). The cognitive impairment is suspected to be the result of injury to commissural tracts, especially the posterior corpus callosum, which are largely concerned with the transfer of cognitive information (60,61).

It is apparent from the preceding discussion that the pathologic sequelae of hypoxic–ischemic damage in premature infants are manifested primarily in the deep areas of the brain. For example, germinal matrix hemorrhage occurs mostly at the heads of the caudate nuclei, and parenchymal damage largely manifests itself as periventricular leukomalacia, which is seen adjacent to the lateral ventricles. Moreover, the degree of enlargement of the ventricles themselves has significant prognostic value. As premature infants have large, open fontanels and the pathologic processes occur in the central areas of the brain, ultrasound is the optimal imaging modality for evaluation of their brains. Sonographic examination is easily performed in the neonatal intensive care unit, using the anterior and posterior fontanels as sonographic windows. Maintenance of body temperature is vital in these infants, and it is difficult to provide adequate warmth and monitoring outside of the neonatal ICU. Therefore, evaluation of these infants by sonography is recommended whenever possible.

In the acute phase after an ischemic injury, sonography will show ventricular compression and mildly increased echogenicity secondary to edema (Fig. 4.14). So-nograms show germinal matrix hemorrhage as a region of increased echogenicity. Images acquired in the coronal plane show a well-defined area of increased echogenicity inferior to the floor of the frontal horn (Fig. 4.15). The sagittal plane is often very useful in differentiating germinal matrix hemorrhage from the echogenic choroid plexus because the choroid plexus does not extend anterior to the foramen of Monro, whereas the caudate heads and the adjacent ganglionic eminence hemorrhage lie immediately anterior to the foramen.

Intraventricular hemorrhage results in filling of a portion or, sometimes, all of the ventricular system with echogenic material. When acute, the intraventricular hemorrhage is extremely echogenic (Fig. 4.14). Over the first few weeks after the acute event, however, the intraventricular clot organizes and becomes well defined and less echogenic. At this stage, it appears as a relatively sonolucent mass within the lateral ventricle, usually in the body or the atrium. The clot is less echogenic than the choroid plexus, which is situated adjacent to the thalamus (Fig 4.15). Hemorrhage can also be detected by CT, on which it appears hyperdense in the acute phase and becomes isodense at 7–10 days after the bleed. The temporal evolution of intraventricular blood in neonates has never been studied by MR. Neonatal intraparenchymal hematomas are iso- to slightly hypointense on T1-weighted images and markedly hypointense on T2- and T2-weighted images in the acute stage (first 3 days). They gradually turn bright on T1-weighted images (while remaining very dark on T2- and T2-weighted images) over the next 3–7 days (Fig. 4.16) (62). Between 7 and 14 days, the hematoma gradually turns bright on T2-weighted images and remains so while slowly turning isointense to CSF on T1-weighted images over the next several months (62).

In the acute phase after intraventricular hemorrhage, ventricular dilatation results from blockage of the arachnoid villi and cerebral aqueduct by hemorrhagic particulate matter; this acute hydrocephalus often resolves and is of no prognostic value. When the hemorrhage is severe, however, it can cause an obliterative arachnoiditis that usually occurs in the cisterna magna. The arachnoidal adhesions block the normal flow of CSF from the fourth ventricle to the basilar cisterns and convexities and therefore necessitate permanent ventriculoperitoneal CSF diversion. The development of this secondary hydrocephalus implies a poorer developmental prognosis for the premature infant (9). Such ventricular dilatation is well demonstrated by transfontanel sonography (Fig. 4.15); the patient should be scanned approximately 1 week after initial documentation of the hemorrhage to exclude subsequent ventricular enlargement.

Grade IV hemorrhages, which are ischemic parenchymal injuries with associated hemorrhage that typically occur in the deep white matter adjacent to the lateral ventricle, are seen on sonography as areas of mixed hy-

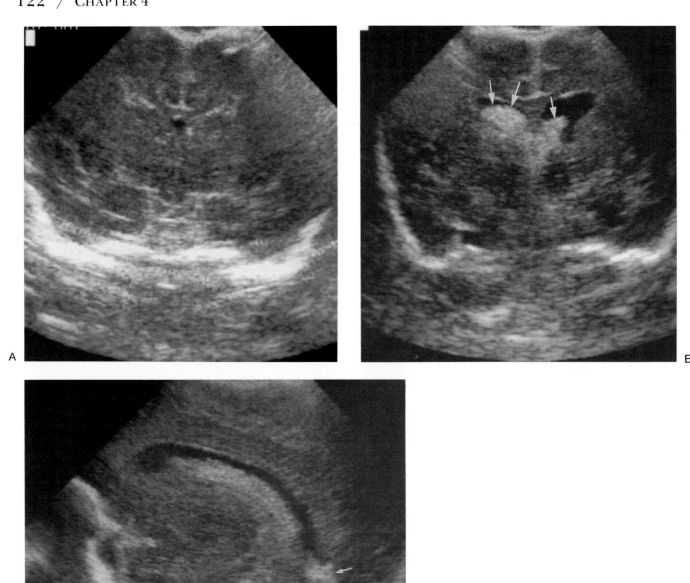

FIG. 4.14. Intraventricular hemorrhage. **A:** Coronal plane sonogram shows cerebral edema, manifest as small lateral ventricles. **B:** Intraventricular hemorrhage is shown as hyperechogenic regions (*arrows*) in the enlarged frontal horns of the lateral ventricles. **C:** Sagittal plane sonogram shows hemorrhage (*arrows*) layering in the occipital horn of the lateral ventricle.

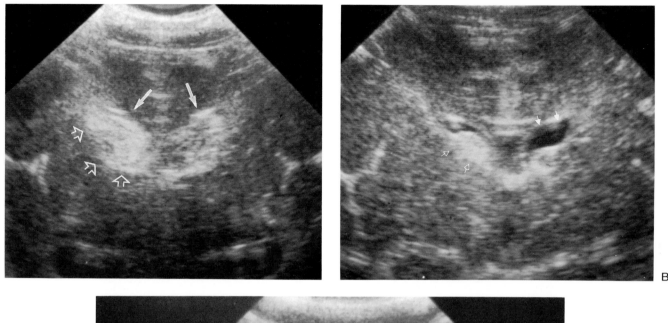

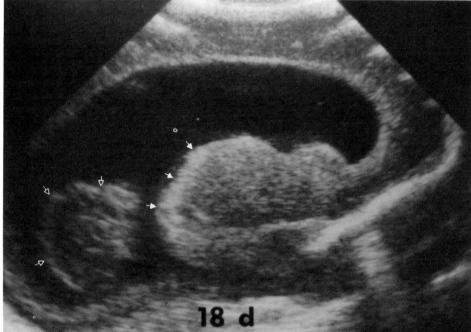

FIG. 4.15. Germinal matrix hemorrhage extending into the ventricles and causing hydrocephalus. **A:** Coronal plane sonogram shows hyperechogenicity (*open arrows*) in the region of the caudate heads with compression of the adjacent frontal horns (*solid arrows*) of the lateral ventricles. **B:** One week later, the hemorrhage (*open arrows*) in the region of the caudate heads is resolving, but the ventricles (*solid arrows*) are starting to enlarge. **C:** Sagittal plane sonogram at age 18 days shows marked ventricular enlargement. A resolving clot (*open arrows*) is present in the ventricular trigone. The clot is less echogenic than, and is situated posteriorly to, the choroid plexus (*solid arrows*).

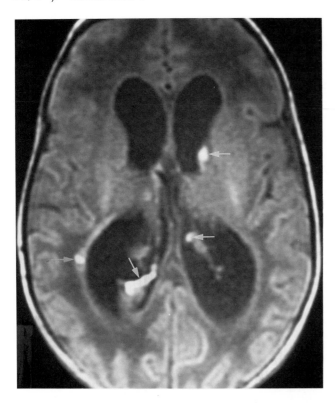

FIG. 4.16. MR of resolving germinal matrix hemorrhage. Axial SE 600/12 image shows foci of methemoglobin (*arrows*) in the germinal zones and choroid plexus. Mild hydrocephalus is present.

per- and hypoechogenicity (Fig. 4.17). It is difficult to determine how much hemorrhage is present based solely on the sonogram. Involved brain regions often undergo liquefaction and end up as large parenchymal cysts (Fig. 4.17).

Periventricular leukomalacia (PVL) has been demonstrated pathologically in 85% of infants with birth weights between 900 and 2,200 g who survived beyond 6 days (63). The two most common locations for PVL are the posterior periventricular white matter adjacent to the lateral aspect of the trigone of the lateral ventricles and the white matter adjacent to the foramina of Monro (1,52,53,64). The lesions are frequently hemorrhagic.

Periventricular leukomalacia should be suspected on ultrasound studies when there is increased echogenicity in the periventricular regions. However, edema also causes increased echogenicity, and edema can resolve without any subsequent brain damage (Fig. 4.18) (65). Moreover, increased echogenicity can be seen in this region in the absence of PVL or edema (66), and normal scans have been reported in infants subsequently proven to have PVL at autopsy (67,68). Therefore, a definitive diagnosis of periventricular leukomalacia by sonography requires demonstration of cavitation and the subsequent formation of cysts in these areas (Fig. 4.19) (69–73). Cavitation occurs 2–6 weeks after injury (74). Severe white matter injury with impending cavitation may be suspected when globular areas of periventricular white matter are more echogenic than the choroid plexus (Fig. 4.19).

PVL can be graded by the characteristics of the periventricular white matter on sonography (75). *Grade I PVL* is defined as periventricular areas of increased echogenicity present for 7 days or more. *Grade II PVL* has periventricular areas of increased echogenicity that evolve into small, localized frontoparietal cysts. In *grade III PVL*, periventricular areas of increased echogenicity evolve into extensive periventricular cystic lesions involving occipital and frontoparietal white matter.

CT and MR do not play a major role in the early diagnosis of PVL because of the difficulty involved in transporting and caring for sick premature neonates. However, if obtained, MR will show signal abnormalities in the periventricular white matter early in the course of the injury (76). Punctate areas of short T1 and T2 are seen in the periventricular white matter for several weeks to months after injury (Fig. 4.19) (76). Gradually, as necrosis of the immediate periventricular tissue occurs and the resulting cysts are incorporated into the lateral ventricles, the areas of signal abnormality come to lie closer and closer to the ventricular wall until they finally disappear (Fig. 4.19). MR and CT are both useful for the diagnosis of end-stage PVL in later infancy and childhood after the fontanels have closed. CT and MR are also useful in making a diagnosis in mild cases of PVL where nonspecific ventriculomegaly is the only detectable abnormality on sonography. The *CT findings of end-stage PVL* are (1) ventriculomegaly with irregular outline of the body and trigone of the lateral ventricles; (2) reduced quantity of periventricular white matter, always

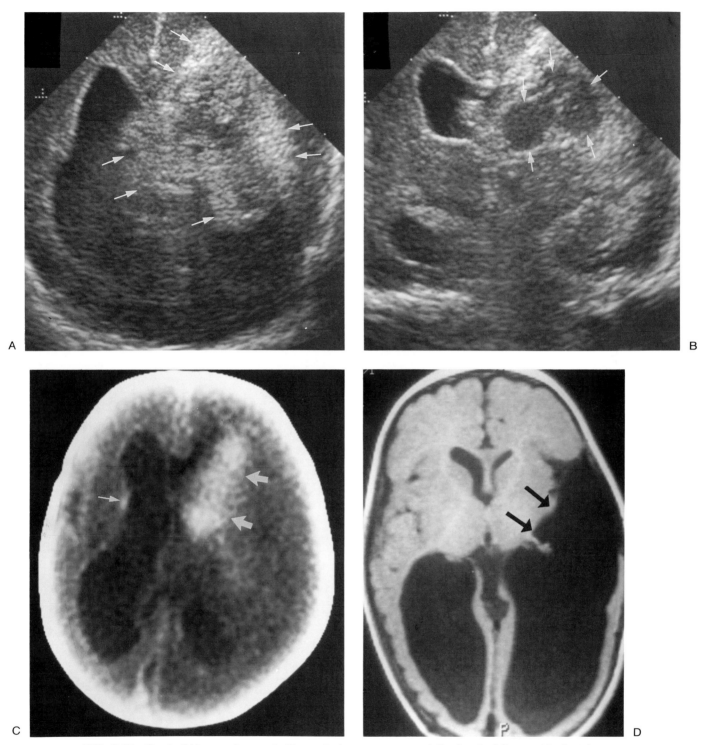

FIG. 4.17. Grade IV hemorrhage. **A:** Coronal plane sonogram at the level of the ventricular trigones shows an echogenic region (*arrows*) adjacent to, and extending into, the trigone of the left lateral ventricle. **B:** At the level of the frontal horns, an area of hypoechogenicity (*arrows*), presumably acute hemorrhage, lies within the larger echogenic zone. **C:** CT image shows hemorrhage (*large arrows*) adjacent to the left frontal horn with abnormally hypodense tissue (presumably infarcted) surrounding it. An area of germinal zone hemorrhage (*small arrow*) is present in the contralateral hemisphere. **D:** Different patient who suffered a grade IV hemorrhage in the past. A large cavity (*arrows*) is present at the site of the hemorrhage.

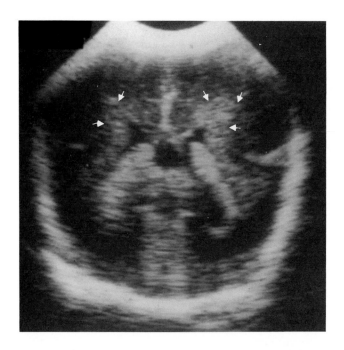

FIG. 4.18. Periventricular hyperechogenicity (*arrows*) in a patient with no neurologic sequelae. This image emphasized that all periventricular hyperechogenicity is not periventricular leukomalacia.

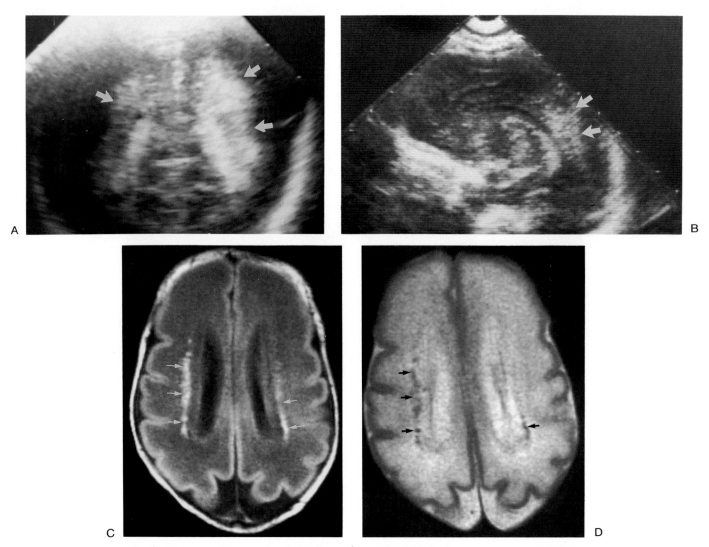

FIG. 4.19. Evolution of periventricular leukomalacia. **A, B:** Coronal and sagittal plane sonograms at 1 week of age show echogenicity (*arrows*) of the periventricular white matter equivalent to that in the choroid plexuses. **C, D:** T1- and T2-weighted MR images at age 3 weeks shows periventricular T1 and T2 shortening (*arrows*), presumably secondary to hemorrhagic necrosis.

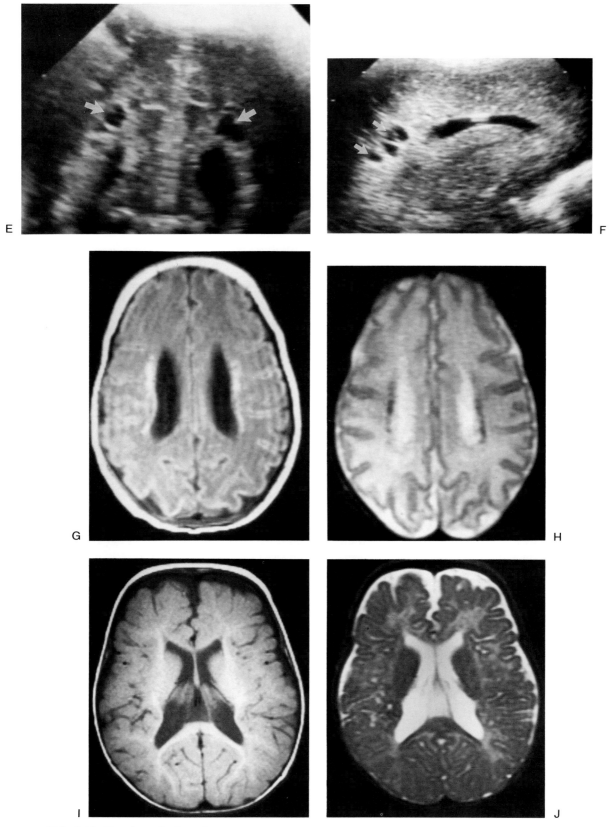

FIG. 4.19. (*Continued.*) **E, F:** Coronal and sagittal sonograms at age 6 weeks shows cavitation (*arrows*) in the hyperechogenic regions of the periventricular white matter. **G, H:** T1- and T2-weighted MR images at age 8 weeks show loss of periventricular white matter. Note that the periventricular T1 and T2 prolongation is closer to the ventricular surface than in (C) and (D). **I, J:** T1- and T2-weighted images at age 7 months show end stage periventricular leukomalacia. The ventricles show irregular enlargement, the cerebral hemispheric white matter is diminished in volume, and the cortex nearly abuts on the ventricular surface.

TABLE 4.1. *Causes of fetal brain perfusion failure*

Maternal Origin
  Maternal shock
  Maternal hypoxia
  Maternal thrombophlebitis
  Maternal abdominal trauma
  Maternal hypo/hypertension
  Fetomaternal transfusion
Fetal Origin
  Fetal infection (arteritis, hypotension)
  Hydrops fetalis
  Fetal embolism (placenta, other)
  Fetofetal transfusion
Placental Origin
  Premature placental separation
  Excessive placental infarction

at the trigones but in severe cases involving the whole centrum ovale; and (3) deep, prominent sulci that abut or nearly abut the ventricles with little or no interposed white matter (52). *MR scans* show these same abnormalities and, in addition, show abnormally increased signal intensity in the periventricular white matter on long TR sequences, most commonly observed in the peritrigonal regions bilaterally (37,53,77) (Fig. 4.20), and delayed myelination (37). The midline, sagittal MR image will often show thinning of the corpus callosum, most commonly the posterior body and splenium, resulting from degeneration of transcallosal fibers (Fig. 4.20).

PVL may look quite similar to the normal areas of slow myelination dorsal and superior to the trigones (see Chapter 2 and Fig. 4.21). The normal regions of unmyelinated white matter, however, will be separated from the ventricular wall by a thin band of normally myelinated white matter in the splenium of the corpus callosum and tapetum, whereas the abnormal signal attributable to PVL directly abuts the ventricular wall. The differentiation is best seen on coronal, long TR sequences; axial views may not depict this finding (77). Moreover, loss of volume of the cerebral white matter is not present on normal scans, as it is in PVL (78), and the ventricular contour in normal patients is smooth, not irregular.

One final comment should be made regarding periventricular leukomalacia. *A finding of periventricular hyperintensity on long TR magnetic resonance images is not specific for hypoxic–ischemic tissue damage in the premature infant.* In fact, periventricular tissue damage can be caused by many different disorders, such as ventriculitis (a common sequelae of meningitis in infants; see Chapter 11), metabolic disorders (see Chapter 3), hydrocephalus (see Chapter 8), and *in utero* events (79,80).

Profound Hypotension or Circulatory Arrest in Premature Infants

A different pattern of brain injury is seen in premature infants who have suffered profound hypotension or cir-

culatory arrest. In these infants, injury is predominantly in the deep gray matter nuclei and brain stem nuclei (Fig. 4.22), although the periventricular white matter may be involved as well (1,38,81). The brain stem and thalami are predominantly injured in the first half of the third trimester, but by the middle of the third trimester, the lentiform nuclei are usually injured as well. The exact reasons for this different pattern are unknown. Most likely, the periventricular pattern seen in hypoxia/ischemia reflects impaired autoregulation whereas the deep gray matter injury in circulatory arrest/anoxia reflects relatively increased metabolic activity in the affected structures compared with the remainder of the brain (related to myelination) or the distribution of N-methyl-D-aspartate receptors (34,44,45). Positron emission tomography studies show that the brain stem and ventrolateral thalami show significant metabolic activity by the beginning of the third trimester, whereas the lentiform nuclei and perirolandic cerebral cortex become more active around the middle of the third trimester (44).

An important concept is that both hypoxia/ischemia and anoxia/arrest can occur *in utero* (Table 4.1). The pattern of brain damage seen in infants who have suffered *in utero* injury is, by imaging criteria, identical to that seen in postnatal infants of the same gestational age (37).

Injury in Term Infants

The problem of perinatal asphyxia in term infants is extremely important for both patient care and medical/legal reasons. It has been estimated that severe asphyxia occurs in between 1 in 100 and 1 in 500 live births (9). Moreover, between 20% and 30% of survivors have some long-term neurologic sequelae. It is therefore important to understand both the pathophysiology of the brain damage in these situations and the pathologic sequelae.

Hypoxia/Ischemia

As discussed in the previous section, the region of the brain that is most susceptible to hypoxic/ischemic damage, resulting primarily from impaired autoregulation, changes as the infant matures. In term infants, the vascular boundary zones ("watershed areas") lie in the regions between the anterior and middle cerebral arteries and between the middle and posterior cerebral arteries. This distribution of tenuous arterial supply has been termed *parasagittal* (Fig. 4.23). Another change that has occurred in the infant brain since the sixth and seventh month of gestation has been the ability of the brain to mount a glial response to injury. The brain of the second-trimester fetus responds to trauma by liquefaction and resorption of the damaged tissue without accompanying gliosis; the more mature brain of the term infant re-

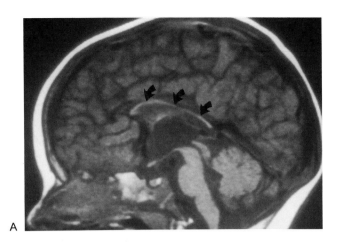

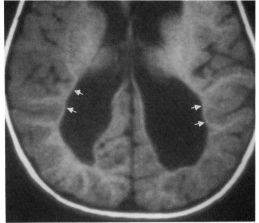

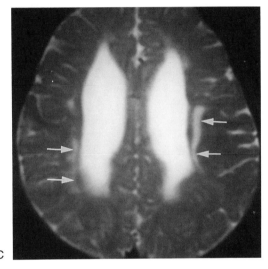

FIG. 4.20. End stage periventricular leukomalacia. A: Sagittal SE 550/16 image shows marked callosal thinning (arrows). B: Axial SE 600/20 image shows enlarged ventricles with irregular ventricular margin (arrows). The cerebral cortex nearly abuts the ventricular surface because of the diminished volume of cerebral white matter. C: Axial SE 3000/120 image shows periventricular T2 prolongation (arrows) in addition to the features of end stage PVL shown in B.

sponds by reactive astrocytosis, more loosely termed *gliosis* (2,5,82).

Pathologically, most asphyxic events in term infants are the result of prolonged hypoxia and result in discrete, often cystic, infarctions in the boundary zones between the major vascular territories. The ischemic lesions are most obvious in the frontal and parieto-occipital regions of the brain. Both the cortex and white matter are usually involved. The parasagittal areas of the brain are difficult to evaluate with sonography because they lie close to the inner table of the skull and angling the transducer to visualize these regions can be difficult. These susceptible areas are also difficult to evaluate with CT in the acute phase because the frontal and parieto-occipital white matter is usually of low attenuation with respect to the remaining brain in the newborn (see Chapter 2) and the cortex may be partially obscured by beam-hardening artifacts from the overlying calvarium. As a result, CT often shows nonspecific edema that may, or may not, evolve into damaged brain (65). Evaluation with MR is, therefore, optimal. Heavily T2-weighted spin echo images or inversion recovery/spoiled gradient echo T1-

weighted sequences are preferred for detecting brain injury in the acute phase (see Chapter 1 for rationale). Edematous brain will appear as areas of low signal intensity in the cortex and subjacent white matter on T1-weighted images when compared with normal white matter (83,84). The white matter edema is more apparent on T1-weighted images than on T2-weighted images because it contrasts with the high signal intensity caused by myelination (myelination changes occur earlier on T1-weighted images than on T2-weighted images; see Chapter 2). In the author's experience, however, heavily T2-weighted images (Fig. 4.24) show the cortical edema better than T1-weighted images, although injury to the underlying white matter is difficult to identify because the high signal intensity of normal white matter is very similar to the high signal of the damaged tissue. The multiplanar imaging capacity of MR also aids detection of ischemic brain damage; the coronal and sagittal planes are best for these high-convexity lesions.

In the subacute phase (several days to weeks after injury), the MR appearance of the injured brain changes; the injured gray matter shows T1 and T2 shortening that

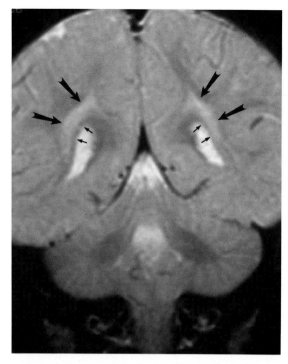

FIG. 4.21. Normal immature periventricular white matter. T2 prolongation in the periventricular white matter (*large arrows*) is not accompanied by any loss of white matter volume. A stripe of normally myelinated white matter (*small arrows*) is present in the immediate periventricular region.

suggests hemorrhage (Figs. 4.9, 4.11) (31). Deeper portions of the cortex are more severely affected than superficial portions. The signal abnormality lasts for weeks to months, as the injured regions of brain undergo progressive atrophy. Changes in gray matter attenuation on CT corresponding to the T1 and T2 shortening on MR are rarely seen.

In the chronic phase, cortical thinning and diminution of the underlying white matter are seen in the parasagittal vascular boundary zones (Figs. 4.24, 4.25). *Ex vacuo* dilatation of the adjacent lateral ventricles can be seen, particularly in the trigones and occipital horns. The parasagittal white matter shows abnormal prolongation of T2 relaxation time, although the abnormal signal intensity of the white matter may not be apparent until T2 shortening, secondary to myelination, has become apparent (85).

A correlation has been shown between the severity of the cortical damage and the severity of the subsequent spastic paresis of the patient (31). The shrunken cortex has a peculiar pattern in which the deep portions of the gyri are more shrunken than the superficial portions, creating mushroom-shaped gyri known as *ulegyria* (1). These peculiarly shaped gyri form because of the unique vascular supply to the gyri in the infant brain. Takashima and Tanaka (86) have shown that, in the newborn, there is greater perfusion to the apices of the gyri than to

the cortex at the depths of sulci. Therefore, when a hypoxic event occurs, the tissue loss is greater in the depths of the sulci, resulting in the characteristic gyral shape (Fig. 4.26). Ulegyria can be identified by MR because of the characteristic gyral pattern and the underlying tissue loss and gliosis (Fig. 4.27). Probably the most important reason to identify this entity is to differentiate it from polymicrogyria, which is an anomaly of neuronal organization and is seen in a number of inherited syndromes. Polymicrogyria (see Chapter 5) appears on MR as an area of thickened and, often, paradoxically smooth cortex. It is not associated with perinatal asphyxia.

Anoxia/Arrest

A different pattern of brain injury is seen in neonates who have suffered profound hypotension or cardiocirculatory arrest, as compared to mild or moderate hypoxia/hypotension (1,34,38,81,87). This group of patients shows injury primarily in the lateral thalami, lentiform nuclei, hippocampi, and corticospinal tracts on MR studies (34). These locations correspond to those regions of brain most metabolically active at the time of birth (44). Some patients will, in addition, show injury in the lateral geniculate nucleus and optic radiations. The cortex is relatively spared, other than the perirolandic gyri. The most severely injured patients in this group have injury to brain stem nuclei; the majority of these brain stem–injured patients probably die and are represented more in pathology reports (1,38,81,87) than in radiology publications.

Patients with the profound asphyxia pattern appear to have different neurologic deficits from those with the moderate hypoxia/hypotension pattern. In contradistinction to the proximal extremity weakness and spasticity seen in patients with "watershed" injuries, patients with the profound asphyxia pattern tend to present with athetosis in addition to long tract signs and symptoms, severe seizure disorders, and mental retardation (88–90). These patients are described in the pathologic literature as having thalamo-putaminal type of athetoid cerebral palsy (88). On pathologic studies, the patients are found to have moderate to severe destruction in the hippocampi, putamina, central gray matter of the midbrain, and ventrolateral nuclei of the thalami (88). Positron emission tomographic studies of patients with athetoid cerebral palsy show normal cortical activity, but diminished metabolism in the thalami and lentiform nuclei (89), consistent with the MR and pathology results.

In the first 2–3 days after anoxia/arrest injuries, ultrasound may show hyperechogenicity in the thalami, globi palladi, putamina, and periventricular white matter (Fig. 4.28). This hyperechogenicity can easily be overlooked if the sonographer is not actively searching for it (91). CT shows hypoattenuation of the thalami and basal ganglia

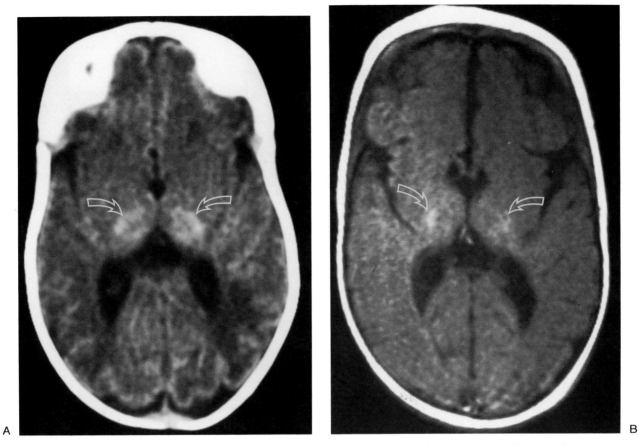

A   B

FIG. 4.22. Profound asphyxia in a 28-week premature infant. **A:** Axial CT image at age 3 weeks shows bilateral thalamic high attenuation (*arrows*), indicating hemorrhage or calcification. **B:** Axial SE 600/15 image at age 2 months shows abnormal blotchy hyperintensity in the lateral thalami (*arrows*).

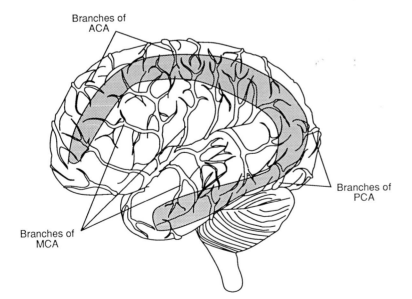

Branches of
ACA

Branches of
PCA

Branches of
MCA

FIG. 4.23. Diagram illustrating the parasagittal boundary zone, or "watershed" zone between the major cerebral artery distributions in term infants. This zone is the primary location of ischemic injury in prolonged partial asphyxia.

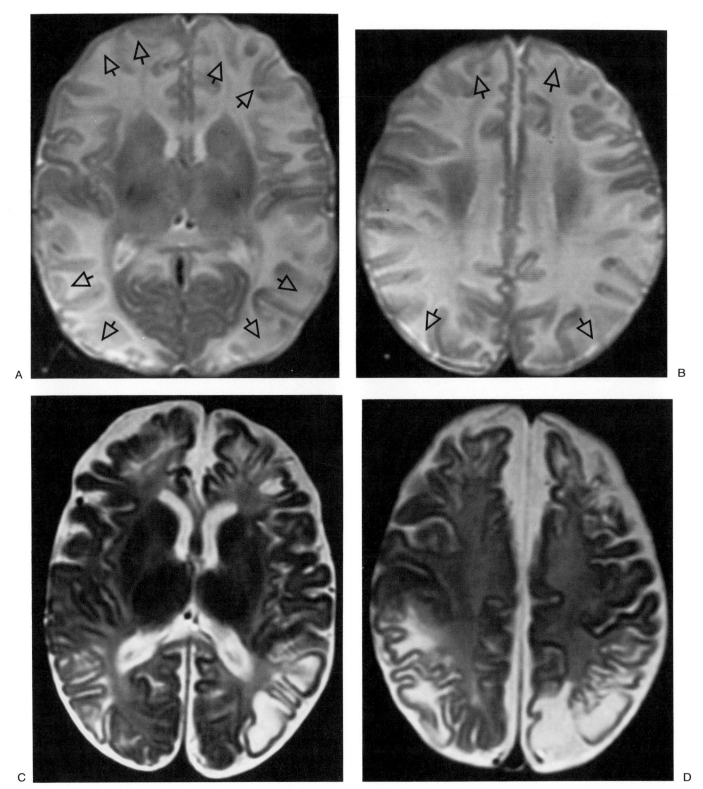

FIG. 4.24. Prolonged partial asphyxia, acute and subacute phases. **A, B:** Axial SE 3000/120 images obtained at age 2 days. The cerebral cortex in the vascular boundary zones (*arrows*) shows abnormally high signal intensity, indicating edema. **C, D:** Axial SE 3000/120 images at age 1 month show significant tissue loss at the areas of injury.

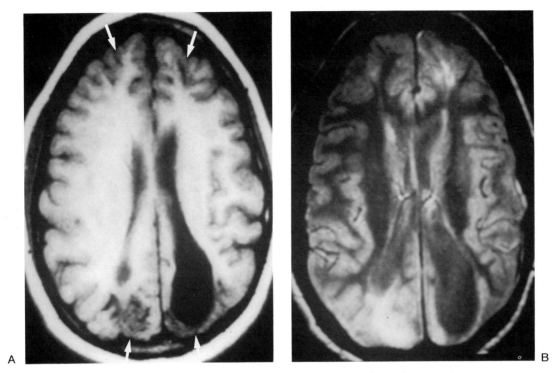

FIG. 4.25. Prolonged partial asphyxia, chronic phase. **A:** Axial SE 600/20 image shows *ex vacuo* enlargement of the lateral ventricles. The cerebral cortex is shrunken (*arrows*) and the volume of white matter diminished in the vascular boundary zones. **B:** Axial SE 2500/30 image shows that the white matter in the boundary zones is abnormally hyperintense.

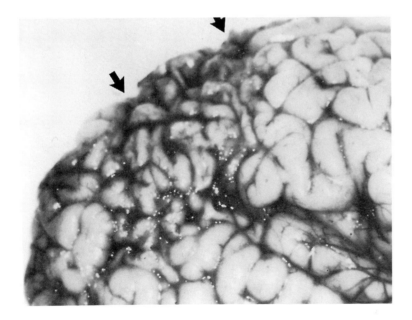

FIG. 4.26. Ulegyria. Anatomic specimen shows the typical appearance of enlarged sulci surrounding somewhat shrunken, mushroom-shaped gyri (*arrows*). The gyral shape results from the relatively greater perfusion to the apices of the gyri as compared to the depth of the sulci.

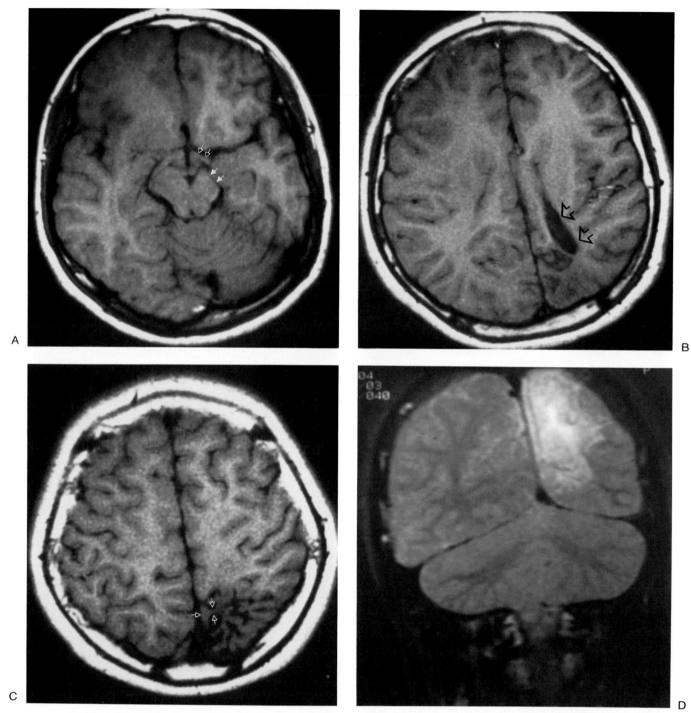

FIG. 4.27. Ulegyria. **A, B:** Axial SE 600/20 images show a small left cerebral peduncle (*solid white arrows*), optic tract (*open white arrows*), and an enlarged left ventricle (*open black arrows*), all secondary to ischemic injury. **C:** Axial SE 600/20 image shows marked loss of cortical and subcortical tissue in the left parieto-occipital region. More tissue is lost from the depth than from the apices of the cortex; this pattern of ulegyria is particularly apparent in the gyrus marked by the *open arrows*. **D:** Coronal SE 2500/70 image shows abnormal hyperintensity in the parieto-occipital region, reflecting tissue damage.

(Fig. 4.28), which can be easily missed, as these gray matter structures become isodense with surrounding white matter (34). The abnormal MR findings are also very subtle in the acute phase, showing symmetric absence of the normal high signal in the posterior limb of the internal capsule on T1-weighted images and patchy or diffuse high signal in the lateral thalami, globi palladi, and posterior putamina (Fig. 4.29) and in deep areas of the cerebral cortex, particularly in the perirolandic area. T2-weighted images may be normal or show patchy high signal in the thalami and putamina.

By 7–10 days after the injury, ultrasound shows better definition of the hyperechogenic areas and some increase in ventricular size as the edema resolves. CT scans may begin to show high signal, probably representing hemorrhage, in the affected gray matter nuclei (34,39). On MR, heterogeneous high signal is seen in the affected struc-tures on T1-weighted images and heterogeneous high and low signal is seen on the T2-weighted images (Fig. 4.28). The extent of injury is variable, being limited to the hippocampi, lateral thalami, and posterior putamina in the least severely injured patients, involving all the deep cerebral nuclei and central mesencephalon in more severely injured patients and involving much of the cerebral cortex, all the deep cerebral nuclei, and many brain stem nuclei in the most severely injured patients (31,34). The extent of involvement is most likely related to the duration of the anoxia/arrest incident. The short T1 and T2 relaxation times slowly fade (Fig. 4.30) as atrophy of the injured tissues develops over the subsequent 6–10 weeks.

In the chronic phase of the injury, the affected areas of brain are shrunken and show T2 prolongation compared to normal brain tissue (Fig. 4.31). The T2 prolongation

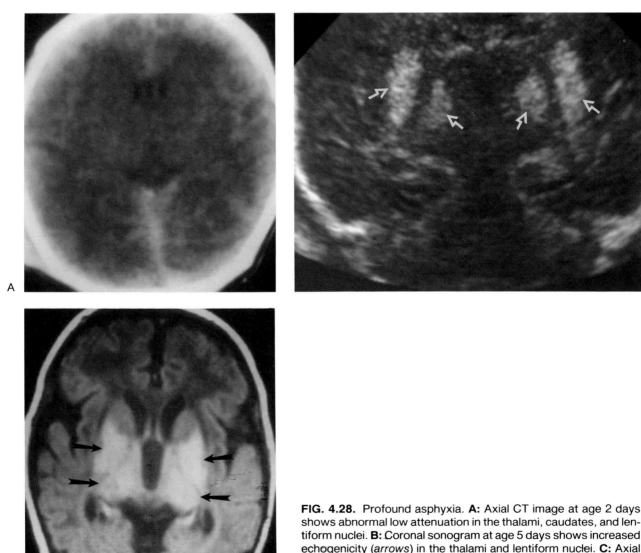

FIG. 4.28. Profound asphyxia. **A:** Axial CT image at age 2 days shows abnormal low attenuation in the thalami, caudates, and lentiform nuclei. **B:** Coronal sonogram at age 5 days shows increased echogenicity (*arrows*) in the thalami and lentiform nuclei. **C:** Axial SE 600/20 image at age 20 days shows marked abnormal hyperintensity (*arrows*) in the thalami and lentiform nuclei bilaterally. (This figure reprinted with permission from ref. 34.)

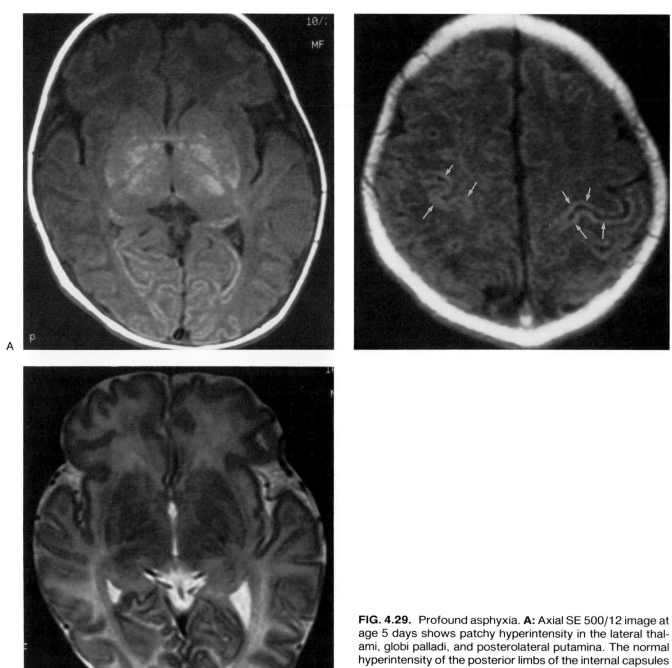

FIG. 4.29. Profound asphyxia. **A:** Axial SE 500/12 image at age 5 days shows patchy hyperintensity in the lateral thalami, globi palladi, and posterolateral putamina. The normal hyperintensity of the posterior limbs of the internal capsules is missing. **B:** Axial SE 500/12 image at the level of the fronto-parietal convexity shows abnormal hyperintensity (*arrows*) at the depth of the central sulcus. **C:** Axial SE 3000/120 image is normal.

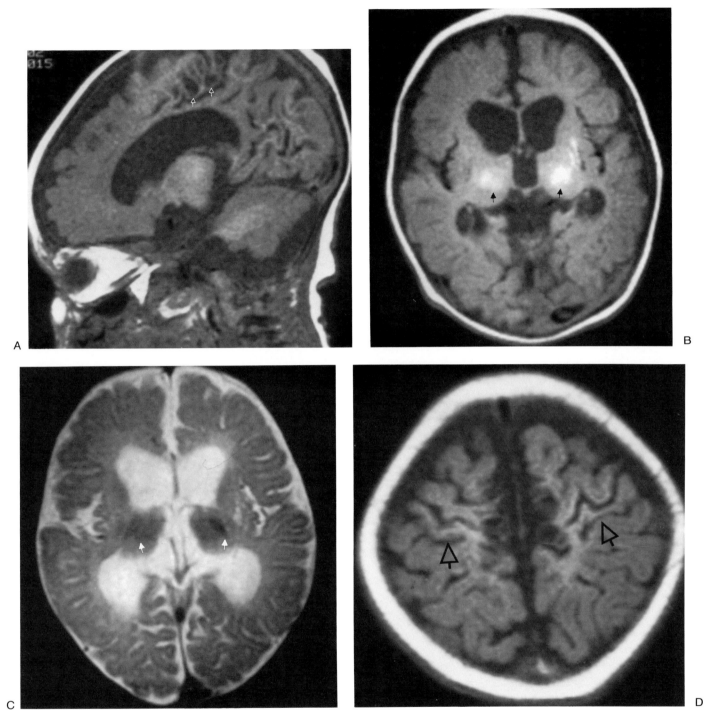

FIG. 4.30. Profound asphyxia, subacute phase. **A:** Sagittal SE 600/20 image shows thinning of cortex (*arrows*) in the region of the central sulcus. **B:** Axial SE 600/20 image shows ventriculomegaly, diminished size of the basal ganglia, and blotchy hyperintensity in the thalami (*arrows*). **C:** Axial SE 3000/120 at the same level as (B) shows that hypointensity is present in the same location as the hyperintensity on the T1-weighted image (*arrow*). This region likely represents calcium or myelin breakdown products. **D:** Axial SE 600/20 image at the frontoparietal convexity shows shrunken gyri (*arrows*) in the perirolandic region.

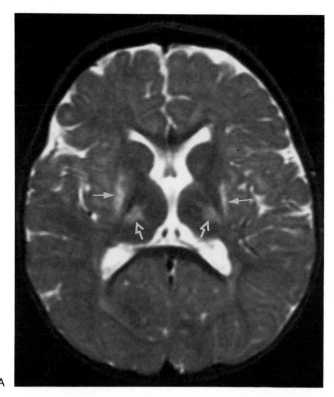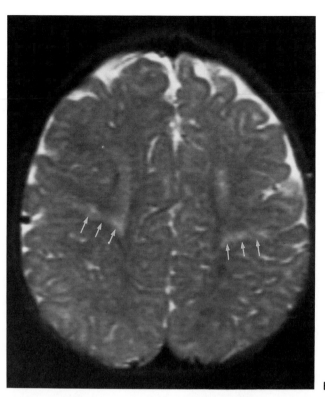

A   B

FIG. 4.31. Profound asphyxia, chronic phase. **A:** Axial SE 2800/70 image shows small basal ganglia and hyperintensity in the thalami (*open arrows*) and putamina (*solid arrows*). **B:** Image at the level of the frontoparietal convexity shows abnormal hyperintensity (*arrows*) along the perirolandic gyri. (This figure reprinted with permission from ref. 34.)

may not become evident in the cerebral white matter, however, until myelination is well under way. It may be seen at ages as young as 8 months (85) or not until 13–14 months, depending on the degree of associated myelination delay. MR is much more sensitive than CT to the damage in the deep cerebral nuclei and corticospinal tracts (34,92) and to the myelination delay that almost invariably accompanies asphyxic brain injury (37,93).

Parenchymal and Intraventricular Hemorrhage in the Term Infant

In contrast to premature infants, in whom germinal matrix hemorrhage fairly commonly extends into the lateral ventricles, intraventricular hemorrhage is uncommon in term infants. Documented sources of intraventricular hemorrhage in this age group include the choroid plexus, residual germinal matrix, vascular malformation, tumor, extension of hemorrhagic cerebral infarction, coagulopathy, and extension of thalamic hemorrhage (9,94,95). *Venous thrombosis* is the most common cause of thalamic [straight sinus thrombosis (Fig. 4.32)], choroid plexus (straight sinus thrombosis), parasagittal (superior sagittal sinus thrombosis), and temporal lobe [vein of Labbé, transverse sinus, or sigmoid sinus thrombosis (Fig. 4.32)] hemorrhage in these

patients. The two most important reasons for differentiating the various sources are that (1) choroid plexus and thalamic hemorrhages are most commonly seen in stressed infants and (2) patients with thalamic hemorrhages have a high incidence of neurologic sequelae, such as spastic paraparesis, hydrocephalus, and seizures (95). The imaging appearance of intraventricular blood was described in the section on premature infants.

Ischemic Injury in Older Children

When hypoxia, ischemia, or circulatory arrest occurs in older children (e.g., after drowning), CT is the initial imaging modality of choice, as the unstable child is easily monitored within the CT scanner. Initial CT images (less than 24 hours) will show subtle hypoattenuation of the basal ganglia and insular cortex; sometimes the cisterns around the midbrain are effaced. Later scans (24–72 hours) will show diffuse cerebral edema, with decreased gray matter–white matter differentiation, effacement of sulci and cisterns, and decreased attenuation of the basal ganglia and cortex (Fig. 4.33) (96,97). Hemorrhage may become apparent in the basal ganglia or cortex by 4–6 days after the injury. An ominous finding is the so-called reversal sign, in which the cerebral hemispheric white matter becomes hyperdense compared to cortex (Fig.

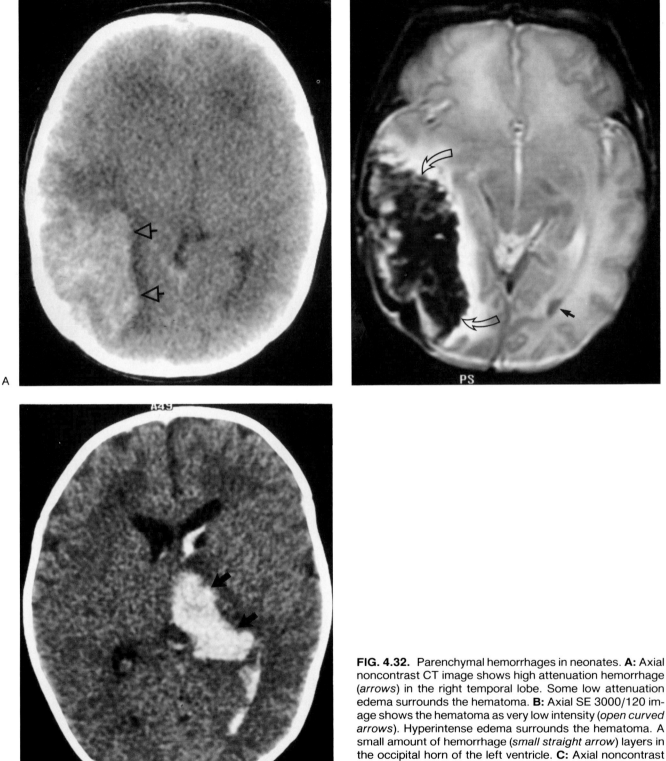

FIG. 4.32. Parenchymal hemorrhages in neonates. **A:** Axial noncontrast CT image shows high attenuation hemorrhage (*arrows*) in the right temporal lobe. Some low attenuation edema surrounds the hematoma. **B:** Axial SE 3000/120 image shows the hematoma as very low intensity (*open curved arrows*). Hyperintense edema surrounds the hematoma. A small amount of hemorrhage (*small straight arrow*) layers in the occipital horn of the left ventricle. **C:** Axial noncontrast CT in a different patient shows left thalamic hemorrhage (*arrows*) with intraventricular extension. Straight sinus occlusion was present.

4.34) (98,99). The reversal sign is believed to result from an accumulation of venous and capillary blood in the white matter; the blood accumulates because venous drainage is impaired by the increased intracranial pressure. The prognosis of children with this sign is dismal (98,99). MR findings of asphyxic injury are very subtle in the first 24–72 hours, consisting of subtle T1 and T2 prolongation in the basal ganglia and insular cortex. An early finding that may be very helpful is the appearance of a curvilinear stripe of T2 prolongation (Figs. 4.10, 4.35) at the cortical–white matter junction, which corresponds to blurring of the cortical-white matter junction on T1-weighted images (Fig. 4.10). This sign, which may represent cortical laminar necrosis, indicates significant cortical damage.

The pattern of brain injury from hypoxic–ischemic injury in children after the neonatal period differs from that seen in neonates. The reasons for this change are not entirely clear, but almost certainly are related to the physiologic and biochemical changes that occur in the brain with maturation; these lead to different patterns in metabolic activity at different ages in the maturing brain (44). In injury from partial hypoxia/ischemia, the differences from the pattern of injury seen in neonates is minor, with some sparing of the immediate periventricular white matter (Fig. 4.36) (37). In profound asphyxia, the difference in injury pattern is more significant. Older

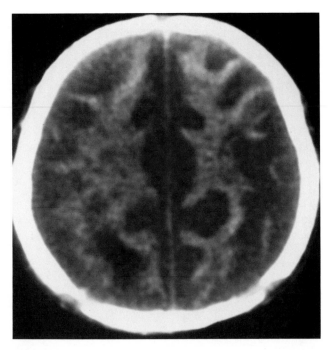

FIG. 4.34. Reversal sign. CT image shows the cerebral white matter is hyperdense compared to the gray matter of the cerebral cortex.

infants and children show involvement of the basal ganglia, with relative sparing of the thalami, and significant cortical involvement with relative sparing of the perirolandic regions (Fig. 4.36) (34). In chronic stages, profound atrophy of the entire cerebrum may be seen (Fig. 4.35).

Ischemia Secondary to Venous Occlusion

Venous sinus thrombosis and venous infarction are discussed in Chapter 11, in the section on complications of meningitis.

Timing of Scans

The subject of optimal timing of scans after asphyxic injury warrants special mention. In the acute phase (24–72 hours) after asphyxia, the brain becomes extremely edematous. CT in the acute phase therefore shows diffuse low signal intensity throughout the cerebral hemispheres, and ultrasound shows diffuse hyperechogenicity; both show diminished ventricular and sulcal size. In this acute phase, it cannot be determined whether brain damage and neurologic sequelae will be severe or minimal unless other associated features, such as focal hemorrhages, are present. Although it is tempting to obtain a follow-up CT at age 1 week in order to see if any brain damage is apparent, *1 week is the worst possible time at which to obtain a follow-up study.* The edema will have

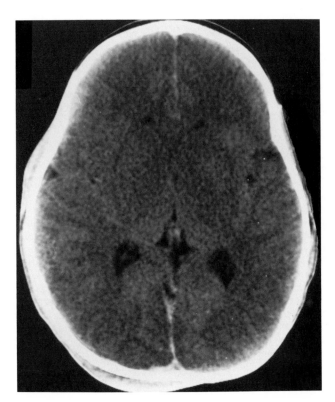

FIG. 4.33. Acute asphyxia. CT image obtained 36 hours after injury shows edema with low attenuation in the basal ganglia and cerebral cortex.

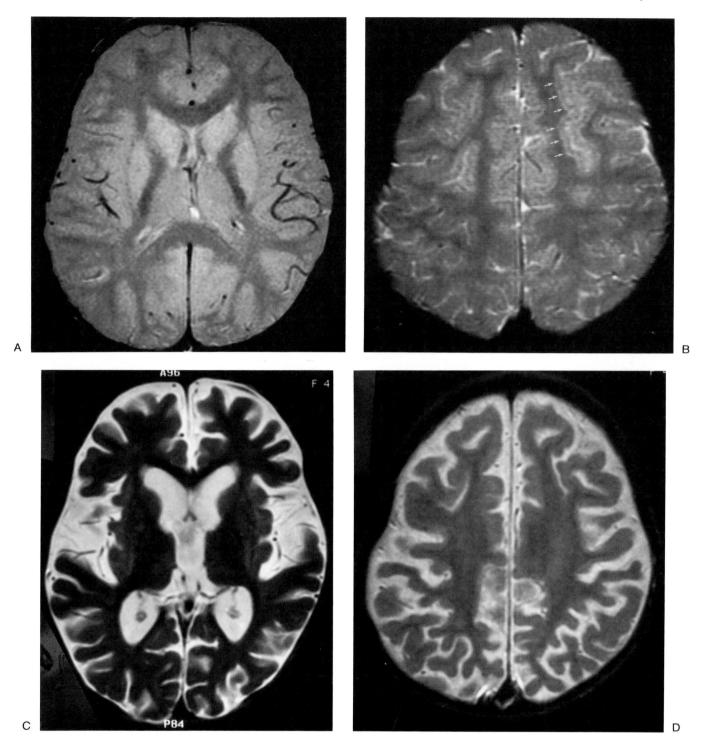

FIG. 4.35. Profound asphyxia in a 2-year-old. Acute and chronic phases. **A:** Axial SE 2500/30 image shows hyperintensity of the putamina and caudates compared with the thalami. The cortex–white matter junction is indistinct. **B:** Axial SE 2500/70 image shows a stripe of hyperintensity (*arrows*) between the cortex and underlying white matter. This can be a useful sign in evaluating asphyxiated children in the first few days after injury. **C, D:** Follow-up images at age 3 years. Marked diffuse atrophy of the cerebrum is present.

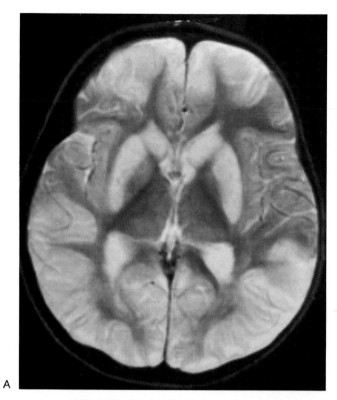
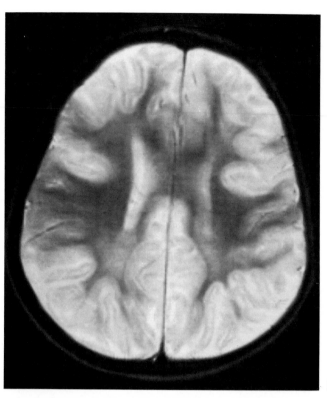

A

B

FIG. 4.36. Profound asphyxia in a 3-year-old. Subacute phase. **A, B:** Axial SE 2500/80 image shows abnormal T2 prolongation in the caudate nuclei, putamina, and cerebral cortex. The cortical involvement spares the perirolandic and perisylvian regions, a characteristic distribution in patients beyond infancy.

resolved, but significant tissue loss will not yet be apparent; therefore, *a follow-up CT at 1 week may look normal, even if significant damage has occurred.* If interpreted as normal, the clinician and parents may be led to believe falsely that the infant has suffered no significant brain damage. Therefore, follow-up scans should be obtained a minimum of 2 weeks after the injury. The repeat scan (preferably an MR, which is considerably more sensitive to detection of damage) in 14 days will show a return to near normal in those patients who will have relatively mild deficits, whereas cystic or hemorrhagic parenchymal degeneration and progressive atrophy indicate a more guarded prognosis. An imaging study at age 3 months will show the full extent of brain injury.

NEONATAL HYPOGLYCEMIA

Neonatal hypoglycemia is probably underrecognized, since common symptoms, such as stupor, jitteriness, and seizures, may be lacking or inconspicuous in many affected neonates; thus, hypoglycemia may remain undetected until seizures develop (100). The definition of hypoglycemia in infants varies with the maturational state of the infant, as less mature infants tolerate lower glucose levels than more mature ones and mature infants

tolerate lower levels than older children and adults. The most widely accepted level defining significant hypoglycemia in the newborn is a whole blood glucose concentration of less than 30 mg/dl in term infants and of less than 20 mg/dl in preterm infants (101,102). Up to 8% of low-risk infants suffer an episode of hypoglycemia using these criteria, typically at 3–4 hours after delivery (103). Reasons for tolerance of low glucose levels by infants include (1) the ability of the newborn brain cells to utilize lactate as an energy source (104,105); (2) low energy requirements of the immature neurons resulting from the low level of neuronal activity (100); and (3) the relatively minor effect of hypoglycemia upon cardiovascular function of the newborn (106).

Imaging studies of patients who have suffered damage from perinatal hypoglycemia reflect the pathologic findings of diffuse brain damage, with the most severe injury localized primarily to the parietal and occipital cortex of the brain (107,108). In the acute phase, edema of the cerebral cortex and underlying white matter is seen (Fig. 4.37). MR shows short T1 and T2 in the cortex in the subacute phase, presumably from petechial hemorrhage. In the chronic phase (Fig. 4.37), the cortex and underlying cerebral white matter become shrunken and atrophic.

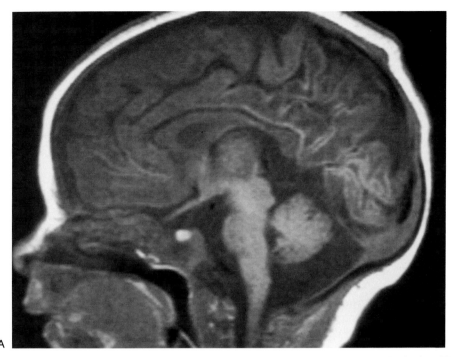

FIG. 4.37. Neonatal hypoglycemia. **A:** Sagittal SE 600/15 image shows abnormal high signal intensity in the cerebral cortex, primarily in the parietal and occipital lobes. (See **B** and **C** on next page.)

BILIRUBIN ENCEPHALOPATHY (KERNICTERUS)

Although the relationship between serum levels of unconjugated bilirubin and brain damage is complicated (109), it is generally accepted that sustained or pronounced neonatal hyperbilirubinemia results in brain damage (109,110). Hyperbilirubinemia may be the result of a number of predisposing factors. Red blood cell hemolysis (secondary to blood group incompatibility, intrinsic defects of the red cell membrane or of hemoglobin, or degradation blood from hematoma formation) is the most common cause. Other causes include polycythemia, inherited or acquired defects of bilirubin conjugation, disorders of gastrointestinal transit, and hormonal disturbances (109,110).

Neonates with bilirubin encephalopathy manifest stupor and hypotonia in the first few days of life; seizures occur in a minority of affected patients. By the middle of the first week, hypertonia, with backward arching of the neck or back, develops. Delayed development becomes apparent during the first postnatal year. Eventually, usually after the age of 1 year, extrapyramidal signs (especially athetosis), abnormalities of vertical and horizontal gaze, and hearing deficits develop (109,111,112).

Pathologic studies of children with chronic bilirubin encephalopathy have demonstrated damage to the globus pallidus, subthalamic nucleus, and the CA2 and CA3 regions of the hippocampus (1,88). On MR, T2 prolongation in the globi pallidi (Fig. 4.38) is the only significant abnormality.

SPECIAL MR STUDIES IN PERINATAL INJURY

A few special MR techniques may be useful in the assessment of neonatal asphyxic brain damage. *MR spectroscopy* using ^{31}P seems to be useful in the acute postinjury phase (113–117). Asphyxiated newborns tend to have lower phosphocreatine/inorganic phosphate (PCr/P$_i$) ratios and lower ATP/total phosphorus ratios than normal patients. Patients with PCr/P$_i$ ratios of less than 0.4 during the first week of life have a very poor prognosis (personal communication, Dr. E. O. R. Reynolds, London). Intracranial acidosis is shown by a shift of the inorganic phosphate peak to the right. Spectra are typically normal on the day of birth and reach minimum PCr/P$_i$ values on day 3 of life.

Proton MRS has also been found to be useful in the subacute and chronic phases (113,114,118,119). The *N*-acetylaspartate (NAA)/choline and NAA/lactate ratios seem to have the greatest predictive value in terms of prognosis. Van der Grond and colleagues (119) have reported that patients with severe asphyxia have NAA/choline values of less than 0.7 and NAA/lactate values less than 2.0. Patients with moderate asphyxia have NAA/choline ratios of 0.7 to 1.0, with absent lactate. Patients who had no neurologic abnormalities and, on imaging studies, no brain damage had NAA/choline values of more than 1 in the first week of life and no lactate.

MR angiography can be useful in the evaluation of infants who have suffered an acute neurologic deficit and have an MR imaging study suggestive of cerebral in-

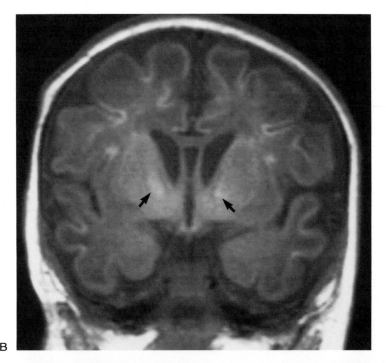

B

C

FIG. 4.37. (*Continued.*) **B:** Coronal SE 600/15 image shows cortical hyperintensity at the depths of the gyri and hyperintensity of the globi palladi (*arrows*). **C:** Follow-up scan 3 weeks after injury shows marked atrophy (*arrows*) in the parietal and occipital cortex.

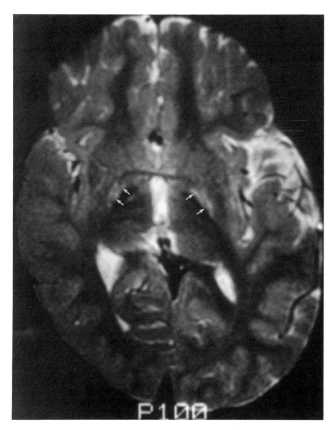

FIG. 4.38. Kernicterus. Axial SE 2800/70 image shows abnormal hyperintensity (*arrows*) of the globi pallidi bilaterally.

farction. Three-dimensional time of flight MRA can detect large thrombi and emboli, as well as vaso-occlusive disease (23,24,26), whereas two-dimensional time of flight MRV can diagnose venous occlusions (120,121). As discussed previously, however, MRA is not sensitive to abnormalities of the medium- and small-caliber vessel; therefore, *a normal MRA should not preclude catheter angiography.*

TRAUMA IN INFANCY AND CHILDHOOD

Pediatric trauma can be divided into two distinct groups. *Birth trauma* is composed of those injuries that occur during and as a result of the birth process. This form of trauma is unique in its pathologic and radiographic manifestations because of the immaturity of the CNS and of the surrounding calvarium and spinal canal. Birth trauma will therefore be dealt with in some detail in this section. Trauma that occurs later in life (*postnatal trauma*) results in a pathologic and radiologic picture that is similar to that in the adult. Since most neuropathology and neuroimaging textbooks discuss the adult type of trauma, only those aspects unique to children,

such as nonaccidental trauma, will be discussed in detail. Birth asphyxia is sometimes considered a form of birth trauma. However, as hypoxic–ischemic injury was discussed earlier in this chapter, its discussion will not be duplicated here.

Birth Trauma

CT and ultrasound are the imaging modalities of choice for the evaluation of birth trauma. (CT is the best for postnatal trauma in the immediate postinjury period). CT and sonography are preferred because the scans can be obtained in a rapid fashion and the patient can be closely monitored during the exam. More important, air and acute blood are easily detected on CT scans. Oxyhemoglobin, the hemoglobin form seen in hyperacute hemorrhage, is difficult to detect by MR. This is particularly true in the subarachnoid space, as the signal intensity of oxyhemoglobin is very close to that of cerebrospinal fluid. The signal void of air is difficult to differentiate from the signal void of cortical bone; because air often lies adjacent to bone, it can be extremely difficult to detect. CT also demonstrates cerebral edema, infarction, and hydrocephalus. In the acute phase, the patient should be scanned with 5-mm slice thickness without the use of IV contrast; at this stage, the major goal is to rule out large, space-occupying hematomas. Acute interhemispheric and posterior fossa subdural hematomas are seen on transfontanel sonography as mildly echogenic fluid collections, and on CT as hyperdense, extra-axial collections. Convexity subdural hematomas are sometimes difficult to see on sonography because of the difficulty in angling the transducer adequately. Cerebral edema and infarcts appear as areas of increased echogenicity in the hemispheric white matter on sonography and as areas of hypoattenuation on CT.

After the patient has stabilized, magnetic resonance is the preferred imaging modality for assessing the full extent of damage to the brain. MR has been proven to be more sensitive than CT in the detection of small extra-axial fluid collections and white matter shearing injuries (122–125). Brain stem injuries, which have important prognostic significance, are more sensitively detected by MR (126). Moreover, MR is extremely sensitive to the presence of hemosiderin from old hemorrhage (127); the presence of old CNS injuries in association with newer ones presents important evidence in the diagnosis of nonaccidental trauma. To detect hemorrhage with maximal sensitivity, gradient echo images should be obtained in all trauma or suspected trauma cases.

Spinal Cord Injury

Various anatomic differences increase the susceptibility of infants to spinal cord injury. The interspinous ligaments, posterior joint capsule, and cartilaginous end-plates are elastic and can be redundant, making the pediatric spine more deformable than the more rigid adult spine. Moreover, the planes of the facet joints are horizontally oriented (in contrast to the more vertically oriented adult facet joint), creating more mobility and less stability. Thus, infants are more susceptible to hyperextension injury, which is most common in the cervical region (128–132). Ligamentous laxity also makes the pediatric spinal cord more susceptible to distraction injuries, as the neonatal spinal column can be stretched 2 inches without structural disruption, whereas the spinal cord ruptures after being stretched 0.25 inch (133); as a result, the neonatal spinal cord may rupture but the spinal column may remain intact (134). Distraction injuries are most common in breech deliveries and tend to occur in the lower cervical and thoracic regions (Figs. 4.39, 4.40), although injury at any level is possible and the involvement of multiple levels is not uncommon (132,133, 135,136). Spinal cord injuries that have been attributed to birth injury include contusions, infarctions, lacerations, transections (Fig. 4.39), dural disruption (Fig. 4.40), and subdural and epidural hematomas (Fig. 4.41) (132,133,137).

The clinical presentation depends upon the level and extent of injury. Severe injuries at the craniovertebral junction cause death immediately. Incomplete injuries may allow survival. Mildly or moderately injured patients may have low Apgar scores, respiratory distress, or hypotonia. Prognosis is related to the severity and level of the injury; high cervical cord injuries carry the worst prognosis because of the effect on diaphragmatic motion and, consequently, ventilation (138). Differential diagnosis includes amyotonia congenita (Oppenheim's disease) or infantile spinal muscular atrophy (Werdnig-Hoffman disease).

When injury to the spinal canal or spinal cord is suspected, MR should be the imaging modality of choice in the acute, subacute, or chronic stage (139). Sagittal, T1-weighted images should be obtained with 3–5-mm slice thickness; these images will show subacute blood and any structural deformity of the cord or the spinal canal (Figs. 4.39–4.41). Sagittal, T2-weighted images should then be obtained using flow compensation and, if possible, cardiac gating. The T2-weighted images will help to identify areas of ischemia, which will have long T2 relaxation time, or areas of hemorrhage, which will have short T2 relaxation time. Gradient echo images, which are the most sensitive to the presence of hemorrhage, should always be obtained. Fast spin echo sequences are relatively insensitive to the presence of hemorrhage and should not be used in the setting of trauma. The worst prognosis for subsequent spinal cord function is in patients who have intramedullary hemorrhage, followed by those with edema over more than one segment. The best prognosis is in those patients without edema or with edema involving one segment or less (140,141). MR performed in the chronic phase, several months after the event, is helpful to determine the full extent of spinal cord damage (Fig. 4.39).

Nerve Root and Brachial Plexus Injuries

Injuries to the nerve roots as they exit the spinal cord are relatively common; although these are generally categorized as brachial plexus injuries, the injury most commonly occurs to the roots that form the trunks of the plexus (9). Injuries range in severity from mild stretching of the nerve, resulting in transient neurologic dysfunction, to complete avulsion from the spinal cord with resultant permanent deficit. Most of these injuries result from traction of the shoulder while delivering the head of an infant in the breech presentation or from turning the head away from the shoulder in a difficult cephalic presentation of a large infant (142,143). Shoulder dystocia and birth weight of greater than 3,500 g are present in more than half of cases (142). Clinically, Erb's palsy (adducted and internally rotated shoulder; extended, pronated elbow; and flexed wrist resulting from injury to C5, C6, and C7 roots) is the most common presentation, with Klumpke's palsy (extended wrist and fingers, often associated with ipsilateral Horner's syndrome resulting from injury to C8 and T1) considerably less common (9,138).

Imaging evaluation of the brachial plexus is performed best by MR, looking for T2 prolongation or discontinuity of the nerves. Avulsion of the roots from the spinal cord is best shown by CT myelography, which will demonstrate empty (without a nerve root) small pseudomeningoceles at the site of the avulsions. Thin section T2- or T2-weighted MR images, obtained in the coronal or axial planes, will show the pseudomeningocele as an ovoid mass of CSF intensity extending through the affected neural foramen (Fig. 4.42). Although MR does not reliably show nerve roots in the pseudomeningocele sac and therefore is not reliable in confirming the avulsion of a root, the presence of the sac is a good indication of nerve root injury (144). Moreover, the presence of the pseudomeningocele implies a poor prognosis for functional recovery (145). Thus, MR imaging, which reliably shows the brachial plexus and pseudomeningocele sac, is the study of choice in affected patients.

Head Trauma

Extracranial Birth Trauma

Caput succedaneum is one of the three major varieties of extracranial hemorrhage, the other two being subga-

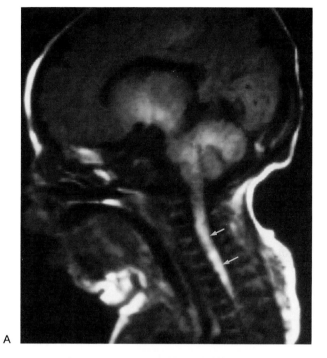

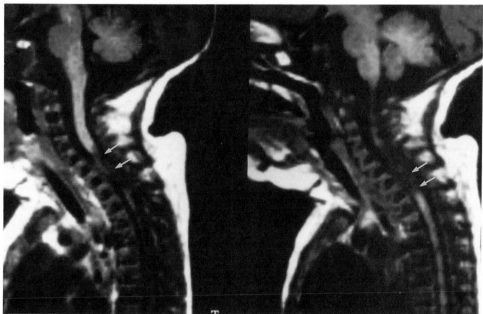

FIG. 4.39. Birth trauma secondary to difficult breech delivery. **A:** Sagittal SE 500/15 image shows abnormal hyperintensity (*arrows*) at the spinal cord at the cervicothoracic junction. **B:** Sagittal SE 500/15 3 weeks later shows that the cord is transected (*arrows*).

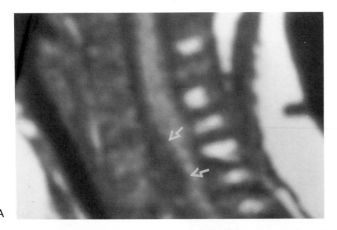

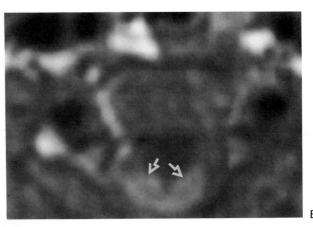

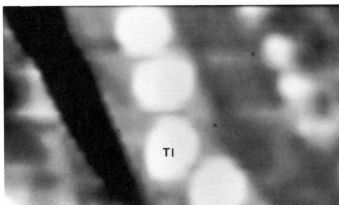

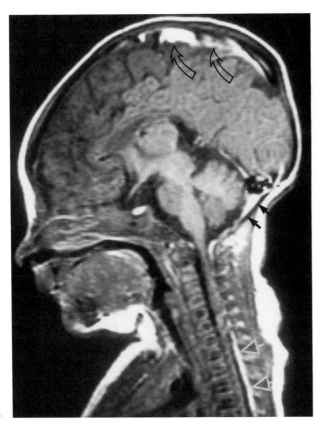

FIG. 4.40. Birth trauma. Difficult delivery secondary to fetal anasarca with vertebral fracture, dural tear, and extradural CSF collection. **A:** Sagittal SE 550/15 image shows an expanded CSF space (*arrows*) ventral to the spinal cord at the cervicothoracic junction. **B:** Axial SE 600/20 image at the T1 level shows the spinal cord (*arrows*) displaced posteriorly by the CSF collection. **C:** Reformation of axial CT scan shows ventral displacement of the T1 vertebral body secondary to ligamentous disruption and fracture.

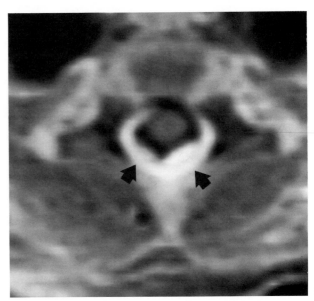

FIG. 4.41. Birth trauma. Spinal and intracranial extraparenchymal hematomas. **A:** Sagittal SE 550/15 image shows hyperintense extraparenchymal blood in the dorsal spine (*open white arrows*), posterior fossa subdural space (*small solid black arrows*) and interhemispheric subdural space (open curved black arrows). **B:** Axial SE 600/15 image shows the blood (*arrows*) in the spinal epidural space. (This case courtesy Dr. Chip Truwit, Minneapolis, MN.)

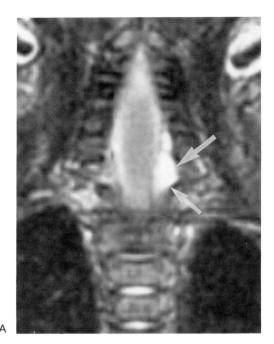

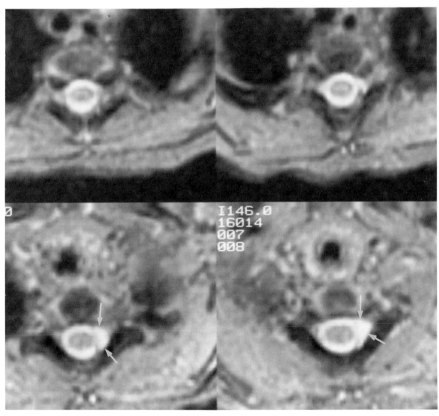

FIG. 4.42. Nerve root avulsion in a neonate. **A:** Coronal FSE 3000/100 image shows a pseudomeningocele (*arrows*) at the left lateral spinal canal. **B:** Axial GE 500/14 images show the pseudomeningocele extending into the left C7–T1 neural foramen.

leal hemorrhage and cephalohematoma. Caput succedaneum refers to hemorrhage and edema beneath the skin that is observed very commonly after vaginal delivery. This edema is soft, superficial, and pitting in nature, and it crosses suture lines. The lesion steadily resolves over the first few days of life. Radiography is neither diagnostic nor necessary (9).

Subgaleal hemorrhage refers to hemorrhage subjacent to the aponeurosis covering the scalp, beneath the occipitofrontalis muscle. Subgaleal hematomas present as firm, fluctuant masses that increase in size after birth; they sometimes dissect into the subcutaneous tissue of the neck. Although patients can become symptomatic from these lesions secondary to blood loss, the lesion usually resolves over 2–3 weeks. Imaging of these lesions is almost never necessary (9).

The term *cephalohematoma* refers to a traumatic subperiosteal hemorrhage; because the blood is beneath the outer layer of periosteum, it is confined by the cranial sutures. Cephalohematomas occur in approximately 1% of live births; the incidence increases markedly with the use of forceps. Cephalohematomas usually increase in size after birth and present as a firm, tense mass; they are rarely of clinical significance, unless a complicating intracranial lesion is present. Resolution occurs in a few weeks to months (9). When seen on CT or MR, cephalohematomas appear as crescent-shaped lesions adjacent to the outer table of the skull. A few may eventually calcify; these gradually disappear over many months of skull growth and remodeling. The MR appearance of these lesions is usually that of subacute blood with a high signal intensity on short TR/TE and long TR/TE images; when imaged more acutely, hypointensity may be seen on long TR images.

Skull Fractures

Although once felt to be an important finding in head trauma, the presence of skull fractures actually has very little prognostic value concerning neurologic damage that results from trauma (146,147). In fact, skull fractures may actually diminish injury to the underlying brain by dispersing the force from the trauma (148). Moreover, the absence of a skull fracture by no means excludes brain damage. Documentation of fractures may be useful in the documentation of nonaccidental trauma, however. When documentation is desired, skull x-rays may be necessary, because some linear skull fractures, especially those in the horizontal plane, can be difficult to detect on routine CT scans. Close examination of the "scout" view can minimize this pitfall. *The "scout" view is extremely valuable for the identification of skull fractures and should be carefully studied in all head trauma cases.*

The most common skull fractures are linear and are most often localized to the parietal or frontal regions of the skull. When the bone is not displaced, the fracture heals spontaneously and no treatment is indicated. In infants, skull fractures may heal in less than 6 months. In older children, fractures generally heal within a year, and in adults, a healing time of 2–3 years is common. As fractures heal, the fracture line on plain films becomes less and less distinct until, eventually, the fracture may be difficult to differentiate from a vascular groove (149).

Depressed skull fractures may result from pressure of the head against the pelvis during the birth process or may be induced by application of forceps (150). Whereas linear fractures of the vault may be adequately visualized by plain films, the amount of displacement in a depressed fracture is more accurately defined by CT. Most important, CT assesses damage to the underlying brain, and plain radiography does not. Depressed skull fractures are most often treated surgically.

Occasionally, skull fractures are associated with tears of the underlying dura. When dural tears occur, meninges and brain tissue can herniate into the diastatic fracture site. The interposition of the meninges between the diastatic bones prevents the osteoblasts from migrating across the fracture site and inhibits healing of the fracture. Moreover, the constant CSF pulsations within the fracture cause enlargement of the fracture and extension of meninges extracranially. This situation has been called a "growing fracture" or a *leptomeningeal cyst* (149,151,152). Leptomeningeal cysts are seen in 0.6% of all fractures, with 90% occurring in patients less than 3 years old (151,152). On imaging studies leptomeningeal cysts have distinct bony margins at the fracture site (149,153), simulating a lytic calvarial lesion if the associated abnormalities of the subarachnoid space and underlying brain are not appreciated (154). Intracranial tissue may be seen extending between the edges of the bone at the fracture site (Fig. 4.43). Encephalomalacia of the underlying brain may or may not be present; if present, it appears as an area of low attenuation on CT and as an area of prolonged T1 and T2 relaxation time on MR (Fig. 4.44).

Traumatic Intracranial Hemorrhage in the Newborn

Mechanical trauma to the infant's brain during delivery may induce lacerations in the tentorium or the falx cerebri, resulting in subdural hemorrhage. MR has greatly increased the knowledge concerning the frequency and severity of subdural hemorrhage in newborns. Whereas it was previously believed that posterior fossa subdural hematomas in infants were rare and often life threatening, we now know that small posterior fossa subdural hematomas are common in the postnatal pe-

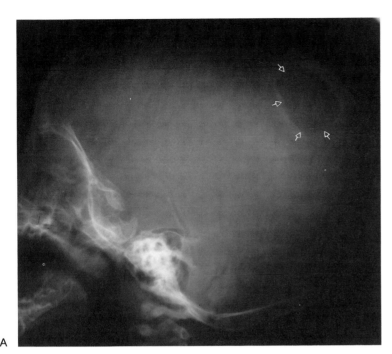
A

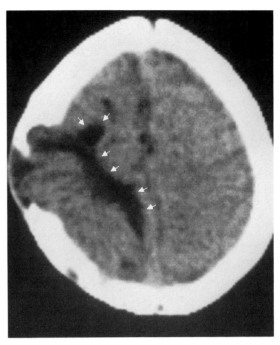
B

FIG. 4.43. Leptomeningeal cyst. **A:** Plain film shows a well-marginated lucency (*arrows*) with a sclerotic border at the site of a previous skull fracture. **B:** Axial CT image shows brain herniating through a dural defect and causing erosive changes in the bone at the fracture site. Encephalomalacia (*arrows*) is present in the underlying brain.

riod (Fig. 4.45). Moreover, they are rarely of clinical importance, becoming significant only if they cause sufficient compression to impair CSF flow or brain stem function (102). There are four major categories of neonatal subdural hemorrhage: (1) tentorial laceration, (2) occipital osteodiastasis, (3) falx laceration, (4) rupture of bridging superficial cerebral veins.

Tentorial Laceration and Occipital Osteodiastasis

Tentorial laceration and occipital osteodiastasis are discussed together because both result in posterior fossa subdural hemorrhage. Large tears of the tentorium result in rupture of the vein of Galen, straight sinus, or transverse sinus; the resulting subdural hemorrhage tends to be massive. The rapidly expanding subdural collection can cause compression of the brain stem and result in death. Lesser degrees of infratentorial subdural hemorrhage may result from smaller tentorial tears or rupture of smaller infratentorial veins without tentorial tears (Fig. 4.45). As stated earlier, these small subdural collections are being recognized more frequently as a result of the increased sensitivity of MR and are usually of no clinical consequence. The falx cerebri or supratentorial veins may be torn at the same time, resulting in simultaneous supratentorial and infratentorial subdural hematomas (Figs. 4.45, 4.46) (102,155).

Occipital osteodiastasis consists of traumatic separation of the squamous portion of the occipital bone and the exoccipital portion of the occipital bone during birth. In severe cases, the dura and occipital sinuses are torn; the result is cerebellar laceration and a massive posterior fossa subdural hemorrhage (9,156). The posterior fossa subdural hematoma lies under the tentorium and extends laterally between the dura and arachnoid overlying the cerebellar hemisphere. The CT appearance of these hemorrhages in the acute phase is that of a high-density thickening of the affected tentorial leaf with the high density extending inferiorly, posterior to the cerebellar hemisphere. These lesions are usually seen better on coronal views; the high-density hematoma is seen immediately beneath the tentorium (149,157). When some supratentorial veins or the falx cerebri are also torn, an interhemispheric subdural hematoma may also be present (Fig. 4.46). In the anemic infant, the acute subdural hematoma may be isodense or even hypodense to brain because of the relatively low protein content of the subdural collection.

Subdural hematomas appear as mildly echogenic extraparenchymal collections on sonography. The MR appearance of subdural hematomas varies with their chronicity. An acute subdural hematoma is isointense to brain on T1-weighted spin echo sequences and hypointense to brain on T2-weighted spin echo and gradient

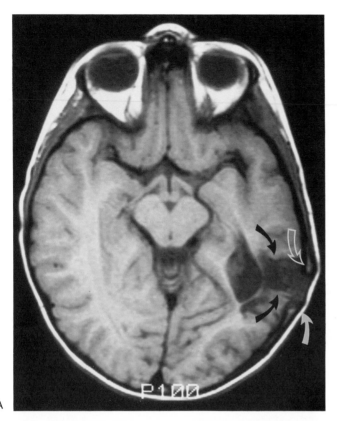

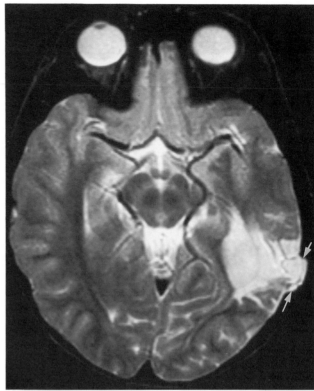

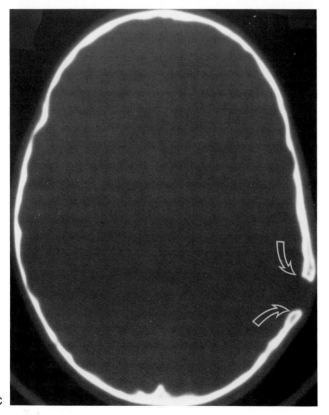

FIG. 4.44. Leptomeningeal cyst. **A:** Axial SE 600/15 image shows encephalomalacia (*curved black arrows*) in the left temporal lobe with a well-demarcated defect (*curved white arrows*) in the adjacent bone. **B:** Axial SE 2500/70 image better demonstrates CSF extending into the fracture site (*arrows*). **C:** Bone window of a CT image shows the heaped-up bone edges (*arrows*) at the fracture site. (This case courtesy Dr. Chip Truwit, Minneapolis, MN.)

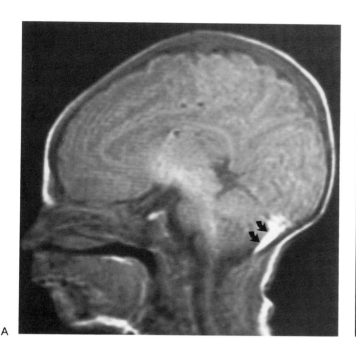

A

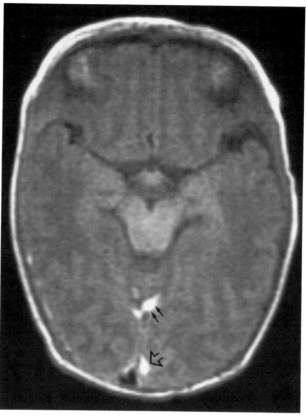

B

FIG. 4.45. Small posterior fossa subdural hematoma in a neonate. Sagittal (A) and axial (B) SE 600/15 images show hyperintense subdural blood posterior to the cerebellum (*curved arrows*) and along the tentorium cerebelli (*small solid arrows*) and posterior falx cerebri (*open arrow*).

echo sequences. This appearance results from the presence of deoxyhemoglobin in the red blood cells (127,158,159). Fast spin echo sequences are less sensitive to the presence of blood products and should not be used in the setting of trauma. As the hematoma evolves, it develops a high signal intensity that starts in the periphery on the T1-weighted spin echo sequences and progresses centripetally toward the center of the hematoma. The high signal intensity, which appears first on T1-weighted spin echo images and later on T2-weighted spin echo images, results from the conversion of deoxyhemoglobin to methemoglobin. Finally, as the blood breakdown products are reabsorbed, signal intensity on the T1-weighted spin echo images diminishes until eventually the subdural collection is isointense with CSF on all sequences. It is important to check the size of the ventricles in these patients because acute hydrocephalus may develop as a result of compression of the fourth ventricle and aqueduct.

Falx Laceration and Superficial Cerebral Vein Rupture

Falx laceration and superficial cerebral vein rupture are discussed together because both result in supraten-

torial subdural hematomas. Laceration of the falx cerebri is much less common than laceration of the tentorium. It usually occurs near the junction of the falx with the tentorium, the source of bleeding, most commonly being the inferior sagittal sinus. The cause of both falx and tentorial tears seems to be excessive vertical molding of the head with frontal-occipital elongation. When laceration of the falx occurs, the subdural hematoma is usually located in the inferior aspect of the interhemispheric fissure over the corpus callosum (9).

Rupture of superficial cortical veins that bridge the dura results in hemorrhage over the cerebral convexity. In this setting, a convexity subdural hematoma results, in contradistinction to the interhemispheric subdural hematoma seen with lacerations of the falx. In contrast to subdural hematomas occurring later in infancy, which are more commonly bilateral, convexity subdural hematomas in the newborn are usually unilateral and accompanied by subarachnoid blood. An underlying cerebral contusion is often present (160).

The CT and MR appearance and evolution of supratentorial subdural hematomas are identical to those previously described for infratentorial subdurals. As with infratentorial subdural hematomas, coronal views are often helpful in assessing the true size and extent of sub-

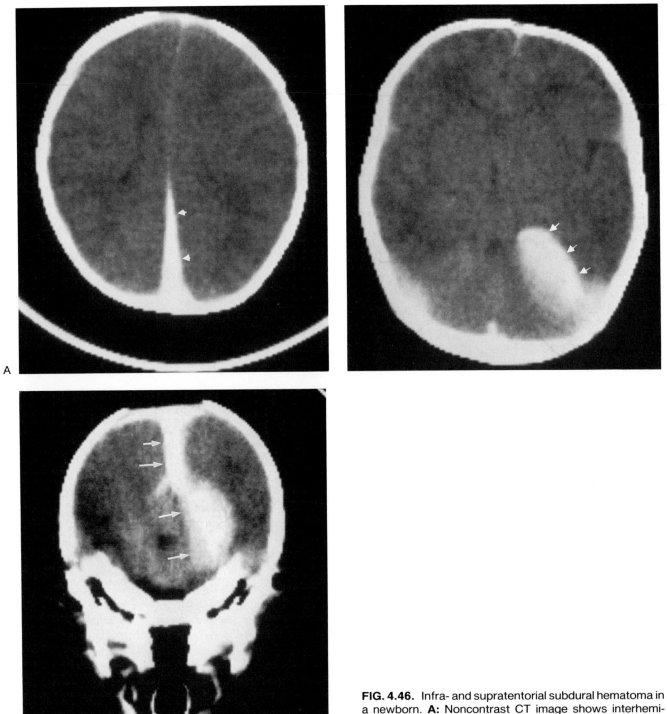

FIG. 4.46. Infra- and supratentorial subdural hematoma in a newborn. **A:** Noncontrast CT image shows interhemispheric subdural hematoma (*arrows*). **B:** A more caudal image shows the high attenuation of the hematoma (*arrows*) along the left leaf of the tentorium. **C:** Coronal image shows the high attenuation hematoma (*arrows*) adjacent to the falx and affected tentorial leaf.

dural collections. For posterior fossa subdural collections, transfontanel ultrasonography is very useful, as both the fluid collection lying beneath the tentorium and the hydrocephalus resulting from compression of the fourth ventricle and aqueduct can be detected. Whereas interhemispheric subdural collections can also be seen relatively easily on sonography, convexity hematomas are more difficult to visualize because of the difficulty involved in angling the transducer to see the convexity region. It is important to note that sonography can be performed in the neonatal ICU and therefore does not necessitate transporting very ill patients.

Postnatal Trauma

Although traumatic brain injury in infants and children is very similar to that in adults, the causes are very different. Severe accidental head trauma, common in older children and adults, is rather uncommon in infants less than 2 years old. In fact, nonaccidental injury (child abuse) is 10–15 times more common than accidental head trauma in infants less than 1 year old (161). Thus, when severe head trauma is found on imaging studies of infants, the suspicion of nonaccidental trauma should always be raised. The imaging findings of trauma in adults are described in a number of publications (153); therefore, characteristics in children that are similar to those in adults will be rather superficially discussed in this book. The differences in imaging findings between children and adults will be emphasized.

Spinal Trauma

Vertebral column fractures and spinal cord injuries in children are less common than in other age groups; however, they are not rare and have received increasing attention in the medical literature since the advent of modern imaging techniques. As discussed in the section on birth trauma, the pediatric spinal column has anatomic characteristics that create different patterns of susceptibility to injury among children, as compared with adults. These include increased elasticity of ligaments and soft tissues, open epiphyses, lack of development of ossification centers, and changes in osseous strength, shape, and size (132,162,163). For example, epiphyseal plates are still open in the vertebral bodies of children; they start to fuse at many levels by age 8 years. Facets are relatively horizontal in infancy, becoming more vertical with ossification between ages 7 and 10 years. Another factor concerns the large head size and the relatively poorly developed paraspinous muscles in infants. This combination, coupled with the increased elasticity of ligaments, creates a relative hypermobility that leads to a predisposition for cervical spinal cord injury without plain film radiologic

abnormality (130,131). Injuries start to approach adult patterns as the spinal column matures, and they reach fully adult patterns at about age 15 (131,132,164).

As infants and young children have a propensity for spinal cord injury, an MR should be obtained in all infants and children in whom spinal injury is suspected, even in the absence of plain film radiologic abnormalities. If plain films are obtained, the radiologist should be aware that plain radiographs of children, especially of the cervical spine, differ from those in adults and that films taken in the "neutral" position can be normal despite significant injury. The mobility of the cervical spine in children is manifest by the large atlantodental space, which can be as wide as 5 mm in children, and "pseudo-subluxation," a term referring to the 4 mm of anterior motion of C2 on C3 and C3 on C4 in up to 40% of children under the age of 8 years (165). Alignment of the spinolaminar line is preserved with pseudosubluxation but malaligned with true subluxation. The size of the prevertebral soft tissues also differs in children, as compared with adults. In children less than 15 years old, the retrotracheal space normally averages 3.5 mm and the retropharyngeal space averages 7–9 mm. The prevertebral soft tissues should not exceed two-thirds of the width of the vertebral body of C2 (132,165). In the adult, the prevertebral distance is normally 5–6 mm at the C3 level (132).

A great deal of literature has been concerned with the concept of spinal cord injury without radiologic abnormality (SCIWORA) in children (130,131). Classification of SCIWORA as a separate entity is unjustified, as long as the radiologist and treating physician recognize the underlying concept that *the immature spinal column allows significant spinal cord injury without plain radiograph abnormalities and that other studies (e.g., flexion-extension views or MR), to look for soft tissue injury, are necessary in appropriate clinical settings.* SCIWORA will not be addressed as a separate entity in this text.

Injuries in Young Children

It is important to remember that young children, through the age of about 8 years, tend to sustain soft tissue injuries without incurring radiologically apparent fractures. Thus, dislocations, ligamentous avulsions, subluxation without fracture, growth plate injuries, and epiphyseal separations are common. Most spinal injuries in this age group involve the cervical spine, particularly the upper segments. These include atlanto-occipital dislocations, which are often fatal (166), and atlantoaxial dislocations, which tend to be less serious because of the more capacious spinal canal at C1 (166). Plain radiographs in flexion and extension (performed *carefully* with physician supervision) will establish the diagnosis;

however, only MR will show whether spinal cord injury has occurred (129,140,141). As discussed in the section on neonatal injury, the MR may show edema, hemorrhage, or atrophy, depending upon the severity and chronicity of the injury. Rotary subluxations accompany rupture of the transverse ligaments and can become fixed. Diagnosis of fixed rotary subluxations is made by performing CT scans with the head turned 45° to the left and then 45° to the right. If the relative alignment of C1 and C2 does not change with head turning, the diagnosis of fixed rotary subluxation is established. Fractures of the atlas and axis are uncommon in younger children.

Fractures involving the thoracic or lumbar spine in children tend to involve the T11–L2 levels, where the more rigid thoracic spine joins the mobile lumbar segments. Soft tissue injuries, involving the ligaments, cartilage, or growth plates, are most common. Seat belt in-juries, secondary to flexion-distraction, usually occur at the L2–L4 levels (Fig. 4.47), lower than in older patients (167). Thirty percent of patients have associated visceral injury (167). These primarily horizontal injuries are difficult to identify on CT (168,169) and are another reason that the combination of flexion–extension plain radiographs and MR is the most useful combination in the diagnosis of spinal trauma.

Adolescent Injuries

Adolescents from ages 9 to 16 years sustain spinal injuries at a rate 10 times that of younger children. The incidence is even higher in the 16–24-year-old age group; in fact, patients from 16 to 24 years of age have the highest incidence of spine trauma of any age group (170). As children get older, they more often injure bone rather

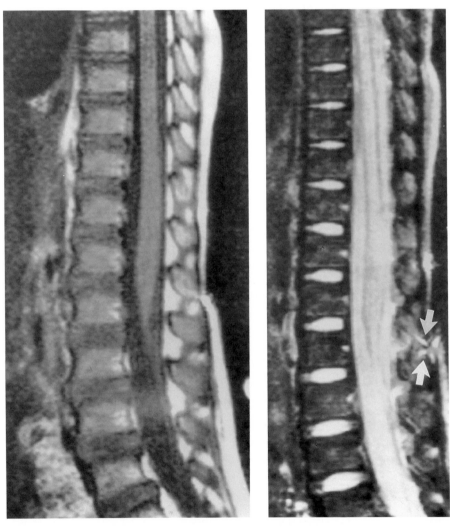

A   B

FIG. 4.47. Spinal cord injury secondary to motor vehicle accident. Plain films were normal. **A:** Sagittal SE 550/15 image shows no significant abnormality. **B:** Sagittal SE 2500/80 image shows diffuse abnormal hyperintensity of the spinal cord. Abnormal hyperintensity is present between the spinous processes of L2 and L3 (*arrows*), indicating ligamentous injury at that site.

than exclusively soft tissues. In addition, injuries tend to be more evenly distributed through the cervical levels, as compared with the predilection for upper cervical injuries in younger children (171). The C5–C6 level is most frequently injured in adolescents (170). Although spinal cord injury can be present without plain radiographic abnormalities in adolescents, bone abnormalities are seen more commonly than not. Moreover, the severity of spinal cord injury in patients without radiographic abnormalities tends to be less than in those with radiograph abnormalities (132).

The radiologic evaluation of adolescents with spine trauma is essentially identical to that of adults with a few exceptions. The treating physicians should remain aware of the possibility of soft tissue injury without associated bone injury and therefore should obtain flexion–extension films, especially in younger adolescents. Also, the radiologist should be aware that traumatic disc herniations in adolescents is frequently associated with fracture of the adjacent vertebral endplate, a finding that is much more easily appreciated on CT and MR than on plain radiographs (172). This finding is important in surgical planning (173). Although plain radiographs and CT are adequate for evaluation of bone injuries, MR is essential to determine the extent of spinal cord injury and, thus, to establish a prognosis (174,175). The presence of hemorrhage (short T2 relaxation time) or long segments (more than one vertebral level) of edema (long T2 relaxation time) implies a poor prognosis for recovery of function (140,141,174,175). MR also shows ligamentous injury, the injured soft tissues appearing abnormally hyperintense on T2-weighted images (153).

Another syndrome that is relatively unique to children and adolescents is posttraumatic spinal cord infarction (176–178). Typically, patients have onset of neurologic signs several hours to several days after the injury. Para- or quadriparesis and dissociated sensory loss then ensue. Prognosis is variable. Plain films and myelography are normal (176,177). MR will show anterior spinal artery infarction, manifest as T2 prolongation in the anterior half to two-thirds of the spinal cord (Fig. 4.48) or as hyperintensity in the ventral gray matter of the cord. Imaging in the subacute phase may show enhancement of the infarcted region.

Patients with certain genetic abnormalities are predisposed to spinal cord injury as a result of ligamentous laxity, spinal stenosis, spinal kyphosis, or stenosis of the foramen magnum. Included in this group are patients with Down's syndrome (see Chapter 5), mucopolysaccharidoses (especially Morquio's syndrome, see Chapter 3), achondroplasia (see Chapter 8), Klippel–Feil syndrome (see Chapter 9), and spondyloepiphyseal dysplasia. These patients should be observed for neurologic dysfunction and neck pain in a longitudinal fashion and should be carefully examined after even minor neck trauma (138,179,180).

Head Trauma

Extraparenchymal Hematomas

Epidural hematomas are uncommon in infants and increase slowly in incidence throughout childhood to peak in adults (138). Epidurals in children differ from those in adults in both pathogenesis and clinical manifestations. In children, epidural hematomas are more commonly the result of tears in the dural veins than of laceration of the middle meningeal artery (181). Moreover, the pediatric skull is more pliable than the adult's and can expand as a posttraumatic hematoma accumulates (182). Therefore, the clinical presentation does not evolve as rapidly. Moreover, in contradistinction to adults, in whom the head injury characteristically induces a loss of consciousness, children more commonly are only stunned by the injury. This necessitates more aggressive, early imaging in the pediatric trauma patient because the clinical manifestations of significant trauma may initially be mild or transient.

The findings of epidural hematomas in children on CT and MR are identical to those of adults. CT will usually reveal a lentiform hyperdense extraparenchymal collection that does not cross cranial sutures. On MR, the acute hematoma is bright on T1-weighted images and dark on T2-weighted images. A fluid–fluid layer may be present secondary to layering of blood cells; the upper layer will be bright on T1- and T2-weighted images, and the lower level will be isointense to brain on T1-weighted images and dark on T2-weighted images (183).

Subdural hematomas are most common in infants and elderly adults and are less common in older children and adolescents (184). They result from tears of cortical veins bridging the subdural space on their way to the dural sinuses. The soft consistency of the unmyelinated brain results in increased brain distortion during trauma and puts increased stress upon these veins (138). In contradistinction to adults, in whom traumatic subdural hematomas are usually unilateral, traumatic subdural hematomas are bilateral in 80% to 85% of infants. The hematomas tend to be located over the frontoparietal convexity. A history of birth trauma or postnatal trauma is usually elicited in these patients. The presence of recent unreported physical trauma or a history of mild trauma that is inconsistent with the severity of the injury suggests child abuse (138,182,185–188). Other factors predisposing to hematomas include blood dyscrasias and prematurity (189). Affected infants present with seizures, vomiting, hyperirritability or lethargy, and progressive head enlargement.

Imaging studies of subdural hematomas in children are identical to those in adults. In the acute phase, CT will show a high attenuation extraparenchymal crescentic fluid collection over the frontoparietal convexities. Within 1–3 weeks after the hemorrhage, the blood be-

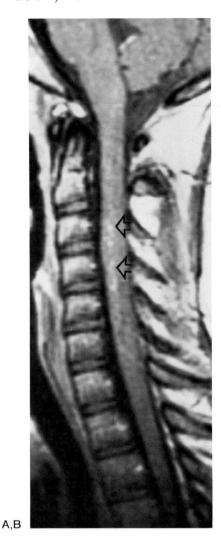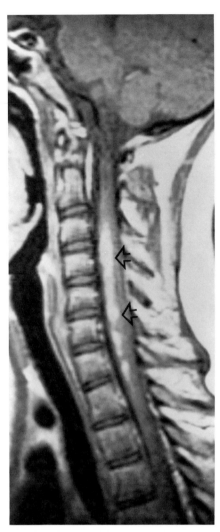

A,B

FIG. 4.48. Spinal cord infarction. **A:** Post-contrast sagittal SE 550/15 image on third day after onset of symptoms shows small foci of hyperintensity (*arrows*) in the anterior half of the spinal cord. **B:** Postcontrast image 1 week later shows significant enhancement within the anterior half of the cord (*arrows*).

comes isodense with brain tissue. At this stage, compression of the ventricles and medial displacement of the gray–white junction with compression of the white matter will indicate presence of the extra-axial fluid collection (Fig. 4.49A). If intravenous contrast is given, the inner and outer membranes of the subdural hematoma will enhance (Fig. 4.49B) (153). It is essential to recognize shift of the ventricles, medial displacement of the corticomedullary junction, and medial displacement of the cortical sulci at this stage (149,190). After 2–3 weeks the density of the hematoma will be lower than that of brain and closer to that of CSF. At this stage, it is usually called a chronic subdural hematoma. Because of the development of fibrovascular granulation tissue in the periphery of the subdural collection, the outer and inner membranes of subacute or chronic subdural hematomas enhance rather densely after IV contrast is given (153). On MR, the signal intensity of the extra-axial fluid collection will evolve as those described for the epidural he-

matoma in the previous section (Figs. 4.50, 4.51). The changes in signal intensity result from the loss of oxygen from hemoglobin followed by the oxidation of hemoglobin to methemoglobin and subsequent breakdown to diamagnetic materials (158). Fluid–fluid layers may be present as a result of layering of the blood cells in the dependent portion of the subdural collection. MR is also useful in the identification of injury to the underlying parenchyma (see subsequent section), such as axonal shearing injuries, contusions, and infarctions, that commonly accompany traumatic subdural hematomas (Fig. 4.50) (148,151,186–188).

Unlike intraparenchymal hematomas, in which the blood-brain barrier inhibits their resorption, hemosiderin and ferritin are not deposited within the wall of the chronic subdural hematoma (153). Therefore, the absence of subdural hemosiderin does not imply that a subdural hematoma is acute or that a prior subdural hematoma has not been present.

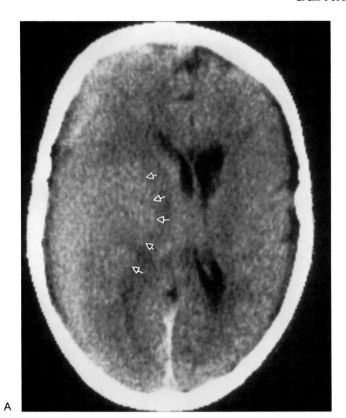
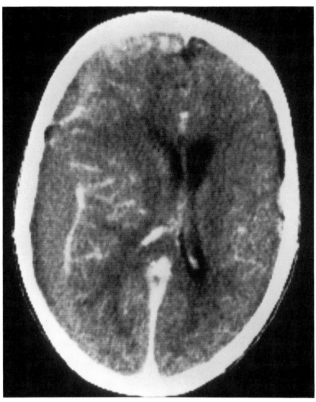

A

B

FIG. 4.49. Subacute (isodense) subdural hematoma. **A:** Axial noncontrast CT image shows compression of the right lateral ventricle and right hemispheric white matter in addition to medial displacement of the gray matter–white matter junction (*arrows*). **B:** After administration of iodinated contrast, part of the inner membrane of the subdural hematoma enhances. In addition, many of the dural veins are seen to be medially displaced by the subdural collection.

Subarachnoid Hemorrhages

Subarachnoid hemorrhage often accompanies intraparenchymal damage in both the child and the adult. In the acute phase after injury, when nonhemorrhagic parenchymal lesions are difficult to identify on CT, subarachnoid hemorrhage may be the harbinger of more severe underlying brain damage (185,190). MR is not useful in the diagnosis of subarachnoid hemorrhage, probably because the hemoglobin is less concentrated than in clotted blood and the high oxygen tension of cerebrospinal fluid inhibits the conversion of hemoglobin to deoxyhemoglobin and methemoglobin (127,191, 192). On CT, subarachnoid hemorrhage appears as increased attenuation in the subarachnoid space. It is most commonly seen in the posterior interhemispheric fissure, adjacent to the falx cerebri (Fig. 4.52), or layering along the tentorium cerebelli (Fig. 4.53). Sometimes this increased attenuation is the only abnormality seen on the CT scan. Blood along the tentorium is best demonstrated by imaging in the coronal plane. When subarachnoid

blood is located along the posterior falx cerebri, the increased density within the interhemispheric fissure is thicker and more irregular than the falx itself. A helpful finding is extension of the blood into the cerebral sulci along the medial aspect of the hemisphere (193) (Fig. 4.53). This thick, dense high signal in the interhemispheric fissure has been called the "falx sign." The reader should note that, even in children, the falx can normally have a high attenuation on CT. The falx itself, however, should be thin and regular in contour, and no extension of the high attenuation into the cortical sulci should be seen.

Lesions of the Cerebral Parenchyma

In the acute phase after either physical trauma or asphyxia, generalized cerebral swelling is seen more commonly in children than in adults with similar types of head injury. This generalized cerebral swelling probably results from edema plus a decrease in cerebrovascular resistance, combining to cause vasodilatation and in-

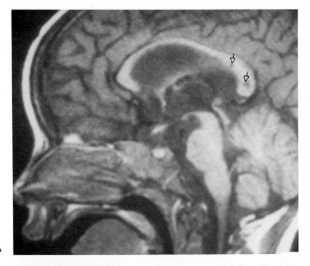

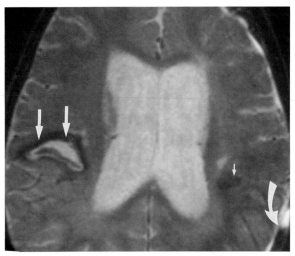

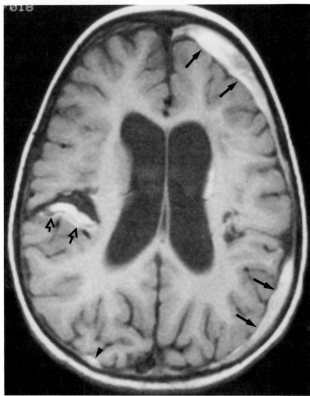

FIG. 4.50. MR of severe head trauma. **A:** Sagittal SE 600/20 image shows two foci of low intensity in the posterior body and splenium of the corpus callosum (*arrows*), secondary to axonal shearing injuries. **B:** Axial SE 600/20 image shows a high-intensity subdural collection (*solid black arrows*) on the left. A hemorrhagic contusion (*open arrows*) is present in the right parietal lobe. A third focus of subacute hemorrhage (*arrowhead*) is seen in the right occipital region. **C:** Axial SE 2800/70 image shows that the left subdural hematoma is hypointense, indicating the presence of intracellular methemoglobin. A fluid–fluid layer (*curved arrow*) is present in the posterior portion of the hematoma. The very-low-signal region (*large straight arrow*) in the right parietal region probably represents hemosiderin or acute hemorrhage. Hemosiderin staining (*small straight arrow*), probably secondary to an axonal shearing injury, is also present in a left hemispheric lesion.

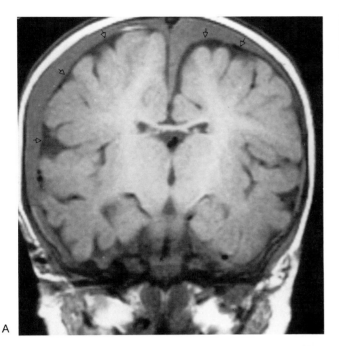

A

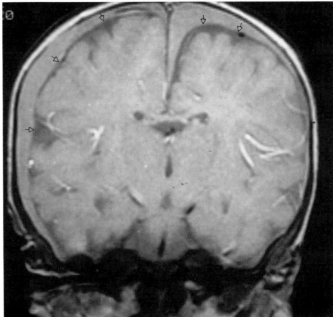

B

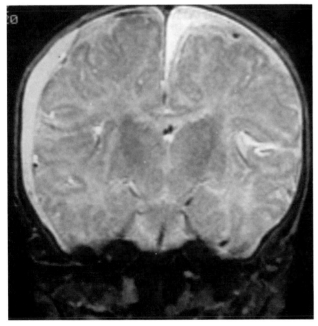

C

FIG. 4.51. Bilateral subdural hematoma. **A:** Coronal SE 800/20 image shows bilateral collections in the subdural space that are hyperintense compared to CSF in the subjacent subarachnoid space (*arrows*). **B:** Coronal SE 2000/40 image shows the CSF in the subarachnoid space remaining hypointense compared to the subdural blood (*arrows*). **C:** SE 2000/80 image shows the CSF and subdural blood to be isointense. The hyperintensity of the subdural fluid and the asymmetry of the subdural collections allow differentiation of subdural hematomas from benign enlargement of the subarachnoid spaces in infancy (see Chapter 8).

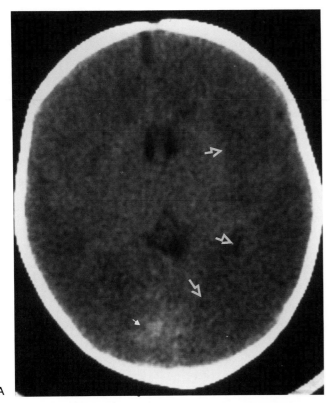
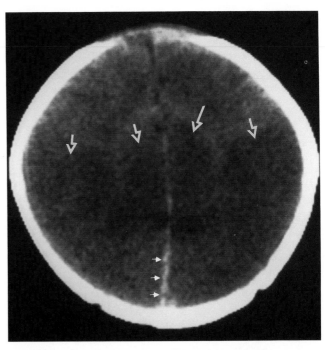

A

B

FIG. 4.52. Subarachnoid hemorrhage and cerebral infarction secondary to nonaccidental trauma. **A:** Axial CT image shows the high attenuation of blood (*small arrow*) in the right occipital lobe secondary to contusion. The middle cerebral distribution of the left hemisphere (*arrows*) is hypodense secondary to infarction. **B:** Axial CT at higher level shows bilateral cerebral infarctions (*large arrows*) and a thick, irregular linear hyperdensity (*small arrows*) representing subarachnoid blood in the posterior interhemispheric fissure.

creased cerebral blood volume (138). If an imaging study is obtained in the first 18 hours after trauma, it is usually normal. By about 24 hours, CT and MR of the brain at this stage show decreased distinction between gray and white matter with compressed, slitlike lateral ventricles (34,185,190). In addition, the cerebral sulci and perimesencephalic cisterns are compressed (Fig. 4.54). Transtentorial herniation of the temporal lobe may cause infarction of the posterior cerebral artery territory by compressing the posterior cerebral artery in the ambient cistern. Stretching of the thalamoperforator arteries during transtentorial herniation may cause thalamic infarcts (194). Subfalcine herniation may cause infarcts in the territory of anterior cerebral artery branches.

Severe swelling of the brain suggests a guarded prognosis (195,196), as does the presence of the "reversal sign" in which cerebral white matter has a higher attenuation than cerebral gray matter (Fig. 4.34) (98,99). It is difficult in this acute phase to detect axonal shearing injuries; therefore, one cannot determine whether diffuse cerebral swelling is the result of increased blood volume

or axonal shearing injuries (138,197). If CT is used as the initial imaging modality, the differentiation of cerebral swelling from nonhemorrhagic axonal injury can only be made on follow-up scans. Atrophy will develop if the brain has suffered significant injury, but the swollen brain will return to a normal appearance if significant neuronal damage has not occurred (138,197). Follow-up MR scans of children with mild head injury will be normal at 3 months after the injury. Of children with moderate to severe closed head injury, and therefore a poorer prognosis, 71% will have parenchymal lesions on MR, predominantly in the frontal lobes, if imaged at least 3 months after the injury. Interestingly, children with frontal lobe lesions were found to be more frequently neurologically and psychologically disabled than those with diffuse injury (198). Proton MR spectroscopy (MRS) may be useful in differentiating swelling secondary to increased blood volume from swelling secondary to shearing injury. Proton MRS is nearly normal in the absence of parenchymal injury but shows decreased NAA and increased lactate if significant injury has occurred.

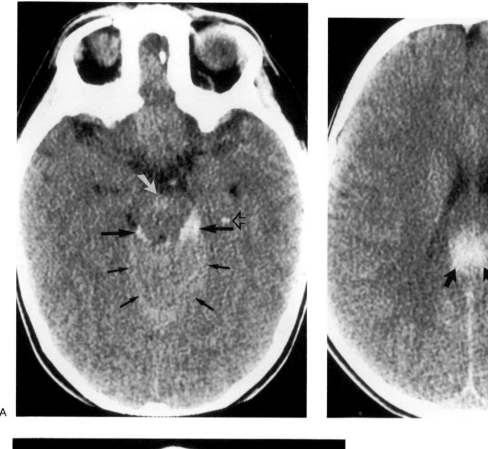

A   B

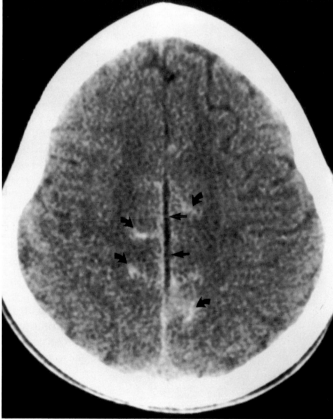

C

FIG. 4.53. Traumatic injury with subarachnoid hemorrhage and parenchymal injury. **A:** Axial CT image shows subarachnoid blood in the ambient cisterns (*large solid black arrows*), in the interpeduncular cistern (*white arrow*), and along the tentorium cerebelli (*small solid black arrows*). Parenchymal hemorrhage (*open arrow*), probably secondary to axonal shear injury, is present in the left temporal lobe. **B:** Image at the level of the corpus callosum shows a large hemorrhage (*arrows*) in the callosal splenium. **C:** Image at the level of the frontoparietal convexities shows subarachnoid blood in medial hemispheric sulci (*curved arrows*) and a widened interhemispheric fissure (*straight arrows*), possible secondary to a dural rent or an adjacent subdural hematoma. (Courtesy of Dr. Alisa Gean, San Francisco).

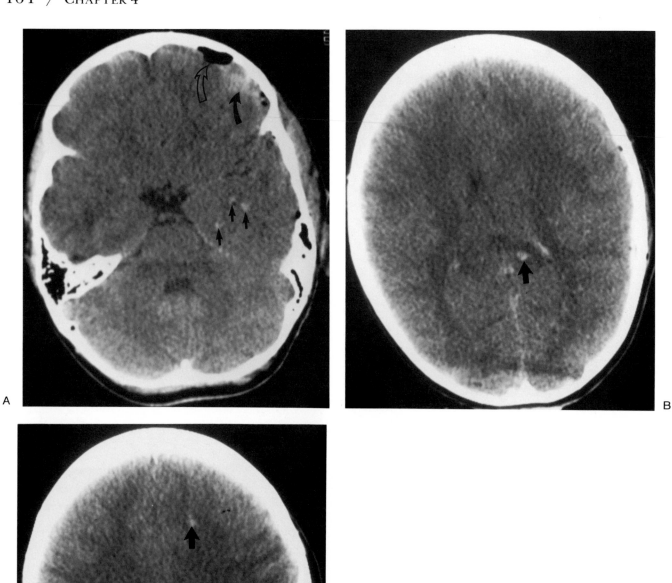

FIG. 4.54. Traumatic brain injury. Images A through C were obtained 20 hours after injury. Images D through F were obtained 2 months later. **A:** Axial CT image shows intracranial air (*open curved arrow*), subdural blood (*solid curved arrow*) and temporal lobe hemorrhages (*solid straight arrows*). **B:** Image at the level of the basal ganglia shows hemorrhage (*arrow*) in the callosal splenium, probably secondary to axonal shearing injury. The left gray matter–white matter junction is medially displaced by an acute subdural hematoma. The ventricles and sulci are compressed. **C:** CT image superior to B shows the subdural hematoma and a left frontal hemorrhage (*arrow*).

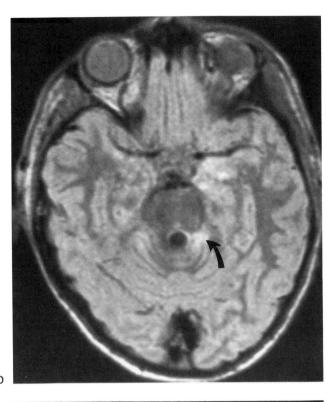

D

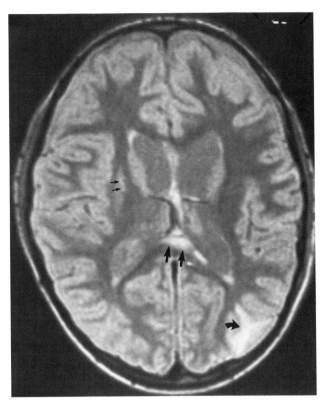

E

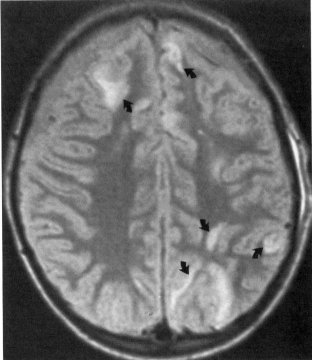

F

FIG. 4.54. (*Continued.*) **D–F:** Axial SE 2500/40 images show generalized atrophy and abnormal hyperintensity, presumably secondary to axonal shearing injuries, in the superior cerebellar peduncle (*large curved black arrow*), callosal splenium (*large straight arrows*), cortex–white matter junctions (*small curved black arrows*), and right putamen (*small straight arrows*).

Parenchymal lesions resulting from head trauma include *cerebral contusions* and *white matter shearing injuries.* Cerebral contusions are bruises of the brain most commonly caused by deceleration injuries in which the brain forcibly contacts the rough edges of the skull in the anterior temporal and orbitofrontal regions (148,199). Shearing injuries result from rotational forces on the skull. When the skull is rapidly rotated, the brain lags behind, causing axial stretching and disruption of nerve fiber tracts. Because the unmyelinated brain is less rigid than the mature brain (and consequently more susceptible to distortion) and because the subarachnoid spaces are more capacious, shearing injuries are a common consequence of rotational injury in infants and young children. Shearing injuries most commonly occur at the junction of the gray and white matter, in the deep white matter of the centrum semiovale, in the corpus callosum, the internal capsule, the basal ganglia, and the brain stem (148,186,200).

CT is sensitive in the diagnosis of hemorrhagic cerebral contusion in the acute phase because it is very sensitive to the presence of acute blood within the brain (186,199) (Fig. 4.52). In addition, CT is sensitive to the accompanying extra-axial hematomas or air that may be present, and the patient is easily monitored during a CT scan. Thus, as stated earlier, it is the imaging study of choice for evaluating acute head injury. However, CT is less sensitive than MR in the detection of nonhemorrhagic contusions and axonal shearing injuries (186). In the subacute or chronic phase, MR is the imaging modality of choice because long TR/TE scans are very sensitive to both the nonhemorrhagic and hemorrhagic injuries that are present at the site of prior contusions and shear injuries (Fig. 4.54) (123,125,186,199). Gradient echo studies with long echo times (20–30 msec), even more sensitive than long TR/TE spin echo studies for detecting products of hemorrhage, are an essential adjunct in the MR examination of trauma victims. CT scans may be normal, even when significant abnormalities can be detected by MR. Subacute injuries will be of high intensity on both long TR and short TR images because of the presence of edema and methemoglobin, respectively (Fig. 4.50). Chronic injuries will appear on long TR/TE images as areas of either high signal intensity (encephalomalacia, which has more water than normal brain (Fig. 4.54)] or low signal intensity [residual blood breakdown products from previous hemorrhage (Fig. 4.55)], or both. Both subacute and chronic hemorrhagic injuries are dark on gradient echo scans with long echo times. Lesions in characteristic locations, the orbitofrontal surface of the frontal lobes and the anterior temporal lobes, are strongly suggestive of prior trauma. Moreover, the location and number of injuries within the brain may be of prognostic value in terms of how

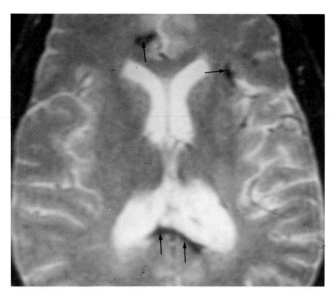

FIG. 4.55. Hemosiderin staining after brain injury. Axial GE 600/30 image shows multiple areas of hemosiderin staining (*arrows*).

much recovery of normal brain function can be expected.

Sequelae of Trauma

The sequelae of trauma include infarction from severe brain edema and vascular injury, infections, leptomeningeal cysts, and hydrocephalus (182). The imaging appearance of these conditions is discussed elsewhere in this book and will not be discussed extensively here.

Infarctions from severe brain edema and *leptomeningeal cysts* secondary to skull fractures are described earlier in this chapter.

Hydrocephalus frequently develops after head injuries, possibly as a result of inflammation and subsequent adhesions caused by subarachnoid blood. In children it is sometimes impossible to differentiate communicating hydrocephalus from cerebral atrophy, which can also result from trauma. Both can appear as dilatation of the cerebral ventricles and sulci on imaging studies, and both can result from severe cerebral injury (201). Differentiation can sometimes be made by careful analysis of the contours of the third ventricle (see Chapter 8). Alternatively, diagnosis can be made by monitoring intracranial pressure or by a radionuclide flow study with technetium-99M DTPA. The technetium compound is injected into the spinal subarachnoid space via lumbar puncture. If flow of the radionuclide upward over the cerebral convexities is not seen by 24 hours after its injection or if the radionuclide is seen within the lateral ventricles at 24 hours after injection, there is very likely a block to CSF flow and hydrocephalus (202,203). Of course, the most important features are clinical. An enlarging head size and sutural splitting indicate hydrocephalus, whereas a decreasing head circumference (compared to the normal distribution on head growth charts) suggests atrophy. Identification of hydrocephalus in this setting is important, as up to 75% of patients with posttraumatic hydrocephalus will show neurologic improvement after placement of a shunt (182).

Vascular complications of head injury include carotid-cavernous fistulas, arterial dissections, and venous sinus occlusions. Carotid cavernous fistulas present with pulsating exophthalmos, deficient ocular motility from multiple cranial nerve palsies and sometimes, blindness or subarachnoid hemorrhage. Catheter angiography is necessary for both diagnosis and treatment (see Chapter 12). Arterial dissections can present with obtundation, mono- or hemiparesis, dysphasia, or Horner syndrome. CT or MR are essential to diagnose cerebral infarction. T1-weighted spin echo MR of the skull base with fat saturation is very sensitive in establishing the diagnosis of dissection. A crescentic rim of hyperintensity, presumably methemoglobin, will be seen in the vessel wall. In some clinical settings, an MR diagnosis of dissection may obviate the need for catheter angiography. Venous sinus occlusion can be diagnosed either by two-dimensional time of flight MR angiography or by intravenous digital subtraction angiography, as described earlier in this chapter ("Ischemia Secondary to Venous Occlusion").

Infection is an uncommon complication of brain injury. When infection does occur, it is usually in the form of meningitis, secondary to bacterial seeding from basilar skull fracture, or cerebritis/abscess from penetrating injuries. The latter is extremely rare in children and is diagnosed from postcontrast CT or MR examinations (see Chapter 11). To diagnose a CSF leak from a basilar skull fracture, 3–5 ml of nonionic iodinated contrast is injected into the subarachnoid space via lumbar or C1–C2 puncture with the patient prone. The patient is then kept prone and tilted 45° (with head down) for 60–90 sec. The patient is maintained in the prone position while being transported to CT, where direct coronal 1.5-mm sections are obtained from the frontal sinuses through the temporal bones. If the patient is actively leaking, contrast will be seen dripping through a defect in the bone of the skull base.

Nonaccidental Trauma

Nonaccidental trauma (child abuse) is an increasing problem in pediatric health care, with an estimated 1.3 million cases every year (204). Of these, nearly half result in disfigurement, permanent neurologic or psychologic deficit, or death (204). Head trauma is the leading cause of morbidity and mortality in the abused child, especially in patients under the age of 2 years (205–207). One prospective study of head injuries in 100 children under the age of 2 years revealed that 24% were victims of abuse; this group had a higher risk of permanent brain damage and death than truly accidental injuries (208). Radiologists have traditionally played an important role in the diagnosis of child abuse by maintaining a high index of suspicion in children who have multiple instances of unexplained trauma. Although the diagnosis has classically been made by the use of bone radiographs, which demonstrate multiple fractures of different ages, brain imaging can make an important contribution. Brain imaging is especially important in the so-called shaken baby syndrome (206,207,209), characterized by retinal hemorrhages, subdural or subarachnoid hemorrhage, cerebral contusion, and diffuse cerebral edema with minimal evidence of external trauma. The injuries in child abuse victims can be the result of direct trauma, shaking injuries, strangulation, or a combination thereof. The direct injuries can result in skull fractures, subdural hematomas, and cerebral contusion of the coup–contrecoup variety. Vigorous shaking often causes axonal shearing injuries in the brain as well as associated subarachnoid and subdural hemorrhage (186–188,190,207,209).

The clinical presentation of the abused child is variable. The most common presentation is that of an irritable or abnormally subdued child who refuses meals and may vomit or have difficulty with respiration or cyanotic attacks (209). The child may present with recurrent encephalopathy, raising suspicion for metabolic disease or encephalitis (210). Another common presentation is seizures; the child may have an isolated seizure secondary to head injury or may present in status epilepticus. If the child presents with a history of head injury, the severity of the injury, typically a fall from a table or down stairs, does not match the severity of the injury.

Skull radiographs are still useful in establishing the diagnosis of child abuse, in that the incidence of skull fractures in affected patients is 45% (187). Multiple fractures, stellate fractures, bilateral fractures, fractures more than 5 mm wide at presentation, and depressed fractures should raise suspicion for nonaccidental trauma (210). Bone scintigraphy is not particularly useful in the diagnosis of linear skull fractures, because the osteoblastic response is limited. Moreover, as mentioned earlier, CT may miss linear skull fractures if they are parallel to the plane of section.

Both CT and MR can be of considerable assistance in the work-up of an abused child, both by confirming the diagnosis and by allowing assessment of the extent of brain injury (186–188,190). CT has advantages in the acute setting, as it is more sensitive in the detection of subarachnoid blood and calvarial fractures and is more easily performed on an unstable, acutely injured child. Often CT provides all the necessary information. MR is most useful when a high clinical suspicion of abuse has not been confirmed by CT.

Subdural hematomas, the most common intracranial manifestations of abuse, *subarachnoid hemorrhage,* and acute *cerebral contusions* (seen as ovoid accumulations of intraparenchymal blood with surrounding edema) can all be visualized by CT, although small subdurals near the base of the brain and vertex and small contusions in the middle cranial fossa may be difficult to detect. As mentioned earlier in the chapter, hemorrhage becomes more difficult to detect by CT after approximately 1 week, as the blood becomes isodense with brain. MR is much more sensitive in diagnosing subacute hematomas, both subdural (Fig. 4.56) and intraparenchymal (Fig. 4.57), and in detecting small hemorrhages at the vertex (Fig. 4.57), in transversely oriented locations (subfrontal, along the tentorium), and in the middle and posterior cranial fossae (186). MR may also allow differentiation of hemorrhages of differing ages (Fig. 4.57); however, caution should be exercised in trying to date

hemorrhages, as the MR appearance of hematomas varies with location, size, and stage of degradation (188).

Shearing injuries to the white matter are more sensitively detected by MR than by CT; they are identified by their characteristic locations (corticomedullary junction, centrum semiovale, corpus callosum) (see Fig. 4.54). The signal intensity of the shear injuries varies, depending upon their ages and the presence or lack of associated blood. As described in prior sections, acute hematomas are isointense with brain on T1-weighted spin echo sequences and hypointense on T2-weighted spin echo and gradient echo sequences. Subacute blood develops high signal intensity, first on short TR/TE and then on long TR/TE spin echo sequences. Old hemorrhage within the brain can be identified by the presence of old blood products, predominantly hemosiderin and ferritin, which appear as ill-defined areas of very low signal intensity on long TR/TE or gradient echo sequences (see Fig. 4.55).

The presence of compartments of subdural hemorrhage of differing ages or the presence of acute and subacute, acute and chronic, or subacute and chronic intraparenchymal hemorrhages is strongly suggestive of nonaccidental trauma (because injuries of different ages

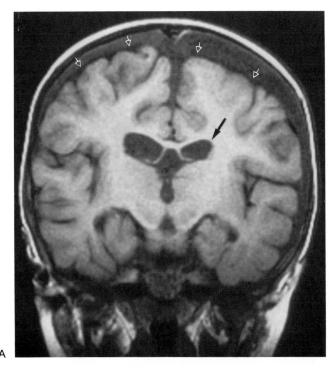

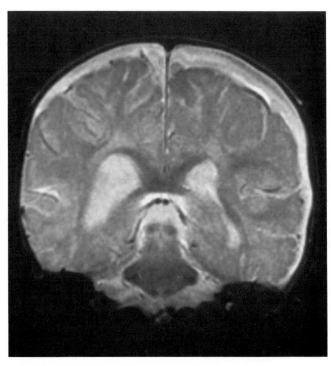

A   B

FIG. 4.56. Bilateral chronic subdural hematomas secondary to nonaccidental trauma. **A:** Coronal SE 600/20 image shows asymmetric subdural fluid collections. If these collections were symmetric, differentiation from benign enlargement of the subarachnoid spaces would be very difficult. However, the asymmetry and the mass effect upon the left lateral ventricle (black arrow) indicate the proper diagnosis. *Open white arrows* point to subarachnoid space. **B:** Coronal SE 2500/70 image fails to differentiate subdural fluid from subarachnoid fluid.

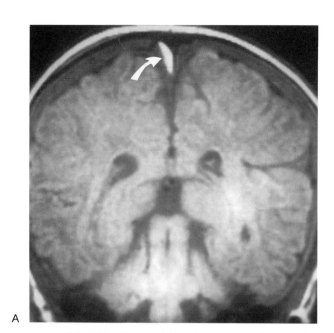
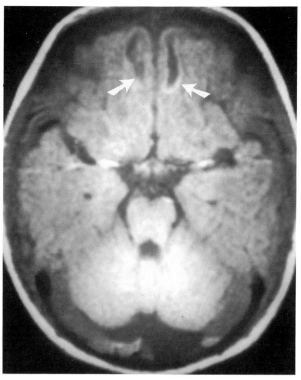

FIG. 4.57. Nonaccidental trauma. **A:** Coronal SE 600/15 image shows bilateral subdural fluid collections that are slightly hyperintense compared to CSF (and therefore likely old hematomas) and a focus (*arrow*) of subacute blood in the interhemispheric subdural space. **B:** Axial SE 600/15 image shows bilateral subacute orbitofrontal hematomas (*arrows*).

suggest repeated trauma). Gradient echo images are especially useful in suspected child abuse cases because of the exquisite sensitivity to regions of different magnetic susceptibilities. Areas of old hemorrhage will be seen on gradient echo images as areas of hypointensity that are larger and much more apparent than on the long TR/long TE spin echo images. (As discussed previously, fast spin echo sequences are rather insensitive to hemorrhage and should not be used in the setting of trauma.) The optimal parameters for the gradient echo images are TR = 100–250 msec, TE = 35 msec, and flip angle = 10°, if single slice acquisitions are used. A longer TR (in the range of 500–750 msec) can be employed if a multislice acquisition sequence is used. These images are obtained in addition to long TR/TE spin echo images, not substituted for them. The information they provide is complementary to that from spin echo images; significant parenchymal injury may be missed when GE sequences are employed exclusively.

Cerebral infarction can also occur in child abuse, as a result of vascular compression resulting from either brain edema or strangulation (211). Typically, the infarct is in the region of the middle cerebral artery distribution or in multiple arterial distributions (Fig. 4.58). When infarction of a large cerebral artery distribution or multiple distributions is seen in conjunction with subdural or subarachnoid hemorrhage in an infant, the possibility of nonaccidental trauma should be raised (211).

It is sometimes difficult to differentiate bilateral chronic subdural hematomas from benign infantile enlargement of the subarachnoid spaces, a condition in which the extra-axial CSF spaces are enlarged as a (presumed) result of immaturity of the arachnoid villi (see Chapter 8). When blood products are present in the subdural collections, the diagnosis of trauma (but not necessarily child abuse) can be confidently made. However, when the extra-axial fluid is nearly isointense with CSF on multiple pulse sequences (Fig. 4.56), differentiation is aided by the presence of asymmetry of the collections (only seen in subdural hematomas) and associated parenchymal injuries. If neither asymmetry nor parenchymal lesions are present, but clinical suspicion of trauma is high, follow-up CT or MR scans should be obtained to look for disappearance of the extra-axial collections that occurs during the second year of life in benign infantile hydrocephalus.

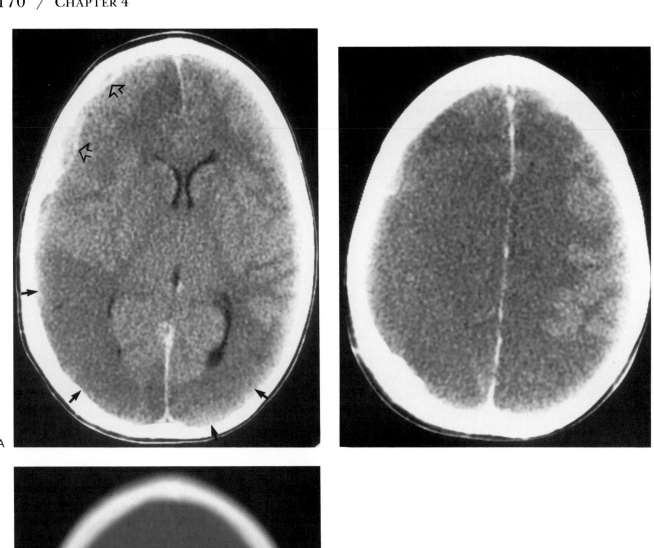

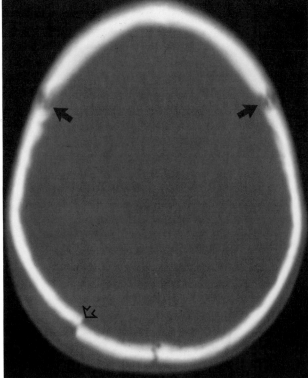

FIG. 4.58. Nonaccidental trauma. **A:** Axial noncontrast CT image shows right-to-left subfalcine shift, right subdural hematoma (*open arrows*), and hypodensity of the posterior cerebral hemispheres bilaterally (*solid arrows*), probably secondary to infarction. **B:** CT image at higher level shows hypodensity of the entire right cerebral hemisphere and the anterior and posterior portions of the left hemisphere. **C:** Bone windows of a CT image superior to B shows a depressed skull fracture (*open arrow*) and splitting of the coronal sutures (*solid arrows*). (Case courtesy of Dr. Alisa Gean, San Francisco).

REFERENCES

1. Friede RL. *Developmental neuropathology*, 2nd ed. Berlin: Springer-Verlag, 1989.
2. Raybaud C. Destructive lesions of the brain. *Neuroradiology* 1983;25:265–291.
3. Yakovlev PI, Wadsworth RC. Schizencephalies. A study of the congenital clefts in the cerebral mantle. 1. Clefts with fused lips. *J Neuropathol Exp Neurol* 1946;5:116–130.
4. Yakovlev PI, Wadsworth RC. Schizencephalies. A study of the congenital clefts in the cerebral mantle. 2. Clefts with hydrocephalus and lips separated. *J Neuropathol Exp Neurol* 1946;5:169–206.
5. Gilles FH. Neuropathologic indicators of abnormal development. In: Freeman JM, eds. *Prenatal and perinatal factors associated with brain disorders*. Bethesda: NIH, 1985:53–107.
6. Probst FP. *The prosencephalies: morphology, neuroradiological appearances and differential diagnosis*. Berlin: Springer-Verlag, 1979.
7. Friede RL, Mikolasek J. Postencephalitic porencephaly, hydranencephaly or polymicrogyria. A review. *Acta Neuropathol* 1978;43:161–168.
8. Warkany J, Lemire RJ, Cohen MM. *Mental retardation and congenital malformations of the central nervous system*. Chicago: Yearbook, 1981.
9. Volpe JJ. *Neurology of the newborn*. Philadelphia: WB Saunders, 1987.
10. Barkovich AJ. Metabolic and destructive brain disorders. In: Barkovich AJ, ed. *Pediatric neuroimaging*. New York: Raven, 1990: 35–75.
11. Young RSK. Neurologic aspects of cardiovascular disease. In: Berg BO, ed. *Neurologic aspects of pediatrics*. Boston: Butterworth-Heinemann, 1992:320–338.
12. Lanska MJ, Lanska DJ, Horwitz SJ, Aram DM. Presentation, clinical course, and outcome of childhood stroke. *Pediatr Neurol* 1991;7:333–341.
13. Bisset GS III, Scjwartz DC, Meyer RA, et al. Clinical spectrum and long-term follow-up of isolated mitral valve prolapse in 119 children. *Circulation* 1980;62:423–427.
14. Shuper Z, Vining EPG, Freeman JM. CNS vasculitis after chickenpox—cause or coincidence? *Arch Dis Child* 1990;65:1245–1248.
15. Liu GT, Holmes GL. Varicella with delayed contralateral hemiparesis detected by MRI. *Pediatr Neurol* 1990;6:131–134.
16. Israels SJ, Seshia SS. Childhood stroke associated with protein C or S deficiency. *J Pediatr* 1987;111:562–564.
17. Heier LA, Carpanzo CR, Mast J, Brill PW, Winchester P, Deck MDF. Maternal cocaine abuse: the spectrum of radiologic abnormalities in the neonatal CNS. *Am J Neuroradiol* 1991;12:951–956.
18. Hoyme HE, Jones KL, Dixon SD, et al. Prenatal cocaine syndrome and fetal vascular disruption. *Pediatrics* 1990;85:743–747.
19. Rossi LN, Penzien JM, Deonna T, et al. Does migraine-related stroke occur in childhood? *Dev Med Child Neurol* 1990;32:1005–1009.
20. Wagle WA, Haller JS, Cousins JP. Cerebral infarction in progeria. *Pediatr Neurol* 1992;8:476–477.
21. Gleuck CJ, Daniels SR, Bates S, et al. Pediatric victims of unexplained stroke and their families: familial lipid and lipoprotein abnormalities. *Pediatrics* 1982;69:308–316.
22. Edwards MSB, Hoffman HJ. *Cerebral vascular disease in children and adolescents*. Baltimore: Williams and Wilkins, 1989.
23. Yamada I, Yoshiharu M, Suzuki S. Moyamoya disease: diagnosis with three-dimensional time-of-flight MR angiography. *Radiology* 1992;184:773–778.
24. Wiznitzer M, Masaryk TJ. Cerebrovascular abnormalities in pediatric stroke: Assessment using parenchymal and angiographic magnetic resonance imaging. *Ann Neurol* 1991;29:585–589.
25. Smith AS, Wiznitzer M, Karaman BA, Horwitz SJ, Lanzieri CF. MRA detection of vascular occlusion in a child with progeria. *Am J Neuroradiol* 1993;14:441–443.
26. Maas KP, Barkovich AJ, Dong L, Edwards MSB, Piecuch RE, Charlton V. Selected indications for and applications of magnetic resonance angiography in children. *Pediatr Neurosurg* 1994;20: 113–125.
27. Mann CI, Dietrich RB, Schrader MT, Peck WW, Demos DS, Bradley WG Jr. Posttraumatic carotid artery dissection in children: evaluation with MR angiography. *Am J Roentgenol* 1993;160:134–136.
28. Del Toro J, Louis PT, Goddard-Finegold J. Cerebrovascular regulation and neonatal brain injury. *Pediatr Neurol* 1991;7:3–12.
29. Hill A. Current concepts of hypoxic–ischemic cerebral injury in the term newborn. *Pediatr Neurol* 1991;7:317–325.
30. Sotrel A, Lorenzo AV. Ultrastructure of blood vessels in the ganglionic eminence of premature rabbits with spontaneous germinal matrix hemorrhages. *J Neuropathol Exp Neurol* 1989;48: 462–482.
31. Steinlin M, Dirr R, Martin E, et al. MRI following severe perinatal asphyxia: preliminary experience. *Pediatr Neurol* 1991;7:164–170.
32. Keeney SE, Adcock EW, McArdle CB. Prospective observations of 100 high-risk neonates by high field (1.5 Tesla) magnetic resonance imaging of the central nervous system: I. Intraventricular and extracerebral lesions. *Pediatrics* 1991;87:421–430.
33. Keeney S, Adcock EW, McArdle CB. Prospective observations of 100 high-risk neonates by high field (1.5 Tesla) magnetic resonance imaging of the central nervous system: II. Lesions associated with hypoxic–ischemic encephalopathy. *Pediatrics* 1991;87: 431–438.
34. Barkovich AJ. MR and CT evaluation of profound neonatal and infantile asphyxia. *Am J Neuroradiol* 1992;13:959–972.
35. Koeda T, Suganuma I, Kohno Y, Takamatsu T, Takeshita K. MR imaging of spastic diplegia: comparative study between preterm and term infants. *Neuroradiology* 1990;32:187–190.
36. Wiklund L-M, Uvebrant P, Flodmark O. Morphology of cerebral lesions in children with congenital hemiplegia: a study with computed tomography. *Neuroradiology* 1990;32:179–186.
37. Barkovich AJ, Truwit CL. MR of perinatal asphyxia: Correlation of gestational age with pattern of damage. *Am J Neuroradiol* 1990;11:1087–1096.
38. Roland EH, Hill A, Norman MG, Flodmark O, MacNab AJ. Selective brainstem injury in an asphyxiated newborn. *Ann Neurol* 1988;23:89–92.
39. Pasternak JF, Predley TA, Mikhael MA. Neonatal asphyxia: vulnerability of basal ganglia, thalamus, and brainstem. *Pediatr Neurol* 1991;7:147–149.
40. McDonald JW, Johnston MV. Physiological and pathophysiological roles of excitatory amino acids during central nervous system development. *Brain Res Rev* 1990;15:41–70.
41. Greenamyre T, Penney JB, Young AB, Hudson C, Silverstein FS, Johnston MV. Evidence for transient perinatal glutamatergic innervation of globus pallidus. *J Neurosci* 1987;7:1022–1030.
42. Bourre J-M. Developmental synthesis of myelin lipids: origin of fatty acids—specific role of nutrition. In: Evrard P, Minkowski A, eds. *Developmental neurobiology*. Nestle nutrition workshop series. New York: Raven, 1989:
43. Dobbing J. Vulnerable periods of brain development. In: Dobbing J, eds. *Lipids, malnutrition and the developing brain*. Amsterdam: Elsevier, 1972:9–23.
44. Chugani HT, Phelps ME, Mazziotta JC. Positron emission tomography study of human brain functional development. *Ann Neurol* 1987;22:487–497.
45. Hasegawa M, Houdou S, Mito T, Takashima S, Asanuma K, Ohno T. Development of myelination in the human fetal and infant cerebrum: a myelin basic protein immunohistochemical study. *Brain Dev* 1992;14:1–6.
46. Kuban KCK, Gilles FH. Human telencephalic angiogenesis. *Ann Neurol* 1985;17:539–548.
47. Nelson MD Jr, Gonzalez-Gomez I, Gilles FH. The search for human telencephalic ventriculofugal arteries. *Am J Neuroradiol* 1991;12:215–222.
48. Van den Bergh R. Centrifugal elements in the vascular pattern of the deep intracerebral blood supply. *Angiology* 1969;20:88–94.
49. Takashima S, Tanaka K. Development of the cerebrovascular architecture and its relationship to periventricular leukomalacia. *Arch Neurol* 1978;35:11–16.
50. DeReuck J. The human periventricular arterial blood supply and

the anatomy of cerebral infarctions. *Europ Neurol* 1971; 5:321–334.

51. Volpe JJ, Herscovitch P, Perlman JM, Raichle ME. Positron emission tomography in the newborn: extensive impairment of regional blood flow with intraventricular hemorrhage and hemorrhagic intracerebral involvement. *Pediatrics* 1983;72:589–595.

52. Flodmark O, Roland EH, Hill A, Whitfield MF. Periventricular leukomalacia: radiologic diagnosis. *Radiology* 1987;162:119–124.

53. Flodmark O, Lupton B, Li D, et al. MR imaging of periventricular leukomalacia in childhood. *Am J Neuroradiol* 1989;10:111–118.

54. Greisen G. Ischemia of the preterm brain. *Biol Neonate* 1992;62:243–247.

55. Hambleton G, Wigglesworth JS. Origin of intraventricular hemorrhage in the pre-term infant. *Arch Dis Child* 1976; 51:651–660.

56. Wigglesworth JS, Pape KE. An integrated model for hemorrhage and ischemic lesions in the newborn brain. *Early Hem Dev* 1978;2:179–199.

57. Gressens P, Richelme C, Kadhim HJ, Gadisseux J-F, Evrard P. The germinative zone produces the most cortical astrocytes after neuronal migration in the developing mammalian brain. *Biol Neonate* 1992;61:4.24.

58. Gould SJ, Howard S, Hope PL, Reynolds EOR. Periventricular intraparenchymal cerebral hemorrhage in preterm infants: the role of venous infarction. *J Pathol* 1987;151:197–202.

59. Van de Bor M, Ens-Dokkum M, Schreuder AM, Veen S, Brand R, Verloove-Vanhorick SP. Outcome of periventricular–intraventricular hemorrhage at five years of age. *Dev Med Child Neurol* 1993;35:33–41.

60. Roth SC, Baudin J, McCormick DC, et al. Relation between ultrasound appearance of the brain of very preterm infants and neurodevelopmental impairment at eight years. *Dev Med Child Neurol* 1993;35:755–768.

61. Ramaekers G. Embryology and anatomy of the corpus callosum. In: Ramaekers G, Njiokikjtien C, eds. *Pediatric behavioural neurology.* Vol. 3: *The child's corpus callosum.* Amsterdam: Suyi, 1991:24.39.

62. Zuerrer M, Martin E, Boltshauser E. MR imaging of intracranial hemorrhage in neonates and infants at 2.35 Tesla. *Neuroradiology* 1991;33:223–229.

63. Shuman RM, Selednik LJ. Periventricular leukomalacia: a one year autopsy study. *Arch Neurol* 1980;37:231–235.

64. Banker BQ, Larroche JC. Periventricular leukomalacia of infancy: a form of neonatal anoxic encephalopathy. *Arch Neurol* 1962;7:386–410.

65. Vannucci RC, Christensen MA, Yager JY. Nature, time-course, and extent of cerebral edema in perinatal hypoxic–ischemic brain damage. *Pediatr Neurol* 1993;9:29–34.

66. Grant EG, Schellinger D, Richardson JD, Coffey ML, Smirniotopoulous JG. Echogenic periventricular halo: normal sonographic finding or neonatal cerebral hemorrhage? *AJNR* 1983;4:43–46.

67. Dipietro MA, Brody BA, Teele RL. Periventricular echogenic "blush" on cranial sonography: pathologic correlates. *AJNR* 1986;7:305–310.

68. Baarsma R, Laurini RN, Baerts W, Okken A. Reliability of sonography in non-hemorrhagic periventricular leucomalacia. *Pediatr Radiol* 1987;17:189–191.

69. Carson SC, Hertzberg BS, Bowie JD, Burger PC. Value of sonography in the diagnosis of intracranial hemorrhage and periventricular leukomalacia: a postmortem study of 35 cases. *Am J Neuroradiol* 1990;11:677–684.

70. Paneth N, Rudelli E, Monte W, et al. White matter necrosis in very low birth weight infants: neuropathologic and ultrasonographic findings in infants surviving six days or longer. *J Pediatr* 1990;116:975–984.

71. Sauerbrei EE. Serial brain sonography in two children with leukomalacia and cerebral palsy. *J Can Assoc Radiol* 1984;35:164–167.

72. Schellinger D, Grant EG, Richardson JD. Cystic periventricular leukomalacia: sonographic and CT findings. *AJNR* 1984;5:439–445.

73. Dubowitz LMS, Bydder GM, Mushin J. Developmental sequence of periventricular leukomalacia: correlation of ultrasound, clinical, and nuclear magnetic resonance functions. *Arch Dis Child* 1985; 60:349–355.

74. Sudakoff GS, Mitchell DG, Stanley C, Graziani LJ. Frontal periventricular cysts on the first day of life: a one year clinical follow-up and its significance. *J Ultrasound Med* 1991;10:25–30.

75. De Vries LS, Eken P, Dubowitz LMS. The spectrum of leukomalacia using cranial ultrasound. *Beh Brain Res* 1992;49:1–6.

76. Schouman-Clays E, Henry-Feugeas M-C, Roset F, et al. Periventricular leukomalacia: correlation between MR imaging and autopsy findings during the first 2 months of life. *Radiology* 1993;189:59–64.

77. Baker LL, Stevenson DK, Enzmann DR. End stage periventricular leukomalacia: MR imaging evaluation. *Radiology* 1988;168:809–815.

78. de la Monte SM, Hsu FI, Hedley-Whyte ET, Kupsky W. Morphometric analysis of the human infant brain: effects of intraventricular hemorrhage and periventricular leukomalacia. *J Child Neurol* 1989;4:101–110.

79. Evrard P, Gadisseux JF, Gerriere G, Lyon G. Le développement prénatal du système nerveux central et ses perturbations. In: Ferriere G, eds. *La déficience mentale: causes, prévention, et traitement.* Brussels: Prodim, 1989:11–93.

80. Evrard P, Belpaire MC, Boog G, et al. Diagnostique anténatal des affections du système nerveux central: résultats préliminaires d'une étude multicentrique européenne. *J Français d'Echographie* 1985;2:123–126.

81. Leech RW, Alvord EC Jr. Anoxic ischemic encephalopathy in the human neonatal period: the significance of brain stem involvement. *Arch Neurol* 1977;34:109–113.

82. Gilles FH, Leviton A, Dooling EC. *The developing human brain.* Boston: John Wright-PSG, 1983.

83. Johnson MA, Pennock JM, Bydder GM, et al. Clinical MR imaging of the brain in children: normal and neurologic disease. *Am J Roentgenol* 1983;141:1005–1018.

84. Johnson MA, Pennock JM, Bydder GM, et al. Serial MR imaging in neonatal cerebral injury. *Am J Neuroradiol* 1987;8:83–92.

85. Byrne P, Welch R, Johnson MA, Darrah J, Piper M. Serial magnetic resonance imaging in neonatal hypoxic–ischemic encephalopathy. *J Pediatr* 1990;117:694.700.

86. Takashima S, Tanaka K. Subcortical leukomalacia, relationship to development of the cerebral sulcus, and its vascular supply. *Arch Neurol* 1978;35:470–476.

87. Schneider H, Ballowitz L, Schachinger H, Hanefeld F, Droszus JU. Anoxic encephalopathy with predominant involvement of basal ganglia, brain stem, and spinal cord in the perinatal period. *Acta Neuropathologica* 1975;32:287–298.

88. Hayashi M, Satoh J, Sakamoto K, Morimatsu Y. Clinical and neuropathological findings in severe athetoid cerebral palsy: a comparative study of globo-luysian and thalamo-putaminal groups. *Brain Dev* 1991;13:47–51.

89. Kerrigan JF, Chugani HT, Phelps ME. Regional cerebral glucose metabolism in clinical subtypes of cerebral palsy. *Pediatr Neurol* 1991;7:415–425.

90. Menkes J, Curran JG. Clinical and magnetic resonance imaging correlates in children with extrapyramidal cerebral palsy. *Am J Neuroradiol* 1994;15:451–457.

91. Phillips R, Brandberg G, Hill A, Roland E, Poskitt K. Prevalence and prognostic value of abnormal CT findings in 100 term asphyxiated newborns. *Radiology* 1993;189P:287.

92. Van Bogaert P, Baleriaux D, Christophe C, Szliwowski HB. MRI of patients with cerebral palsy and normal CT scan. *Neuroradiology* 1992;34:52–56.

93. Van de Bor M, Guit GL, Schreuder AM, et al. Does very preterm birth impair myelination of the central nervous system? *Neuropediatrics* 1990;21:37–39.

94. Mitchell W, O'Tuama L. Cerebral intraventricular hemorrhages in infants: a widening age spectrum. *Pediatrics* 1980;65:35–39.

95. Roland EH, Flodmark O, Hill A. Thalamic hemorrhage with intraventricular hemorrhage in the full-term newborn. *Pediatrics* 1990;85:737–742.

96. Fitch SJ, Gerald B, Magill HL, Tonkin ILD. Central nervous system hypoxia in children due to near drowning. *Radiology* 1985;156:647–650.

97. Kjos BO, Brant-Zawadzki M, Young RG. Early CT findings of

global central nervous system hypoperfusion. *AJR* 1983;141: 1227–1232.

98. Bird CR, Drayer BP, Gilles FH. Pathophysiology of reverse edema in global cerebral ischemia. *AJNR* 1989;10:95–98.

99. Han BK, Towbin RB, De Courten-Myers G, McLaurin RL, Ball WS Jr. Reversal sign on CT: effect of anoxic/ischemic cerebral injury in children. *Am J Neuroradiol* 1989;10:1191–1198.

100. Volpe JJ. Hypoglycemia and brain injury. In: Volpe JJ, eds. *Neurology of the newborn*. Philadelphia: WB Saunders, 1987:364.385.

101. Cornblath M, Schwartz P. *Disorders of carbohydrate metabolism in infancy*. Philadelphia: WB Saunders, 1976.

102. Huang C-C, Shen E-Y. Tentorial subdural hemorrhage in term newborns: ultrasonographic diagnosis and clinical correlates. *Pediatr Neurol* 1991;7:171–177.

103. Sexson WR. Incidence of neonatal hypoglycemia: a matter of definition. *J Pediatr* 1984;105:149–153.

104. Vannucci RC, Randis EE, Vannucci SJ. Cerebral metabolism during hypoglycemia and asphyxia in newborn dogs. *Biol Neonate* 1980;38:276–283.

105. Hernandez M, Vannucci R, Salcedo A, Brennan R. Cerebral blood flow and metabolism during hypoglycemia in modern dogs. *J Neurochem* 1980;35:622–626.

106. Vannucci RC, Nardis EE, Vannucci SJ, Campbell PA. Cerebral carbohydrate and energy metabolism during hypoglycemia in newborn dogs. *Am J Physiol* 1981;240:192–198.

107. Banker BQ. The neuropathological effects of anoxia and hypoglycemia in the newborn. *Dev Med Child Neurol* 1967;9:544.550.

108. Anderson JM, Milner RDG, Strich SJ. Effects of neonatal hypoglycaemia on the nervous system: a pathological study. *J Neurol Neurosurg Psychiatr* 1967;30:295–310.

109. Volpe JJ. Bilirubin and brain injury. In: Volpe JJ, ed. *Neurology of the newborn*. Philadelphia: WB Saunders, 1987:386–408.

110. Maisels MJ. Jaundice in the newborn. *Pediatr Rev* 1982;3:305–313.

111. Jones M, Sands R, Hyman C, et al. Longitudinal study of the incidence of central nervous system damage following erythroblastosis fetalis. *Pediatrics* 1954;14:346–354.

112. Van Praagh R. Diagnosis of kernicterus in the neonatal period. *Pediatrics* 1961;28:870–874.

113. Peden CJ, Cowan F, Bryant KJ, Cox IJ, Menon DK, Young IR. Proton and phosphorus MR spectroscopy of infants with hypoxic—ischemic brain injury. *Radiology* 1990;177P:123.

114. Moorcraft J, Bolas NM, Ives NK, et al. Spatially localized magnetic resonance spectroscopy of the brains of normal and asphyxiated newborns. *Pediatrics* 1991;87:273–282.

115. Laptook AR, Corbett RJT, Nguyen HT, Peterson J, Nunnally RL. Alterations in cerebral blood flow and phosphorylated metabolites in piglets during and after partial ischemia. *Pediatr Res* 1988;23:206–211.

116. Laptook AR, Corbett RJ, Uauy R, Mize C, Mendelsohn D, Nunnally RL. Use of 31P magnetic resonance spectroscopy to characterize evolving brain damage after perinatal asphyxia. *Neurology* 1989;39:709–712.

117. Azzopardi D, Wyatt JS, Cady EB, et al. Prognosis of newborn infants with hypoxic–ischemic brain injury assessed by phosphorus magnetic resonance spectroscopy. *Pediatr Res* 1989;25:445–451.

118. Peden CJ, Cowan FM, Bryant DJ, et al. Proton MR spectroscopy of the brain in infants. *J Comput Assist Tomogr* 1990;14:886–894.

119. Van der Grond J, Veenhoven RH, Groenendaal F, de Vries LS, Mali WP. MR spectroscopy in full-term infants with perinatal asphyxia. (abs.) *Radiology* 1992;185(P):185.

120. Mattle HP, Wentz KU, Edelman RR, et al. Cerebral venography with MR. *Radiology* 1991;178:453–458.

121. Chakeres DW, Schmalbrock P, Brogan M, Yuan C, Cohen L. Normal venous anatomy of the brain: demonstration with gadopentetate dimeglumine in enhanced 3-D MR angiography. *AJNR* 1990;11:1107–1118.

122. Kelly AB, Zimmerman RD, Snow RB, Gandhi SE, Heier LA, Deck MDF. Head trauma: comparison of MR and CT—experience in 100 patients. *AJNR* 1988;9:699–708.

123. Han JS, Kaufman B, Alfidi RJ, et al. Head trauma evaluated by magnetic resonance and computed tomography: a comparison. *Radiology* 1984;150:71–77.

124. Gentry LR, Godersky JC, Thompson B, et al. Prospective comparative study of intermediate-field MR and CT in the evaluation of closed head trauma. *Am J Neuroradiol* 1988;9:101–110.

125. Snow RB, Zimmerman RD, Gandy SE, Deck MDF. Comparison of MRI and CT in the evaluation of head injury. *Neurosurgery* 1986;18:45–52.

126. Gentry LR, Godersky JC, Thompson BH. Traumatic brain stem injury: MR imaging. *Radiology* 1989;171:177–187.

127. Barkovich AJ, Atlas SW. MRI of intracranial hemorrhage. *Radiol Clin N Am* 1988;26:801–820.

128. Sullivan CR, Bruwer AJ, Harris LE. Hypermobility of the cervical spine in children: a pitfall in the diagnosis of cervical dislocation. *Am J Surg* 1958;95:636–640.

129. Rossitch E Jr, Oakes WJ. Perinatal spinal cord injury: clinical radiographic and pathologic features. *Pediatr Neurosurg* 1992;18:149–152.

130. Osenbach RK, Menezes AH. Spinal cord injury without radiographic abnormality in children. *Pediatr Neurosci* 1989;15:168–174.

131. Pang D, Wilberger JE Jr. Spinal cord injury without radiographic abnormalities in children. *J Neurosurg* 1982;57:114.129.

132. Dickman CA, Rekate HL, Sonntag VKH, Zabramski JM. Pediatric spinal trauma: vertebral column and spinal cord injuries in children. *Pediatr Neurosci* 1989;15:237–256.

133. Leventhal HR. Birth injuries of the spinal cord. *J Pediatr* 1960;56:447–453.

134. Byers RK. Spinal cord injuries during birth. *Dev Med Child Neurol* 1975;17:103–110.

135. Koch BM, Eng GM. Neonatal spinal cord injury. *Arch Phys Med Rehabil* 1979;60:378–381.

136. Ford FR. Breech delivery in its possible relations to injury of the spinal cord, with special reference to infantile paraplegia. *Arch Neurol Psychiatr* 1925;14:742–750.

137. Towbin A. Spinal cord and brain stem injury at birth. *Arch Pathol* 1964;77:620–632.

138. Edwards MSB, Cogen PH. Craniospinal trauma in children. In: Berg BO, ed. *Neurological aspects of pediatrics*. Boston: Butterworth-Heinemann, 1992:595–613.

139. Castillo M, Quencer RM, Green BA. Cervical spinal cord injury after traumatic breech delivery. *Am J Neuroradiol* 1989;10:S99.

140. Kulkarni MV, McArdle CB, Kopanicky D, et al. Acute spinal cord injury: MR imaging at 1.5T. *Radiology* 1987;164:837–843.

141. Schaefer DM, Flanders AE, Osterholm JL, Northrup BE. Prognostic significance of magnetic resonance imaging in the acute phase of cervical spine injury. *J Neurosurg* 1992;76:218–223.

142. Gordon M, Rich H, Deutschberger J, Green M. The immediate and long term outcome of obstetric birth trauma. I. Brachial plexus paralysis. *Am J Obstet Gynecol* 1973;117:51–61.

143. Eng GD. Brachial plexus palsy in newborn infants. *Pediatrics* 1971;48:18–26.

144. Hashimoto T, Mitomo M, Hirabuki N. Nerve root avulsion of birth palsy: comparison of myelography with CT myelography and somatosensory evoked potential. *Radiology* 1991;178:841–845.

145. Miller S, Glasier C, Griebel M, Boop F. Brachial plexopathy in infants after traumatic delivery: evaluation with MR imaging. *Radiology* 1993;189:481–484.

146. Thornbury JR, Campbell JA, Masters SJ, Fryback DG. Skull fracture and the low risk of intracranial sequelae in minor head trauma. *Am J Roentgenol* 1984;143:661–664.

147. Masters SJ, McClean PM, Arcarese JS, et al. Skull x-ray examination after head trauma: recommendations by a multidisciplinary panel and validation study. *N Engl J Med* 1987;316:84.91.

148. Lindenberg R. Pathology of craniocerebral injuries. In: Newton TH, Potts DG, eds. *Anatomy and pathology*. In: Newton TH, Potts DG, eds. *Radiology of the skull and brain*. St Louis: CV Mosby, 1977:3049–3087.

149. Chuang SH, Fitz CR. CT of head trauma. In: Gonzales CF, Grossman CB, Masdeu JC, eds. *CT of the head and spine*. New York: Wiley, 1985:523–536.

150. Harwood-Nash DC, Hendrick EB, Hudson AR. The significance

of skull fracture in children. A study of 1187 patients. *Radiology* 1971;101:151–160.

151. Adams JH. Head injury. In: Adams JH, Corsellis JAN, Duchen LW, eds. *Greenfield's neuropathology.* New York: Wiley, 1984: 85–124.

152. Eames FA, Waldman JB. CT of posttraumatic intradiploic meningocele of the skull base: a case report. *AJNR* 1991;12:985–987.

153. Gean A. *Imaging of head trauma.* New York: Raven, 1994.

154. Numerow LM, Krcek JP, Wallace CJ, Tranmer BI, Auer RN, Fong TC. Growing skull fracture simulating a rounded lytic calvarial lesion. *AJNR* 1991;12:783–784.

155. Koch TK, Jahnke S, Edwards MSB, Davis RL. Posterior fossa hemorrhage in term newborns. *Pediatr Neurol* 1985;1:96–102.

156. Hernansanz J, Munoz F, Rodriquez M, et al. Subdural hematomas of the posterior fossa in normal-weight newborns. *J Neurosurg* 1984;61:972–977.

157. Lau LSW, Pike JW. The CT findings of peritentorial subdural hemorrhage. *Radiology* 1983;146:699–701.

158. Gomori JM, Grossman RI, Goldberg HI, Zimmerman RA, Bilaniuk LP. Intracranial hematomas: Imaging by high field MR. *Radiology* 1985;157:87–93.

159. Hayman LA, Taber KH, Ford JJ, Bryan RN. Mechanisms of MR signal alteration by acute intracerebral blood: old concepts and new theories. *Am J Neuroradiol* 1991;12:899–907.

160. Schreiber MS. Some observations on certain head injuries in infants and children. *Med J Aust* 1957;2:930–936.

161. Rivera FP, Kamitsuka MD, Quan L. Injuries to children younger than one year of age. *Pediatrics* 1988;81:93–97.

162. Wilberger JE Jr. *Spinal cord injuries in children.* Mt Kisco, NY: Futura, 1986.

163. Hadley MN, Zabramski JM, Browner CM, Rekate H, Sonntag VKH. Pediatric spinal trauma. Review of 122 cases of spinal cord and vertebral column injuries. *J Neurosurg* 1988;68:18–24.

164. Anderson JM, Schutt AH. Spinal injury in children. A review of 156 cases seen from 1950 through 1978. *Mayo Clin Proc* 1980;55: 499–504.

165. Cattell HS, Filtzer DL. Pseudosubluxation and other normal variations in the cervical spine in children. A study of one hundred and sixty children. *J Bone Joint Surg* 1965;47A:1295–1309.

166. Fielding JW. Cervical spine injuries in children. In: The Cervical Spine Research Society, eds. *The cervical spine.* Philadelphia: JB Lippincott, 1983:268–281.

167. Johnson DL, Falci S. The diagnosis and treatment of pediatric lumbar spine injuries caused by rear seat lap belts. *Neurosurgery* 1990;26:434.441.

168. Sivit CJ, Taylor GA, Newman KD, et al. Safety belt injuries in children with lap-belt ecchymosis: CT findings in 61 patients. *Am J Roentgenol* 1991;157:111–114.

169. Taylor GA, Eggli KD. Lap-belt injuries of the lumbar spine in children: a pitfall in CT diagnosis. *Am J Roentgenol* 1988;150: 1355–1358.

170. Kraus JF. Epidemiological aspects of acute spinal cord injury. A review of incidence, prevalence, causes, and outcome. In: Becker DP, Povlishock JT, eds. *Central nervous system trauma status report.* Bethesda, MD: NIH, 1985:313–322.

171. Hill SA, Miller CA, Kosnik EJ, Hunt WE. Pediatric neck injuries. A clinical study. *J Neurosurg* 1984;60:700–706.

172. Banerian KG, Wang A-Y, Samberg LC, Kerr HH, Wesolowski DP. Association of vertebral end plate fracture with pediatric lumbar intervertebral disk herniation: value of CT and MR imaging. *Radiology* 1990;177:763–765.

173. Gennuso R, Humphries RP, Hoffman HJ, Hendrick EB, Drake JM. Lumbar intervertebral disc disease in the pediatric population. *Pediatr Neurosci* 1992;18:282–286.

174. Flanders AE, Schaefer DM, Doan HT, Mishkin MM, Gonzalez CF, Northrup BE. Acute cervical spine trauma: correlation of MR imaging findings with degree of neurologic deficit. *Radiology* 1990;177:25–33.

175. Hackney DB. Denominators of spinal cord injury. *Radiology* 1990;177:18–20.

176. Blennow G, Starck L. Anterior spinal artery syndrome: report of seven cases in childhood. *Pediatr Neurosci* 1987;13:32–37.

177. Choi J-U, Hoffman HJ, Hendrick EB, Humphreys RP, Keith WS. Traumatic infarction of the spinal cord in children. *J Neurosurg* 1986;65:608–610.

178. Ahmann PA, Smith SA, Schwartz JF, et al. Spinal cord infarction due to minor trauma in children. *Neurology* 1975;25:301–307.

179. Hecht JT, Butler IJ. Neurologic morbidity associated with achondoplasia. *J Child Neurol* 1990;5:84.97.

180. Kao SCS, Waziri MH, Smith WL, Sato Y, Yuh WTC, Franken EA Jr. MR imaging of the craniovertebral junction, cranium, and brain in children with achondoplasia. *Am J Roentgenol* 1989;153:565–569.

181. Menkes J. *Textbook of child neurology.* Philadelphia: Lea & Febiger, 1985.

182. Humphries RP. Complications of pediatric head trauma. *Pediatr Neurosurg* 1991–1992;17:274–278.

183. Fobbin J, Grossman R, Atlas S. MR characterization of subdural hematomas and hygromas at 1.5T. *Am J Neuroradiol* 1989;10: 687–693.

184. Luerssen TG, Klauber MR, Marshall LF. Outcome from head injury related to the patients's age. *J Neurosurg* 1988;68:409–416.

185. Merten DF, Osborne DRS, Radkowski MA, et al. Craniocerebral trauma in the child abuse syndrome: radiological observations. *Pediatr Radiol* 1984;14:272–277.

186. Sato Y, Yuh WTC, Smith WL, Alexander RC, Kao SCS, Ellerbroek CJ. Head injury in child abuse: Evaluation with MR imaging. *Radiology* 1989;173:653–660.

187. Harwood-Nash DC. Abuse to the pediatric central nervous system. *Am J Neuroradiol* 1992;13:569–575.

188. Ball WS Jr. Nonaccidental craniocerebral trauma (child abuse): MR imaging. *Radiology* 1989;173:609–610.

189. Moyes PD. Subdural effusions in infancy. *Can Med Assoc J* 1969;100:231–235.

190. Zimmerman RA, Bilaniuk LT, Bruce D, et al. Computed tomography of cerebral injury in the abused child. *Radiology* 1979;130: 687–690.

191. Grossman RI, Gomori JM, Goldberg HI, et al. MR imaging of hemorrhagic conditions of the head and neck. *Radiographics* 1988;8:441–454.

192. Gomori JM, Grossman RI, Steiner I. High-field magnetic resonance imaging of intracranial hematomas. *Isr J Med Sci* 1988;24: 218–223.

193. Dolinskas C, Zimmerman RA, Bilaniuk LT. A sign of subarachnoid bleeding on cranial computed tomography of pediatric head trauma patients. *Radiology* 1978;126:409–411.

194. Endo M, Ichikawa F, Miyasaka Y, Yada K, Ohwada T. Capsular and thalamic infarction caused by tentorial herniation subsequent to head trauma. *Neuroradiology* 1991;33:296–299.

195. Levin H, Aldrich E, Saydjari C, et al. Severe head injury in children: experience of the traumatic coma data bank. *Neurosurgery* 1992;31:435–444.

196. Aldrich EF, Eisenberg HM, Saydjari C, et al. Diffuse brain swelling in severely head-injured children: a report from the NIH Traumatic Coma Data Bank. *J Neurosurg* 1992;76:450–454.

197. Bruce DA, Alavi A, Bilaniuk L, et al. Diffuse cerebral swelling following head injuries in children: the syndrome of "malignant brain edema." *J Neurosurg* 1981;54:170–178.

198. Mendelsohn D, Levin HS, Burce D, et al. Late MRI after head injury in children: relationship to clinical features and outcome. *Childs Nerv Syst* 1992;8:445–452.

199. Hesselink JR, Dowd CF, Healy ME, et al. MR imaging of brain contusions: a comparative study with CT. *Am J Neuroradiol* 1988;9:269–278.

200. Gentry LR, Godersky JC, Thompson B. MR imaging of head trauma: review of the distribution and radiopathologic features of traumatic lesions. *Am J Neuroradiol* 1988;9:101–110.

201. Fitz CR, Harwood-Nash DC. CT of hydrocephalus. *Comput Tomogr* 1978;2:91–108.

202. Guertin SR. Cerebrospinal fluid shunts. Evaluation, complications, and crisis management. *Pediatr Clin North Am* 1987;34: 203–217.

203. Howman-Giles R, McLaughlin A, Johnston I, Whittle I. A radionuclide method of evaluating shunt function and CSF circulation in hydrocephalus. Technical note. *J Neurosurg* 1984;61:604.605.

204. Child Protection Division of the American Humane Association.

National analysis of official child neglect and abuse reporting, 1982. Denver: American Humane Association, 1982.

205. Kempe CH, Silverman FN, Steele BF, et al. The battered child syndrome. *JAMA* 1962;181:17–24.

206. Caffey J. On the theory and practice of shaking infants: its potential residual effects of permanent brain damage and mental retardation. *Am J Dis Child* 1972;124:161–169.

207. Caffey J. The whiplash shaken infant syndrome: manual shaking by the extremities with whiplash induced intracranial hemorrhage linked with residual permanent brain damage and mental retardation. *Pediatr* 1974;54:396–403.

208. Duhaime A, Alario A, Lewander W, et al. Head injury in very young children: mechanisms, injury types, and ophthalmological findings in 100 hospitalized patients younger than 2 years. *Pediatrics* 1992;90:179–185.

209. Duhaime A-C, Gennarelli TA, Thibault LE, Bruce DA, Margulies SS, Wiser R. The shaken baby syndrome: a clinical, pathological, and biomechanical study. *J Neurosurg* 1987;66:409–415.

210. Brown J, Minns R. Non-accidental head injury, with particular reference to whiplash shaking injury and medicolegal aspects. *Dev Med Child Neurol* 1993;35:849–869.

211. Bird CR, McMahan JR, Gilles FH, Senac MO, Apthorp JS. Strangulation in child abuse: CT diagnosis. *Radiology* 1987;163:373–375.

CHAPTER 5

Congenital Malformations of the Brain and Skull

BASIC CONCEPTS: EMBRYOLOGY OF THE BRAIN

Concepts

As will become evident in the sections that follow, most structures of the brain (including the cerebral cortex, corpus callosum, cerebellum, and deep cerebral nuclei) form at about the same time. Therefore, an injury to the developing brain often results in anomalies of more than one structure. For example, cerebellar anomalies may have associated anomalies of neuronal migration, cephaloceles often have associated anomalies of the corpus callosum, and holoprosencephalies frequently have associated anomalies of the corpus callosum and the cerebral cortex. The reader should keep this high incidence of multiple anomalies in mind when reviewing imaging studies: If you find one anomaly, you should start to look hard for a second and a third.

One result of the simultaneous formation of the structures that form the brain is a difficulty in the classification of anomalies of the structures. Any attempt to classify brain anomalies into a few large groups based on embryology or morphology runs into difficulties because of the frequency of multiple anomalies. Should cephaloceles with heterotopic gray matter and callosal agenesis be classified as a disorder of neural tube closure, of neuronal migration, or of commissuration? Because of this difficulty of classification, this chapter is largely descriptive. I describe anomalies of the various structures of the brain (i.e., corpus callosum, cerebral cortex) and discuss the embryology of those structures but do not attempt to group the disorders otherwise, as was done in Chapter 9, on anomalies of the spine.

One final important concept concerns the causes of brain anomalies. In discussing the various brain anomalies, I often discuss the time during which the affected portion of the brain forms. An injury (of any type) to the brain at the time a particular structure is forming will result in an anomaly of that structure. A genetic defect can cause an identical anomaly if the gene is coding for the formation of the same structure at that same time. Because the product of a single gene may be involved in the formation of different structures at different times, a single genetic defect may cause anomalies of structures that form at different times. Eventually, brain anomalies will be classified by a system that accounts for both the timing of injury and the defective expression of genes.

Early Brain Development

On about the 15th day of life, ectodermal cells proliferate along the surface of the embryo to form a plate of tissue, the primitive streak. A rapidly proliferating group of cells, known as *Hensen's node*, forms at one end of the primitive streak and defines its cephalic end. From Hensen's node, cells that will form the notochord migrate rostrally and induce differentiation of dorsal midline ectoderm into neuroectoderm. This platelike condensation of neuroectoderm is known as the *neural plate*.

At about 17 days, the lateral aspects of the neural plate begin to thicken. Actin myofibrils located within these thickened folds contract, bending the neural folds medially and causing the edges to approach each other in the midline. At about 20 days, these folds meet in the midline at the level of the rhombencephalon. This junction of the neural folds begins the formation of the *neural tube* (1–3).

As the neural tube closes, the neuroectoderm, which will form the central nervous system, separates from the overlying ectoderm, which will become the skin. Until recently, most experts believed that neural tube closure proceeds cranially and caudally in a zipperlike fashion. Recent evidence, however, indicates that the neural tube may have as many as five independent closure sites (4–6). If substantiated, this information may provide a unifying concept of some developmental malformations, especially cephaloceles. The cephalic end of the neural tube, the anterior neuropore, completely closes at about 25 days of gestation. The caudal end of the neural tube, the posterior neuropore, closes at about 27–28 days of gestation. At the time of closure of the anterior neuropore, three dilations or brain vesicles develop in the rostral cavity of the neural tube. These three early subdivisions are the *prosencephalon* (forebrain), the *mesencephalon* (midbrain), and the *rhombencephalon* (hindbrain) (Fig. 5.1). The rhombencephalon is separated from the mesencephalon by the cephalic flexure, and from the cervical spinal cord by the cervical flexure. At the time of closure of the anterior neuropore, the optic vesicles have already begun to bud from the diencephalic portion of the prosencephalon. The prosencephalon divides into the *diencephalon*–which will be composed of the thalami, hypothalami, and globi pallidi–and the *telencephalon*, which will form the cerebral hemispheres, putamina, and caudate nuclei. The cells that compose the diencephalon arise from the germinal matrix in the wall of the area that will become the third ventricle; those of the telencephalon arise from the germinal matrix in the walls of the future lateral ventricles (7–11). As the telencephalon develops, the cerebral hemispheres grow posteriorly to cover the mesencephalon and portions of the rhombencephalon (Fig. 5.1). Further details of the development of the telencephalon will be discussed in the sections on anomalies of neuronal migration and holoprosencephalies.

The rhombencephalon will eventually divide into the *myelencephalon*, which will form the pons and medulla, and the *metencephalon*, which will form the cerebellar hemispheres and vermis. This process of development

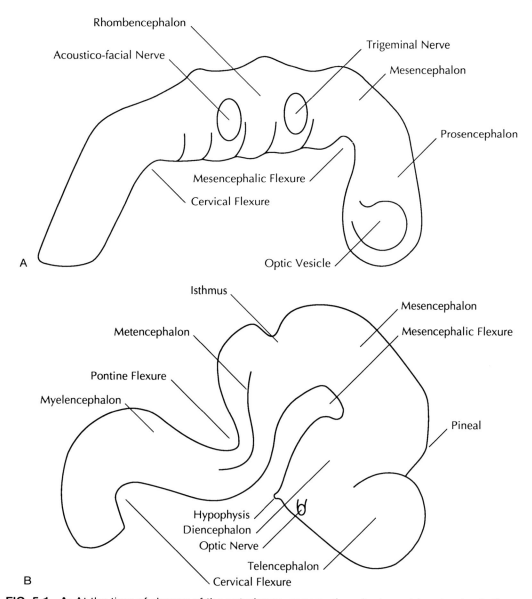

FIG. 5.1. A: At the time of closure of the anterior neuropore, three brain vesicles develop in the rostral cavity of the neural tube. These three subdivisions are the prosencephalon, the mesencephalon, and the rhombencephalon. The rhombencephalon is separated from the mesencephalon by the cephalic flexure and from the cervical spinal cord by the cervical flexure. **B:** The pontine flexure, which is very important in the development of the cerebellum, develops after the cervical and cephalic flexures. The fourth ventricle will develop at the site of the pontine, or rhombic, flexure. (See **C** on next page.)

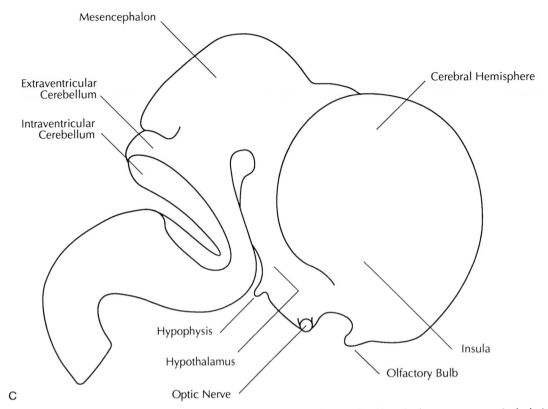

Mesencephalon

Extraventricular Cerebellum

Intraventricular Cerebellum

Cerebral Hemisphere

Hypophysis

Hypothalamus

Optic Nerve

Insula

Olfactory Bulb

C

FIG. 5.1. (*Continued.*) **C:** As the telencephalon develops, the cerebral hemispheres grow posteriorly to cover the midbrain and portions of the hindbrain. The cerebellar hemispheres grow from the rhombic lips, which sit at the cranial edge of the developing fourth ventricle (the site of the pontine flexure).

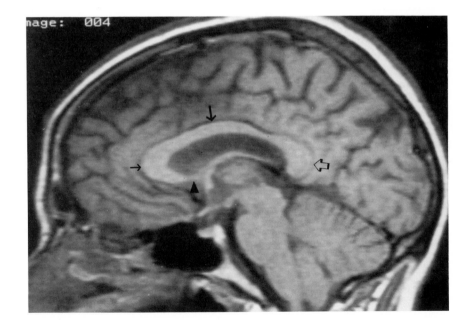

FIG. 5.2. The normal corpus callosum is composed of the rostrum (*arrowhead*), genu (*small arrow*), body (*large arrow*), and splenium (*open arrow*).

will be discussed further in the section on anomalies of the hindbrain.

ANOMALIES OF THE CORPUS CALLOSUM

Embryology

The corpus callosum is composed of four sections: the rostrum, genu, body, and splenium (Fig. 5.2). To understand callosal anomalies it is essential to understand the basics of its development. During the seventh week of gestation, the dorsal portion of the lamina terminalis (at the rostral-most end of the neural tube) undergoes a generalized thickening. This thickened portion has been called the lamina reuniens, or commissural plate (Fig. 5.3) (12). The lamina reuniens develops a groove in its ventral surface, which becomes filled with cellular material that originates in the developing subarachnoid space (meninx primitiva) and in the developing cerebral hemispheres (Fig. 5.4). This groove (the sulcus medianus telencephali medii) is then bridged superiorly by a glial bridge or "sling" (12,13). The cells that compose the "sling" express surface molecules and secrete chemicals into the extracellular space that help to guide axons across the midline (14). These axons form the cerebral commissures, the anterior commissure, the hippocampal commissure, and the corpus callosum (15). It is important to realize that this process does not happen simultaneously throughout the entire corpus callosum. In fact, while the initial pioneer axons are beginning to cross in the posterior portion of the genu, the glial "sling" is just beginning to form in the anterior body, while the sulcus medianus telencephali medii is forming in the posterior body (Fig. 5.4) (15,16). Appreciation of this anterior to posterior sequence of development is important because if any injury occurs to the developing brain during formation of the corpus callosum, the anterior portion of the corpus callosum will be formed but the posterior portion will not. The exceptions to this anterior-to-posterior sequence of development are the late formation of the anterior portion of the genu and of the callosal rostrum, the thin portion of the corpus that runs from the genu to the lamina terminalis. The anterior portion of the genu forms at approximately the same time as the posterior callosal body, and the rostrum forms last, slightly after the splenium (15).

If the normal developmental process is disturbed, the corpus callosum may be completely absent or partially formed (hypogenetic). When the corpus is hypogenetic, it is the posterior portion that is nearly always affected. In other words, in a partially formed corpus callosum, the genu will nearly always be present, with the body less commonly so, and the splenium and rostrum will frequently be small or absent. This concept is important in differentiating a hypogenetic corpus from one that is secondarily destroyed: A small or absent genu or body is almost certainly the result of a secondary destructive process when the splenium and rostrum are intact. A few exceptions have been observed in which the callosal genu or body may be absent despite the presence of a normal splenium (17,18). Callosal anomalies are atypical in holoprosencephaly, where the splenium may be present without formation of a normal genu or body, or the callosal body and splenium may be present in the absence of a genu (18). Very rarely, in the variety of holoprosencephaly known as middle interhemispheric fusion, the genu and splenium may be present without a normal callosal body (17). The callosal anomalies seen in holoprosencephaly represent truly "dysgenetic" (defectively developed) corpora callosi, distinct from the more common "hypogenetic" corpora that are merely incompletely formed. Examples are shown in the holoprosencephaly section of this chapter. The other exceptions to the "front-to-back" rule are those situations in which the region of brain that sends axons through a specific

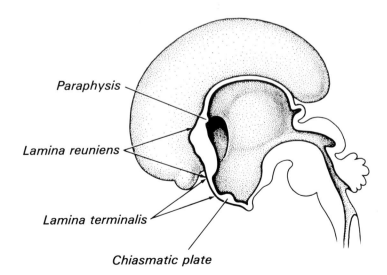

FIG. 5.3. Schematic of the rostral midline telencephalon at approximately 7 weeks gestational age. The thickening of the dorsal aspect of the thin rostral wall of the telencephalon (the primitive lamina terminalis) represents the lamina reuniens of Rakic, which will eventually form the precursors of the corpus callosum and the anterior commissure.

Paraphysis

Lamina reuniens

Lamina terminalis

Chiasmatic plate

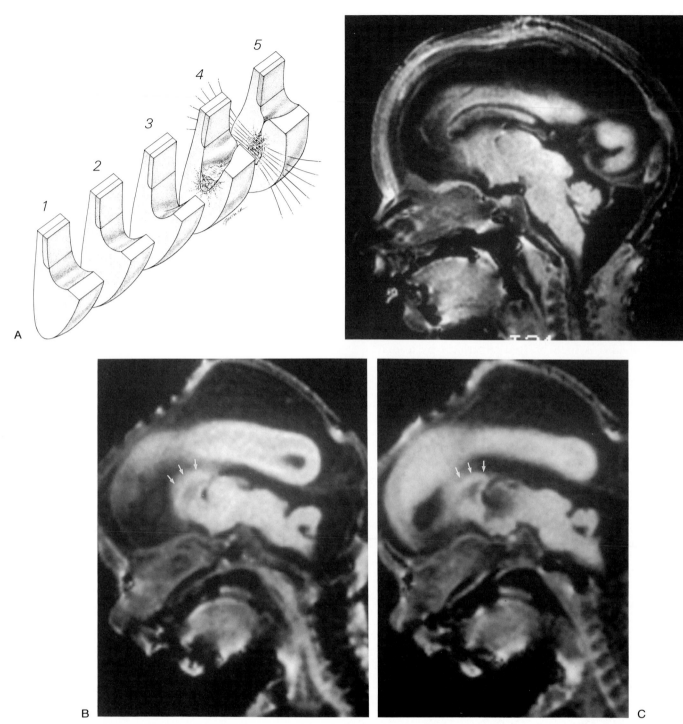

FIG. 5.4. Formation of the corpus callosum. **A:** Schematic. Initially, a thickening of the dorsal lamina terminalis forms the lamina reuniens (1). A groove develops in the superior aspect of the lamina reuniens, forming the sulcus medianus telencephali medii (SMTM) (2,3). Cells from the cerebral hemisphere on either side migrate into the SMTM (4), which is filled by these cells and eventually obliterated as the superior banks fuse, forming the commissural plate. The plate becomes the bed for ingrowing fibers of the developing cerebral hemispheres (5) forming the corpus callosum. These steps occur sequentially in the developing corpus callosum as it forms in a ventral to dorsal direction. Thus, an insult to the developing corpus will result in dysgenesis of portions dorsal to those formed (or almost formed) at the time of the insult. **B, C:** Sagittal T1-weighted MR images from an anatomy specimen estimated at 13–14 weeks. Only a small portion of the corpus callosum is formed (*arrows*), primarily in the region of the posterior genu and anterior body. **D:** In an 18-week specimen, most of the corpus is formed other than the rostrum.

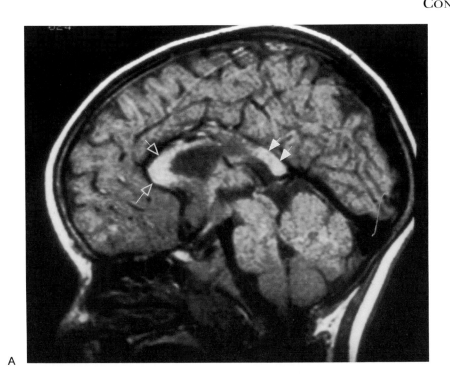

A

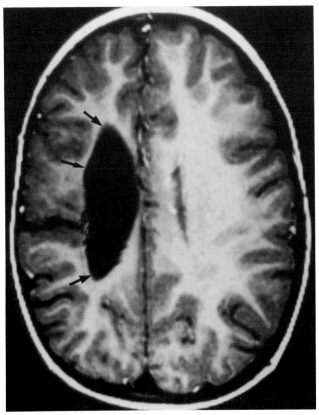

B

FIG. 5.5. Central callosal defect secondary to parenchymal injury. **A:** Sagittal T1-weighted image shows presence of the genu (*open arrows*) and splenium (*closed arrows*) of the corpus. The callosal body is absent. **B:** Axial T1-weighted image shows destruction of most of the white matter in the middle portion of the right cerebral hemisphere, with *ex vacuo* dilatation of the right lateral ventricle (*arrows*). Destruction of the white matter includes destruction of the transcallosal axons.

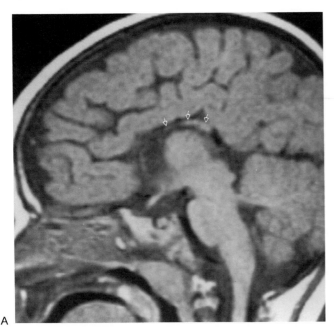
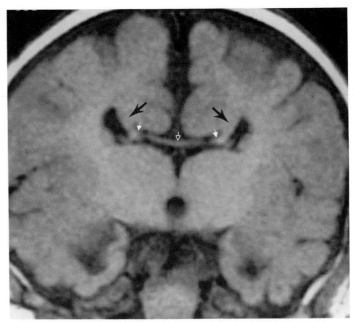

A

B

FIG. 5.6. Callosal agenesis with enlarged hippocampal commissure mimicking splenium. **A:** Sagittal T1-weighted image shows apparent formation of the splenium in the absence of formation of the anterior corpus. **B:** Coronal image shows that the commissure connects the fornices and is therefore a hippocampal commissure, not the splenium of the corpus callosum. (Reprinted with permission from ref. 18.)

region of the corpus is destroyed [e.g., porencephalies and schizencephalies (Fig. 5.5)]. Those patients who have had corpus callosotomies for seizure surgery (19) or transcallosal surgical approaches to the lateral or third ventricles (20) have callosal defects that may mimic congenital callosal defects if the surgical history is not known.

Occasionally, the hippocampal commissure will be enlarged in patients with hypogenesis or agenesis of the corpus callosum (16). The enlarged commissure may mimic a callosal splenium on midline sagittal images. Analysis of coronal images will show that the commissure connects the fornices, and not the cerebral hemispheres (Fig. 5.6).

Associated Anomalies and Syndromes

The formation of the corpus callosum and its precursors occurs between about 8 weeks and 20 weeks of gestational age (12,21). Most of the cerebrum and cerebellum form at the same time. Therefore, anomalies of the corpus callosum are often associated with other brain anomalies, most commonly the Dandy-Walker malformation, anomalies of neuronal migration and organization, encephaloceles, and midline facial anomalies (16,22,23). Isolated agenesis of the corpus callosum is usually asymptomatic and can only be detected by sophisticated neurologic testing. When patients with callosal hypogenesis or agenesis are symptomatic, the associated anomalies are the cause of the symptoms (most commonly, seizures, macrocephaly, mental retardation, or hypothalamic dysfunction) (24,25).

Callosal anomalies are part of many syndrome complexes (22,25–27); the most frequently mentioned of these is *Aicardi's syndrome* (26). Aicardi's syndrome is an X-linked dominant disorder consisting of infantile spasms, callosal agenesis or hypogenesis, chorioretinopathy, and an abnormal EEG. The syndrome occurs almost exclusively in females [affected patients must have two X chromosomes, so patients with Kleinfelter's syndrome (47XXY) can also have it] with no family history of ophthalmologic or neurologic disease. The mutation forms a spontaneous balanced translocation of the X chromosome. Intracranial anomalies include callosal hypogenesis (typically associated with interhemispheric cysts), gray matter heterotopia, cortical dysplasia, posterior fossa cysts, cerebellar hypoplasia, choroid plexus papillomas, and microphthalmia. Ophthalmologic exam reveals characteristic chorioretinal lacunae, which result from retinal dysplasia, and ocular colobomata. Myelination may be delayed (26,28–30). A complete list of syndromes with callosal anomalies is beyond the scope of this text.

Anatomic Sequelae of Callosal Anomalies

When the corpus callosum is absent, the axons that would normally course into the contralateral hemisphere through the corpus instead turn at the interhemispheric fissure and run parallel to that fissure, forming the longitudinal callosal bundles of Probst (Fig. 5.7). The Probst bundles lie lateral to the cingulate gyri; their inferomedial borders merge with rudimentary fornices. Because of their location, the bundles of Probst invaginate the me-

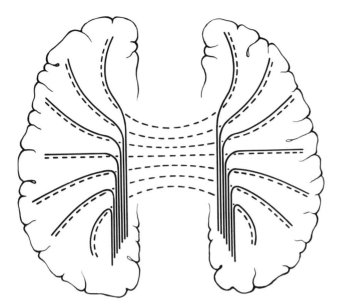

FIG. 5.7. Formation of the lateral callosal bundles (of Probst). Because of lack of induction by the massa commissuralis, axonal fibers from the cerebral hemispheres fail to cross the midline. Instead, these fibers reach the medial hemispheric wall and turn, coursing parallel to the interhemispheric fissure and indenting the medial walls of the lateral ventricles. Broken lines represent fibers of corpus callosum in the normal brain. Solid lines represent fibers that fail to cross where the dysgenetic corpus callosum is present.

dial borders of the lateral ventricles, giving them a crescentic shape that is most pronounced frontally (Fig. 5.8, 5.9B) (12,15,16). The third ventricle is located higher than normal, between the lateral ventricles. The foramina of Monro tend to be enlarged. The formation of the corpus callosum is associated with an inversion of the cingulate gyri, resulting in the formation of the cingulate sulcus, superior to the gyrus. When the corpus callosum does not form, the cingulate gyri remain everted and the cingulate sulcus remains unformed (16). Persistent eversion of the cingulate gyri results in extension of the sulci

of the medial hemisphere all the way into the third ventricle (Fig. 5.9). This radiation of the medial hemispheric sulci into the third ventricle is one of the hallmarks of absence of the corpus callosum; it is especially helpful when evaluating newborns, in whom the corpus is thin and can be difficult to see.

The corpus callosum is the most tightly packed bundle of axons in the brain. This compactness makes the corpus a very firm structure and gives the adjacent lateral ventricles their shape; moreover, the firmness of the corpus helps the ventricles to maintain their normal size, especially posteriorly. The firm caudate heads and lentiform nuclei keep the size of the frontal horns relatively small, even in the absence of the corpus callosum (although, when the genu is absent, the frontal horns are convex laterally instead of concave, as in the normal case) (Fig. 5.9, 5.10). Posteriorly, however, only loose white matter surrounds the ventricles when the callosal splenium is absent. In the absence of the splenium, therefore, the ventricles expand into the soft white matter surrounding them, resulting in dilatation of the trigones and occipital horns of the lateral ventricles. This condition is known as colpocephaly (Figs. 5.9C, 5.10). The temporal horns also frequently enlarge, probably as a result of associated limbic system anomalies (31,32). The bodies of the lateral ventricles are affected when the callosal body is absent, with the result being straight, parallel ventricles (Fig. 5.9B). Rarely, hypertrophy of the hippocampal or anterior commissures accompanies callosal agenesis or hypogenesis (Fig. 5.6) (18).

In the absence of a complete corpus callosum, the third ventricle tends to be widened and extends superiorly into the interhemispheric fissure, forming an interhemispheric CSF collection, generally referred to as an *interhemispheric cyst* (Fig. 5.11). The cyst may communicate with the third ventricle and one or both of the lateral ventricles. Typically, the interhemispheric cyst is multiloculated. One or more of the loculations of the in-

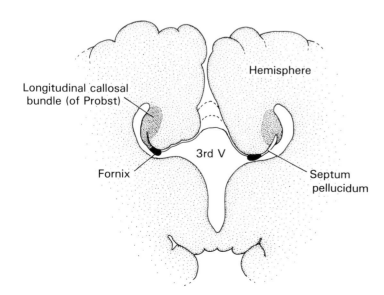

Fig 5.8. Schematic illustrating the findings in callosal agenesis. The lateral ventricles have a crescentic shape secondary to the medially located bundles of Probst. The third ventricle extends upward between the lateral ventricles into the interhemispheric fissure. The cingulate gyri remain everted and the cingulate sulci do not form. (Reprinted with permission from ref. 18.)

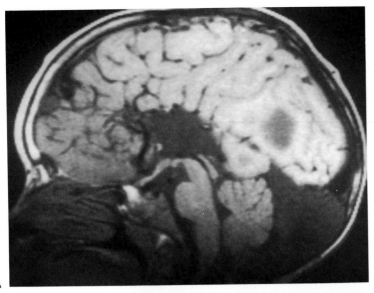

A

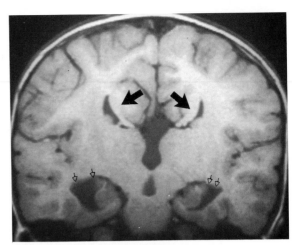

B

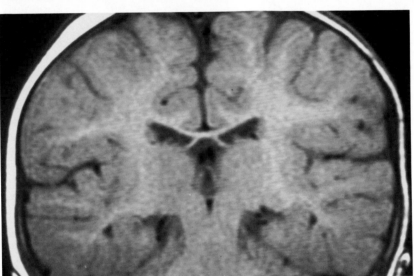

C

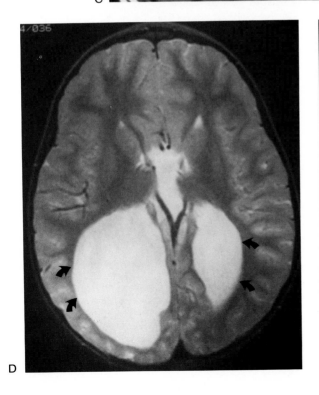

D

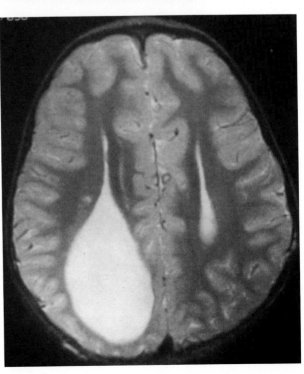

E

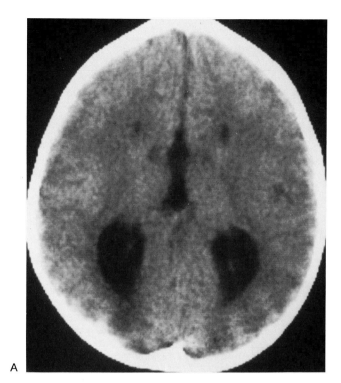
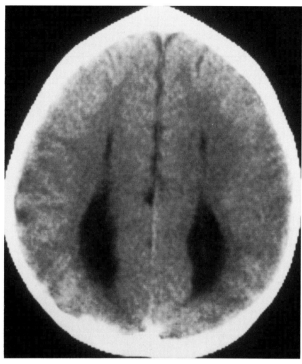

A

B

FIG. 5.10. Agenesis of the corpus callosum. **A:** Axial CT image shows continuity of the third ventricle with the interhemispheric fissure and lateral convexity of the frontal horns. **B:** Higher axial CT image shows parallel lateral ventricles and dilated posterior ventricles.

terhemispheric cyst may grow and compress the ventricular system, resulting in hydrocephalus. Under these circumstances it is important to establish which of the loculations are in communication with one another and with the ventricles, in order to plan properly which compartments should be shunted and in what order. A CT cisternogram or ventriculogram is performed after nonionic iodinated contrast is introduced into the cyst(s) to establish which of the CSF collections communicate. The prognosis for patients with callosal agenesis and interhemispheric cysts is good if the cysts are adequately shunted and no associated brain anomalies are identified (33).

Imaging of Callosal Anomalies

Agenesis of the corpus callosum can be detected on images obtained in the axial plane, although the sagittal and coronal planes are better for showing the associated anatomic deformities. The characteristic lateral convexity of the frontal horns, parallel lateral ventricles, colpocephaly, upward extension of the third ventricle into the interhemispheric fissure between the lateral ventricles, and communication of the third ventricle with the interhemispheric fissure anteriorly can all be identified in the axial plane (Fig. 5.10). Milder callosal anomalies, however, are difficult to identify with axial images. As it allows images to be easily obtained in all planes, MR shows all variations of callosal anomalies exquisitely. The exact extent of callosal hypogenesis or dysgenesis is well seen on the midline sagittal images (Figs. 5.11, 5.12). As mentioned earlier, when the corpus is hypogenetic, the posterior portions and the rostrum are usually absent. Therefore, a hypogenetic corpus callosum may include the genu; genu and part of the body; genu and entire body; or genu, body, and splenium (without the rostrum).

FIG. 5.9. Agenesis of the corpus callosum. **A:** Sagittal SE 600/20 image shows medial hemispheric sulci radiating into the third ventricle because of lack of inversion of the cingulate gyrus. **B:** Coronal image shows high third ventricle, crescentic lateral ventricles compressed by Probst bundles (*large arrows*), and large temporal horns (*small open arrows*) secondary to hypoplasia of the hippocampi. Also note the persistent eversion of the cingulate gyri and the continuity of the third ventricle with the interhemispheric fissure. **C:** Coronal SE 550/15 image from a patient with a normal corpus callosum shows normally inverted cingulate gyri and normal formation of cingulate sulci. **D:** Colpocephaly secondary to large trigones and occipital horns (*arrows*). **E:** Bodies of lateral ventricles are parallel.

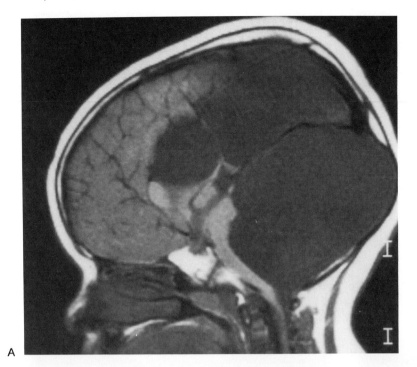

FIG. 5.11. Dandy-Walker malformation with hypogenesis of the corpus callosum and interhemispheric cyst. **A:** Sagittal T1-weighted image reveals an enlarged posterior fossa containing a huge cyst and absence of the cerebellar vermis, compatible with a Dandy-Walker malformation. Only the genu of the corpus callosum is present. A large CSF-intensity region is seen dorsal and superior to the genu. **B:** Axial T1-weighted image reveals a large cystic midline CSF intensity structure displacing the medial aspect of the left cerebral hemisphere to the left. Both lateral ventricles can be identified (*open arrows*) and are separate from the cyst. **C:** Axial T2-weighted image reveals the cyst extending up to the top of the cerebral hemispheres. These so-called interhemispheric cysts may or may not communicate with the third ventricle. They generally extend on one or the other side of the falx cerebri. Only rarely do they straddle the falx.

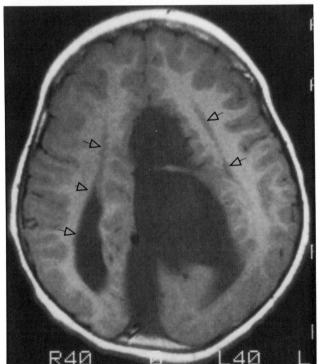

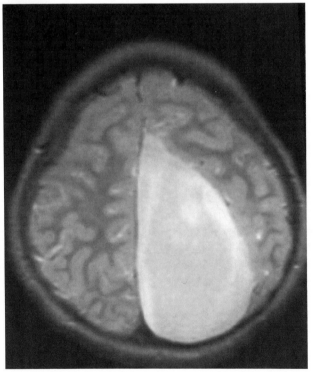

Other MR findings in the absence of a corpus callosum include persistent eversion of the cingulate gyri (with the medial hemispheric sulci extending all the way into the third ventricle), crescent-shaped lateral ventricles (caused by an impression upon the medial walls of the ventricles by the medially positioned bundles of Probst), incomplete inversion of the hippocampal formation in the medial temporal lobes, and extension of the third ventricle into the interhemispheric fissure (Figs. 5.8–5.10).

MR imaging has revealed a much higher incidence of callosal anomalies than was previously suspected. It is only since the advent of MR imaging that the high percentage of callosal anomalies associated with the Chiari II malformation (80% to 85%) has been appreciated, for example (16).

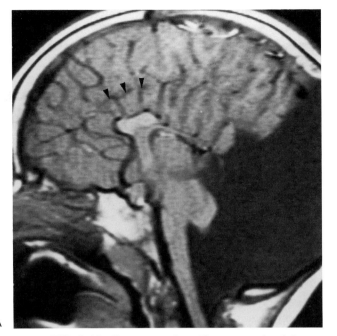

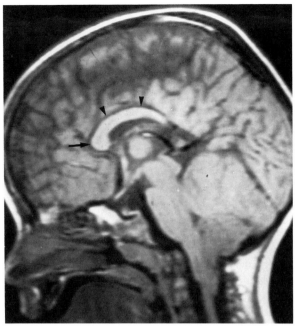

A B

FIG. 5.12. Two examples of hypogenesis of the corpus callosum. A: Patient with Dandy-Walker malformation. In this patient only the genu of the corpus callosum is present. The arrowheads show the cingulate sulcus, which is only present where the callosal fibers have crossed. B: Patient with a Chiari II malformation and hypogenesis of the corpus callosum. The genu (arrow) and body (arrowheads) are present, but the rostrum and splenium have not formed.

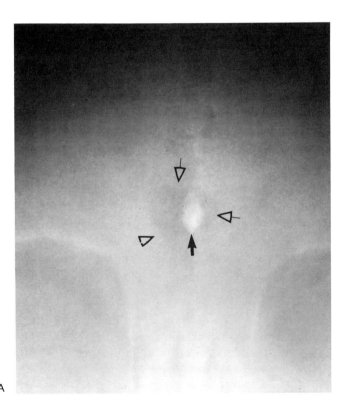

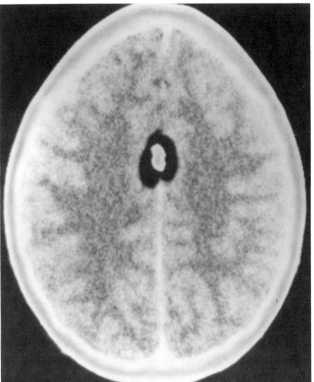

A B

FIG. 5.13. Interhemispheric lipoma. A: Anteroposterior plain film shows midline lucency (open arrows) with central calcification (closed arrow). B: Axial CT scan through the lipoma shows a lucent area in the interhemispheric fissure immediately superior to the corpus callosum with a focal calcification within it.

INTRACRANIAL LIPOMAS

Intracranial lipomas are malformations believed to result from abnormal differentiation of the meninx primitiva, the undifferentiated mesenchyme that surrounds the developing brain (34–36). Normally, the meninx primitiva differentiates into the leptomeninges and the subarachnoid space. For some as yet unknown reason, meninx differentiates into fat in some patients, forming intracranial lipomas. As a result of their formation from the meninx, intracranial lipomas almost always are located in the subarachnoid space. As they are malformations, not neoplasms, lipoma cells do not multiply (they will hypertrophy, like other normal fat cells, when patients gain weight) and almost never exert mass effect on adjacent structures. Moreover, because lipomas are maldifferentiated subarachnoid space, blood vessels and cranial nerves almost always course through them. Therefore, surgical treatment has a high morbidity and is essentially always contraindicated. The most common locations for intracranial lipomas are the deep interhemispheric fissure (40% to 50%), the quadrigeminal plate/supracerebellar cisterns (20% to 30%), the suprasellar/interpeduncular cisterns (10% to 20%), the cerebellopontine angle cisterns (~10%), and the Sylvian cisterns (5%) (36).

Interhemispheric lipomas (commonly called *callosal lipomas* or *lipomas of the corpus callosum* despite the fact that they are separate from the corpus) are almost always associated with hypogenesis or agenesis of the corpus callosum. Encephaloceles and cutaneous lipomas are sometimes associated, as well, usually in the frontal region. In fact, a spectrum of midline developmental disorders appears to have lipomas of the interhemispheric fissure as a part of the syndrome. Many of these are associated with midline facial clefts, a condition known as *midline craniofacial dysraphism* (see the next section, on cephaloceles) (37,38).

Skull x-rays of patients with intracranial lipomas may be normal or, in large interhemispheric lipomas, may reveal punctate or curvilinear midline calcifications with adjacent lucencies of fat density (Fig. 5.13) (23). On CT, lipomas are sharply demarcated areas of marked hypodensity in affected cisterns. Interhemispheric cistern lipomas may extend inferiorly between the ventricles or anteriorly in front of the callosal genu. Calcification is often present in interhemispheric lipomas, most commonly within a fibrous capsule surrounding the lipoma (39). The calcification may be curvilinear, extending around the periphery of the lipoma, or may be nodular, within the center of the lipoma (Fig. 5.13). Calcification is less common in lipomas in other locations. The full extent of the lipoma and associated callosal hypogenesis can only be fully appreciated on MR.

The MR appearance of a lipoma is that of a hyperintense mass on T1-weighted sequences, becoming hypointense on long TR images as the TE increases (Fig. 5.14). Large lipomas will show chemical shift artifact, resulting from the different chemical shifts of water and fat protons. Application of a fat saturation pulse will make the lipoma isointense to gray matter. Lipomas in the suprasellar (Fig. 5.15) and quadrigeminal plate cisterns are typically small and may not show obvious chemical shift artifact. In contrast, lipomas in the interhemispheric fissure and Sylvian fissure may be quite large. Interhemispheric fissure lipomas may involve the area of the lamina terminalis or fornix (36,39). The adjacent corpus callosum is essentially always hypogenetic, with lipoma extending around the posterior portion of the corpus; no callosal fibers are seen dorsal or posterior to the lipoma (Figs. 5.14, 5.16). Occasionally, the fat from the lipoma can be seen extending through the choroidal fissure into the choroid plexuses of the lateral ventricles. Branches of the pericallosal artery frequently appear as curvilinear flow voids coursing through the lipoma; at times, they can be difficult to differentiate from calcium or chemical shift artifact by MR alone. When affected patients have associated facial dysmorphism, computed tomography is extremely helpful for the evaluation of the bony craniofacial anomalies and the planning of surgical reconstruction.

CEPHALOCELES AND OTHER CALVARIAL AND SKULL BASE DEFECTS

Definition and Classification

The term *cephalocele* refers to a defect in the skull and dura with extracranial extension of intracranial structures. Cephaloceles are divided into four types (40). *Meningoencephaloceles* are herniation of CSF, brain tissue, and meninges through the skull defect. *Meningocele* refers to herniation of the meninges and CSF only. *Atretic cephaloceles* are formes frustes of cephaloceles consisting of dura, fibrous tissue, and degenerated brain tissue; they are most common in the parieto-occipital area. *Glioceles* consist of a glial lined cyst containing CSF. The skull defect and herniation most commonly occur in the midline. The etiology of the cephalocele varies with its location. Those extending through the skull base, which is formed of enchondral bone, are usually caused by either failure of induction of the bone resulting from faulty closure of the neural tube (41,42) or failure of the basilar ossification centers to unite (43). Cephaloceles through the calvarium, which is composed of membranous bone, may be secondary to defective induction of the bone, pressure erosion of the bone by an intracranial mass or cyst (41,44,45), or failure of closure of one of the sites of primary neural tube closure (5).

Cephaloceles are named for the location of the bone defects through which they course. The categories of cephaloceles include (1) occipitocervical (involving the

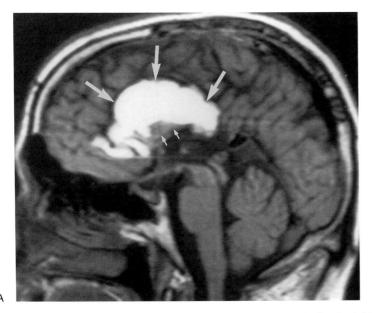
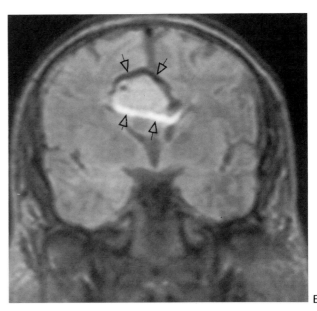

A

B

FIG. 5.14. Large interhemispheric lipoma. **A:** Sagittal SE 500/11 image shows a large lobulated hyper-intense mass (*large arrows*) adjacent to a hypogenetic corpus callosum (*small arrows*). **B:** Coronal SE 2500/20 image shows marked chemical shift artifact (*arrows*) around the lipoma.

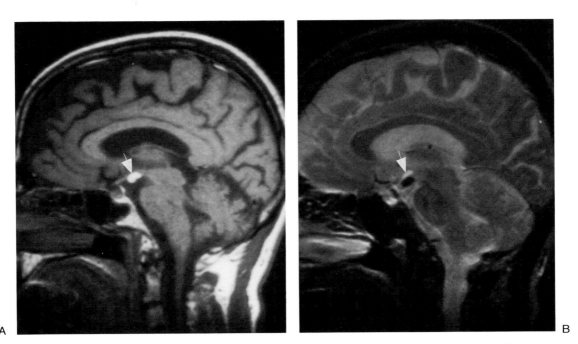

A

B

FIG. 5.15. Hypothalamic, interpeduncular cistern lipoma. T1-weighted **(A)** and T2-weighted **(B)** images show the small lipoma (*arrows*). Some chemical shift artifact is seen on the T2-weighted image.

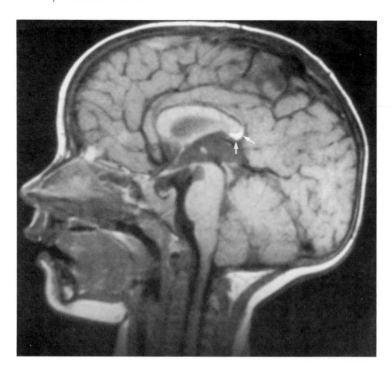

FIG. 5.16. Small callosal lipoma. A very small lipoma (*arrows*) is present at the dorsal aspect of the corpus callosum. Note that the corpus callosum does not extend dorsal to the lipoma and the splenium has not formed. The rostrum is absent.

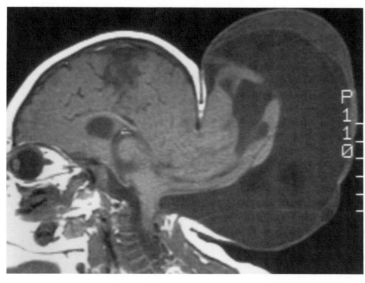

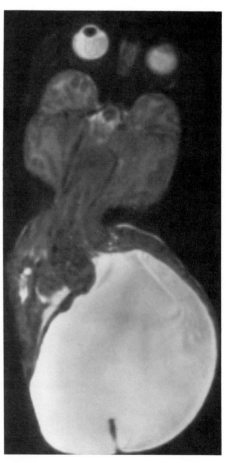

FIG. 5.17. Occipital cephalocele. **A:** Sagittal SE 500/11 image shows a large occipital cephalocele. Both supra- and infratentorial brain tissue, in addition to CSF from cisterns and the fourth ventricle, enter the cephalocele. Note the deformation of the brain as it "stretches" into the cephalocele sac. **B:** Axial SE 2800/80 image shows the supra- and infratentorial structures stretching into the cephalocele sac.

occipital bone, foramen magnum, and posterior arches of upper cervical vertebrae); (2) occipital; (3) parietal; (4) frontal; (5) temporal (along the superior surface of the petrous ridge); (6) frontoethmoidal (between nasal bones and ethmoid bone); (7) sphenomaxillary (through orbital fissures into pterygopalatine fossa); (8) spheno-orbital (through defect in sphenoid bone or optic canal/orbital fissure into orbit); (9) nasopharyngeal (through ethmoid, sphenoid, or basiocciput into nasal cavity or pharynx; and (10) lateral (along coronal or lambdoid sutures) (46). A complete discussion of cephaloceles in all these locations is beyond the scope of this book. The embryology is complex and may differ for different types of cephaloceles. Moreover, theories of cephalocele embryogenesis are changing as new theories of neural tube development are proposed (5). This section discusses the four most common and therefore most important locations in which cephaloceles occur; then it discusses the imaging appearance of other lesions that may mimic cephaloceles clinically. Nasal dermoids and nasal gliomas are included in the section on frontoethmoidal cephaloceles, as the clinical presentation can be very similar. Finally, this section includes a discussion of calvarial dermoids and other masses that present as calvarial masses in childhood and that may therefore mimic cephaloceles.

Occipital Cephaloceles

The occipital bone is the most common location for cephaloceles in the white populations of Europe and

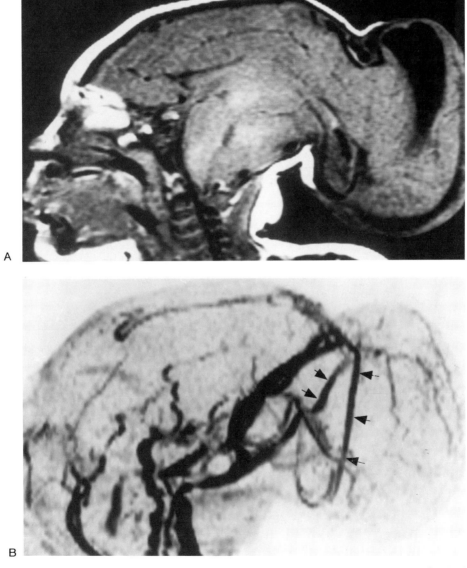

FIG. 5.18. Use of MR venography to demonstrate dural sinuses in cephalocele sac. **A:** Sagittal SE 500/11 image shows the occipital cephalocele. **B:** 2D TOF venogram shows dural venous sinuses (*arrows*) in the cephalocele sac. This is important information for the surgeon.

North America, accounting for approximately 80% of cephaloceles in that group. Supratentorial and infratentorial structures are involved with equal frequency. Not uncommonly, supratentorial structures, infratentorial structures, and the tentorium are all included within the cephalocele. Both the occipital horn of the lateral ventricle and the fourth ventricle may extend into the sac. The diagnosis is usually obvious clinically, and imaging studies are ordered to answer two major questions: (1) "Are other severe brain anomalies present?" and (2) "Do the dural venous sinuses (superior sagittal sinus, straight sinus, and transverse sinuses) course within the cephalocele?" MR is the modality of choice to answer these questions. Routine MR imaging studies (Fig. 5.17) will show the amount of brain tissue versus fluid in the cyst in addition to demonstrating associated callosal anomalies, anomalies of neuronal migration, Chiari malformations, or Dandy-Walker malformations, all of which have higher frequencies in patients with cephaloceles

(40,41,45). The course of the dural venous sinuses can be demonstrated by the use of MR venography (47), acquired at the time of the MR imaging study (Fig. 5.18). 2D time of flight acquisition in the coronal plane is optimal for the venogram (47).

Frontoethmoidal Cephaloceles, Nasal Dermoids, and Nasal Gliomas

Embryology

Frontoethmoidal cephaloceles, nasal gliomas, and nasal dermoids are included in the same section because all three can present as congenital midline nasal masses (48). Moreover, all three are believed to have a similar embryologic derivation, resulting from a lack of normal regression of a projection of dura that extends through the embryologic foramen cecum, between the develop-

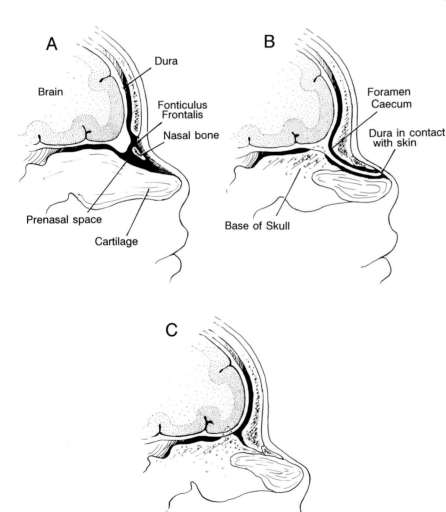

FIG. 5.19. Embryology of the frontoethmoidal region. Nasal dermoids, frontoethmoidal cephaloceles, and nasal gliomas all are believed to have similar embryologic derivations. Frontal cephaloceles presumably result from lack of closure of the fonticulus frontalis **(A):** with herniation of brain tissue or dura through the calvarial opening. Normally, a projection of dura extends through the embryologic foramen cecum **(B):** between the developing nasal cartilage and nasal bone. Normal regression leads to a normal skull base and frontonasal region, as in **(C):** Lack of regression leads to frontonasal pathology, as in the following examples. (Reprinted with permission from ref. 48.)

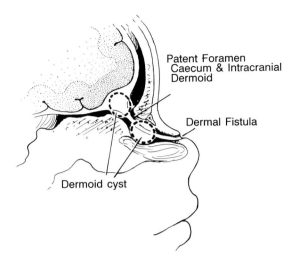

FIG. 5.20. Formation of nasal dermal sinuses. If the dural projection (Fig. 5.19B) remains adherent to the skin, a small dimple will develop on the surface of the nose. The dimple is the orifice of a dermal sinus tract that can extend superiorly along the path of the dural projection for any distance, including all the way into the cranial vault through the foramen cecum. Dermoids or epidermoids may develop anywhere along the tract. (Reprinted with permission from ref. 48.)

ing nasal cartilage and nasal bone (Fig. 5.19) (43,48). If the dural projection remains adherent to the skin, a small dimple will develop on the surface of the nose. The dimple is the orifice of a *dermal sinus tract* that can extend superiorly along the path of the dural projection for a variable distance, including all the way into the cranial vault through the foramen cecum (Fig. 5.20). Dermoid or epidermoid tumors can develop anywhere along the dermal sinus tract. *Cephaloceles* presumably result from

herniation of intracranial tissues into the dural projection through the foramen cecum (Fig. 5.21) (43,48). *Nasal gliomas* (nasal cerebral heterotopias) are accumulations of dysplastic brain tissue in the nasal cavity or subcutaneous tissue that are separate from intracranial contents (Fig. 5.22). They are postulated to result from herniation of brain tissue into the dural projection with subsequent regression of the more superior portion of the projection (43,48).

Clinical and Imaging Aspects

Frontoethmoidal encephaloceles are the most common variety in southeast Asia (40,41,49,50). They are subdivided by location into three subtypes. In the *nasofrontal* group, the defect is located between the frontal and nasal bones. *Nasoethmoidal* cephaloceles extend through a defect between the nasal bones and the nasal cartilage. The defect in *naso-orbital* cephaloceles is bordered anteriorly by the frontal process of the maxilla and posteriorly by the lacrimal bone and the lamina papyracea of the ethmoid bone (50). Clinical presentation of frontoethmoidal cephaloceles, nasal dermoids, and nasal gliomas is similar, usually nasal stuffiness or a nasal mass (42,49). If examination reveals a nasal dimple, establishing the diagnosis of dermal sinus, an imaging study is required to search for an associated (epi)dermoid tumor. If no dimple is seen, an imaging study is usually ordered to establish the presence or absence of a connection of the mass with intracranial contents.

CT and MR appear to be equivalent in the evaluation of nasal dermal sinuses (48). CT will show the dermal sinus as it courses through the nasal septum more accu-

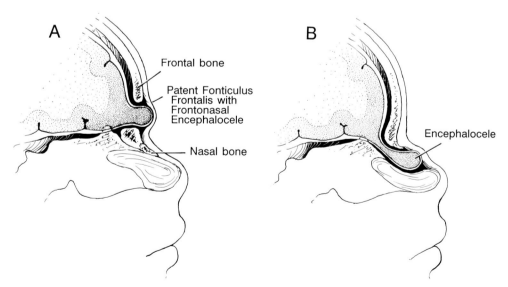

FIG. 5.21. Formation of frontoethmoidal cephaloceles. Cephaloceles presumably result from herniation of intracranial tissues into the dural projection through the fonticulus frontalis **(A)** or foramen cecum **(B)**. (Reprinted with permission from ref. 48.)

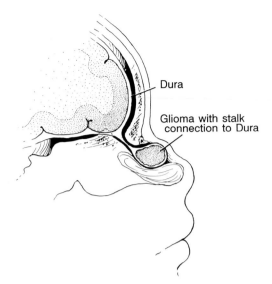

FIG. 5.22. Formation of nasal gliomas (nasal cerebral heterotopia). These accumulations of dysplastic brain tissue in the nasal cavity or subcutaneous tissue are postulated to result from herniation of brain tissue into the dural projection (Fig. 5.19B) with subsequent regression of the more superior portion of the projection. (Reprinted with permission from ref. 48.)

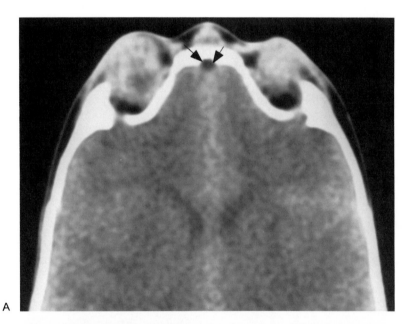

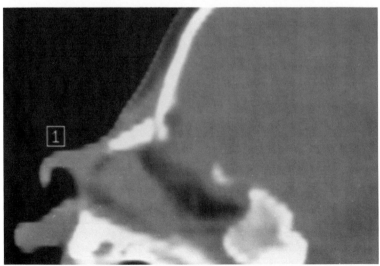

FIG. 5.23. Nasal dermal sinus with intracranial dermoid. **A:** Axial CT after intrathecal injection of iodinated contrast shows a filling defect (*arrows*) superior to the foramen cecum. **B:** Sagittal reformation shows erosion of the adjacent inner table of the frontal bone by the dermoid. (Reprinted with permission from ref. 48.)

rately than MR, but both modalities will show associated intracranial dermoids with equal accuracy. CT should be performed using 1.5-mm slice thickness; subarachnoid infusion of iodinated contrast helps to detect intracranial masses (Fig. 5.23). MR should be obtained using T1 weighting and 3-mm image thickness in the sagittal, coronal, and axial planes. (Epi)dermoids will be isointense to hyperintense compared to brain (Fig. 5.24). Care should be taken not to mistake normal marrow in the crista galli or the nasal process of the frontal bone (see Fig. 2.19B) for a dermoid tumor. Gradient echo images with gradient spoilers can be used to obtain thinner slices but may be degraded by susceptibility artifact from interfaces of intracranial contents with bone and air.

MR is superior to CT in the evaluation of cephaloceles and nasal gliomas because it directly shows the extension of brain tissue through the bone defect (Figs. 5.25–5.27) in cephaloceles and the lack thereof in nasal gliomas. Imaging in the sagittal plane is optimal for this determination. In difficult cases, acquisition of CT images through the defect after intrathecal contrast administration can be helpful to determine whether the soft tissue mass is continuous with the subarachnoid space; sagittal reformations of 3-mm images are optimal. MR is also superior to CT in showing the presence or absence of associated brain anomalies (Fig. 5.26), the presence of which has profound prognostic implications. Hypogenesis of

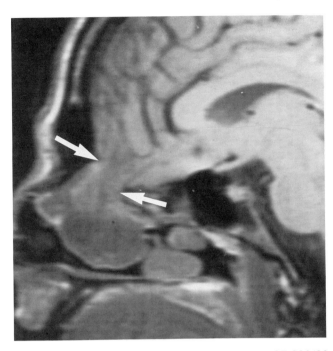

FIG. 5.25. Frontoethmoidal cephalocele. Sagittal SE 600/20 image shows extension of brain tissue and CSF through a defect (*arrows*) in the skull base in the region of the cribriform plate and crista galli. The cephalocele sits within the ethmoid air cells and nasal cavity. (Reprinted with permission from ref. 48.)

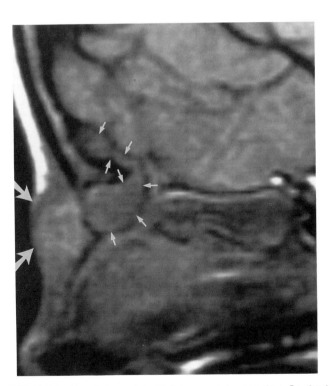

FIG. 5.24. Nasal dermoid with intracranial extension. Sagittal SE 550/15 image shows a glabellar mass (*large arrows*) and a (epi)dermoid tumor (*small arrows*) extending from the glabellar region superiorly through the foramen cecum into the intracranial cavity.

the corpus callosum, interhemispheric lipomas, and anomalies of neuronal migration frequently accompany nasofrontal encephaloceles. Frontoethmoidal encephaloceles are not uncommonly seen in association with craniofacial anomalies, often in the form of the midline craniofacial dysraphisms mentioned earlier (Fig. 5.28) (37,38,40). Hypertelorism is common in all cephaloceles in this group and in nasal gliomas because of separation of midline structures by the herniating brain tissue.

Parietal and Atretic Cephaloceles

Parietal cephaloceles are uncommon, comprising approximately 10% of cephaloceles (40). They are usually associated with significant underlying brain anomalies and, consequently, have poor prognoses. Among the most common associated anomalies are the Dandy-Walker malformation, callosal agenesis, the Chiari II malformation, and holoprosencephaly (44,46,51). Because of the proximity of parietal cephaloceles to the superior sagittal sinus, it is particularly important to locate the position of the sinus with respect to the cephalocele in these patients (Fig. 5.29). Neurosurgical repair is much more difficult when the sinus is located within the cephalocele.

A high percentage of parietal cephaloceles falls into the category of atretic cephaloceles (44,51). *Atretic parietal*

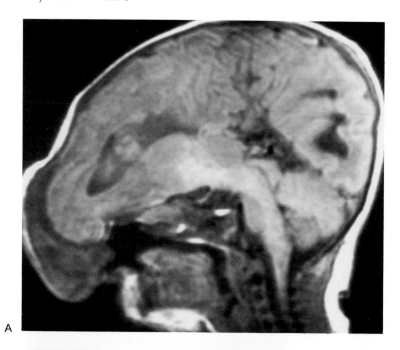

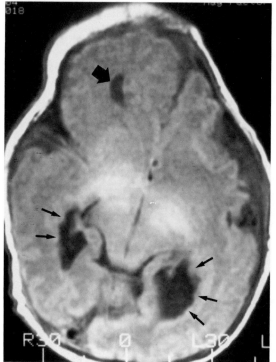

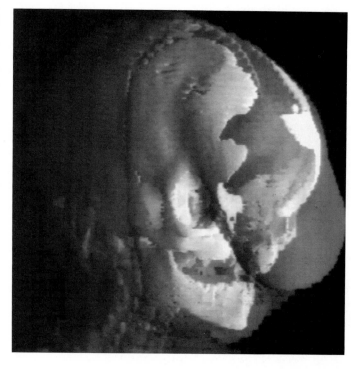

FIG. 5.26. Frontal cephalocele. **A:** Sagittal SE 600/20 image shows a large protrusion of frontal lobe extending into the facial region. **B:** Axial SE 600/20 image shows the right frontal horn (*large arrow*) extending into the cephalocele. Note the nodular subependymal heterotopia (*small arrows*) in the trigones. **C:** Three-dimensional reformation from a CT aids surgeons in the cephalocele repair.

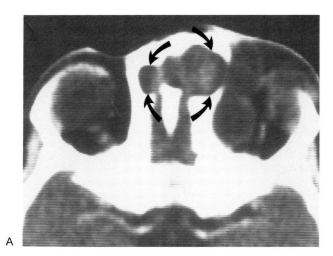
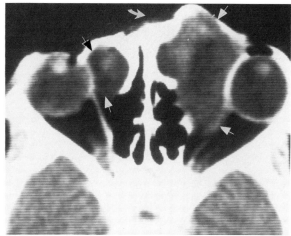

FIG. 5.27. Fronto-orbital cephalocele. **A, B:** Axial noncontrast CT images show bilateral extensions of tissue (*arrows*) into the orbits through medial orbital defects bordered anteriorly by the frontal process of the maxilla and posteriorly by the lachrymal bone and the lamina papyracea of the ethmoid bone. (Reprinted with permission from ref. 48.)

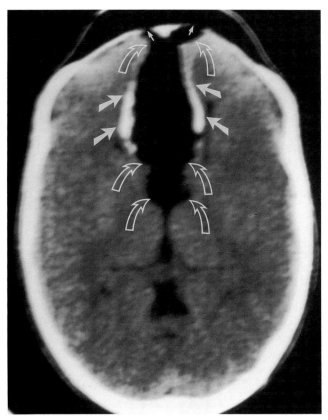
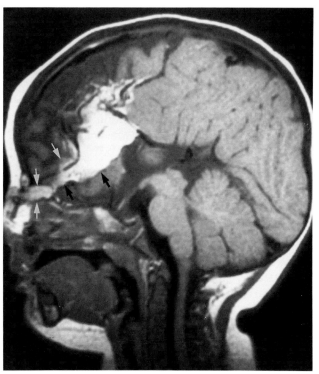

FIG. 5.28. Midline cranio-facial dysraphism. **A:** Axial CT shows lipoma (*open curved arrows*) with peripheral calcification (*solid arrows*) extending through a frontal calvarial defect. **B:** Sagittal SE 600/20 image shows the interhemispheric lipoma extending from the posterior frontal region down through the crista galli into the nasofrontal area (*arrows*). The corpus callosum is agenetic.

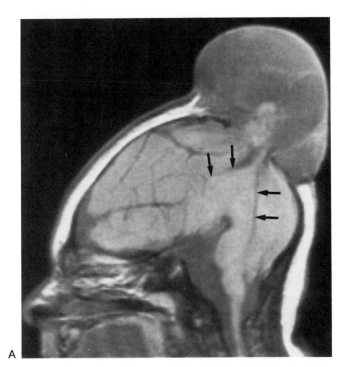
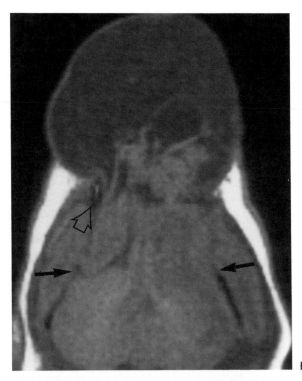

FIG. 5.29. Parietal cephalocele. **A:** SE 600/20 image shows the acallosal brain stretched toward a large parietal calvarial defect. Notice, in particular, the displacement and distortion of the midbrain (*arrows*). **B:** Coronal SE 800/20 image shows elevation of the cerebellum through the widened tentorial incisura (*closed arrows*). The superior sagittal sinus (*open arrow*) is identified within the calvarium, not in the sac.

cephaloceles usually present as small (5–15 mm), hairless midline masses near the vertex (44). A sharply marginated calvarial defect is present below the skin lesion, through which the cephalocele communicates with the intracranial cavity (Fig. 5.30). The calvarial defect may be too small to see on standard spin echo MR images; thin-section gradient echo (with gradient spoiler) MR images or thin CT images may be necessary to establish the communication. Atretic parietal cephaloceles have a very high incidence of associated midline anomalies [100% in Yokota's series (44)], including porencephalies, interhemispheric cysts, and callosal agenesis (40).

Atretic occipital cephaloceles (Fig. 5.31) usually present as nodular, small (less than 15 mm) masses just above the external occipital protuberance (44). They enter the calvarium through a small calvarial defect and then penetrate the dura immediately below the torcula, which is typically located higher than usual. The tracts typically terminate in the falx cerebri or tentorium. Patients with atretic occipital cephaloceles appear to have a low incidence of associated anomalies and a good prognosis for normal development (44).

Nasopharyngeal Cephaloceles

Nasopharyngeal encephaloceles are also very uncommon. They are important, however, as they are occult encephaloceles; they are not obvious on clinical examination. In contrast to encephaloceles in other locations, which are diagnosed at birth, nasopharyngeal encephaloceles usually present toward the end of the first decade of life. The usual clinical presentation is that of persistent nasal stuffiness or excessive "mouth breathing" by the child secondary to obstruction of the nasopharynx (41,42). Clinical examination will reveal a nasal or pharyngeal mass that increases in size with Valsalva maneuver. Associated intracranial anomalies are common. Agenesis of the corpus callosum is seen in approximately 80% of affected patients (Fig. 5.32). Hypoplasia of the optic discs is seen on ophthalmologic exam. Diminished visual acuity and hypothalamic–pituitary dysfunction are common because the inferior third ventricle, hypothalamus, and optic chiasm are stretched as they extend into the sac (Fig. 5.32) (41,42).

The diagnosis of nasopharyngeal cephalocele can be made by plain film or imaging studies. On a submento-vertex plain film, a hole of variable diameter with well-defined sclerotic margins is seen in the sphenoid, ethmoid, or, rarely, basioccipital bone. Imaging studies demonstrate a large sac of CSF extending through this bone defect into the nasopharynx. In large encephaloceles, erosive changes will be seen in the hard palate. When the defect is in the ethmoid or sphenoid bone, the third ventricle, hypothalamus, pituitary gland, optic

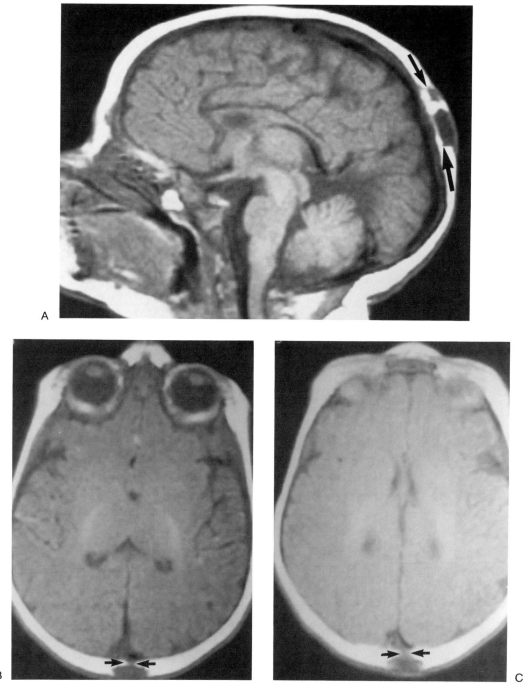

FIG. 5.30. Atretic parietal cephalocele. **A:** A subcutaneous mass (*arrows*) is present in the parietal region. It is difficult to determine whether the mass continues through the calvarium. **B, C:** Axial SE 600/20 images more clearly show continuity (*arrows*) of the subcutaneous mass with the intracranial space.

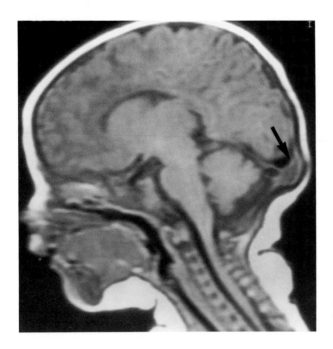

FIG. 5.31. Atretic occipital cephalocele. A nodular, small mass (*arrow*), just above the external occipital protuberance, enters the calvarium through a small calvarial defect. This mass terminated in the dura of the tentorium.

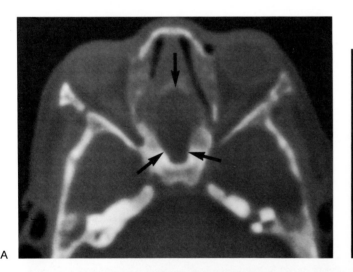

A

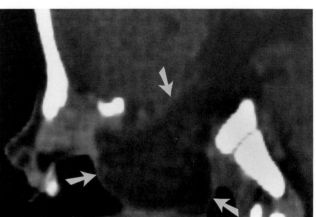

B

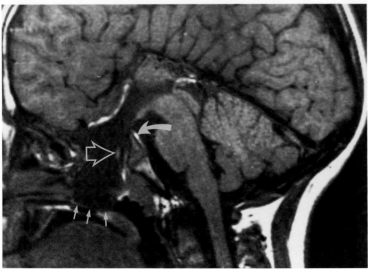

C

FIG. 5.32. Sphenoidal cephalocele. **A:** Axial CT image shows large, sharply marginated hole (*arrows*) in the sphenoid bone. **B:** Sagittal CT reformation shows the large bony defect with CSF (*arrows*) herniating within it. **C:** Sagittal SE 600/20 image reveals the encephalocele extending down through the sphenoid bone into the nasopharynx and impression upon the posterior hard palate (*small arrows*). The dorsum sellae (*curved arrow*) remains intact. The optic chiasm (*open white arrow*) runs through the encephalocele. The corpus callosum is absent.

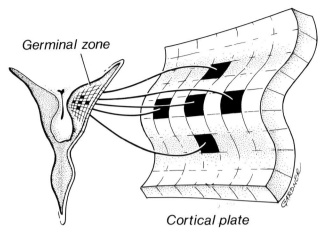

Germinal zone

Cortical plate

FIG. 5.35. Schematic drawing shows the relationship of the germinal matrix and the wall of the lateral ventricle to the developing cortical plate. There is a 1:1 correspondence between the site of cell proliferation within the germinal zone and its eventual destination within the cortical plate. The corresponding regions are connected by radial glial cells that span the entire thickness of the hemisphere.

ment and migration (61); neurons migrate from the germinal zone to the cortex in an "inside out" sequence. Those destined for the deepest cortical layer (layer 6) migrate early, followed by those destined for layer 5, layer 4, layer 3, and, finally, layer 2. The exception to the "inside-out" rule of neuronal migration is that those neurons destined for the molecular layer (layer 1) seem to be the first to arrive in the cortex (59,62,63). The fact that the molecular layer forms first has led to speculation that the molecular layer in some way interacts with the subsequently migrating neurons of the lower layers in order to facilitate their separation from the radial glial fibers at the end of their migration (59,62,63). After their arrival in the cortex, neurons become arranged in discrete lamina and establish synaptic contacts with local and distant neurons in a process known as cortical *organization* (15,64,65).

Any event that inhibits neuronal migration or subsequent cortical organization can cause a cortical anomaly. These can include destructive events, such as infections or ischemia that damage the radial glial fibers, the molecular layer, or the overlying "pial–glial barrier," or the introduction of toxins (exogenous, from ingestion of toxic substances, or endogenous, from metabolic disorders) that may inhibit chemotaxis of the neurons along the glial fibers (64,65). All anomalies of neuronal migration and organization are, by definition, hamartomas in that the abnormalities are composed of normal neurons located in abnormal places. Because the neurons are normal, the malformations that result from their abnormal location usually have a normal signal intensity on imaging studies; that is, the signal intensity is isointense to normal gray matter. A few exceptions to this rule are seen in the cortical dysplasias and will be discussed in that section.

The neuronal migration anomalies are divided into several categories, depending upon the timing and the severity of the injury and the appearance of the resulting anomaly. Developmental anomalies of the cerebral neocortex occur in a number of different syndromes, many of which are listed in Table 5.1. The details of most of these syndromes will not be elaborated upon in this chapter, as they are more appropriately discussed in a genetics text. Only a few well-known, common, or particularly instructive syndromes will be elaborated upon.

Lissencephalies

The term *lissencephaly* means "smooth brain" and refers to a paucity of gyral and sulcal development on the surface of the brain. *Agyria* is defined as an absence of gyri on the surface of the brain and is synonymous with "complete lissencephaly," whereas *pachygyria* is defined as the presence of a few broad, flat gyri and is used interchangeably with the term *incomplete lissencephaly*. Children with lissencephaly are typically severely disabled, both physically and intellectually, although some variability in clinical course is seen in patients with less severe cortical involvement. Lissencephalies can be divided into a number of subcategories based upon the

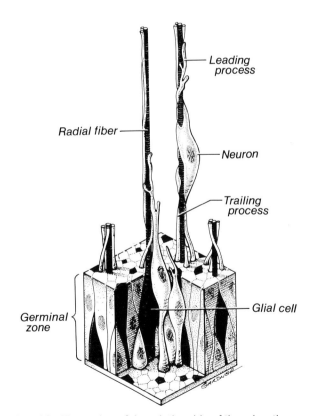

Leading process

Radial fiber

Neuron

Trailing process

Glial cell

Germinal zone

FIG. 5.36. Illustration of the relationship of the migrating neurons to fibers of the radial glial cells. A migrating neuron is seen ascending the radial glial fiber. Any damage to the radial glial fiber or alteration of the molecules on the surface of either the migrating neuron or the radial glial cell will cause an arrest of cell migration.

morphology of the smooth brain and the associated brain anomalies.

Type I Lissencephaly (The Agyria–Pachygyria Complex)

Children with type I lissencephaly are variably microencephalic and retarded, depending upon the severity of the cortical anomaly (66–68); many have a defect of chromosome 17 at locus 17p13.3 (69). A subset of this group with characteristic facies is classified as having the Miller–Dieker syndrome (68,70). Patients with complete lissencephaly are typically hypotonic at birth, gradually developing appendicular and oropharyngeal spasticity as their nervous system matures (66,71). Patients with incomplete lissencephaly have less severe motor abnormalities and hypotonia (66). Infantile spasms are common in severely affected infants. The development of medically refractory epilepsy at a very early age, with increasingly complex seizure disorders, is characteristic. Systemic anomalies, particularly those of the ears, eyes, heart, and kidney, are present in the more severely affected patients (66,68,70,72,73).

Most patients in this group have areas of both agyria and pachygyria (i.e., incomplete lissencephaly). The areas of agyria are most frequently parieto-occipital in location, whereas the pachygyric areas are more common in the frontal and temporal regions (66,71,74), although exceptions to this pattern occur. Microscopically, the cerebral cortex is composed of a thin outer layer of neurons, a cell sparse zone, and a thick inner layer of neurons (Fig. 5.37). The inner layer of neurons is thought to represent young neurons that were prematurely stopped during their migration to the cortex. Presumably, a molecular marker on the surface of the radial glial cells (or, perhaps, on the migrating neurons) is either abnormal or deficient (59,64,66,71,74); alternatively, the arrest of neuronal migration may reflect some abnormality of the fetal ependyma (75,76). Whatever the cause, the last phase of neuronal migration to the cerebral cortex is impaired.

Imaging studies of patients with type I lissencephaly reveal a smooth brain surface with diminished white matter and shallow, vertically oriented Sylvian fissures (Fig. 5.38) (64,66,68,71,77,78). A thin outer cortical layer is separated from a thick deeper cortical layer by a zone of white matter (the "cell-sparse zone") that seems to myelinate normally (Fig. 5.38). The gross appearance of the brain resembles that of the fetus prior to 23 or 24 gestational weeks, when sulci normally begin to form (see the section on normal brain development in Chapter 2 and Fig. 5.39). The cerebrum has a figure-of-eight appearance on axial images as a result of the shallow, vertical Sylvian fissures (Fig. 5.38). In cases of severe agyria, sagittal images may show callosal hypogenesis (Fig. 5.40). The ventricular trigones and occipital horns are enlarged, mostly because of underdevelopment of the calcarine sulci (71); hypoplasia of the callosal splenium may play a role in some patients. The brain stem often appears hypoplastic, probably because many of the corticospinal and corticobulbar tracts do not form.

Areas of pachygyria also have a thickened cortex, but broad gyri and shallow sulci are present. Pachygyria can be focal or diffuse. When focal (Fig. 5.41), it can occur in any part of the brain. When diffuse (Fig. 5.42), it is often associated with regions of agyria and tends to be more severe in the parieto-occipital region of the brain (and least severe in the frontal and temporal lobes). This has led some people to hypothesize a vascular etiology for retardation of neuronal migration with the most severe migration anomaly being in the watershed area between the anterior and posterior circulations of the brain (74). The vascular hypothesis is not widely accepted at the present time (64,69,71).

Type II Lissencephaly (Walker-Warburg Syndrome, Fukuyama's Congenital Muscular Dystrophy, and Related Syndromes)

Patients with type II lissencephaly classically present with the *Walker-Warburg syndrome* (68,72,79). Affected patients are obviously abnormal at birth and may have severe congenital eye malformations, posterior cephaloceles, congenital hydrocephalus, or congenital hypotonia (68,80). The hypotonia is usually profound and unchanging, with most patients dying in the first year of life secondary to recurrent aspiration and respiratory illnesses.

On imaging studies, patients with Walker-Warburg syndrome have a thickened cortex with shallow sulci (which may appear intermediate between type I lissencephaly and diffuse polymicrogyria), microphthalmia (which may be unilateral or bilateral), hydrocephalus, callosal hypogenesis, and hypomyelination (Fig. 5.43) (81). The appearance of the cortex is quite distinctive, with an irregular gray matter–white matter junction (Fig. 5.43), possibly reflecting the extension of bundles of disorganized cortical neurons into the underlying white matter (64). More severe cases will have vermian hypogenesis, cerebellar polymicrogyria, and occasionally an occipital cephalocele.

Some authors (68,80,82–86) have pointed out similarities and apparent overlap of Walker-Warburg syndrome with *Fukuyama's congenital muscular dystrophy* (FCMD), a condition seen primarily in children of Japanese ancestry (87,88). Overlapping features include the presence of congenital muscular dystrophy in some patients with the Walker-Warburg syndrome (83) and the presence of diffuse cortical dysplasia (84), type II lissencephaly (Dr. K. Takada, personal communication), hypomyelination (86), and ocular dysplasias (85) in Fukuyama's congenital muscular dystrophy. A family has

TABLE 5.1. *Syndromes associated with neuronal migration/organization disorders*

Metabolic syndromes
Zellweger's syndrome
Neonatal adrenoleukodystrophy
Glutaric aciduria II
Menke's kinky hair disease
Gm2 gangliosidosis

Neuromuscular syndromes
Walker-Warburg syndrome
Fukuyama's congenital muscular dystrophy
Myotonic dystrophy
Anterior horn arthrogryposis

Neurocutaneous syndromes
Incontinentia pigmenti
Type I neurofibromatosis
Hypomelanosis of Ito
Encephalocranial cutaneous lipomatosis
Tuberous sclerosis
Linear sebaceous nevus syndrome

Multiple congenital anomalies syndromes
Smith-Lemli-Opitz syndrome
Potter syndrome
Cornelia de Lange syndrome
Meckel-Gruber syndrome
Oro-Facio-Digital syndrome
Coffin-Siris syndrome
Bergeron syndrome
Short-Small syndrome

Chromosomal syndromes
Trisomy 13
Trisomy 18
Trisomy 21
Deletion 4p
Deletion 17p 13 (Miller-Dieker syndrome)

Skeletal dysplasias
Thanatophoric dysplasia

Other CNS dyplasias
Aicardi syndrome
Joubert syndrome
Rhombencephalosynapsis
Idiopathic lissencephaly sequence
Hemimegalencephaly

Twin syndromes
Parabiotic twin syndrome

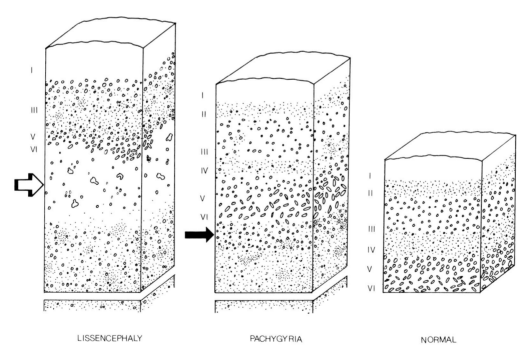

LISSENCEPHALY   PACHYGYRIA   NORMAL

FIG. 5.37. Cortical architecture in agyric (labeled lissencephaly) and pachygyric regions of the brain as compared with normal cortical architecture. In the agyric cortex there is a large cell-sparse layer (*open arrow*) that separates a disorganized cortex (outer cellular layer) from a thick layer of ectopic neurons located medially. The pachygyric cortex is better organized and the cell-sparse layer (*closed arrow*) is thinner and populated by more cells.

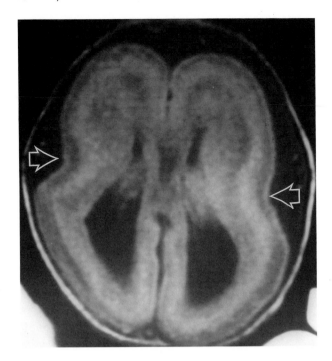

FIG. 5.38. Lissencephaly. Axial SE 550/15 image shows the thin outer cortical layer separated from layer of arrested neurons by normal white matter. The shallow, vertically oriented Sylvian fissures (*arrows*) are open laterally, giving the brain a figure-of-eight appearance.

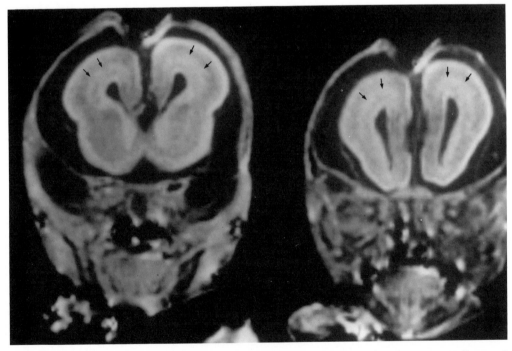

FIG. 5.39. Normal 18-week fetal brain shows agyric surface. Layer of migrating neurons (*arrows*) can be seen between the germinal zone and cortex. (Reprinted with permission from ref. 64.)

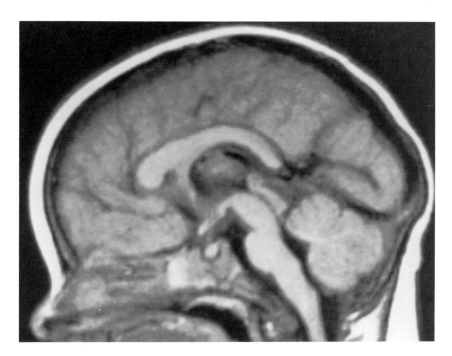

FIG. 5.40. Lissencephaly. Sagittal SE 500/25 image shows a hypogenetic corpus callosum with small splenium and absent rostrum.

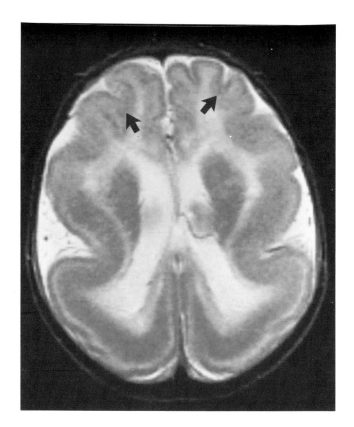

FIG. 5.41. Incomplete lissencephaly. Axial SE 3000/120 image shows nearly complete agyria posteriorly. The vertical, shallow Sylvian fissures and arrested layer of neurons can be seen. Frontally (*arrows*), the cortex abruptly becomes mildly pachygyric.

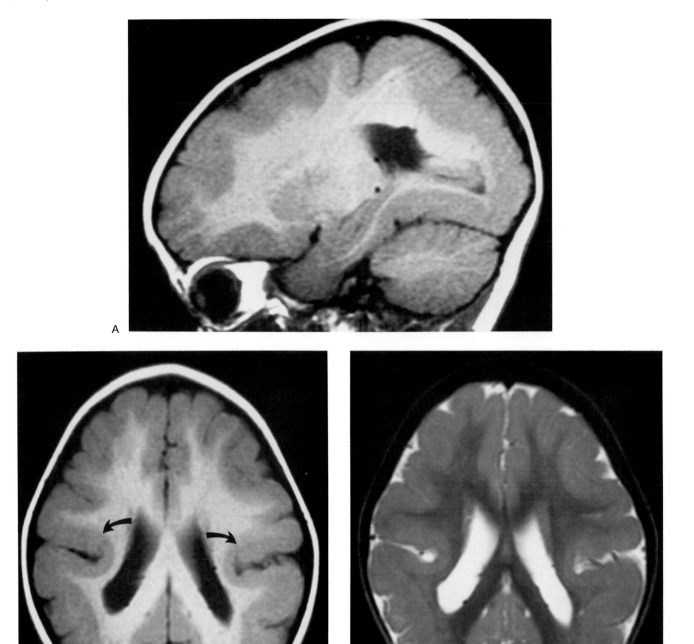

FIG. 5.42. Diffuse pachygyria. **A:** Parasagittal SE 500/16 image shows thickened cortex with relatively few and large gyri and sulci. **B:** Axial SE 550/16 image shows that the pachygyria is more severe in the parietal and occipital lobes than in the frontal lobes. The Sylvian fissures (*arrows*) are abnormally vertical. **C:** Axial SE 2800/80 image shows hyperintensity (*arrows*), possibly the cell-sparse zone, in the occipital lobe.

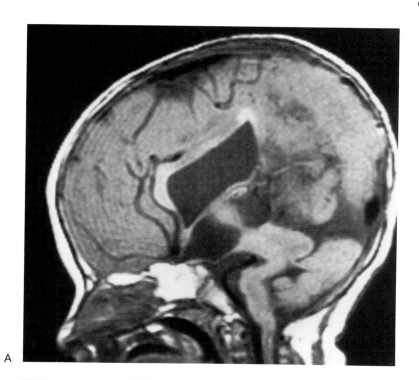

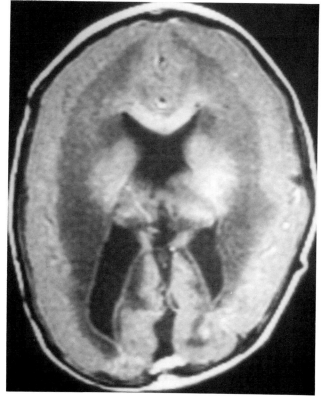

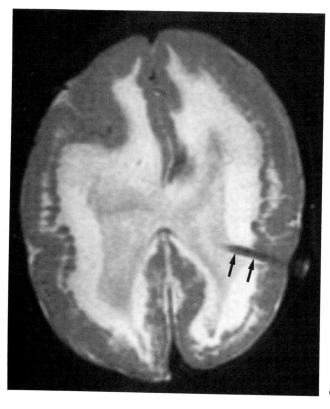

FIG. 5.43. Walker-Warburg syndrome. **A:** Sagittal SE 550/15 image shows agyria, callosal hypogenesis, and distortion of the brain stem secondary to a forme fruste occipital cephalocele. **B:** Axial SE 600/15 image shows nearly complete agyria and profound hypomyelination. **C:** Axial SE 3000/120 image shows a left ventriculostomy tube (*arrows*), marked hypomyelination, and irregular projections of cortex into the underlying white matter, a pattern characteristic of type 2 lissencephaly.

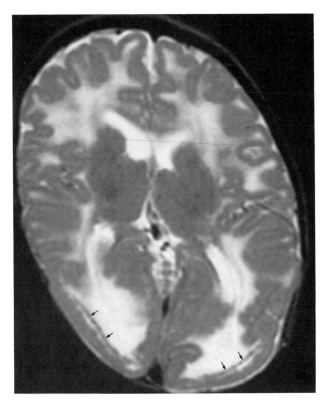

FIG. 5.44. Fukuyama's congenital muscular dystrophy. Axial SE 3000/120 image shows agyria in the occipital lobes with a thin layer of gray matter (*arrows*) deep to the cortex. The white matter shows marked hypomyelination.

been reported in which one sibling has FCMD and another has the Walker-Warburg syndrome (89). Imaging findings are similar as well, as MR studies of patients with Fukuyama's CMD show type II lissencephaly or polymicrogyria, delayed myelination, cerebellar polymicrogyria, and enlarged cerebral ventricles (although not frank hydrocephalus) (Fig. 5.44) (86). Some authors have proposed that the Walker-Warburg syndrome and Fukuyama's congenital muscular dystrophy are part of a spectrum of pathology with an intermediate form (muscle–eye–brain disease) consisting of congenital muscular dystrophy, congenital retinal dysplasia, hydrocephalus, hypomyelination of the white matter, and cerebral cortical dysplasia (82,90–93).

Type III Lissencephaly (Microcephalia Vera)

The term *microcephalia vera* describes several genetic and sporadic diseases (94,95). Typically, patients present with moderate developmental delay but no focal neurologic findings. Histologic examination of the cerebral cortex reveals severe depletion of the neurons of layers 2 and 3. Histopathologic examination of one entire brain revealed no migratory disorder and no heterotopias, but a depleted germinal zone at a gestational age of 26 weeks (96) [which is the age of maximal volume in the germinal zone in normal fetuses (97)], raising the possibility that the disorder is caused by early exhaustion of the germinal zone (95). On gross pathologic examination, these brains have thin cortices, shallow sulci, and markedly diminished callosal fibers (which originate and terminate in the outer cortical layers) (96). One case of presumed microcephalia vera studied by MR showed a dramatically small brain with lissencephaly and an extremely thin cortex (Fig. 5.45) (64).

Type IV Lissencephaly (Radial Microbrain)

The term *radial microbrain* has been used to describe a group of patients that were born at term and had markedly reduced brain size despite normal gyral patterns, ab-

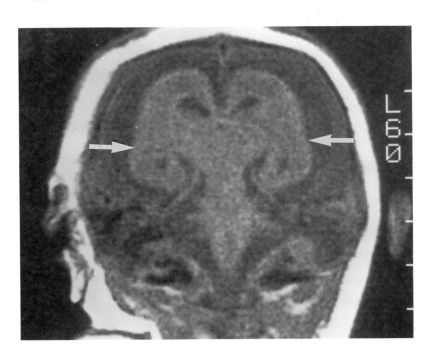

FIG. 5.45. Presumed microcephalia vera. Coronal SE 600/20 image shows a very small, agyric brain with a very thin cortex (*arrows*). The extra-axial fluid may be in the subarachnoid or subdural space.

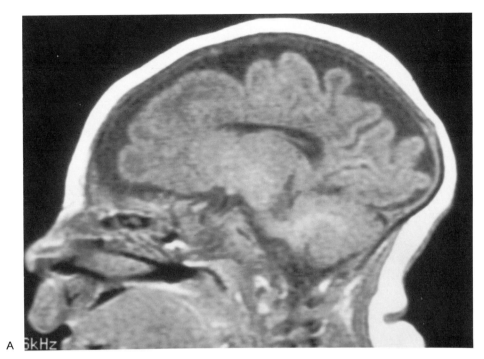

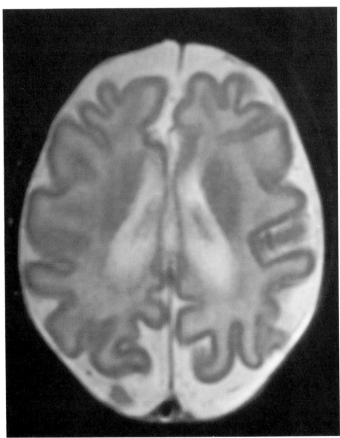

FIG. 5.46. Presumed radial microbrain. **A:** Sagittal SE 500/11 image shows very small brain with simplified gyral pattern. (Reprinted with permission from ref. 64.) **B:** Axial SE 3000/120 image shows hypomyelination and simplified gyral pattern.

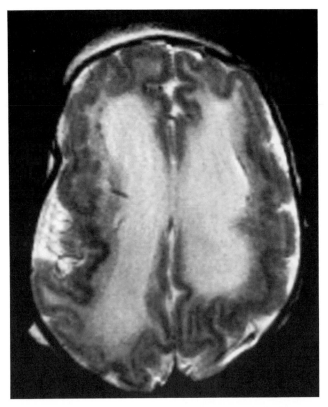

FIG. 5.47. Lissencephaly from congenital cytomegalovirus infection. The gyral pattern is diffusely abnormal, with shallow sulci and broad, irregular gyri. Pathologically, these patients are found to have polymicrogyria.

sence of destruction or gliosis, normal cortical thickness, and normal cortical lamination (98). However, the number of neocortical neurons was only 30% of normal. All affected patients had profound microcephaly and extra–central nervous system anomalies, such as nephropathy and acromicria. MR scans show microcephaly, delayed myelination, and a slightly immature gyral pattern (Fig. 5.46). I suspect the myelination delay comes from lack of production of oligodendrocyte precursors by the depleted germinal zones.

Type V Lissencephaly (Diffuse Polymicrogyria)

The final type of lissencephaly is a diffusely smooth brain caused by abnormal organization of cortical neurons, resulting in diffuse cortical dysplasia, or polymicrogyria (Fig. 5.47) (99). This is the type of lissencephaly seen in patients with cortical involvement from congenital cytomegalovirus infection (see Chapter 11).

Heterotopia

Gray matter heterotopia are collections of nerve cells in abnormal locations secondary to arrest of radial migration of neurons. (Note that the word *heterotopia* is plural; the singular form of the noun is *heterotopion*.) Heterotopia can be isolated or can be seen in association

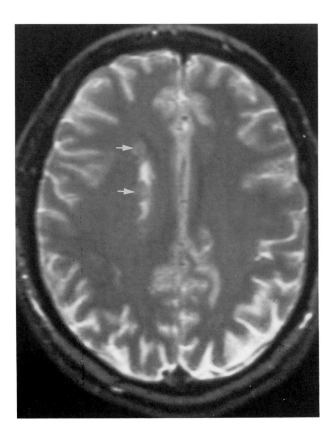

FIG. 5.48. Subependymal heterotopia. Axial SE 2500/70 image shows two subependymal nodules (*arrows*) of gray matter.

with other structural anomalies. In a broad sense, all anomalies of neuronal migration are heterotopia in the sense that all are composed of normal nerve cells in abnormal locations; however, the term *heterotopia* is reserved for cases in which the ectopic neurons are localized in an area other than the cortex.

Patients with heterotopic gray matter almost always present with a seizure disorder (77,100,101). For the purposes of clinical evaluation and prognostication, it is useful to divide heterotopia into three groups: (1) subependymal heterotopia; (2) focal subcortical heterotopia; and (3) diffuse heterotopia (100). Patients with *subependymal heterotopia* usually manifest mild clinical symptoms, with normal development, normal motor function, and onset of seizures during the second decade of life. Seizures are typically mixed partial complex and tonic–clonic (100). Patients with *focal subcortical heterotopia* have variable motor and intellectual disturbances, depending upon the size of the heterotopion and the effect on the overlying cortex. Patients with large, thick subcortical heterotopia present with moderate to severe developmental delay and hemiplegia, whereas those with smaller or thinner subcortical heterotopia may have normal motor function and normal development (100). Finally, patients with *diffuse gray matter heterotopia* (also referred to as "*band heterotopia*" (102) or "*double cortex*" (103,104) typically present with moderate to severe developmental delay and mixed seizure

disorders that are usually refractory to medical therapy (102–104). Livingston and colleagues (103), however, report two patients with "double cortex" and relatively mild clinical manifestations, indicating some variability in clinical presentation.

MR is much more sensitive than CT in the detection of heterotopia (101). Heterotopia appear as nodular or broad regions in the subependymal, periventricular, or subcortical areas that are isointense with gray matter on all imaging sequences. The most important features in distinguishing heterotopia from tumors are that heterotopia lack surrounding edema, remain isointense with gray matter on all imaging sequences and with all imaging modalities, and do not enhance after administration of contrast agents (77,100,101). *Subependymal heterotopia* are smooth, ovoid masses (Figs. 5.48, 5.49) that grow into the adjacent lateral ventricle, often causing the ventricle to appear compressed. They are differentiated from the subependymal hamartomas of tuberous sclerosis by their shape [hamartomas of tuberous sclerosis are irregular and often elongated (105–107)], their signal intensity [subependymal hamartomas of tuberous sclerosis are usually iso- to hypointense compared to mature white matter (107,108), not isointense with gray matter], and the fact that they do not enhance after intravenous infusion of paramagnetic contrast (105,109). *Focal subcortical heterotopia* will sometimes appear to contain vessels or cerebrospinal fluid, thereby mimicking tu-

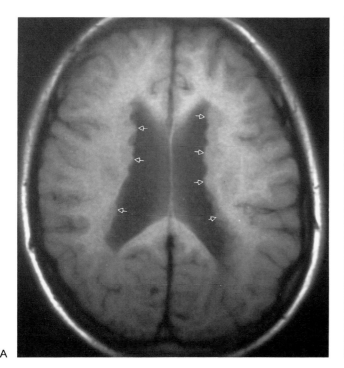 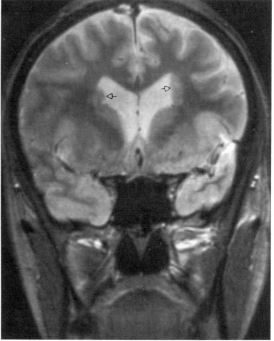

A   B

FIG. 5.49. Subependymal heterotopia. **A:** Axial SE 600/20 image reveals multiple nodular masses lining the lateral ventricles (*arrows*). The key to identifying these as heterotopia is their isointensity with cortical gray matter. **B:** Coronal SE 2500/70 image reveals that the heterotopia (*arrows*) remain isointense with cortical gray matter on all imaging sequences, assuring the diagnosis.

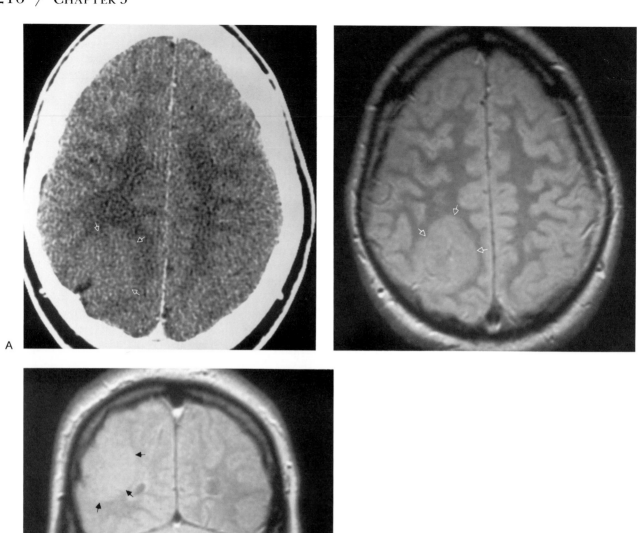

FIG. 5.50. Subcortical heterotopia. **A:** Axial CT shows a nodular mass of gray matter in the left parieto-occipital region (*arrows*). **B, C:** Axial SE 2800/70 (B) and coronal SE 2800/30 (C) images show that the mass (*arrows*) remains isointense with gray matter on all sequences.

mors. Closer examination in these cases will show that the vessels and cerebrospinal fluid are within infoldings of the cortex adjacent to the heterotopia (Figs. 5.50, 5.51) (100). Thus, these patients may, in fact, be better classified as having convoluted regions of cortical dysplasia. Patients with large subcortical heterotopia may show thinning of the overlying cortex. The heterotopia may appear to exert mass effect on the adjacent ventricle or the interhemispheric fissure. Further scrutiny of the images, however, will show the affected hemisphere to be small and that the apparent mass effect is actually distortion of the hemisphere caused by the dysplasia. Thus, heterotopia can be differentiated from tumors, which will enlarge the affected hemisphere. Finally, *diffuse gray matter heterotopia (band heterotopia)* appear as a cir-

cumferential band of gray matter that is deep to the cerebral cortex and separated from the cortex by a layer of normal-appearing white matter (Fig. 5.52). The overlying cortex may appear normal, may have normal thickness with shallow sulci, or may be pachygyric. The degree of cortical gyral dysplasia seems to be related to the thickness of the band heterotopia (i.e., the thicker the band of heterotopic gray matter, the more anomalous the overlying cortex).

When studied by PET using [^{18}F]-fluorodeoxyglucose, heterotopia are found to have a glucose uptake that is similar to normal cortex (110,111). This finding contrasts with the hypometabolism found in cortical dysplasias (see the next section) and in most epileptogenic foci. Morrell and colleagues (112) have found epileptiform

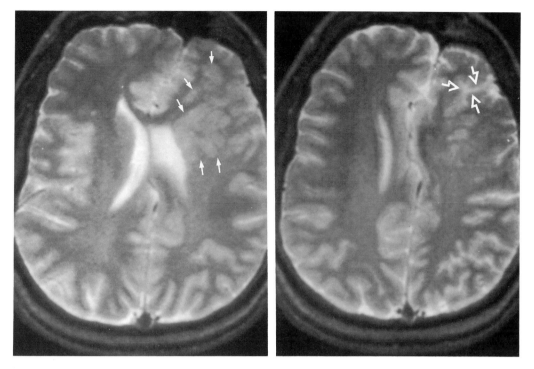

FIG. 5.51. Subcortical heterotopia. Axial SE 2500/70 images show gray matter nodules (*arrows*) in the left frontal lobe. The left hemisphere is smaller than the right. The subarachnoid space (*open arrows*) extends into the ectopic gray matter.

discharges emanating from the band, suggesting that it is the source of the seizure activity in affected patients.

The deep neuronal layer of band heterotopia is identical to the layer of heterotopic neurons seen in type I lissencephaly, in that both are layers of neurons that have been arrested during their migration to the cortex (104).

Band heterotopia, therefore, appear to be the mildest end of a spectrum of disorders that includes the type I lissencephalies. It appears that both the degree of pachygyria and the degree of mental and developmental retardation in affected patients are related to the thickness of the band (unpublished observations). Therefore, band heterotopia are perhaps better classified among lissencephalies.

Polymicrogyria (Cortical Dysplasia)

Polymicrogyria is an anomaly of migration in which the neurons reach the cortex but distribute abnormally, resulting in the formation of multiple small gyri; technically, it is more correctly classified as a disorder of neuronal organization. Polymicrogyria has a range of histologic appearances, all having in common a derangement of the normal six-layered lamination of the cortex (64); thus, the term *cortical dysplasia* may be more appropriate. Small or large portions of the hemisphere can be involved. The most common location is around the Sylvian fissure, particularly the posterior aspect of the fissure. However, any area, including the frontal, occipi-

tal, and temporal lobes, can be affected (19,99,113–115). Patients may present at any age. The severity of the clinical presentation depends upon the extent of cortical involvement. Bilateral involvement and involvement of more than half of a single hemisphere are poor prognostic indicators, portending moderate to severe developmental delay and significant motor dysfunction (99). Cortical dysplasia is a common brain manifestation of congenital cytomegalovirus infection (CMV, see Chapter 11). Many infants with congenital CMV present at birth with a variety of visceral and CNS abnormalities. In the absence of congenital infection, patients typically present with seizures or motor dysfunction, and some exhibit developmental delay; they cannot be differentiated from patients who have cortical dysplasia from other causes (19,99,115,116). A specific *syndrome of bilateral opercular cortical dysplasia* has been described in which patients present with a syndrome of developmental pseudobulbar palsy (oropharyngeal dysfunction and dysarthria) and epilepsy (117,118). Another syndrome with cortical dysplasia, best known as *Aicardi's syndrome*, was discussed in the section on callosal anomalies.

Grossly, cortical dysplasia has a variable pattern. It can have an irregularly bumpy surface or be paradoxically smooth because the outer cortical (molecular) layer fuses at the microsulci. Although the dysplastic cortex typically shows an irregular, bumpy inner and outer cortical surface on CT and MR (Fig. 5.53), it may have the ap-

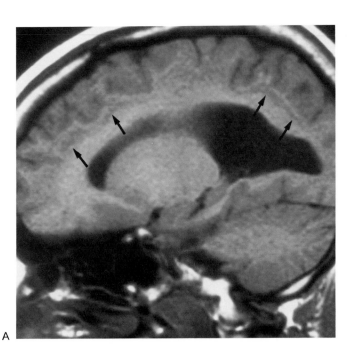
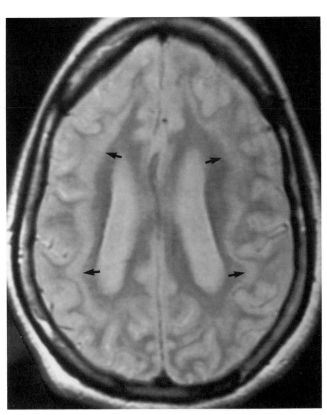

FIG. 5.52. Band heterotopia. **A:** Sagittal SE 600/20 image shows a thin layer of heterotopic neurons (*arrows*) deep to a normal-appearing cortex. **B:** Axial SE 2500/30 image shows a continuous layer of gray matter (*arrows*) separated from the cortex by a layer of myelinated white matter. The cortex is mildly pachygyric.

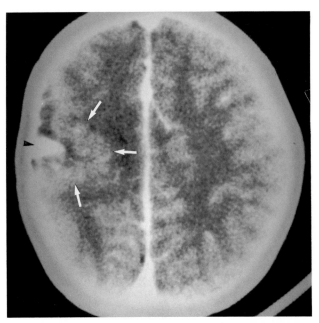
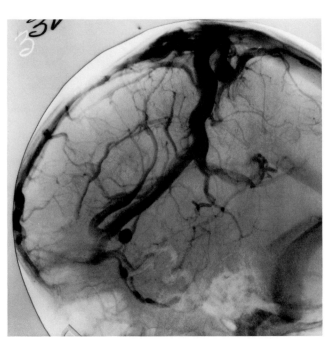

FIG. 5.53. Cortical dysplasia with anomalous venous drainage. **A:** Contrast-enhanced CT shows a very large vessel (*arrowhead*) coursing through an infolding of irregular, thickened gray matter (*white arrows*). **B:** Lateral view from venous phase of a right internal carotid arteriogram. The large vessel seen on CT scan is shown to be a large superficial vein that drains the majority of superficial veins in the hemisphere (no arteriovenous shunting and no abnormal tangles of vessels were noted on previous films in this sequence).

pearance of pachygyria, with broad, thickened gyri (Fig. 5.54) (77,99,114), or it may look normal. Because the gyri are so small, polymicrogyria may not be detected on routine spin echo images. Volume 3D gradient echo acquisition with thin partition size (1.5 mm or less) and evaluation in three planes is often necessary to detect subtle irregularities of the gray matter–white matter junction, often the only evidence of dysplastic brain (Fig. 5.55). These volume acquisitions can be displayed as three-dimensional images (Fig. 5.56), aiding in surgical therapy.

Dysplastic cortex can be flat and congruent to the arc of normal cortex (Fig. 5.57), or the dysplastic cortex may extend centripetally, appearing as if the cortex were buckled or folded inward (Fig. 5.58). The infolding of cortex may be small or large; when it extends all the way to the lateral ventricle and communicates with the ventricle, it is called a schizencephaly (see the next section). The character of the cortex in these regions of infolding is similar to that in superficial cortical dysplasia, with bumpy, irregular inner and outer cortical surfaces.

Typically, dysplastic cortex is isointense to normal cortex on imaging studies (Figs. 5.53, 5.54). Occasionally, however, the imaging appearance is atypical. Prolonged T2 relaxation time is present in the white matter subjacent to dysplastic cortex in about 20% of patients (19,99,115), possibly caused by the same insult that resulted in the disorganization of the cortex. A small proportion of cortical dysplasias, probably less than 5%, will be calcified (Fig. 5.59). Finally, it is important to realize that anomalous venous drainage is common in areas of dysplastic cortex (119). Large vessels are especially common in regions where there is a large infolding of thickened cortex (Figs. 5.53, 5.54). Such large vessels, when seen in association with an abnormal, thickened cortex, should not be mistaken for vascular malformations. Angiography is not indicated.

A number of articles have indicated that [18]FDG–PET scanning or [99m]Tc HmPAO SPECT scanning (120) may be useful in detecting small areas of cortical dysplasia (121,122). Typically, interictal PET scans show hypometabolism in dysplastic areas, including some that are cryptic to MR imaging, whereas SPECT studies show decreased perfusion (120–122). Intraictal or immediate postictal studies may show increased activity (120–122). However, PET and SPECT are nonspecific, and correlative MR imaging is always needed. Our approach is to use PET scanning in those patients who have some localization to their seizure disorder and a normal initial MR scan. If the PET study shows an area of hypometabolism, a high-resolution 3D gradient echo MR scan with gradient spoilers is performed with partition size of less than 1 mm through the region of abnormality. The cortex in that area is then closely scrutinized for any irregularity of the cortical surface or gray–white junction.

Schizencephaly

Schizencephaly, also called agenetic porencephaly, is the term used to describe gray matter–lined clefts that extend through the entire hemisphere, from the ependymal lining of the lateral ventricles to the pial covering of the cortex (123,124). The gray matter lining these clefts is dysplastic and does not exhibit normal cortical lamination. The clefts can be unilateral or bilateral and are most commonly located near the pre- and postcentral gyri. In fact, the locations in which they occur are nearly identical to those in which cortical dysplasia occurs (99,113). It has been proposed, and is likely, that schizencephaly is merely an extreme variant of cortical dysplasia, in which the infolding of cortex extends all the way into the lateral ventricle (99,113). I prefer to classify schizencephaly as a different disorder from cortical dysplasia (and, for that matter, a separate disorder from porencephaly; see Chapter 4) because of the unique imaging appearance of the gray matter–lined cleft that extends into the ventricle. For prognostic purposes, schizencephaly is divided into clefts with fused lips and those with separated lips. In the clefts with fused lips, the walls appose one another directly, obliterating the CSF space within the cleft at that point (Figs. 5.60, 5.61). When the lips are separated, CSF fills the cleft all the way from the lateral ventricle to the subarachnoid spaces surrounding the hemispheres (Figs. 5.62, 5.63) (113,123–125).

Affected patients typically present with seizures, hemiparesis, and variable developmental delay. The severity of the patient's symptoms is related to the amount of involved brain (113,126,127). Those patients with a single cleft with fused lips generally have epilepsy and may have a mild hemiparesis but are otherwise developmentally normal. Patients with unilateral clefts with separated lips usually present with epilepsy, hemiparesis, and a mild to moderate developmental delay, depending upon the location of the cleft within the brain. Patients with bilateral clefts tend to be severely retarded with early onset of epilepsy, severe motor anomalies, and frequently, blindness. The blindness often results from optic nerve hypoplasia, which is seen in up to one-third of patients with schizencephaly (77,125,128,129). The optic nerve hypoplasia, in conjunction with a high incidence of absence of the septum pellucidum, results in the classification of many affected patients in the category of septo-optic dysplasia (129).

Imaging studies of schizencephaly show a full-thickness cleft through the affected hemisphere; gray matter, typically characterized by a bumpy outer surface and an irregular gray matter–white matter junction, lines the cleft (77,78,113,125,127). The gyral pattern of the cortex adjacent to the cleft is usually abnormal, demonstrating cortical dysplasia. The gray matter in the cleft may extend into the ventricle in the form of subependy-

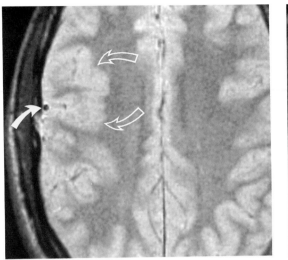 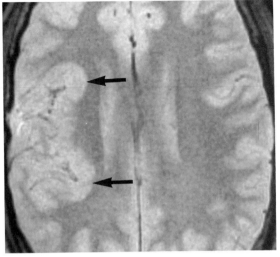

A   B

FIG. 5.54. Cortical dysplasia. **A:** Axial SE 2500/30 image shows abnormally thick cortex (*open arrows*) with irregular gray–white junction. A large vessel (*closed arrow*) lies within the adjacent sulcus. **B:** Image 12 mm below (A) shows thickened, abnormally high Sylvian fissure (*arrows*) on the right. The Sylvian cortex and adjacent cortex are the most common locations involved by polymicrogyria.

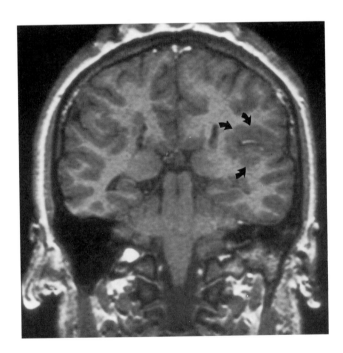

FIG. 5.55. Cortical dysplasia. Note thickened cortex (*arrows*) with irregular gray matter–white matter junction.

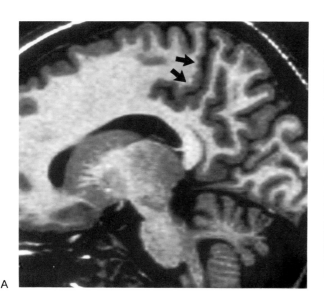

A

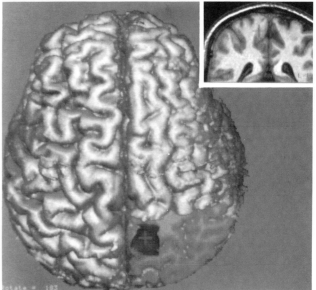

B

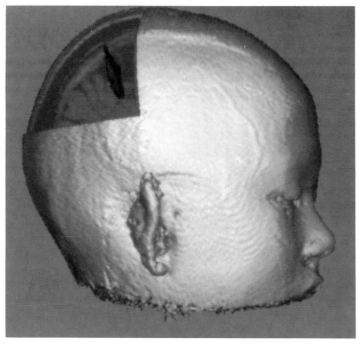

C

FIG. 5.56. Cortical dysplasia. A: Parasagittal reformation from volume gradient echo acquisition shows irregular gray matter–white matter junction (*arrows*). B, C: Three-dimensional reformation shows location of dysplastic cortex with relation to the surface of the brain and external landmarks.

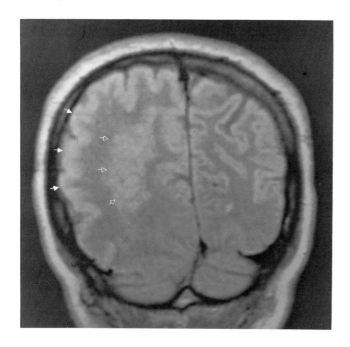

FIG. 5.57. Superficial (flat) cortical dysplasia with underlying gliotic white matter. Coronal SE 2500/35 image shows the polymicrogyria (*closed arrows*) and some gliotic white matter/ heterotopic white matter (*open arrows*) in the deep white matter.

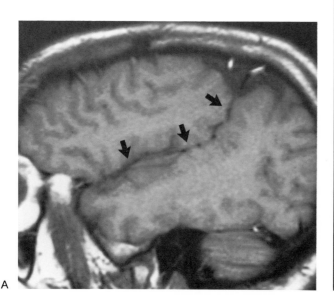

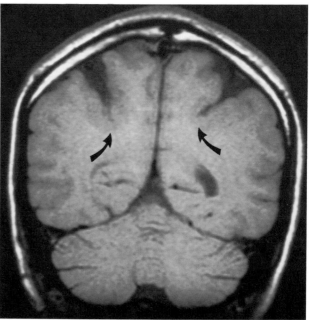

A

B

FIG. 5.58. Infolded cortical dysplasia. **A:** Parasagittal SE 600/20 image shows continuity of the Sylvian fissure (*arrows*) with a deep postcentral sulcus. **B:** Coronal SE 600/20 image shows bilateral, symmetrical infoldings of cortical dysplasia (*arrows*), with thick cortex and irregularity of gray matter–white matter junction. (Reprinted with permission from ref. 99.)

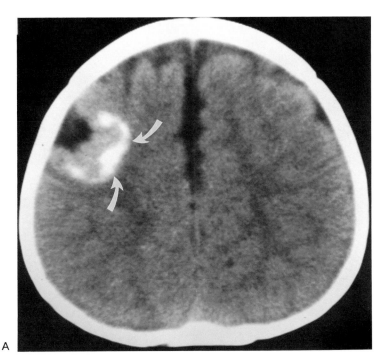

A

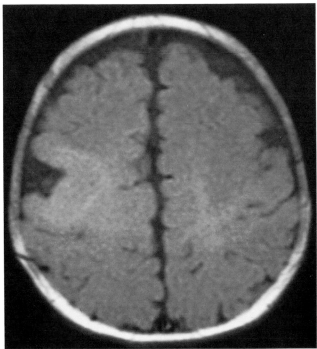

B

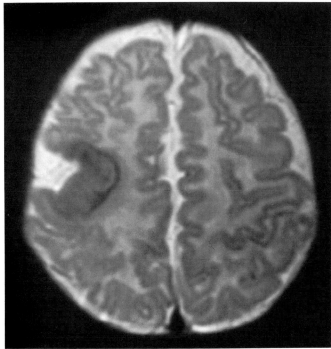

C

FIG. 5.59. Calcified cortical dysplasia. **A:** Axial CT shows area of calcified cortex (*arrows*) in the right frontal lobe. **B:** Axial SE 550/16 image shows some T1 shortening in the affected cortex. **C:** Axial SE 3000/120 image shows T2 shortening in the involved region.

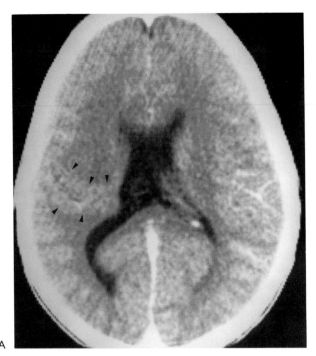
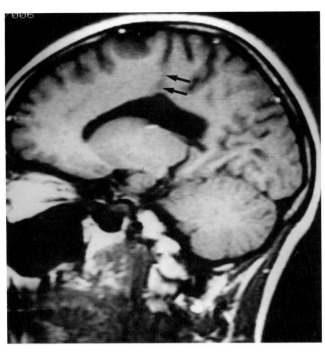

A   B

FIG. 5.60. Closed lip schizencephaly. **A:** Contrast-enhanced CT scan reveals a strip of gray matter (*arrowheads*) extending from the cortex to the lateral wall of the body of the lateral ventricle. The septum pellucidum is absent, as is the case in approximately 80% of patients with schizencephaly. **B:** Parasagittal SE 600/20 image shows a vertical holohemispheric cleft (*arrows*) extending into the lateral ventricle. (Reprinted with permission from ref. 113.)

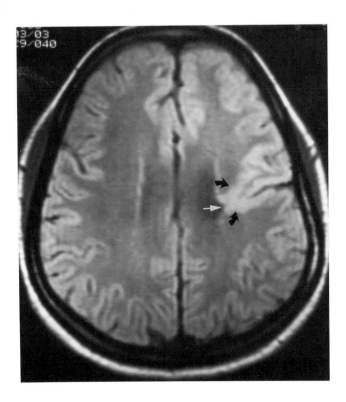

FIG. 5.61. Closed-lip schizencephaly. Axial SE 2500/20 image shows irregular gray matter (*curved black arrows*) extending from the cortex to the ventricular surface. A dimple (*white arrow*) in the ventricular wall shows the opening of the cleft into the ventricle.

mal heterotopia (Fig. 5.62). If the cleft has narrow open lips or closed lips, a dimple is usually seen in the wall of the lateral ventricle where the cleft communicates (Fig. 5.61). The dimple is often a helpful sign of continuity of the cleft with the ventricle when the lips of the cleft are fused. The reader should be aware that clefts with fused lips can be missed if the imaging plane is parallel to the plane of the cleft. For that reason, imaging should always be performed in at least two planes in patients who present with seizures or developmental delay. Cortical dysplasia may be present in the hemisphere contralateral to a unilateral schizencephaly (Fig. 5.64) (99,113); thus, the contralateral hemisphere should always be scrutinized. The septum pellucidum is absent in 80% to 90% of patients with schizencephaly.

The calvarium is often expanded over the opening of an open lip schizencephaly (Figs. 5.62, 5.64). The expansion is believed to result from CSF pulsations that emanate from the lateral ventricles and propagate through the cleft. When plagiocephaly is severe, the insertion of a ventriculoperitoneal shunt may help to dampen the pulsations and partially reverse the cranial asymmetry.

Unilateral Megalencephaly

Unilateral megalencephaly is the name given to a hamartomatous overgrowth of all or part of a cerebral hemisphere with neuronal migration defects in the affected hemisphere (77,130–133). The brain can be affected in isolation or can be associated with hemihy-

pertrophy of part or all of the ipsilateral body. Pathologically, affected hemispheres contain areas of pachygyria, polymicrogyria, and heterotopias, as well as gliosis of the hemispheric white matter (133,134). Patients present with an intractable seizure disorder that begins at a very early age (usually before the first birthday), hemiplegia, and severe developmental delay (131–134). A high incidence of hemimegalencephaly seems to occur in the linear sebaceous nevus syndrome (135,136). Other associated conditions include unilateral hypomelanosis of Ito (137) and neurofibromatosis type I (138).

On CT and MR, the involved hemisphere is moderately to markedly enlarged. The cortex is typically dysplastic, with broad gyri, shallow sulci, and cortical thickening (Fig 5.65); however, the gyral pattern may appear grossly normal or may be frankly agyric (Fig. 5.66). In severely affected patients, the usually sharp border between the cortex and the subcortical white matter may blur or disappear altogether (131,132). The white matter is of abnormally low signal on CT and usually shows prolonged T1 and T2 relaxation times on MR studies (Figs. 5.65, 5.67), representing heterotopia and gliosis. The configuration of the lateral ventricle on the affected side is quite characteristic. This lateral ventricle is enlarged in proportion to the enlargement of the affected hemisphere. Moreover, the frontal horn of the ipsilateral ventricle is almost straight, pointing superiorly and anteriorly (Fig. 5.65) (131). Rarely, the affected portion of the brain has a bizarre, hamartomatous appearance (Fig. 5.68) (131,132). In this situation, the malformation is

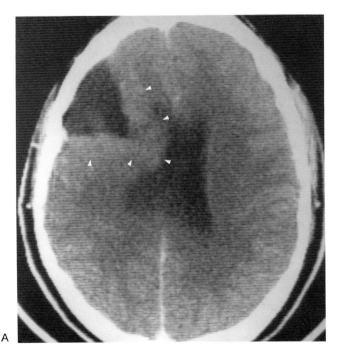
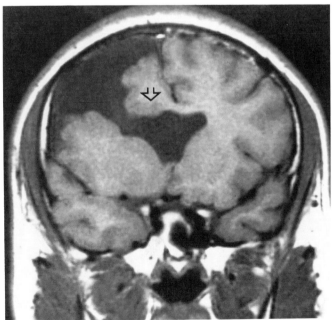

A

B

FIG. 5.62. Unilateral schizencephaly with separated lips. **A:** Contrast-enhanced axial CT scan shows a deep infolding of cortex in the right frontal region, apparently pressing upon the right lateral ventricle (*arrowheads*). **B:** Coronal SE 600/20 MR image shows this infolding to be a large cleft in continuity with the lateral ventricle. Continuity of gray matter through the cleft is clearly shown, as is the focus of heterotopic gray matter along the roof of the right lateral ventricle (*open arrow*).

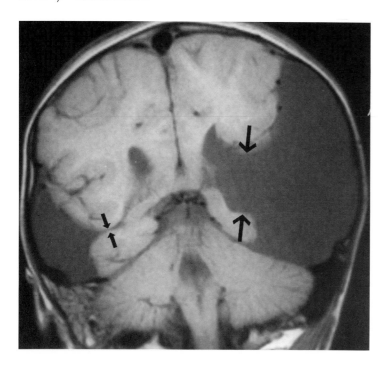

FIG. 5.63. Bilateral open-lip schizencephaly. Coronal SE 700/20 image shows the bilateral open lip schizencephalies (*arrows*). This child was severely retarded, as is usually the case with bilateral schizencephalies.

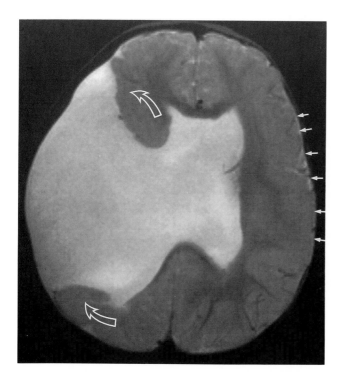

FIG. 5.64. Unilateral schizencephaly with contralateral cortical dysplasia. Axial SE 2800/80 image shows a large right schizencephaly (*open curved arrows*) with expansion of the overlying calvarium. Cortical dysplasia, with thickened cortex and shallow sulci (*small arrows*) is seen in the left hemisphere. (Reprinted with permission from ref. 113.)

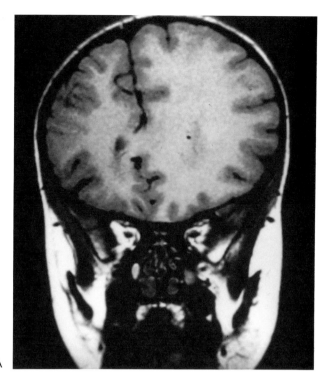

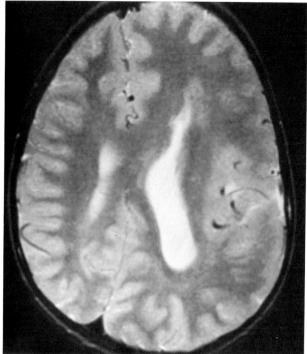

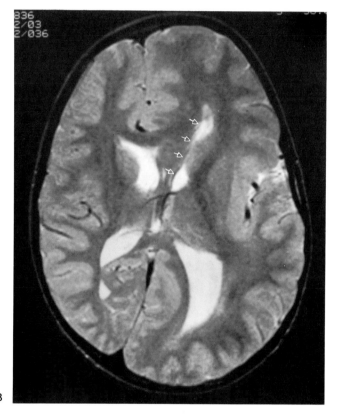

FIG. 5.65. Unilateral megalencephaly. **A:** Coronal SE 600/20 image reveals marked enlargement of the left cerebral hemisphere as compared to the right. The left frontal cortex has a pachygyric appearance. **B, C:** Axial SE 2800/70 images reveal straightening of the left frontal horn and high signal intensity from gliosis in the white matter surrounding the enlarged lateral ventricle. Notice the indistinct gray–white matter distinction in the left parietal region. The left frontal and parietal cortices are pachygyric.

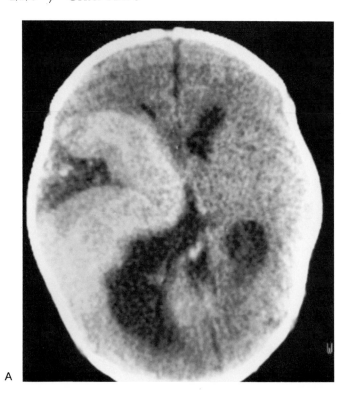

A

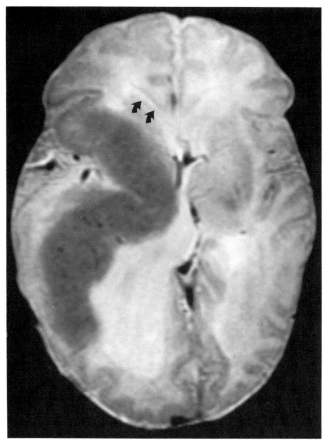

FIG. 5.66. Unilateral megalencephaly. A: CT scan in this infant shows a relatively normal left hemisphere. The right hemisphere is enlarged with a normal-appearing cortex in the frontal polar region. The posterior frontal region and the remainder of the hemisphere, however, have a primitive lissencephalic appearance with a shallow, vertical Sylvian fissure and a smooth cortex. The cortex appears calcified. The ipsilateral lateral ventricle is enlarged. B, C: Axial SE 2800/30 (B) and 2800/70 (C) images again reveal the enlarged ipsilateral ventricle, the calcified, thickened, smooth cortex; and the characteristic straightening of the frontal horn on the affected side (arrows).

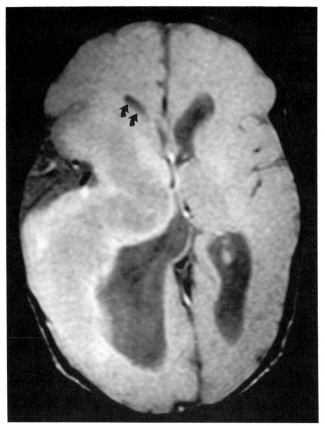

B

C

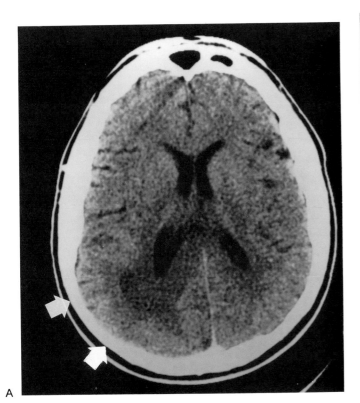

A

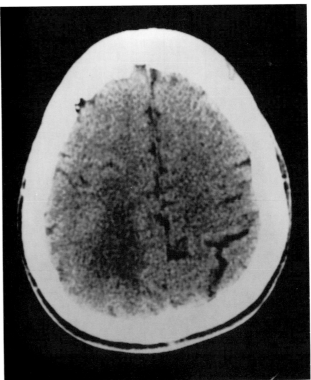

B

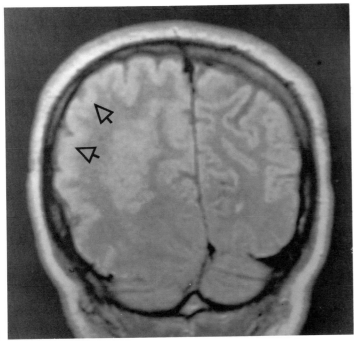

C

FIG. 5.67. Localized megalencephaly. **A, B:** Axial CT images show focal enlargement (*arrows*) of the right parietal and occipital regions with enlargement of the right ventricular trigone and hypoattenuation of adjacent white matter. **C:** Coronal SE 2500/20 image shows localized cortical dysplasia (*arrows*) in the megalencephalic region.

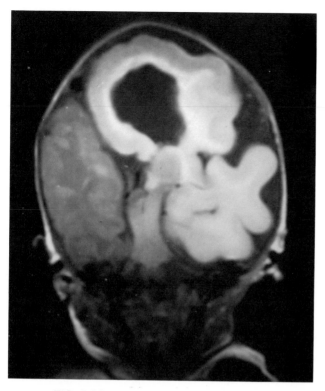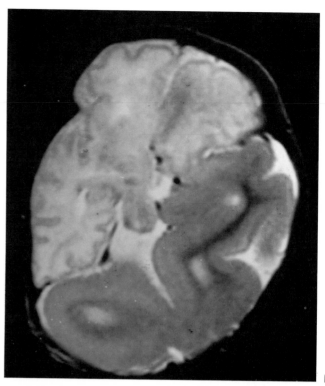

A

B

FIG. 5.68. A,B: Unilateral megalencephaly with bizarre, hamartomatous enlargement of the left hemisphere. Cortex is thick and convoluted. Myelination appears abnormally advanced.

recognized by the characteristic enlargement of the affected brain and ipsilateral ventricle.

The affected portion of the hemisphere has essentially no function in these patients save for acting as a seizure focus. Partial or complete hemispheric resection may therefore be indicated if the seizure disorder is intractable and the contralateral hemisphere is normal (139).

HOLOPROSENCEPHALY

The holoprosencephalies are a group of disorders that are characterized by a failure of differentiation and cleavage of the prosencephalon. In the normal embryo, a single prosencephalic vesicle is established at the rostral end of the neural tube between days 22 and 24 of gestation by closure of the anterior neuropore. As the prosencephalon grows, thickenings occur in the walls of the prosencephalic vesicle; these are the germinal matrices, which will produce all the cells that make up the cerebral hemispheres and deep cerebral nuclei (2,3,9). Most of the neurons that will form the diencephalon (the thalamus, hypothalamus, and globus pallidus) form in a region of the germinal zone at the base of the lateral ventricles, lateral to what will become the third ventricle (7,8,10,11). The cells that will form the telencephalon (the caudate, putamen, and cerebral hemispheres) form in the remainder of the germinal matrix. In the normal brain, the germinal matrices that will form the telencephalon and the diencephalon have separated by approximately day 32, re-

sulting in a discernible telencephalic–diencephalic junction. The cerebral hemispheres begin to evaginate on day 35 (8,11,140). Between days 32 and 34, the region of the midline between the developing hemispheres differentiates into an inactive lamina terminalis anteriorly and the active lamina reuniens (which will develop into the interhemispheric commissures) posteriorly (12). There-

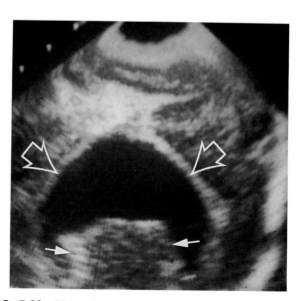

FIG. 5.69. Alobar holoprosencephaly. Transfontanel sonogram shows no definable interhemispheric fissure. The falx cerebri is completely absent. A crescent-shaped holoventricle (*open arrows*) surrounds fused thalami (*closed arrows*).

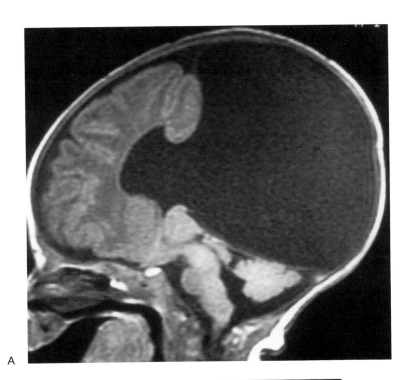

A

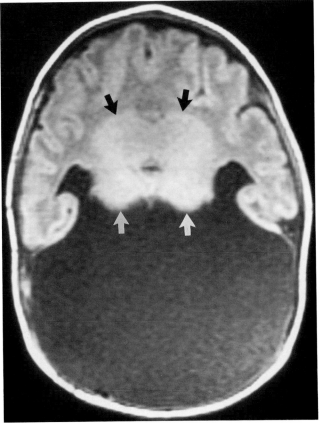

B

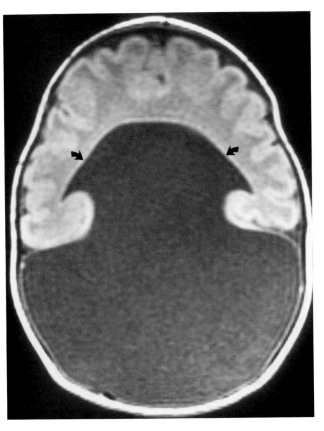

C

FIG. 5.70. Alobar holoprosencephaly. **A:** Sagittal SE 500/11 image shows a pancake of brain anteriorly. The holoventricle leads into a large dorsal cyst. **B:** Axial SE 600/15 image shows fused basal ganglia (*black arrows*) and thalami (*white arrows*). **C:** Image slightly superior to (B) shows the crescent-shaped holoventricle (*arrows*) leading into the dorsal cyst.

fore, both the differentiation of the telencephalon from the diencephalon and the separation of the telencephalon into two cerebral hemispheres are in progress by day 35, the end of the fifth week of gestation (8,11,141–143). In holoprosencephaly, the cerebrum fails to cleave laterally into distinct cerebral hemispheres and fails to cleave transversely into a diencephalon and telencephalon. In severe cases, the premaxillary segments of the face are hypoplastic as well.

Holoprosencephaly has an equal gender incidence and can be seen in several syndromes, most commonly in trisomy 13 and, less commonly, in trisomy 18. Facial dysmorphism, particularly hypotelorism and midline facial clefts, are frequently seen in the more severe forms (143–146). Clinical presentation depends upon the severity of the malformation.

DeMyer has divided holoprosencephaly into three subcategories: alobar, semilobar, and lobar holoprosencephaly (145,146). These categories are useful for classifying holoprosencephalies of different severities. The reader should be aware, however, that the holoprosencephalies represent a continuum of forebrain malformation (with the anterior portions of the brain most severely affected and the posterior parts of the brain least severely affected), that no clear distinction between the different categories exists, and that other classification systems have been suggested (143,145,146).

The embryogenesis of holoprosencephaly has not been clearly elucidated. The disorder is postulated to result from a deficient or defective cranial mesenchyme, with subsequent lack of induction of neural differentiation (17,140,147). The deficiency of mesenchyme may be responsible for the hypoplasia of the premaxillary segments of the face and the falx cerebri, the lack of differentiation of the telencephalon from the diencephalon, the lack of separation of the telencephalon into two hemispheres, and the common lack of cortical organization in those regions where the cortex is formed (17,140,143,145–147). Others suggest that the pathogenesis is related to a primary disturbance of the lamina terminalis (75).

Alobar Holoprosencephaly

Alobar holoprosencephaly is the most severe form of holoprosencephaly. In affected patients, the thalami are fused, resulting in absence of the third ventricle. No interhemispheric fissure, falx cerebri, or corpus callosum can be identified. Most commonly, the cerebrum is composed of a pancakelike mass of tissue in the rostralmost portion of the calvarium. A crescent-shaped holoventricle is continuous with a large dorsal cyst, which usually occupies most of the volume of the calvarium (Figs. 5.69, 5.70). Patients with alobar holoprosencephaly usually

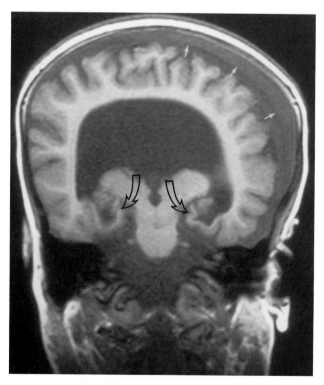

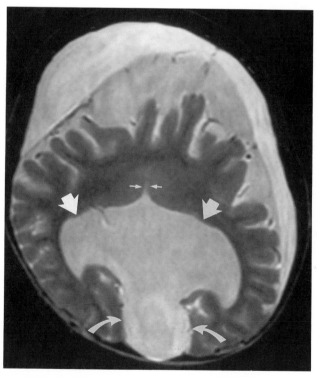

A

B

FIG. 5.71. Semilobar holoprosencephaly. **A:** Coronal SE 600/20 image shows an abnormal gyral configuration, absence of the corpus callosum and interhemispheric fissure, a crescent-shaped holoventricle, and a small third ventricle (*arrows*). The hippocampi (*open curved arrows*) are incompletely formed. A small subdural hematoma (*arrows*) is present. **B:** Axial SE 2500/70 image reveals absence of an interhemispheric fissure. The telencephalic ventricle (*large arrows*) is continuous with the third ventricle (*small arrows*) and the dorsal cyst (*medium, curved arrows*).

have severe midline facial deformities and hypotelorism, resulting from absence or hypoplasia of the premaxillary segment of the face. In the extreme forms, the orbits and globes are fused, resulting in cyclopia. The anterior cerebral arteries are nearly always azygous, with a single arterial trunk supplying branches to anterior cerebral artery territories in both cerebral hemispheres. Alobar holoprosencephaly is the most common form of holoprosencephaly diagnosed by prenatal ultrasound (148, 149). Most affected infants are stillborn or have a very short life span, and it is somewhat unusual for them to be imaged by computed tomography or magnetic resonance.

Semilobar Holoprosencephaly

In the semilobar form of holoprosencephaly the brain is less dysmorphic than in the alobar form. The interhemispheric fissure and falx cerebri are usually partially formed in the posterior portions of the brain; however, the anterior (frontal) regions of the brain remain fused and underdeveloped. The thalami are partially separated, resulting in a small third ventricle. Rudimentary temporal horn formation is seen, although the hippocampus is incompletely formed (Fig. 5.71). The septum pellucidum is absent in all forms of holoprosencephaly. The callosal splenium is present without a callosal body

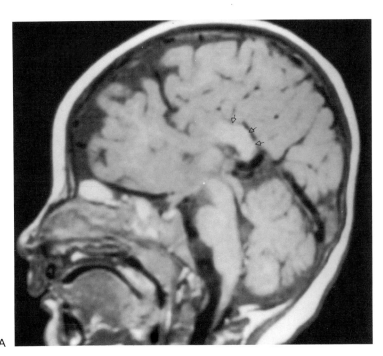

A

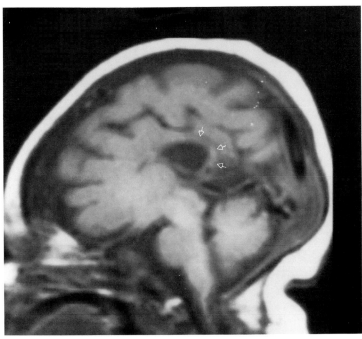

B

FIG. 5.72. Corpus callosum in semilobar holoprosencephaly. **A, B:** Sagittal T1-weighted images show presence of a callosal splenium in the absence of a rostrum, genu, and body (*arrows*). Holoprosencephaly is the only condition in which this occurs.

or genu in many patients with semilobar holoprosencephaly (Fig. 5.72) (16,18,143). *Holoprosencephaly is the only brain anomaly described in which the posterior corpus callosum forms in the absence of anterior callosal formation.* As the spectrum of holoprosencephaly is observed from the most poorly differentiated alobar brain to the most differentiated lobar brain, we see a gradient of development in which the separation of the hemispheres, development of the falx cerebri, and development of the cerebral hemispheres progress from the occipital pole to the frontal pole of the cerebrum. Because

the severity of holoprosencephaly is related to how completely the anterior (frontal) regions of the brain are developed, the anterior extent of callosal formation, which reflects the anterior extent of cerebral development, can be used as an approximate marker of brain development in holoprosencephalic patients. In other words, the further anterior the corpus forms, the better developed the brain (Figs. 5.72, 5.73). Patients with semilobar holoprosencephaly usually have mild facial anomalies or normal facies (143–147).

A few cases have been described in which the inter-

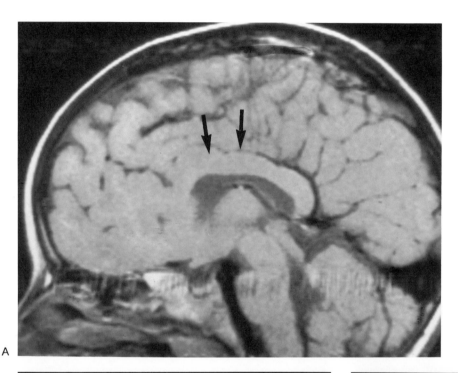

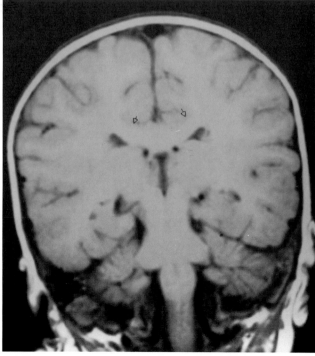

FIG. 5.73. Lobar holoprosencephaly. **A:** Sagittal SE 550/15 image shows a normal posterior corpus callosum; the corpus seems to fade in the region of the anterior body and genu (*arrows*), however. **B:** Coronal SE 600/20 image shows a normal interhemispheric fissure and posterior callosal body (*arrows*). **C:** Axial SE 2800/80 image shows a normal appearing splenium (*large closed arrows*), normal third ventricle (small *closed arrows*), and rudimentary frontal horns (*small open arrows*). The anterior interhemispheric fissure is unformed, and the anterior cerebral artery (*curved black arrow*) is azygous. (Reprinted with permission from ref. 18.)

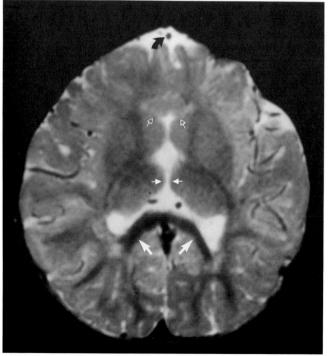

A

B

C

hemispheric fissure is formed frontally and occipitally but the hemispheres are fused in the posterior frontal and parietal regions (17). This condition is termed *holoprosencephaly with middle interhemispheric fusion.* I consider it a form of semilobar holoprosencephaly. It is one of the few conditions in which the callosal genu and splenium appear normally formed in the absence of the callosal body (see the section on callosal anomalies earlier in this chapter and Fig. 5.74.)

Lobar Holoprosencephaly

The point at which a brain is identified as being a lobar, in contrast to a semilobar, holoprosencephaly is poorly defined. If the third ventricle is fully formed, some frontal horn formation is present, and the posterior half of the callosal body is formed (in addition to the splenium), the holoprosencephaly can be classified as lobar (Fig. 5.73). In these patients, the interhemispheric fissure

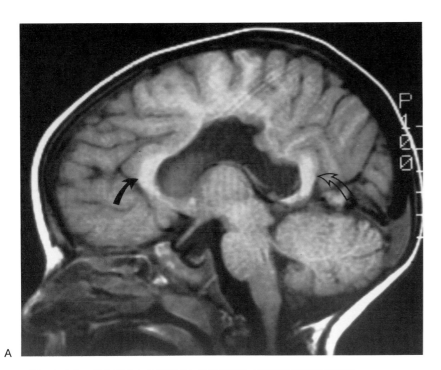

A

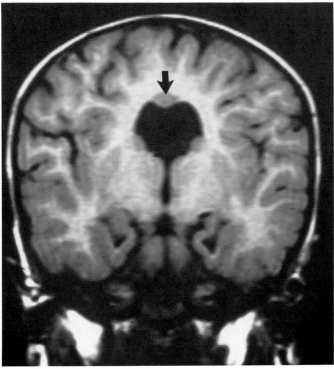

B

FIG. 5.74. Middle interhemispheric fusion variant of holoprosencephaly. **A:** Sagittal T1-weighted image shows an apparently normal callosal splenium (*open curved arrow*) and genu (*closed curved arrow*) but an absent callosal body. **B:** Coronal SE 550/15 image shows absence of the interhemispheric fissure at the site of the missing corpus. A focus of gray matter (*arrow*) sits on the roof of the telencephalic ventricle. (Reprinted with permission from ref. 17.)

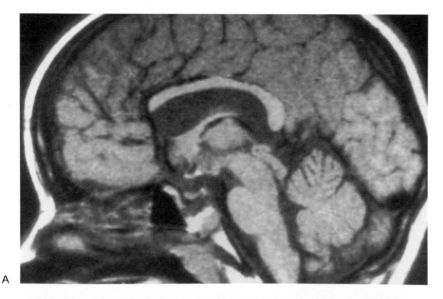

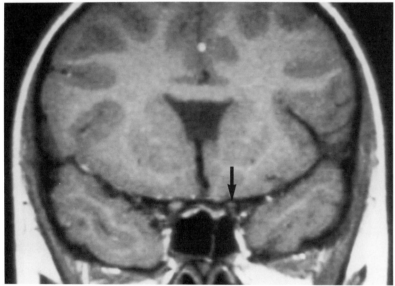

FIG. 5.75. Septo-optic dysplasia with dysgenesis of corpus callosum. **A:** Sagittal SE 550/15 image shows lack of formation of the callosal genu despite a normal body and splenium. **B:** Coronal SE 650/15 image shows absence of the septum pellucidum and hypoplasia of the left optic nerve (*arrow*).

and falx cerebri extend into the frontal area of the brain, although the anterior falx may be hypoplastic. The septum pellucidum is absent, and the frontal lobes (and frontal horns of the ventricles) are typically hypoplastic (Fig. 5.73). The hippocampal formations are normal or nearly normal, and the temporal horns and third ventricles are better defined than in the semilobar brains (143–147). There is some evidence that some patients with lobar holoprosencephaly fall into the spectrum of septo-optic dysplasia (129,144). This concept will be elaborated upon in the next section (see Fig. 5.75). Patients with lobar holoprosencephaly typically present with mild or moderate developmental delay, hypothalamic–pituitary dysfunction, or visual problems.

SEPTO-OPTIC DYSPLASIA

The syndrome of septo-optic dysplasia, named by de Morsier in 1956, consists of hypoplasia of the optic nerves and hypoplasia or absence of the septum pellucidum (150). Approximately two-thirds of affected patients have hypothalamic–pituitary dysfunction (151–155). The clinical presentation is variable. Visual symptoms may include nystagmus and diminished visual acuity; however, the patients can have normal vision (152). Occasionally, hypotelorism is present. When hypothalamic–pituitary dysfunction is present, it is usually manifested as growth retardation secondary to deficient secretion of growth hormone and thyroid-stimulating hormone (151,154,155). The diagnosis is made by ophthalmologic examination in conjunction with neuroimaging. When hypoplasia of the optic discs is seen in association with partial or complete absence of the septum pellucidum, the diagnosis of septo-optic dysplasia is made.

The combination of optic nerve hypoplasia and septal hypoplasia or aplasia should not be regarded as a homogeneous entity; in all probability the "syndrome" of septo-optic dysplasia is the end result of several different genetic abnormalities and *in utero* injuries, among them ischemic injuries in the first or second trimester (causing anomalies of neuronal migration and organization) and mesenchymal deficiencies (causing an anomaly that probably overlaps with lobar holoprosencephaly) (129,156–158). Those patients with neuroradiologic findings limited to isolated optic nerve hypoplasia or optic nerve hypoplasia in conjunction with partial or complete absence of the septum seem to have a good developmental prognosis, whereas those with hemispheric anomalies or posterior pituitary ectopia have more guarded prognoses (156).

Imaging studies show hypoplasia or complete absence of the septum pellucidum, resulting in boxlike frontal horns (129,144,159,160). One can often observe hypoplasia of the optic nerve and optic canals in severe cases; however, determining mild hypoplasia of the optic nerves, chiasm, and tracts is extremely difficult and, in fact, is seen in only about 50% of affected patients (129). Severe optic nerve hypoplasia is best identified on sagittal and coronal MR images (Fig. 5.75). Hypoplasia of the optic chiasm and hypothalamus sometimes results in bulbous dilatation of the anterior recess of the third ventricle and a large suprasellar cistern.

At least two distinct MR appearances are identified in patients with septo-optic dysplasia (129,156). One group shows a high incidence of neuronal migration anomalies [especially schizencephaly and gray matter heterotopia (129,156)], partial absence of the septum pellucidum, and hypothalamic dysfunction (Fig. 5.76). A second subset, believed to be a mild form of lobar holoprosencephaly, has findings of complete absence of the septum pellucidum and hypoplasia of the cerebral white matter, resulting in ventriculomegaly (Figs. 5.75, 5.77), but normal cerebral cortex. Some patients in this second subset have hypoplasia of the anterior falx cerebri or the genu of the corpus callosum (Fig. 5.75), further supporting the hypothesis that some patients with septo-optic dysplasia have a mild form of holoprosencephaly. A third subset of septo-optic dysplasia may be composed of patients with posterior pituitary ectopia (156,161).

Isolated absence of the septum pellucidum is a relatively rare structural anomaly that may have no neurologic manifestations. Because isolated septal agenesis is rare, the brain should be carefully scrutinized for associated anomalies when the septum is absent. Possible causes of septal absence include holoprosencephaly, callosal agenesis, septo-optic dysplasia, schizencephaly, chronic severe hydrocephalus, and Chiari II malformations (160).

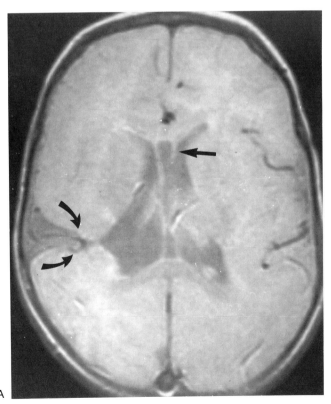

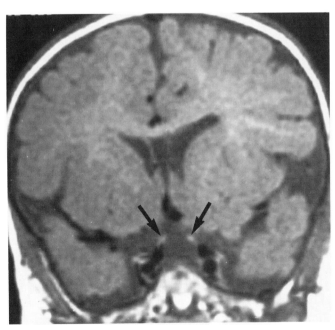

A

B

FIG. 5.76. Septo-optic dysplasia with schizencephaly and partial absence of the septum. **A:** Axial SE 2800/30 image through the lateral ventricles. There is schizencephaly (*curved arrows*) involving the posterior right lateral ventricle. The right leaf of the septum pellucidum is intact. Only a small portion of the left septal leaf is present (*straight arrow*). **B:** Coronal SE 600/20 image reveals a cavum septi pellucidi and partial destruction of the left septal leaf. The intracranial optic nerves (*arrows*) are hypoplastic.

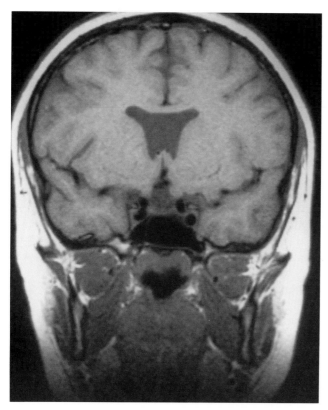

FIG. 5.77. Septo-optic dysplasia. Coronal SE 600/20 image reveals complete absence of the septum and thinning of the cerebral white matter. The intracranial optic nerves are too small to be visible at the level of the anterior clinoid processes.

THE CHIARI MALFORMATIONS

In 1891, Chiari (162) described three malformations of the hindbrain, all of which were associated with hydrocephalus. These three malformations will be discussed in the order in which they were described.

Chiari I

The Chiari I malformation is defined as caudal cerebellar tonsillar ectopia; that is, caudal extension of the cerebellar tonsils below the foramen magnum. Mild cerebellar tonsillar ectopia (less than 5 mm below a line from the basion to the opisthion in adults) appears to be of no clinical significance (163–165). When the tonsils extend more than 5 mm below the foramen magnum (Fig. 5.78), however, clinical symptoms are more likely to develop. The extent of asymptomatic tonsillar descent below the foramen magnum appears to be age dependent. Children between the ages of 5 and 15 years have slightly greater tonsillar ectopia than adults or children less than 5 years old. Tonsillar herniation of 6 mm should not be considered pathologic in patients between the ages of 5 and 15 years (164,166).

A number of subgroups of Chiari I malformations can be identified. In some patients, intrauterine hydrocephalus causes tonsillar herniation. Because the tonsils were low at the time of myelination, they retain a pointed configuration and a low-lying position (57). Patients with this subgroup of Chiari I malformation tend to present in childhood with hydrocephalus and, often, accompanying hydromyelia. A second group of patients with Chiari I malformation are those with craniocervical dysgenesis. This group also frequently has platybasia, occipitalization of the atlas, lack of segmentation of cervical vertebrae (Klippel-Feil anomalies), and other abnormalities of C1 and C2 (Fig. 5.78). Affected patients present clinically with occipital headaches (especially when straining), cranial nerve palsies, or dissociated anesthesia of the extremities secondary to syringohydromyelia. A third group of patients with Chiari I malformation are those with acquired deformities of the foramen magnum, such as basilar invagination. These patients, nearly always adults, also present with headaches, cranial neuropathies, or syringohydromyelia. A fourth subgroup, actually mislabeled as Chiari I malformations, are patients with myelomeningoceles and mild hindbrain anomalies, consisting primarily of tonsillar ectopia [2% of myelomeningocele patients in Emery's series of 100 autopsies of patients with myelomeningoceles had tonsillar ectopia as their only hindbrain anomaly (57)]. The patients in this subgroup have myelomeningoceles at birth; often have supratentorial anomalies, such as hypogenesis of the corpus callosum, mild tectal beaking, and fenestrations of the falx; and probably should be classified as Chiari II malformations with mild hindbrain manifestations. In all patients with Chiari I malformations, the cervical spine should be imaged to look for concurrent syringohydromyelia (Fig. 5.78), which has an estimated incidence of 20% to 25% (165,167,168). Syringohydromyelia is discussed in Chapter 9, as are the CSF flow studies used to determine flow dynamics at the level of the foramen magnum.

Chiari I malformations are most commonly isolated but can be seen in any anomalies that lead to small posterior fossae, such as occipital encephaloceles after repair, multiple craniosynostosis syndromes, syndromes that result in a small skull base (169), and syndromes that cause hydrocephalus. Chiari I malformations frequently develop as a consequence of lumbar peritoneal shunting (170,171); the tonsillar herniation may reverse after removal of the shunt.

Chiari II

The Chiari II malformation is a complex malformation involving the hindbrain, spine, and mesoderm of the skull base and spinal column (172). Affected patients have a high incidence of associated supratentorial anomalies. Virtually all patients with Chiari II malformations present at birth with myelomeningoceles. After closure of the myelomeningocele (usually within the first 48 hours of life), they nearly always develop hydrocephalus;

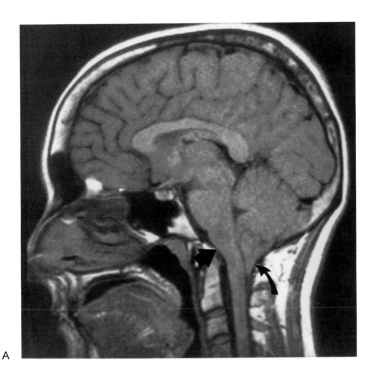

A

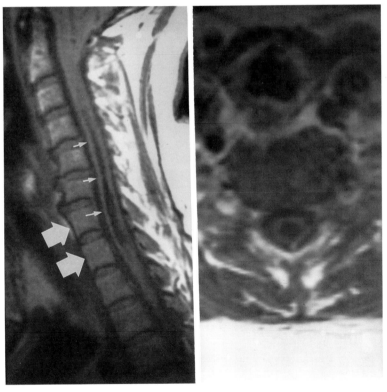

B,C

FIG. 5.78. Chiari I malformation. **A:** The cerebellar tonsil (*curved black arrow*) is enlarged and extends more than 1.5 cm below the bottom of the foramen magnum. Notice that there is also some compression of the inferior medulla by the odontoid (*straight black arrow*). The posterior fossa is normal in size. The corpus callosum is intact, and no supratentorial anomalies were present. **B:** Sagittal SE 500/15 image shows cervical hydromyelia (*small arrows*) and lack of complete segmentation (*large arrows*) of C7 and T1. **C:** Axial SE 700/16 image shows that the central canal of the cord is dilated, confirming hydromyelia.

it is in the evaluation of the hydrocephalus that the radiologist is most often exposed to these patients. Less commonly, they are evaluated for compression of the brain stem at the foramen magnum or C1 level; in these circumstances, the patients typically present with difficulty swallowing, stridor, apneic spells, weak cry, or arm weakness (173).

Although many theories have been proposed to explain the development of Chiari II malformations in association with myelomeningoceles, the best theory at present suggests that the underlying problem is the lack of expression of specific surface molecules (carbohydrates) on neurons in the developing neural tube. These molecules are required for neural tube closure and for the development of focal expansions of the central canal of the developing neural tube that will eventually form the cerebral ventricles (174). When these surface molecules are incorrectly expressed, (1) the posterior neuro-

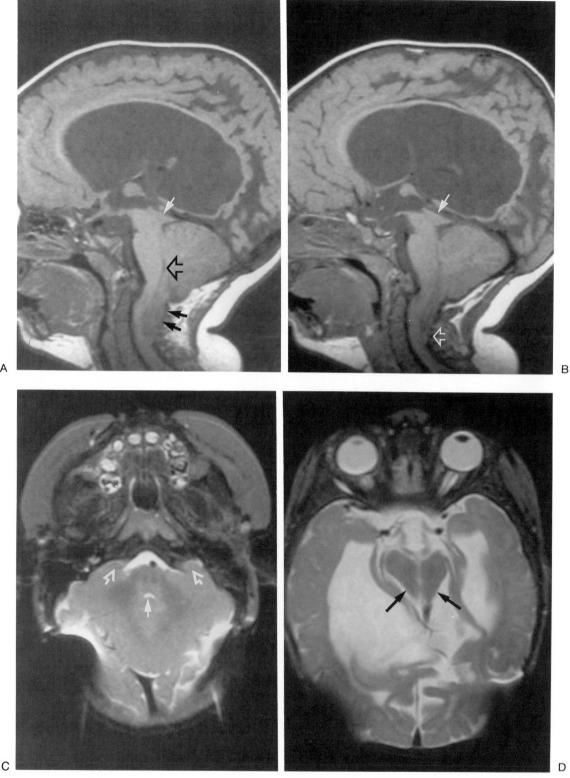

FIG. 5.79. Chiari II malformation. **A, B:** Sagittal SE 600/15 images show multiple findings that are characteristic of this malformation. The patient has severe hydrocephalus. The quadrigeminal plate is stretched inferiorly and posteriorly, having a somewhat triangular shape (*closed white arrows*). The fourth ventricle is narrow in its AP diameter and lies somewhat low in the posterior fossa (*open black arrows*). The medulla is low lying; its most inferior aspect is signaled by the characteristic cervicomedullary kink (*open white arrow*). The cerebellar vermis is herniated into the cervical spinal canal (*closed black arrows*). **C:** Axial SE 2800/70 image shows the cerebellar hemispheres extending anterior to the pons (*open arrows*) and the small fourth ventricle (*closed arrow*). **D:** Axial SE 2800/70 image shows the "beaked" tectum (*arrows*) and dysplasia of the medial occipital cortex.

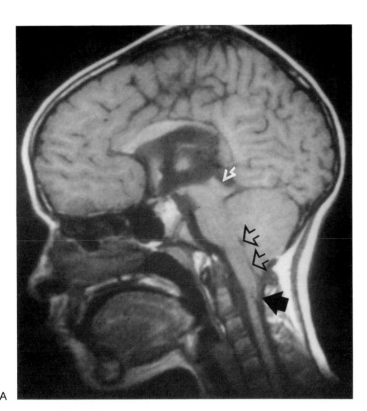

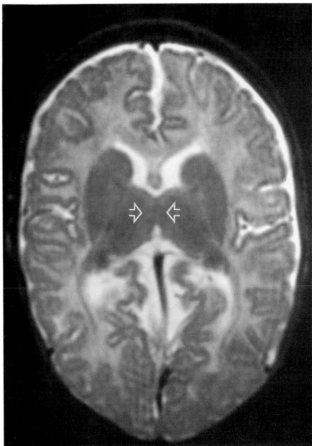

A

B

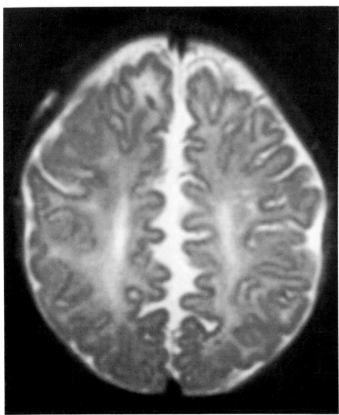

C

FIG. 5.80. Chiari II malformation. **A:** Sagittal SE 600/20 image shows mild beaking of the tectum (*open white arrow*). The fourth ventricle (*open black arrows*) is extremely narrow in its AP diameter and extends down into the foramen magnum. The corpus callosum is hypogenetic with absence of the splenium and rostrum. The cervicomedullary kink (*closed black arrow*) is present at the C2–C3 level. **B:** Axial SE 3000/120 image shows the large massa intermedia (*arrows*). **C:** Axial SE 3000/120 shows widened interhemispheric fissure.

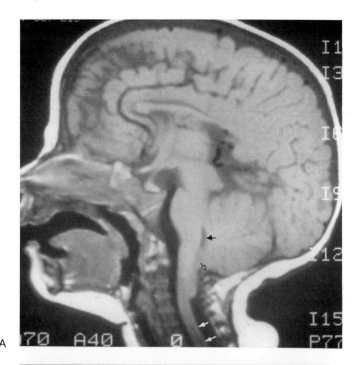

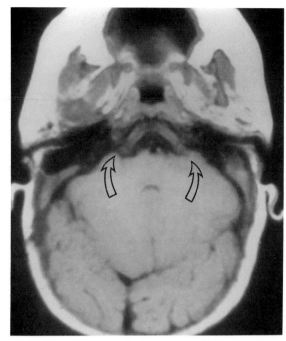

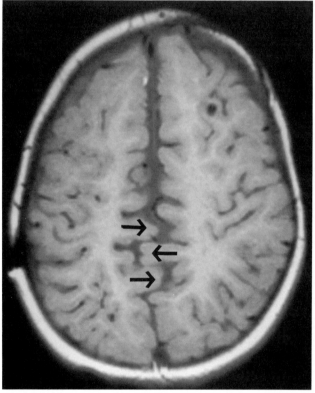

FIG. 5.81. Chiari II malformation. **A:** Sagittal SE 600/16 image shows the abnormal tectum, small fourth ventricle (*closed black arrow*), and herniation of cerebellar contents into the cervical subarachnoid space. The open black arrow points to the posterior arch of C1, which is indenting the herniated cerebellum. Cervical hydromyelia (*white arrows*) is present. **B:** Axial SE 600/16 image reveals the cerebellar hemispheres extending laterally around the brain stem and actually in front of the brain stem (*curved black arrows*). **C:** Axial SE 600/16 image shows interdigitation of gyri (*arrows*) across the interhemispheric fissure.

pore fails to close and (2) the cerebral ventricles fail to expand sufficiently for a normal-sized posterior fossa to form and for the thalami to be normally separated.

The hindbrain findings of the Chiari II malformation are best explained by the theory of McLone and Knepper (174). This theory allows us to conceptualize the hindbrain disorder as resulting from a normal-sized cerebellum developing in an abnormally small posterior fossa with a low tentorial attachment. Consequently, the cerebellum is "squeezed" out of the posterior fossa as it grows. The cerebellum is indented superiorly by the tentorium and inferiorly by the foramen magnum or, more commonly, the posterior arch of C1. The pons is stretched inferiorly and narrowed in its anterior–posterior diameter (Figs. 5.79, 5.80). The medulla is also stretched inferiorly and extends below the foramen magnum. The cervical spinal cord is stretched inferiorly as well. The dentate ligaments, which attach to the lateral aspects of the spinal cord and hold it in place, allow a variable amount of caudal displacement of the cervical spinal cord; however, caudal displacement of the cord is eventually restricted by the ligaments. If the medulla stretches down further than the dentate ligaments will allow the spinal cord to move, a characteristic cervicomedullary kink is formed (Figs. 5.79, 5.80). This kink is seen in approximately 70% of patients with the Chiari

II malformation (57,172). The cerebellum sometimes extends anterolaterally into the cerebellopontine and cerebellomedullary angles, wrapping around the brain stem (Fig. 5.81). The fourth ventricle is low in position, vertically oriented, and narrowed in its anterior–posterior diameter (Figs. 5.79–5.81). The cerebellar vermis is usually herniated into the cervical spinal canal. The herniated cerebellum often degenerates; when this degeneration is severe, virtually no cerebellum may be present (Fig. 5.82) (172). Occasionally, the fourth ventricle can herniate posteriorly and inferiorly, behind the medulla and beneath the vermis; this condition is known as "an encysted fourth ventricle" (172). The fourth ventricle may also be isolated or "trapped" (see Chapter 8) as a result of a combination of aqueductal narrowing (or scarring) and diminished CSF flow through the fourth ventricular outflow foramina or the basilar cisterns (Fig. 5.83).

Because the normal fourth ventricle in the patient with a Chiari II malformation is so small, the isolated fourth ventricle may not look enlarged on casual observation; a "normal-sized" fourth ventricle in a patient with a Chiari II malformation should initiate a search for hydrocephalus. When affected patients have hydrocephalus or an isolated fourth ventricle, the spine should be examined because of a high incidence of associated syringo-

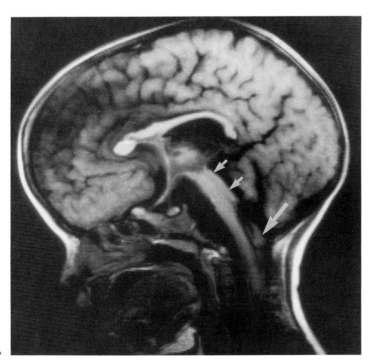 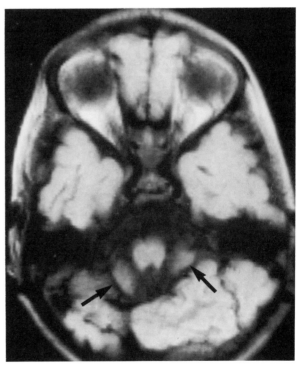

A   B

FIG. 5.82. Chiari II malformation. **A:** Sagittal SE 500/20 image reveals a tectum that is markedly stretched inferiorly (*small arrows*). The pons is narrowed in its AP diameter and inferiorly displaced; it is difficult to identify the upper and lower levels of the pons accurately. Only a small amount of cerebellar vermis can be identified (*large arrow*). **B:** Axial 2000/30 image slightly above the skull base shows the two small remnants of the cerebellar hemispheres (*arrows*). The cerebellum in patients such as these has presumably degenerated as a result of pressure necrosis from herniation through the foramen magnum.

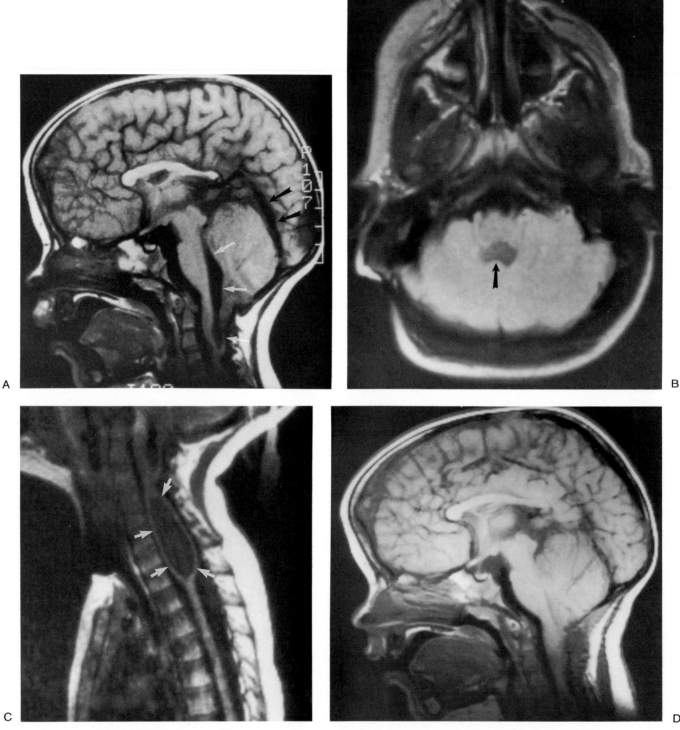

FIG. 5.83. Chiari II malformation with isolated fourth ventricle. **A:** Sagittal SE 600/20 image reveals a dysgenetic corpus callosum with hypoplastic splenium and posterior body and absent rostrum. The mesencephalic tectum is nearly normal. The straight sinus (*black arrows*) angles too steeply toward the torcula. The fourth ventricle (*white arrows*) is much too large in its AP diameter for a patient with the Chiari II malformation. (Compare with Figs. 5.79–5.81.) **B:** Axial SE 2500/20 image. In this patient with a relatively normal-sized cerebellum, the trapped fourth ventricle (arrow) looks normal on axial images. **C:** Sagittal SE 600/20 through the cervical and thoracic spinal cord shows a focal syringohydromyelia (*arrows*) extending from approximately C4 to T2. Syringohydromyelia is often seen in association with an isolated fourth ventricle or a nonfunctioning ventriculoperitoneal shunt in patients with a Chiari II malformation. **D:** After diversion of CSF from the encysted fourth ventricle, the ventricle assumes a more normal appearance (for a Chiari II hindbrain malformation).

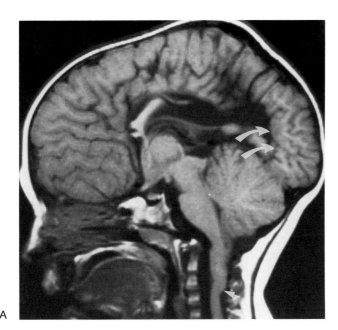 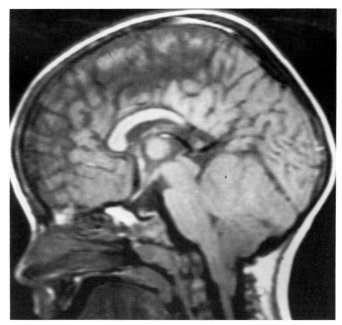

FIG. 5.84. Hypogenesis of the corpus callosum and stenogyria in the Chiari II malformation. **A:** Sagittal SE 600/20 image shows presence of only the genu and anterior body of the corpus callosum, tectal beaking, cervicomedullary kink (*straight arrow*), and stenogyria (*curved arrows*) of the occipital lobe. **B:** Sagittal SE 600/20 image shows callosal hypogenesis; mild tectal beaking; a low, narrow fourth ventricle; low medulla; and occipital stenogyria.

hydromyelia (Fig. 5.83). Conversely, when worsening syringohydromyelia develops in patients who have had myelomeningocele repairs (almost all of whom will have a Chiari II malformation), the head should be studied to look for worsening hydrocephalus or a trapped fourth ventricle.

The mesencephalic tectum (quadrigeminal plate) is often distorted in patients with the Chiari II malformation, probably secondary to compression by the temporal lobes, which are expanded as a result of hydrocephalus, and the cerebellar hemispheres, which surround the brain stem because of the small volume of the posterior fossa. The tectum is therefore stretched posteriorly and inferiorly (Figs. 5.79–5.82) (175). This appears on axial CT and MR scans as "beaking" of the tectum and on sagittal images as posterior and inferior stretching of the quadrigeminal plate. Another finding that may be present on axial CT is a posterior concavity of the petrous bones and, less commonly, clivus, probably resulting from pressure effects of the cerebellum and brain stem in the small posterior fossa (176). This "scalloping" of the petrous bones is more difficult to appreciate on MR.

Supratentorially, abnormalities of the corpus callosum are seen in 80% to 90% of these patients. The abnormality usually consists of hypoplasia or absence of the splenium of the corpus callosum and absence of the rostrum (Figs. 5.80, 5.81, 5.84) (16). Enlargement of the caudate heads is frequently seen, as is enlargement of the massa intermedia (177). The falx cerebri is usually fenestrated; interdigitation of gyri across the interhemispheric

fissure may be seen at the sites of fenestration (Fig. 5.82). Prominence of the occipital horns is common and can remain even after shunting (177). Also after shunting, the medial walls of the ventricular trigones often appear dysplastic and a large CSF-containing structure may appear between the atria and occipital horns of the lateral ventricles. This large midline CSF space is most likely a result of the dysplastic adjacent cortex rather than a dilated suprapineal recess of the third ventricle (172). The gyral pattern is often abnormal in the medial aspect of the occipital lobe on sagittal MR images, having the appearance of multiple small gyri (Fig. 5.84). This pattern is not polymicrogyria, because the cortex is of normal thickness, but may be secondary to shunting of the hydrocephalus or to the dysplasia in the hemisphere medial to the atria and occipital horns. This appearance has been called *stenogyria* (178,179).

When very young patients with the Chiari II malformation are imaged on CT, irregularity of the surfaces of the inner and outer table of the skull is frequently seen. This lacunar skull, or *luckenschädel,* appearance is explained by McLone and Knepper as being the result of incomplete expansion of the calvarium *in utero,* with resultant disorganization of the collagenous outer meninges from which the membranous calvarium forms (174). It is of no diagnostic significance in the era of CT and MR.

The multiple findings described earlier are present in a variable proportion of patients (Table 5.2). It is unusual to see all the cerebral and cerebellar manifestations of the

TABLE 5.2. *Frequency of brain and spine anomalies in patients with Chiari II malformations*

Anomaly	Frequency
Myelomeningocele	Always
Hydrocephalus	Almost always
Dysplastic tentorium	Almost always
Small posterior fossa	Almost always
Lückenshadel	Almost always
Caudal displacement of brain stem	Usually
Cervicomedullary kink	Usually
Upward Cb herniation	Usually
Large massa intermedia	Usually
Elongated cranial nerves	Usually
Tectal beak	Usually
Callosal hypogenesis	Usually
Syringohydromyelia	~50%
Neuronal migration anomalies	Occasionally
Aqueductal stenosis	Occasionally

Chiari II malformation in a single patient. The hindbrain deformity can be extremely severe, with near total absence of the cerebellum, or it can be relatively mild, with only cerebellar tonsillar ectopia. The patients with mild hindbrain deformities are often included under the classification of a Chiari I malformation; however, the presence of supratentorial anomalies and myelomeningocele suggests that these patients belong in the Chiari II classification. It should be noted that the term *Arnold-Chiari malformation* is only properly applied to the Chiari II malformation.

Chiari III

The Chiari III malformation is a condition characterized by herniation of posterior fossa contents (the cerebellum and, sometimes, brain stem) through a posterior spina bifida at C1–C2. This is an extremely rare condition, and only two such cases have been seen by the author.

EMBRYOLOGIC DEVELOPMENT OF THE CEREBELLUM

During the fifth week of gestation, a thickening occurs bilaterally in the alar plate of the rhombencephalon, forming the rhombic lips, which are the primordia of the cerebellar hemispheres. The glial and neuronal cells that compose the cerebellum migrate to their final location in the cerebellar hemispheres by two general pathways. The neurons that will form the deep cerebellar nuclei and the Purkinje layer of the cerebellar cortex migrate radially outward from the germinal matrix in the wall of the fourth ventricle (180–182). Generation of these neurons in the germinal matrix seems to occur between 9 and 13 weeks of gestation (182). The neurons that will form the granular layer of the cerebellar cortex, in contrast, have a more complicated journey. At 11–13 weeks, these cells begin to migrate tangentially from a germinal zone (in the lateral portion of the rhombic lips) over the cerebellar surface, forming the transitory external granular layer (182). The cells in this external layer then proliferate at a high rate as the cerebellum begins a rapid growth period (commencing in the 13th gestational week and continuing until the seventh postnatal month). The proliferation of the external granule cells continues while, at 16 weeks, daughter cells begin to migrate inward. Some of the daughter cells form the basket and stellate cells of the outer (molecular) layer of the cerebellar cortex. Others continue their migration and move inward past the Purkinje cells to form the inner granular layer of the cortex (Fig. 5.85). The external granular layer attains maximum cell number in the first few postnatal months and then diminishes in size as the granule cells migrate inward. By the end of the first postnatal year, the external granular layer has essentially disappeared and the cerebellar cortex achieves its adult three-layered histologic composition with an outer molecular layer, middle Purkinje layer, and inner granular layer (182).

The afferent and efferent connections of the cerebellar cortex consist of fibers that synapse with the deep cerebellar nuclei and fibers that communicate with the rest of the central nervous system via the superior, middle, and inferior cerebellar peduncles. Cortical, afferent, and efferent white matter tracts seem to form even if the migration of some of the cerebellar cortical components is interrupted (182,183). As a result of the formation of these white matter tracts, the cerebellum is grossly normal in appearance (with a cortex and medulla that are roughly proportionate to those in a normal cerebellum), in spite of the developmental insult. The cerebellum appears merely small, no matter what type of insult occurs (183).

The cerebellar vermis forms from the fusion of the developing hemispheres. The fusion begins when the hemispheres meet superiorly in the midline during the ninth gestational week, and it continues inferiorly as the hemispheres grow. The entire vermis is formed by the end of the 15th week (184). As a result of this mechanism of formation, the vermis cannot form in the absence of formation of the cerebellar hemispheres.

One other important concept in the development of the cerebellum as it relates to posterior fossa cysts is the complex development of the roof of the fourth ventricle. Bonnevie and Brodal (185) have shown that the roof of the fourth ventricle of the mouse is divided by a ridge of developing choroid plexus into the anterior and posterior membranous areas on the 11th gestational day (Fig. 5.86). By the end of the 11th day, the anterior membranous area (above the choroid ridge) is incorporated into the developing choroid plexus. The posterior membranous area (below the ridge of choroid) remains; an area

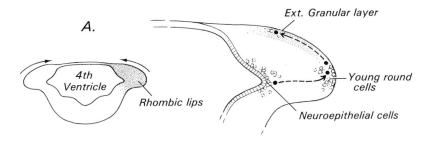

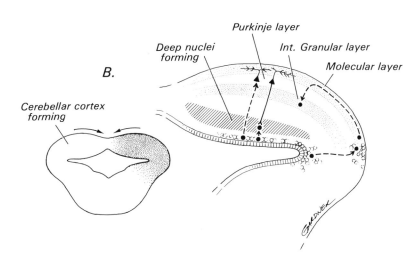

FIG. 5.85. Schematic showing normal formation of the cerebellum. During the fifth week of gestation **(A)**, a thickening occurs bilaterally in the alar plate of the rhombencephalon, forming the rhombic lips, which are the primordia of the cerebellar hemispheres. At 11–13 weeks, cells that will form the granular layer of the cerebellar hemisphere begin to migrate tangentially from a germinal zone in the lateral portion of the rhombic lips to the cerebellar surface, forming the transitory external granular layer (*dotted arrow*). At approximately 16 weeks of gestation **(B)**, cells of the external granular layer begin to migrate inward to form the internal granular layer of the cerebellar cortex. These cells will eventually synapse with cells within the deep cerebellar nuclei. Cells that will form the Purkinje layer of the cerebellar cortex and the deep cerebellar nuclei originate in the wall of the fourth ventricle. These cells migrate directly from the germinal matrix to their final destinations within the cerebellar hemispheres. Cortical afferent and efferent white matter tracts seem to form even if migration of some of the cerebellar cortical components is interrupted. As a result of the formation of these white matter tracts, the cerebellum is grossly normal in appearance (but hypoplastic) even if a developmental insult occurs.

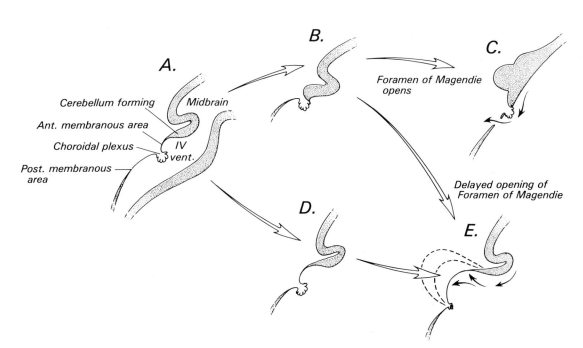

FIG. 5.86. Schematic showing normal and abnormal development of the fourth ventricle. Early in gestation, the roof of the fourth ventricle is divided by a ridge of developing choroid plexus into anterior and posterior membranous areas. **A:** Normally, the anterior membranous area is incorporated into the developing choroid plexus. **B:** The posterior membranous area remains and eventually cavitates to form to the midline foramen of Magendie. **C:** If the anterior membranous area is not incorporated into the developing choroid plexus. **D:** If there is delayed opening of the foramen of Magendie, the roof of the fourth ventricle can balloon posteriorly to form a fourth ventricular–cisterna magna cyst. **E** is identical to what is seen in the Dandy-Walker malformation.

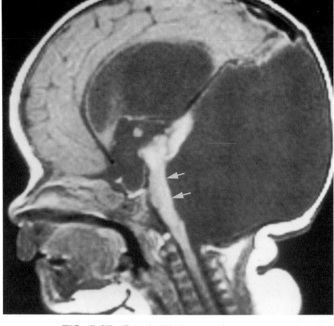

A

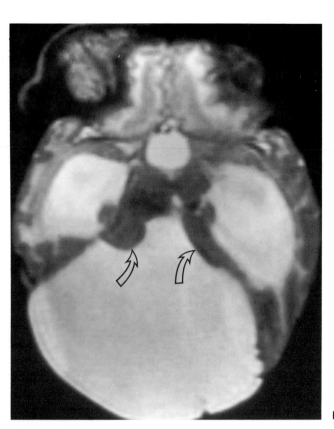

B

FIG. 5.87. Dandy-Walker malformation. **A:** Sagittal SE 500/11 image shows the classic findings of a Dandy-Walker malformation. Marked hydrocephalus is present. The tentorium is elevated and the posterior fossa is markedly enlarged. The vermis is hypogenetic. The enlarged posterior fossa is filled with a large cyst that is actually a huge fourth ventricle. The brain stem (*arrows*) is compressed against the clivus. **B:** Axial SE 600/16 image through the mid-fourth ventricle shows continuity of the large cyst with the fourth ventricle. The cerebellar hemispheres (*arrows*) are hypoplastic and are pushed superiorly and laterally by the cyst.

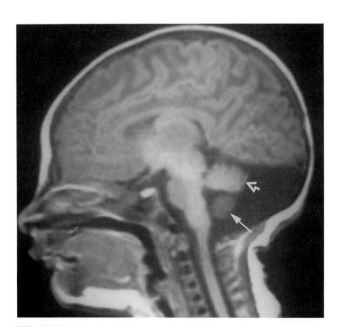

FIG. 5.88. Dandy-Walker variant. Sagittal SE 600/20 image shows a small, hypogenetic cerebellar vermis (*open arrow*). The posterior fossa is normal to slightly enlarged. The closed arrow points to the bottom of the cerebellar hemisphere, located beneath the vermis.

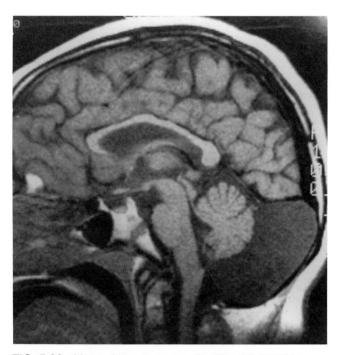

FIG. 5.89. Mega cisterna magna. Sagittal SE 600/20 image shows a normal cerebellar vermis associated with an enlarged cisterna magna that is causing some scalloping of the inner table of the occipital bone and enlargement of the posterior fossa. Supratentorial structures are normal.

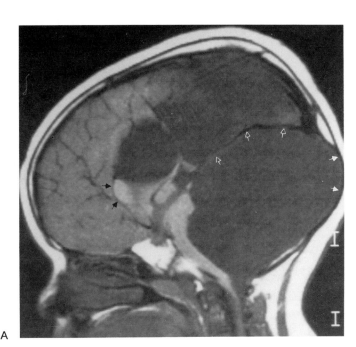

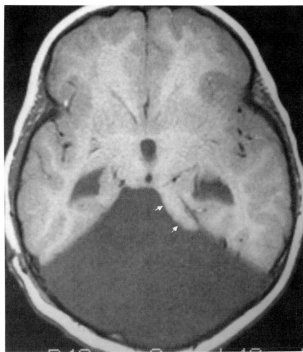

FIG. 5.90. Dandy-Walker malformation with hypogenesis of the corpus callosum and interhemispheric cyst. **A:** Sagittal SE 600/20 image reveals a large posterior fossa cyst elevating the tentorium (*open arrows*) and causing scalloping of the inner table of the expanded occipital bone (*closed white arrows*). The corpus callosum is dysgenetic with only the genu (*black arrows*) present. There is a large supratentorial CSF collection. Note the compression of the brain stem against the clivus by the posterior fossa cyst. **B:** Axial SE 600/20 image at the level of the superior aqueduct reveals the Dandy-Walker cyst causing superior displacement of the markedly hypoplastic left cerebellar hemisphere (*arrows*). The right cerebellar hemisphere, not seen at this level, was even smaller. Note the dilated temporal horns of the lateral ventricles, indicative of hydrocephalus.

within it eventually cavitates to form the midline foramen of Magendie. The lateral foramina of Luschka open at some later, as yet unknown, time.

POSTERIOR FOSSA CYSTIC MALFORMATIONS

The Dandy-Walker Complex

Classically, posterior fossa cystic malformations have been divided into the Dandy-Walker malformation, the Dandy-Walker variant, and the mega cisterna magna (186,187). (Arachnoid cysts, which are unrelated, are discussed in Chapter 8.) The *Dandy-Walker malformation* consists of an enlarged posterior fossa with a high position of the tentorium, hypogenesis or agenesis of the cerebellar vermis, and a cystic dilatation of the fourth ventricle that fills nearly the entire posterior fossa (Fig. 5.87) (186,187). The *Dandy-Walker variant* consists of a hypogenetic cerebellar vermis and a cystic dilatation of the fourth ventricle without enlargement of the posterior fossa (Fig. 5.88). The *mega cisterna magna* consists of an enlarged posterior fossa, secondary to an enlarged cis-

terna magna, but a normal cerebellar vermis and fourth ventricle (Fig. 5.89). Patients with any of these anomalies can present with developmental delay, enlarged head circumference, or signs and symptoms of hydrocephalus (186–189). The degree of developmental delay seems to be related to the level of control of hydrocephalus and to the extent of supratentorial anomalies (188,190,191). Seizures, hearing or visual difficulties, systemic abnormalities, and CNS abnormalities are associated with poor intellectual development. The presence of two of these four risk factors identifies patients with borderline or less intelligence 94% of the time (188).

Hydrocephalus is unusual at birth but is present by 3 months of age in approximately 75% of patients; hydrocephalus is present in about 90% of affected patients at the time of diagnosis (189). The most common accompanying cerebral anomaly is callosal hypogenesis, present in as many as 32% of affected patients (188). The callosal anomaly generally consists of either complete agenesis or presence of only the genu (Fig. 5.90) of the corpus callosum. Polymicrogyria or gray matter heterotopia are seen in 5% to 10% of affected patients. Occipital encephaloceles are present in up to 16% of patients with the Dandy-Walker malformation (188). Of the associ-

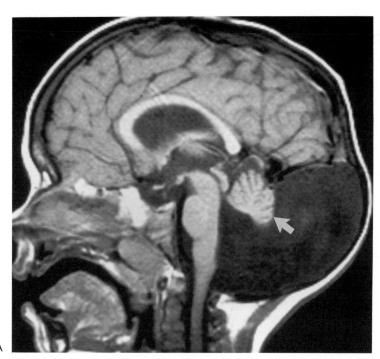
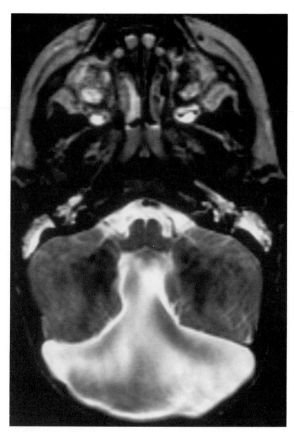

FIG. 5.91. Dandy-Walker malformation with mild hypoplasia of the cerebellum. **A:** Sagittal SE 550/15 image shows the enlarged posterior fossa with a mildly hypogenetic vermis (*arrow*). **B:** Axial SE 2500/ 80 image shows that the cerebellar hemispheres are only mildly hypoplastic. The low signal in the cyst results from misregistration artifact and indicates that the cyst fluid is circulating freely from the fourth ventricle into the cyst.

ated systemic anomalies, polydactyly and cardiac anomalies are the most common (187).

On imaging studies, the classic Dandy-Walker malformation is identified by hypoplasia or absence of the cerebellar vermis, hypoplasia of the cerebellar hemispheres, a large fluid-filled fourth ventricle–cisterna magna complex, and a large posterior fossa (high tentorium) (192). The cerebellum may be markedly (Figs. 5.87, 5.90) or mildly (Fig. 5.91) hypoplastic. The Dandy-Walker variant differs in that the vermis is typically less hypoplastic and the posterior fossa less enlarged. However, it is not possible to define an exact characteristic that separates the classic malformation from the variant; as with so many other malformations, they represent a continuum. The mega cisterna magna may be differentiated by the presence of an intact or nearly intact vermis; again, however, no precise characteristic allows separation of the mega cisterna magna from the Dandy-Walker variant. Thus, the concept of a continuum of posterior fossa cystic anomalies (referred to as the Dandy-Walker com-

plex), in which the prognosis is related not to the extent of cerebellar anomaly but to the extent of associated cerebral anomalies and the control of hydrocephalus, is attractive. This concept is expanded upon in the following section.

With all the anomalies in this group, the cerebellar hemispheres may appose each other inferiorly after the posterior fossa cyst has been shunted; midline sagittal images may then simulate the appearance of an intact vermis (Fig. 5.92). Axial or coronal images will show the cerebellar hemispheres in apposition without intervening vermis. It is important to look for associated supratentorial anomalies because the prognosis for these patients is much better in the absence of such anomalies.

ANOMALIES FEATURING HYPOGENESIS OF CEREBELLAR STRUCTURES

The major traditional classification system for the categorization of anomalies featuring hypogenesis of cere-

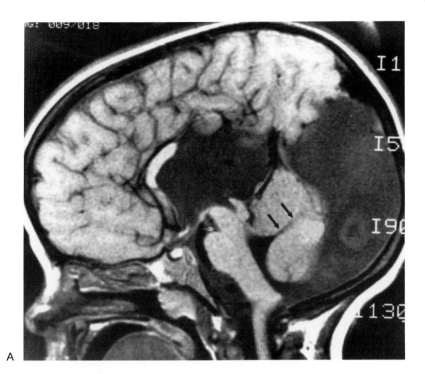

A

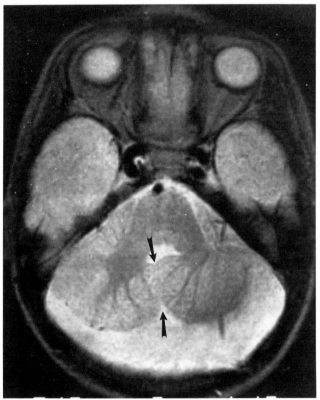

B

FIG. 5.92. Dandy-Walker malformation after shunting of the posterior fossa cyst. **A:** The corpus callosum is dysgenetic with only the genu present. The posterior fossa is enlarged as a result of a high tentorium. On first glance, the vermis looks intact. However, closer inspection shows a hypoplastic vermis with cerebellar hemispheres in the position beneath the vermis. Arrows mark the lower limits of the vermis. The cerebellar tissue below these arrows is composed of the inferior cerebellar hemispheres, which are in apposition as a result of diversion of CSF by the shunt. **B:** Axial SE 2500/70 image at the level of the inferior fourth ventricle shows the cerebellar hemispheres in apposition (*arrows*) without an intervening vermis.

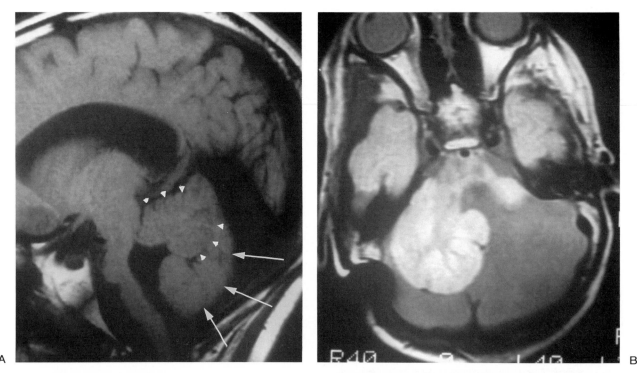

FIG. 5.93. Cerebellar anomaly. According to the traditional classification, this would be considered left lateral cerebellar hypoplasia. It can also be considered a part of the Dandy-Walker complex. **A:** SE 600/20 sagittal image shows upward rotation of the cerebellar vermis (*arrowheads*) and a slightly enlarged posterior fossa. The cerebellar hemisphere (*long arrows*) is seen beneath the vermis. There is indentation of the back of the brain stem by the posterior fossa cyst. **B:** Axial SE 2500/35 image through the mid-fourth ventricle shows marked hypoplasia of the left cerebellar hemisphere and mild hypoplasia of the right cerebellum.

bellar structures divides them into (1) total or subtotal agenesis, (2) lateral aplasia, (3) median aplasia, and (4) hypoplasias (divided into total, lateral, and medial hypoplasia) (193). Unfortunately, this classification is not particularly helpful for the radiologist or the treating clinician in that it is descriptive but lacks any underlying embryologic basis. Moreover, poor correlation is found between the severity of the cerebellar deformity and the severity of the clinical syndrome. Finally, it is often difficult, on the basis of imaging studies, to differentiate CSF collections that are encysted and under pressure from those that are secondary to cerebellar hypoplasia.

Recently, as alluded to earlier, evidence has been presented that the Dandy-Walker malformation, Dandy-Walker variant, and mega cisterna magna represent regions on a spectrum of posterior fossa cystic malformations that result from insults to the developing fourth ventricle and cerebellum. Moreover, these anomalies can be differentiated from cerebellar atrophies on the basis of MR findings (194). It is postulated that the mega cisterna magna results from an insult primarily to the developing fourth ventricle, the Dandy-Walker variant results from an insult primarily to the developing cerebellar hemispheres, and the full-blown Dandy-Walker

malformation results from a more extensive insult involving both the developing cerebellum and the fourth ventricle. This classification is attractive because it simplifies decisions about treatment. The only treatment for these malformations is CSF diversion, which is performed only if hydrocephalus or mass effect on adjacent structures is present. Moreover, because prognosis is related to the severity of associated supratentorial anomalies in all the posterior fossa cystic malformations, the extent of cerebellar hypoplasia is unimportant. Finally, the traditional classification system of cerebellar anomalies (Figs. 5.93, 5.94) is purely descriptive and has no embryologic basis. Therefore, it is lacking in conceptual value. I believe that these malformations should be united under the title of the Dandy-Walker Complex. Combining the posterior fossa cystic malformations in this way simplifies both diagnosis and treatment.

JOUBERT SYNDROME

In 1969 Joubert (195) reported five children with episodic hyperpnea, abnormal eye movements, ataxia, and mental retardation. His report and subsequent communications (196–198) have shown that this clinical syn-

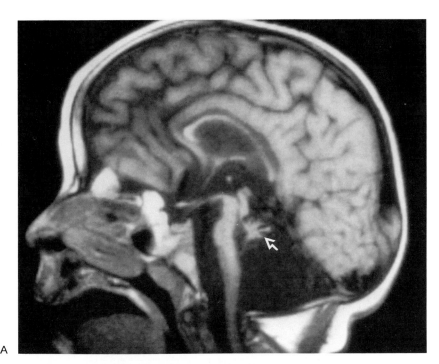

A

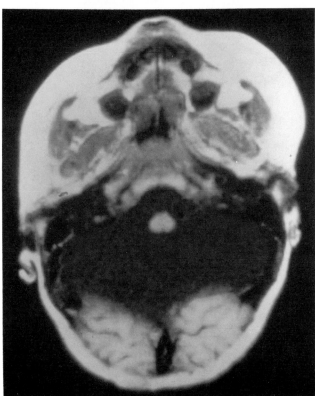

B

FIG. 5.94. Cerebellar anomaly. By the traditional classification, this is considered median cerebellar hypoplasia. It can also be considered part of the Dandy-Walker complex. **A:** Sagittal SE 600/20 image shows a small posterior fossa with a tiny vermis (*arrow*) and pons. **B:** Axial SE 600/20 shows essentially no cerebellum at the level of the medulla.

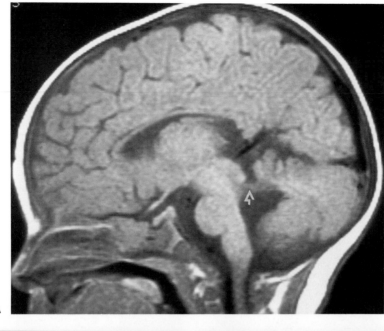

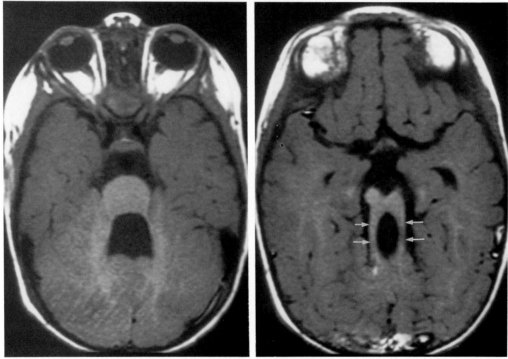

FIG. 5.95. Joubert syndrome. **A:** Sagittal SE 550/16 image shows absence of normal vermian folia. The horizontal superior cerebellar peduncle (*arrow*) is well seen on this image. **B:** Axial image at the level of the pons shows the "bat-wing" appearance of the fourth ventricle. **C:** Axial image at the midbrain level shows the superior cerebellar peduncles well because of their horizontal course and the absence of the vermis (*arrows*).

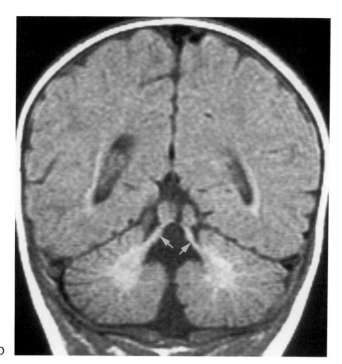

FIG. 5.95. (*Continued.*) **D:** Coronal image clearly shows the superior cerebellar peduncles because of the absence of the vermis (*arrows*).

drome is associated with characteristic pathologic findings. Patients with the Joubert syndrome have nearly total aplasia of the cerebellar vermis, dysplasias and heterotopias of cerebellar nuclei, near total absence of the pyramidal decussation, and anomalies in the structure of the inferior olivary nuclei, descending trigeminal tract, solitary fascicle, and dorsal column nuclei (179).

The imaging studies of patients with Joubert syndrome are quite characteristic (197). Sagittal images show a complete or nearly complete lack of the normal vermian folia (Fig. 5.95) (a portion of the superior vermis may be present). Absence of the vermis results in a triangular-shaped mid-fourth ventricle and a "batwing"-shaped fourth ventricle superiorly (Figs. 5.95, 5.96). The two cerebellar hemispheres appose one another in the midline. The superior cerebellar peduncles are nearly horizontal and can be clearly seen as they extend anteriorly toward the midbrain, surrounded by CSF (Figs. 5.95, 5.96). Associated supratentorial anomalies are uncommon, but cerebral cortical dysplasia and gray matter heterotopia have been reported.

RHOMBENCEPHALOSYNAPSIS

Rhombencephalosynapsis, originally described by Obersteiner in 1914 (199), is an anomaly characterized by fusion of the cerebellar hemispheres and absence of the cerebellar vermis. Clinical presentation is variable and seems to be related to the presence and severity of associated supratentorial anomalies. The brain anomalies that are most commonly present are fusion of the cerebellar dentate nuclei, superior cerebellar peduncles, and thalami; absence of the septum pellucidum; olivary hypoplasia; anomalies of the limbic system; and hydrocephalus (179,200). A wide range of other associated supratentorial, infratentorial, and nonneurologic anomalies has been reported in association with the classic cerebellar deformity (179,200).

Imaging studies show the characteristic appearance of dorsal fusion of the cerebellar hemispheres, hypogenesis or agenesis of the vermis, fusion of the superior cerebellar peduncles, and absence of the septum pellucidum, usually in association with ventriculomegaly (Fig. 5.97). The cerebellar anomaly may be difficult to detect on CT but may be suggested if posterior pointing of the fourth ventricle is detected in a patient with large lateral ventricles and absence of the septum pellucidum. The diagnosis is most easily established on MR by the observation that the cerebellar folia appear continuous across the midline without intervening vermis (Fig. 5.97). Once the diagnosis is established, the cerebral cortex, ventricles, and limbic system should be carefully evaluated.

LHERMITTE-DUCLOS SYNDROME (DYSPLASTIC CEREBELLAR GANGLIOCYTOMA)

Also known as diffuse hypertrophy of the cerebellar cortex and dysplastic cerebellar gangliocytoma, Lhermitte-Duclos syndrome was first reported by Lhermitte and Duclos in 1920 (201). It consists of focally enlarged cerebellar cortex that is sharply marginated. Typically, a portion of one cerebellar hemisphere is involved; the process may extend into the vermis or, rarely, the contralateral hemisphere (179). Microscopically, the disorder consists of a thick layer of abnormal ganglion cells replacing the granular layer of the cerebellar cortex, a thick hypermyelinated marginal layer, and a thin Purkinje cell layer (179). Patients may become symptomatic because of mass effect from the lesion, with resultant intracranial hypertension and cerebellar signs and symptoms (202–204). Alternatively, the anomaly may be discovered incidentally at autopsy or when imaging for an unrelated condition (202–204).

CT scans show the presence of a nonspecific hypodense cerebellar mass (205). MR shows a sharply marginated cerebellar mass with T1 and T2 prolongation; coursing through the mass are curvilinear structures of gray matter intensity that appear to be the cerebellar cortex (Fig. 5.98). In apparent contradiction of pathologic findings, the cortical ribbon appears of normal or slightly less than normal thickness. Pial enhancement is seen after administration of paramagnetic contrast (Fig. 5.99).

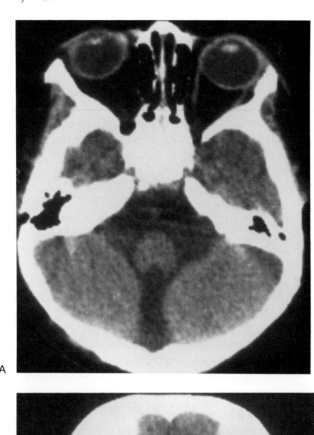

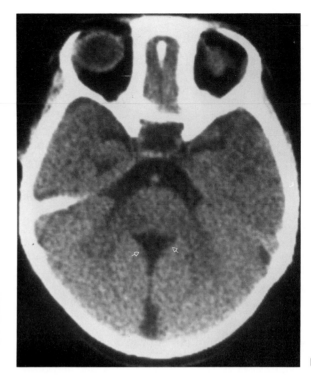

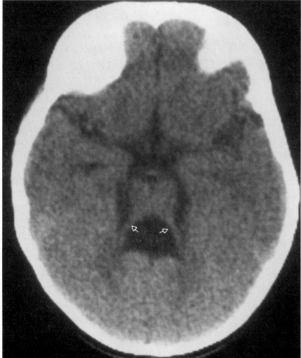

FIG. 5.96. Joubert syndrome. **A:** Axial CT through the level of the inferior fourth ventricle reveals normal-sized cerebellar hemispheres but complete absence of the cerebellar vermis. **B:** Axial CT image at the mid-fourth ventricle level shows a fourth ventricle with the appearance of an inverted triangle (*arrows*). **C:** Near the pontomesencephalic junction, the superior cerebellar peduncles are bordered by CSF and are therefore extremely well seen (*arrows*). The top of the fourth ventricle at this level has the appearance of a bat wing.

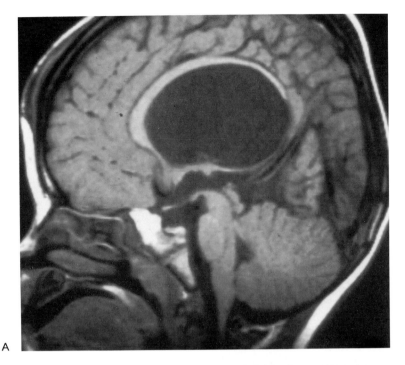

A

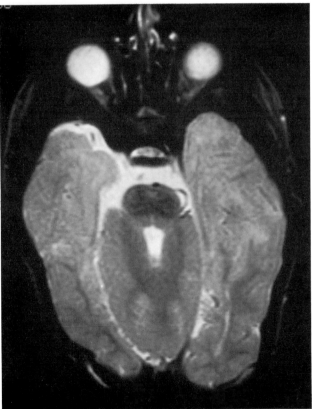

B

C

FIG. 5.97. Rhombencephalosynapsis. **A:** Sagittal SE 600/20 image shows enlarged lateral ventricles and an abnormal appearance of the cerebellar vermis. **B:** Coronal SE 600/20 image shows absence of the septum pellucidum, enlarged lateral ventricles, and fusion of the cerebellar hemispheres without intervening vermis. **C:** Axial SE 2800/70 image shows fusion of the cerebellar hemispheres without intervening vermis, with pointing of the posterior fourth ventricle.

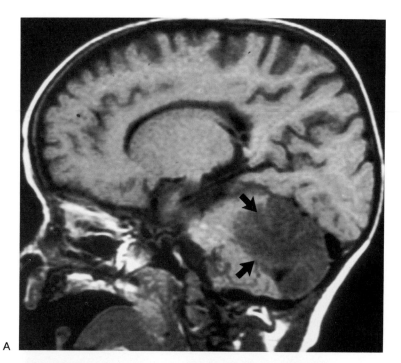

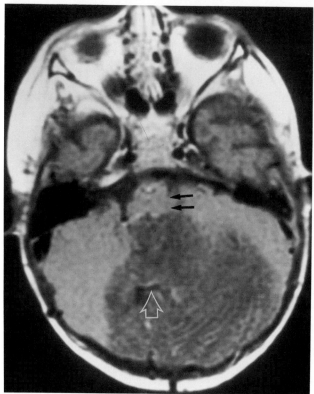

FIG. 5.98. Lhermitte-Duclos syndrome. **A:** Sagittal SE 600/15 image shows hypointensity (*arrows*) of the posterior left cerebellar hemisphere. **B:** Axial SE 600/15 image shows the hypodense region has mass effect, displacing fourth ventricle (*white arrow*) and medulla (*black arrows*).

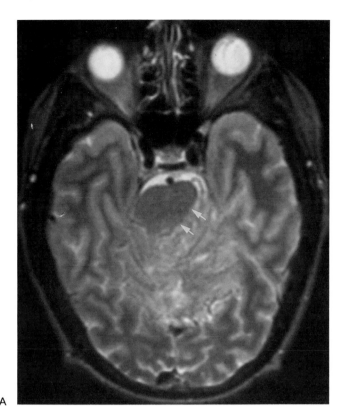
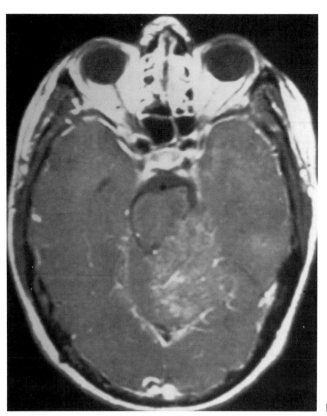

A

B

FIG. 5.99. Lhermitte-Duclos syndrome. **A:** Axial SE 2800/70 image shows heterogeneous hyperintensity in the cerebellum with mass effect (*arrows*) upon the pons. **B:** Postcontrast image shows heterogeneous, pial enhancement of the malformation.

ANOMALIES OF THE HYPOTHALAMIC–PITUITARY AXIS

Embryology

Between 28 and 32 days of embryonic life, a shallow vesicle known as Rathke's pouch or Rathke's cleft appears on the roof of the foregut, immediately rostral to the notochord. Traditionally, Rathke's pouch has been considered to arise from the buccal cavity; however, recent evidence supports origin from neuroectoderm (206). Whatever the origin, Rathke's pouch contacts and comes to lie anterior to a downward extension of the embryonic hypothalamus known as the *neurohypophysis*, or posterior pituitary lobe (Fig. 5.100). The connection of Rathke's pouch with the buccal cavity then undergoes obliteration, although portions of it may persist as the craniopharyngeal canal or as nests of ectopic pituitary tissue in the nasopharynx or sphenoid sinus. After its connection to the buccal cavity is obliterated between 42 and 44 days gestational age, Rathke's pouch becomes known as the *adenohypophysis*, or anterior pituitary lobe (207,208).

Between 37 and 42 days gestational age, lateral lobes form in the developing adenohypophysis. These lobes, known as the tuberal processes, will differentiate into the *pars tuberalis*. Between 42 and 44 days, the tuberal pro-

cesses surround the infundibulum and developing neurohypophysis laterally and give some definition to the developing hypophysis. Between 44 and 48 gestational days, the midline anterior lobe cells that are in close approximation to the posterior lobe differentiate into the primordium of the *pars intermedia*. All the components of the mature hypothalamic–pituitary axis are now in place and will slowly evolve into the mature system (207,208).

Pituitary Absence, Hypoplasia, and Duplication

Absence or hypoplasia of the pituitary gland is a rare anomaly that involves absence or hypoplasia of both the anterior and posterior lobes and, in many cases, the pituitary stalk (179). When present, other congenital anomalies are nearly always associated. Most commonly, the adrenal glands, thyroid, testes, ovaries, and penis are hypoplastic. The sella is small and flat, and sometimes is covered by a layer of dura. Although pituitary aplasia is nearly always fatal at birth, patients with pituitary hypoplasia can survive with hormonal replacement therapy (179,184). These patients may have short stature as a result of deficiency of growth hormone and, therefore, fall into the category of pituitary dwarfism.

Very rarely, the hypothalamus and pituitary gland

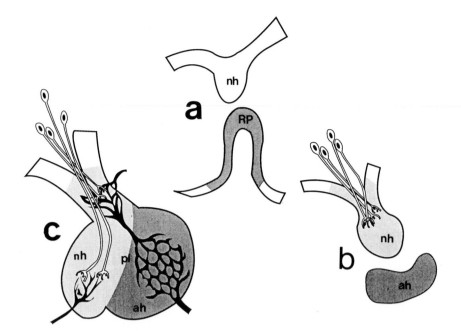

FIG. 5.100. Formation of the pituitary gland. **A:** Between 28 and 32 days of embryonic life Rathke's pouch (RP) appears on the roof of the foregut, immediately rostral to the notochord. Rathke's pouch contacts and comes to lie anterior to a downward extension of the embryonic hypothalamus known as the *neurohypophysis*, or posterior pituitary lobe (nh). **B:** The connection of Rathke's pouch with the buccal cavity undergoes obliteration between 42 and 44 days of gestational age, at which time Rathke's pouch becomes known as the *adenohypophysis*, or anterior pituitary lobe (ah). **C:** Between 44 and 48 gestational days, the midline anterior lobe cells that are in close approximation to the posterior lobe differentiate into the primordium of the *pars intermedia* (pi). All of the components of the mature hypothalamic–pituitary axis are now in place and will slowly evolve into the mature system.

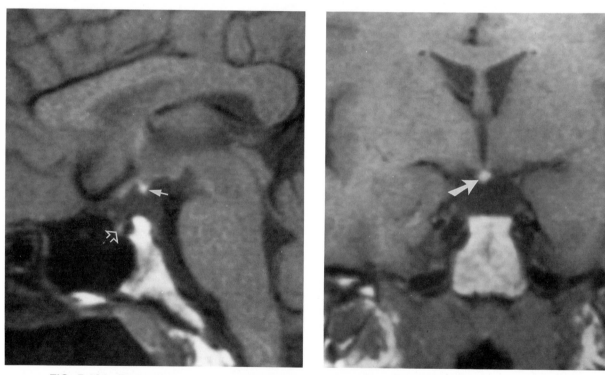

FIG. 5.101. Pituitary hypoplasia. **A:** Sagittal SE 550/16 image shows a diminutive sella (*open white arrow*), unidentifiable infundibulum, and ectopic posterior pituitary gland (*closed white arrow*). **B:** Coronal SE 550/16 image shows the ectopic posterior pituitary gland (*arrow*) located within the tuber cinereum of the hypothalamus.

may be duplicated. Agenesis of the corpus callosum and other brain anomalies are almost always present (209).

Pituitary Dwarfism

Pituitary dwarfism is a heterogeneous group of diseases caused by growth hormone deficiency and characterized by short stature, slow growth, defective dentition, and delayed skeletal maturation. Males are affected twice as commonly as females. The hormonal deficiency may be limited to growth hormone or may involve multiple adenohypophyseal and neurohypophyseal hormones. Diagnosis is usually suspected if a patient is exceptionally short for age according to standard growth charts, is growing poorly for age without evidence of any other disorder, or has short stature and any signs or symptoms of CNS abnormality (210). Imaging studies show a range of characteristic features, including a diminutive sella and pituitary gland, hypoplasia or absence of the pituitary stalk, and presence of the high-intensity posterior lobe of the pituitary gland in the median eminence of the hypothalamus ("ectopic bright spot") (Fig. 5.101) (211–213). Only about 40% of patients with pituitary dwarfism will have the full spectrum of imaging features; those patients with the full spectrum are likely to have multiple hormone deficiencies and lower levels of growth hormone (212,213). MR scans of patients with less severe hormonal disturbances typically show only a small or normal gland.

Kallmann Syndrome (Hypogonadotropic Hypogonadism)

Kallmann syndrome (214) is a genetic disorder of neuronal migration in which olfactory cells and cells that normally express luteinizing hormone releasing hormone (LHRH) fail to migrate from the olfactory placode into the forebrain. Normally, both of these cell types originate in the olfactory placode (in the nasal fossa) and migrate superiorly and anteriorly toward the developing cerebral hemispheres (215). The migration is facilitated by the recognition of specific neural cell adhesion molecules (N-CAMs) on the surface of cells along the pathway of migration (216,217). In Kallmann syndrome, the gene controlling the expression of the N-CAM is deleted; as a result, the cells generated in the olfactory placode remain in the nasal cavity (218).

Patients with Kallmann syndrome typically present with anosmia or hyposmia and, in older patients, with hypogonadism. Establishing the proper diagnosis is important, as hormonal treatments can restore reproductive function and patients can lead relatively normal life-styles (219). MR imaging can be important in establishing the diagnosis (220), as it allows assessment of the formation of the olfactory sulcus, which is hypoplas-

tic or absent in Kallmann syndrome. Although axial images can suggest the absence of the olfactory sulcus (220,221), coronal scans will show the anatomy more definitively (Fig. 5.102). Moreover, the olfactory bulbs, which are normally seen on good coronal MR images (Fig. 5.102E), are hypoplastic and usually not apparent in patients with Kallmann syndrome. If the hypothalamic hypofunction is severe, sagittal images may show a small pituitary gland.

CRANIOFACIAL ANOMALIES

The category of craniofacial anomalies includes those disorders in which the face and the skull develop abnormally. From an embryologic perspective, most of these disorders are believed to result from insufficient formation of, or inadequate migration of, mesenchyme (primarily neural crest cells) to the skull base and the face (222,223). A discussion of the full spectrum of craniofacial malformations is well beyond the scope of this book; therefore, this chapter discusses those aspects of craniofacial anomalies that are of concern in neuroradiology. This topic was discussed briefly in regard to cephaloceles, frontonasal dermoids, and midline craniofacial dysraphism in "Cephaloceles and Other Anomalies of the Skull Base and Calvarium" earlier in this chapter. The present section discusses craniosynostosis syndromes, their diagnosis, and the brain anomalies that may be associated with them.

Diagnosis of Craniosynostosis

Craniosynostosis can be broadly grouped into two categories. *Primary craniosynostosis* refers to premature fusion of one or more cranial sutures as a developmental error. The cause is thought to be a developmental anomaly of the skull base. *Secondary synostosis* refers to premature sutural closure resulting from other causes, such as intrauterine compression of the skull, the effect of teratogens, or lack of brain growth. The condition may be seen in otherwise normal individuals and as a part of syndromes associated with other developmental anomalies (224–226).

Isolated Synostosis

When isolated to a single suture, craniosynostosis is usually sporadic and presents as an abnormally shaped head. Isolated sagittal synostosis causes a long, narrow head shape (*scaphocephaly* or *dolichocephaly*, Fig. 5.103); isolated metopic synostosis causes a prominent, wedge-shaped forehead (*trigonocephaly*; Fig. 5.104), and isolated unilateral coronal or lambdoid synostosis causes cranial asymmetry (*plagiocephaly*, Fig. 5.105). Isolated sagittal, metopic, or unilateral coronal synostosis is diag-

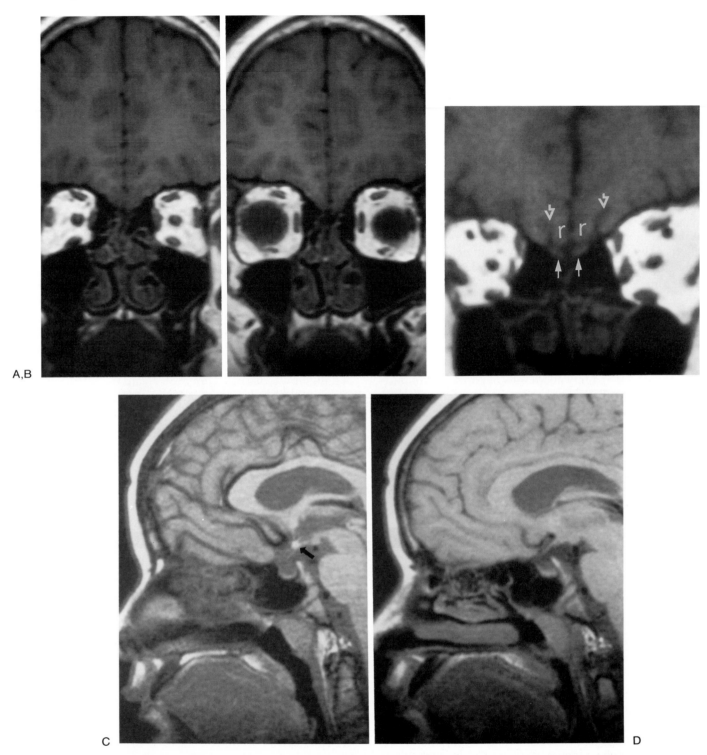

FIG. 5.102. Kallmann syndrome. **A, B:** Coronal SE 600/15 images show absence of the normal olfactory sulci separating the gyri recti from the medial orbital gyri. **C, D:** Sagittal SE 550/15 images show pituitary hypoplasia and ectopia of the posterior pituitary (*arrow*). **E:** Normal patient. Olfactory sulci (*open arrows*) separate gyri recti (r) from medial orbital gyri. The olfactory bulbs (*closed arrows*) can often be seen.

nosed clinically and confirmed by plain films of the skull. The characteristic findings on skull films are available in any standard text on pediatric radiology.

Imaging is performed in patients with isolated sutural synostosis primarily to look for underlying brain anomalies. For example, isolated unilateral lambdoid synostosis can usually be diagnosed on physical examination by observation of unilateral flattening of the back of the head. However, some patients develop unilateral flattening of the occipital region secondarily, as a result of extended periods of lying on their backs, primarily on one side; this group often has an underlying brain abnormality (either metabolic or anatomic) that may be identified by imaging. Moreover, secondary flattening resulting from lack of infant movement may not be associated with synostosis. As plain skull films are not helpful in diagnosing lambdoid synostosis, CT is the modality of choice. We perform CT with 3 mm contiguous axial slices, using a soft tissue algorithm to evaluate the brain and a bone algorithm to evaluate the skull. It is impor-

tant to realize that the suture may only be closed in a single spot and that the suture is therefore open throughout most of its extent. In patients with lambdoid synostosis, the affected lambdoid suture may be overgrown compared to the contralateral side; this is the radiologic equivalent of the sutural "ridging" found on physical exam. Occasionally, a thin line of bridging hyperdensity, possibly representing periosteum, will be seen across the suture. Compensatory enlargement of the anterior portion of the ipsilateral middle cranial fossa is usually seen and is an important finding. The CT will show elevation of the orbit and increased lateral convexity of the squamous portion of the ipsilateral temporal bone (Fig. 5.105).

Occasionally, the diagnosis of coronal synostosis is indeterminate by clinical and plain film examinations. In such cases, CT may be useful. CT findings in isolated coronal synostosis are narrowing of the sphenopetrosal angle, contralateral bulging of the frontal calvarium, and decreased size of the ipsilateral frontal fossa.

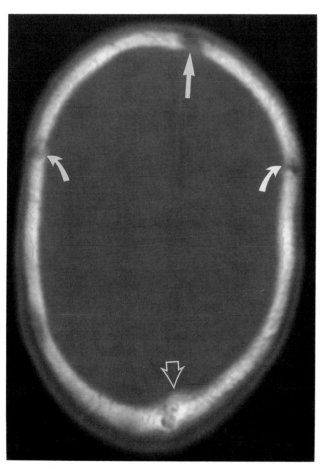

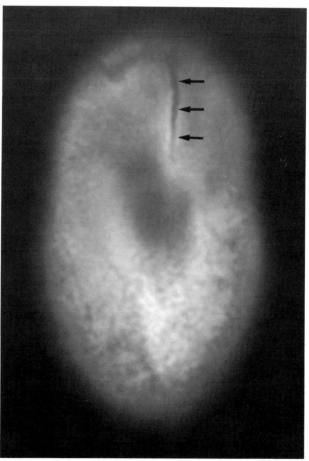

A

B

FIG. 5.103. Scaphocephaly secondary to sagittal suture synostosis. **A:** Axial CT image shows open metopic suture (*straight arrow*) and coronal sutures (*curved arrows*). The sagittal suture (*open arrow*) is fused, Note the ridging at the site of the closed suture. **B:** At the level of the vertex, the sagittal suture is open anteriorly (*arrows*) but closed posteriorly, resulting in continuity of the calvarium across the midline.

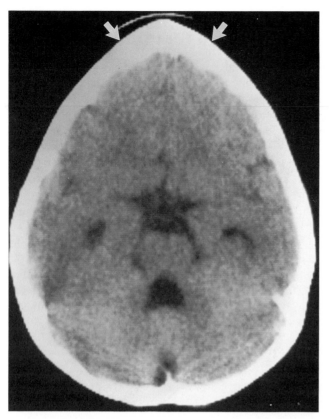

FIG. 5.104. Trigonocephaly. Axial CT shows a pointed frontal region (*arrows*) secondary to premature closure of the metopic suture.

Multiple Synostosis Syndromes

A number of genetic syndromes result in multiple sutural synostoses (Table 5.3). Bilateral coronal synostosis (Fig. 5.106) is the most common combination, but bilateral coronal and bilateral lambdoid synostosis or a combination of bilateral coronal synostosis and sagittal synostosis can be seen, among others. When the sagittal suture is synostotic in conjunction with both coronal sutures (and sometimes both lambdoid sutures), the membranous bone of the calvarium expands between the sutures but not at them, resulting in a characteristic lobulated skull configuration known as *cloverleaf skull or Kleebatshädl* (Fig. 5.107). Multiple synostosis syndromes may be isolated but are more commonly associated with syndactactyly, polydactyly, or other somatic anomalies (Table 5.3)(224–226).

Anomalies of the underlying brain are present in a significant number of affected patients (224,227,228), and their identification is the primary reason for obtaining imaging studies. Ventriculomegaly is very common, probably as a result of the small skull base and increased resistance to venous outflow (Fig. 5.107) (227,229). The differentiation of benign ventriculomegaly from hydrocephalus can be difficult, as discussed in Chapter 8, and is dependent upon assessment of subtle features, such as the degree of enlargement of the anterior recesses of the third ventricle. Other common anomalies include corti-

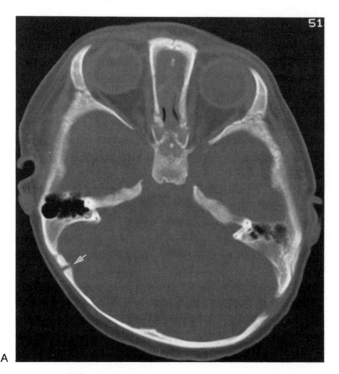

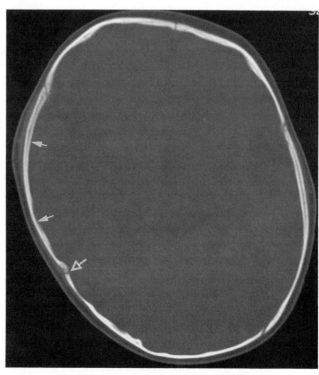

FIG. 5.105. Plagiocephaly. A: Axial CT image shows anteriorly positioned right lateral orbital wall, right ear, and right petrous bone. The right lambdoid suture (*arrow*) shows slight ridging. B: At a higher level, the right posterior skull is flattened, the squamous portion of the temporal bone (*closed arrows*) is expanded, and the lambdoid suture (*open arrow*) is narrowed.

TABLE 5.3. *Inherited forms of craniosynostosis*

Syndromes	Classification	Essential features	Inheritance
Apert, Apert-Crouzon	Acrocephalosyndactyly I, II	Craniosynostosis, severe syndactyly of hands and feet, down-turned mouth, hypertelorism	Autosomal dominant
Saethre-Chotzen	Acrocephalosyndactyly III	Craniosynostosis, facial asymmetry, low-hairline ptosis, deviated nasal septum, syndactyly of second, third fingers	Autosomal dominant
Pfeiffer, Noack	Acrocephalopolysyndactyly I, V	Craniosynostosis, malformed enlarged thumb and great toe, soft tissue syndactyly of second, third digits, normal intelligence	Autosomal dominant
Carpenter, Summitt, Goodman, Sakati-Nyhan	Acrocephalopolysyndactyly II, III, IV	Craniosynostosis, preaxial polydactyly, soft tissue syndactyly, malformed ears, obesity, hypogenitalism, variable mental retardation	Autosomal recessive
Crouzon, craniofacial dysostosis	Craniosynostosis with other somatic abnormalities	Craniosynostosis, maxillary hypoplasia, shallow orbits with proptosis, bifid uvula or cleft palate	Autosomal dominant
Craniosynostosis, fibular aplasia, Lowry	Craniosynostosis with other somatic abnormalities	Craniosynostosis and fibular aplasia	Autosomal recessive
Craniosynostosis, foot defects, Jackson-Weiss	Craniosynostosis with other somatic abnormalities	Craniosynostosis, varus deformity of great toes and tarsal fusion	Autosomal dominant
Craniosynostosis, mental retardation clefting	Craniosynostosis with other somatic abnormalities	Craniosynostosis, cleft lip and palate, choroidal coloboma, mental retardation	Autosomal recessive
Craniosynostosis, radial aplasia, Baller-Gerold	Craniosynostosis with other somatic abnormalities	Synostosis of one or more sutures, bilateral radial aplasia	Autosomal recessive
Craniosynostosis, arachnodactyly hernia, Shprintzen-Goldberg	Craniosynostosis with other somatic abnormalities	Synostosis of multiple sutures, mandibular and maxillary hypoplasia, multiple abdominal hernias, exophthalmos, mental retardation	Autosomal dominant

cal dysplasias, callosal agenesis or hypogenesis, agenesis or hypogenesis of the septum pellucidum, and cephaloceles (224,227,228). CT of the skull in affected patients shows a dysplastic calvarium with thin, irregular bone that is difficult to separate from the underlying dura. The patients have hypertelorism and shallow orbits with marked proptosis (Figs. 5.106,5.107).

CHROMOSOMAL ANOMALIES

Chromosomal anomalies have only recently been systematically catalogued and characterized with respect to their pathologic and neuroradiologic findings (230). The field is rapidly evolving as the genetic bases of many anomalies are elucidated. It is interesting to note that many sets of siblings have identical dysmorphic features and brain anomalies (Fig. 5.108) that fit no known genetic syndrome. As genetic evaluations become more common and more precise, the chromosomal abnor-

malities that cause these disorders will most likely be discovered.

A partial list of known genetic disorders that affect the brain, together with a list of the associated brain anomalies, is presented in Table 5.4. More complete lists can be found in standard pediatric texts and texts of chromosomal alterations in humans. More important, essentially all the brain anomalies that result from genetic disorders are described in this chapter, along with the imaging characteristics of the anomalies. When the information in this chapter is used in conjunction with lists of chromosomal disorders, the imaging studies of such disorders should be interpreted easily. This section concentrates on the well-defined trisomies, those of chromosomes 13, 18, and 21.

Down Syndrome

Down syndrome, caused by trisomy of chromosome 21, is the most common chromosomal disorder, with an

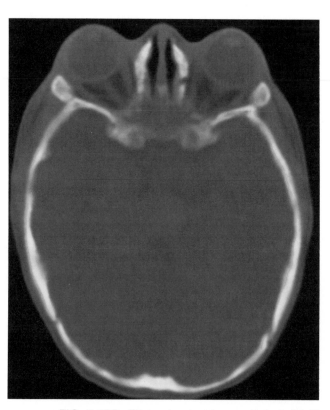
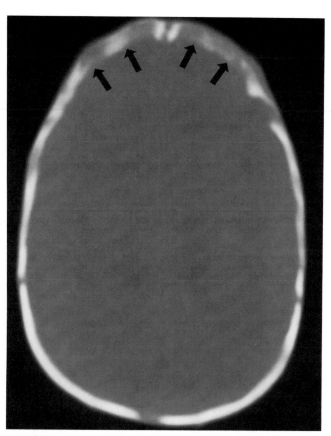

FIG. 5.106. Bilateral coronal synostosis in Pfeiffer syndrome. **A:** Axial CT image at the orbital level shows shallow orbits. **B:** At a higher level, the frontal bones (*arrows*) are dysplastic and the coronal sutures fused.

TABLE 5.4. *Some genetic syndrome and their associated brain anomalies*

Disorder	Brain anomalies
Down syndrome (Trisomy 21)	Small frontal lobes Hypoplastic inf. frontal gyrus
Edwards syndrome (Trisomy 18)	Immature cerebral gyral pattern Hypoplastic cerebellum Callosal hypogenesis Hippocampal dysplasia
Patau syndrome (Trisomy 13)	Holoprosencephaly Callosal hypogenesis Olfactory hypoplasia Cerebellar vermian hypoplasia
Trisomy 9 (240)	Dandy-Walker malformation Callosal hypogenesis Pachygyria Hippocampal hypoplasia
Wolfe syndrome (Deletion short arm 4)	Neuronal migration anomalies Callosal hypogenesis Cerebellar vermian hypoplasia
Cri du chat syndrome (Deletion short arm 5)	Microcephaly Hypertelorism
Prader-Willi syndrome (Deletion long arm 15)	Hypothalamic–pituitary hypoplasia
Miller-Dieker syndrome (Deletion short arm 17)	Lissencephaly type I Characteristic facies
Fragile X syndrome (Fragile long arm X)	Anomalies of neuronal migration Cerebellar vermian hypoplasia

incidence of about 1 in 1,000 live births (231). The disorder is a leading cause of mental retardation, with 80% of affected patients being severely retarded (IQ less than 50). Although examination of the brain at autopsy shows many abnormalities—including senile plaques and neurofibrillary tangles at an early age, reduced brain weight, a narrow superior temporal gyrus, and hypoplastic inferior frontal gyrus—imaging studies are not dramatic. Patients are brachycephalic, with a short, round brain; reduced anteroposterior diameter of the frontal lobes; a narrow superior temporal gyrus; small cerebellum and pons; and forward kinking of the brain stem (232).

Cervical spine abnormalities are common in Down syndrome. The most common anomaly is atlantoaxial subluxation, presumably as a result of ligamentous laxity, which has a prevalence of 10% to 22% (233,234). Ligamentous laxity may also contribute to the increased incidence of atlanto-occipital subluxation (235,236). Superimposed upon the ligamentous laxity, a high incidence of bony anomalies of the upper cervical spine puts the affected child in even greater jeopardy of spinal cord injury with relatively minor trauma. Odontoid anomalies, such as hypoplasia and dysplasia of the odontoid and os odontoideum, have been described (237,238). Patients may also have hypoplasia of the posterior arch of C-1 (233), and they can develop progressive basilar invagination (237). The craniocervical junction should al-

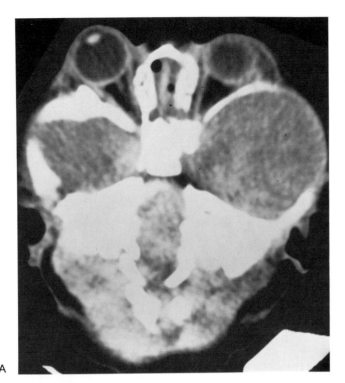

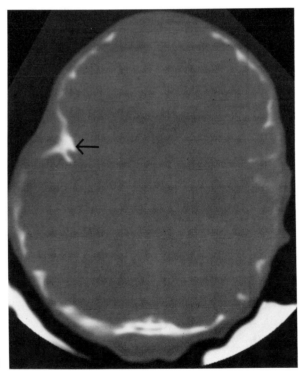

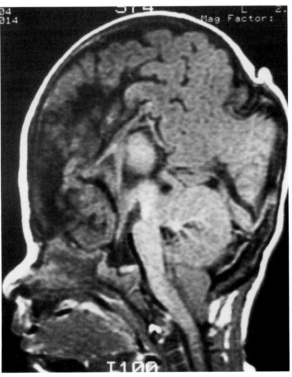

FIG. 5.107. Kleebatshädl in patient with Apert syndrome. **A:** Axial CT image shows markedly shallow orbits with resultant proptosis. The anterior middle cranial fossae are markedly expanded secondary to the bilateral lambdoid synostosis. **B:** Bone windows at a higher level show the bizarre appearance of the inner table of the calvarium. Note the indentation of the calvarium (*arrow*) at the site of the coronal suture. **C:** Sagittal SE 600/20 image after ventriculoperitoneal shunt shows tiny skull base resulting in Chiari I malformation and compression of the brain stem. The corpus callosum is hypogenetic.

A

B

C

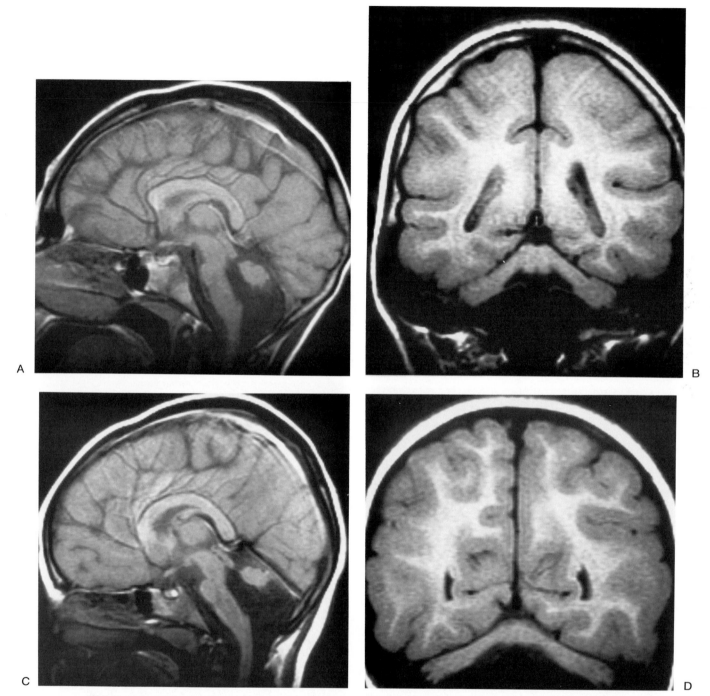

FIG. 5.108. Siblings with unknown genetic abnormality. **A, B:** Sagittal and coronal images show pachygyria with pontine and cerebellar hypogenesis. **C, D:** Sibling of patient in (A,B) shows identical brain anomalies.

ways be closely scrutinized in patients with Down syndrome, and, as stated in Chapter 4, these patients should be observed regularly for neurologic dysfunction and neck pain and should be examined carefully after even minor neck trauma. Plain film radiographs of the cervical spine with flexion and extension views are adequate for patients without neurologic deficits. However, patients with neurologic signs or symptoms or with a history of signs or symptoms referable to craniocervical junction anomalies should undergo MR imaging with sagittal flexion and extension T1-weighted images. T2-weighted images should also be obtained to look for areas of high signal within the cord, indicative of prior injury.

Trisomy 18

Trisomy 18, also known as Edwards's syndrome, is the second most commonly encountered trisomy encountered in newborns, occurring in about 1 in 5,000 live births. Patients are dolichocephalic with malformed, low-set ears; micrognathia; short upper lip; short palpebral fissures; epicanthal folds; midline facial clefts; ptosis; corneal opacities; and microphthalmos. Characteristic hand and foot anomalies, where the fingers flex and over-

ride (most commonly, the index finger overlaps the long finger and the small finger overlaps the ring finger) and the great toe is dorsiflexed, are common. Anomalies of the cardiac, gastrointestinal, and urogenital systems are common (179,231,239).

The most consistently identified neuropathologic findings are anomalies of the cerebral gyral pattern, hypoplasia of the cerebellum and basis pontis, hypogenesis or agenesis of the corpus callosum, and dysplasia of the hippocampus, lateral geniculate body, and inferior olivary nucleus (179). CT may show dolichocephaly and cerebellar hypoplasia but is not as useful as MR in demonstrating the gyral anomalies, callosal hypogenesis, and hippocampal dysplasia (Fig. 5.109) (231,232).

Trisomy 13

Trisomy 13, also known as Patau syndrome, occurs in about 1 in 6,000 live births. The clinical features include microcephaly, severe mental retardation, absent eyebrow, shallow supraorbital ridges, anophthalmia, microphthalmia with coloboma, micrognathia, cleft palate, malformed ears, and cardiac anomalies. Anomalies of the brain are characterized by holoprosencephaly, which

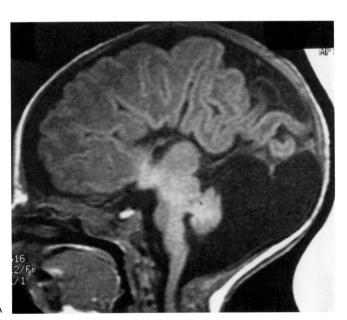
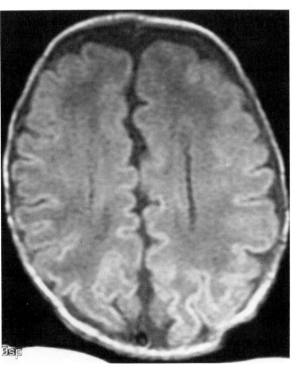

FIG. 5.109. Trisomy 18. **A:** Sagittal SE 550/15 image shows callosal agenesis, a simplified cerebral cortical gyral pattern, pontine hypoplasia, and cerebellar hypoplasia with a large posterior fossa (Dandy-Walker complex). **B:** Axial SE 600/16 image shows shallow sulci and a simplified cortical gyral pattern.

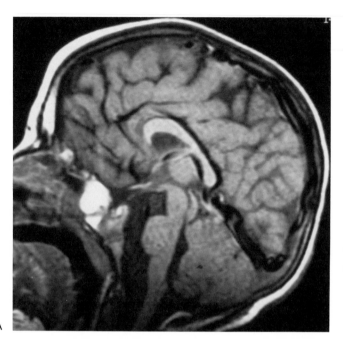

A

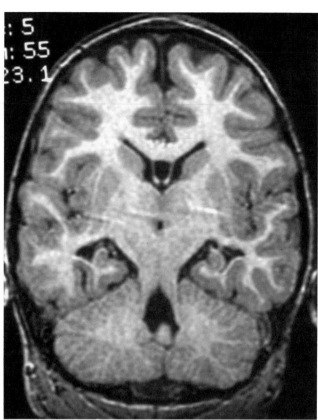

B

FIG. 110. Trisomy 13. **A:** Sagittal SE 500/11 image shows mild callosal hypogenesis and mild vermian hypogenesis. **B:** Oblique coronal image shows bilateral hippocampal hypoplasia.

occurs in 80% of affected infants. In those patients without holoprosencephaly, reported anomalies include callosal agenesis, olfactory hypoplasia, cerebellar cortical dysplasias, and inferior vermian hypoplasia (Fig. 5.110) (231,239).

REFERENCES

1. Müller F, O'Rahilly R. The first appearance of the human nervous system at stage 8. *Anat Embryol* 1981;163:1–13.
2. Müller F, O'Rahilly R. The first appearance of the major divisions of the human brain at stage 9. *Anat Embryol* 1983;168:419–432.
3. Müller F, O'Rahilly R. The first appearance of the neural tube and optic primordium in the human embryo at stage 10. *Anat Embryol* 1985;172:157–169.
4. Golden J, Chernoff G. Intermittent pattern of neural tube closure in two strains of mice. *Teratology* 1993;47:73–80.
5. Van Allen M, Kalousek D, Chernoff G, et al. Evidence for multi-site closure of the neural tube in humans. *Am J Med Genet* 1993;47:723–743.
6. O'Rahilly R, Müller F. *Neurulation in the normal human embryo.* Presented at CIBA Foundation Symposium No. 181, May 1993.
7. Rakic P. Cell migration and neuronal ectopias in the brain. *Birth Defects* 1975;11:95–129.
8. Sidman RL, Rakic P. Development of the human central nervous system. In: Haymaker W, Adams RD, eds. *Histology and histopathology of the nervous system.* Springfield, IL: Thomas, 1982:73.
9. Müller F, O'Rahilly R. The development of the human brain and the closure of the rostral neuropore at stage 11. *Anat Embryol* 1986;175:205–222.
10. Müller F, O'Rahilly R. The development of the human brain, the closure of the caudal neuropore, and the beginning of secondary neurulation at stage 12. *Anat Embryol* 1987;176:413–430.
11. Müller F, O'Rahilly R. The first appearance of the future cerebral hemispheres in the human embryo at stage 14. *Anat Embryol* 1988;177:495–511.
12. Rakic P, Yakovlev PI. Development of the corpus callosum and cavum septae in man. *J Comp Neurol* 1968;132:45–72.
13. Silver J, Lorenz SE, Wahlsten D, Coughlin J. Axonal guidance during development of the great cerebral commissures: descriptive and experimental studies, *in vivo,* on the role of preformed glial pathways. *J Comp Neurol* 1982;210:10–29.
14. Zaki W. Le processus dégénératif au cours du développement du corps calleux. *Archiv Anat Micr Morphol Expér* 1985;74:133–149.
15. Barkovich AJ, Lyon G, Evrard P. Formation, maturation, and disorders of white matter. *AJNR* 1992;13:447–461.
16. Barkovich AJ, Norman D. Anomalies of the corpus callosum: correlation with further anomalies of the brain. *AJNR* 1988;9:493–501.
17. Barkovich AJ, Quint D. Middle interhemispheric fusion: an unusual variant of holoprosencephaly. *Am J Neurorad* 1993;14:431–440.
18. Barkovich AJ. Apparent atypical callosal dysgenesis: analysis of MR findings in six cases and their relationship to holoprosencephaly. *AJNR* 1990;11:333–340.
19. Palmini A, Andermann F, Olivier A, Tampieri D, Robitaille Y. Focal neuronal migration disorders and intractable partial epilepsy: results of surgical treatment. *Ann Neurol* 1991;30:750–757.
20. Petrucci RJ, Buchheit WA, Woodruff GC, Karian JM, DeFilipp

GJ. Transcallosal parafornicial approach for third ventricle tumors: neuropsychological consequences. *Neurosurgery* 1987;20:457–464.

21. Barkovich AJ, Kjos BO. Normal postnatal development of the corpus callosum as demonstrated by MR imaging. *AJNR* 1988;9:487–491.
22. Parrish ML, Roessmann U, Levinsohn MW. Agenesis of the corpus callosum: a study of the frequency of associated malformations. *Ann Neurol* 1979;6:349–354.
23. Kendall BE. Dysgenesis of the corpus callosum. *Neuroradiology* 1983;25:239–256.
24. Byrd S, Radkowski M, Flannery A, McLone D. The clinical and radiologic evaluation of absence of the corpus callosum. *Eur J Radiol* 1990;10:65–73.
25. Ettlinger G. Agenesis of the corpus callosum. In: Vinicken PJ, Bruyn GW, eds. *Handbook of clinical neurology,* vol 30. Amsterdam: North-Holland, 1977:285–297.
26. Aicardi J, Lefebre J, Lerrique-Koechlin A. A new syndrome: spasm in flexion, callosal agenesis, ocular abnormalities. *Electroencephalogr Clin Neurophysiol* 1965;19:609–610.
27. Pappas CTE, Rekate HL. Cervicomedullary junction decompression in a case of Marshall-Smith syndrome. *J Neurosurg* 1991;75:317–319.
28. Baierl P, Markl A, Thelen M, Laub MC. MR imaging of Aicardi syndrome. *AJNR* 1988;9:805–806.
29. Hall-Craggs MA, Harbord MG, Finn JP, et al. Aicardi syndrome: MR assessment of brain structure and myelination. *AJNR* 1990;11:532–536.
30. Igidbashian V, Mahboubi S, Zimmerman RA. CT and MR findings in Aicardi syndrome. *J Comput Assist Tomogr* 1987;11:357–358.
31. Baker LL, Barkovich AJ. The large temporal horn: MR analysis in developmental brain anomalies versus hydrocephalus. *AJNR* 1992;13:115–122.
32. Atlas SW, Zimmerman RA, Bilaniuk LT, et al. Corpus callosum and limbic system: neuroanatomic MR evaluation of developmental anomalies. *Radiology* 1986;160:355–362.
33. Young JN, Oakes WJ, Hatten HP. Dorsal third ventricular cyst: an entity distinct from holoprosencephaly. *J Neurosurg* 1992;77:556–561.
34. Osaka k, Handa R, Matsumoto S, Yasuda M. Development of the cerebrospinal fluid pathway in the normal and abnormal human embryos. *Childs Brain* 1980;6:26–38.
35. O'Rahilly R, Müller F. The meninges in human development. *J Neuropathol Exp Neurol* 1986;45:588–608.
36. Truwit CL, Barkovich AJ. Pathogenesis of intracranial lipoma: an MR study in 42 patients. *AJNR* 1990;11:665–674.
37. Naidich TP, McLone DG, Bauer BS, Kernahan DA, Zaparackas ZG. Midline craniofacial dysraphism: midline cleft upper lip, basal encephalocele, callosal agenesis, and optic nerve dysplasia. *Concepts Pediatr Neurosurg* 1983;4:186–207.
38. Naidich TP, Osborn RE, Bauer B, Naidich MJ. Median cleft face syndrome: MR and CT data from 11 children. *J Comput Asst Tomogr* 1988;12:57–64.
39. Dean B, Drayer BP, Beresini DC, Bird CR. MR imaging of pericallosal lipoma. *AJNR* 1988;9:929–931.
40. Naidich TP, Altman NR, Braffman BH, McLone DG, Zimmerman RA. Cephaloceles and related malformations. *AJNR* 1992;13:655–690.
41. Diebler C, Dulac O. Cephaloceles: clinical and neuroradiological appearance. *Neuroradiology* 1983;25:199–216.
42. Yokota A, Matsukado Y, Fuwa I, Moroki K, Nagahiro S. Anterior basal encephalocele of the neonatal and infantile period. *Neurosurgery* 1986;19:468–478.
43. Sessions RB. Nasal dermal sinuses—new concepts and explanations. *Laryngoscope* 1982;92 (suppl. 29):1–28.
44. Yokota A, Kajiwara H, Kohchi M, Fuwa I, Wada H. Parietal cephalocele: clinical importance of its atretic form and associated malformations. *J Neurosurg* 1988;69:545–551.
45. Chapman PH, Swearingen B, Caviness VS. Subtorcular occipital encephaloceles: anatomical considerations relevant to operative management. *J Neurosurg* 1989;71:375–381.
46. Simpson DA, David DJ, White J. Cephaloceles: treatment, outcome and antenatal diagnosis. *Neurosurgery* 1984;15:14–21.

47. Maas KP, Barkovich AJ, Dong.L, Edwards MSB, Piecuch RE, Charlton V. Selected indications for and applications of magnetic resonance angiography in children. *Pediatr Neurosurg* (in press).
48. Barkovich AJ, Vandermarck P, Edwards MB, Cogen PH. Congenital nasal masses: CT and MR imaging features in 16 cases. *Am J Neuroradiol* 1991;12:105–116.
49. Suwanwela C, Sukabote C, Suwanwela N. Frontoethmoidal encephalomeningocele. *Surgery* 1971;69:617–625.
50. Suwanwela C, Suwanwela N. A morphological classification of sincipital encephalomeningoceles. *J Neurosurg* 1972;36:201–211.
51. Curnes JT, Oakes WJ. Parietal cephaloceles: radiographic and magnetic resonance imaging evaluation. *Pediatr Neurosci* 1988;14:71–76.
52. Martinez-Lage JF, Capel A, Costa TR, Perez-Espejo MA, Poza M. The child with a mass on its head: diagnostic and surgical strategies. *Childs Nerv Syst* 1992;8:247–252.
53. Pannell BW, Hendrick EB, Hoffman HJ, Humphreys RP. Dermoid cysts of the anterior fontanelle. *Neurosurgery* 1982;10:317–323.
54. Kaplan SB, Kemp SS, Oh KS. Radiographic manifestations of congenital anomalies of the skull. *Radiol Clin North Am* 1991;29:195–218.
55. Schut L, Sutton LN, Bruce DA. Vascular malformations of the scalp and skull. In: Edwards MSB, Hoffman HJ, eds. *Cerebral vascular disease in children and adolescents.* Baltimore: Williams and Wilkins, 1988:411–422.
56. Bollar A, Allut A, Prieto A, Gelabert M, Becerra E. Sinus pericranii: radiological and etiopathological considerations. *J Neurosurg* 1992;77:469–472.
57. Emery JL, MacKenzie N. Medullo-cervical dislocation deformity (Chiari II deformity) related to neurospinal dysraphism (myelomeningocele). *Brain* 1973;96:155–162.
58. Rakic P. Neuronal migration and contact guidance in the primate telencephalon. *Postgrad Med J* 1978;54:25–40.
59. Caviness VS Jr. Normal development of the cerebral neocortex. In: Evrard P, Minkowski A, eds. *Developmental neurobiology.* Nestle nutrition workshop series. New York: Raven, 1989:1–10.
60. O'Rourke NA, Dailey ME, Smith SJ, McConnell SK. Diverse migratory pathways in the developing cerebral cortex. *Science* 1992;258:299–304.
61. McConnell S, Kaznowski C. Cell cycle dependence of laminar determination in the developing cerebral cortex. *Science* 1991;254:282–285.
62. Marin-Padilla M. Structural organization of the human cerebral cortex prior to the appearance of the cortical plate. *Anat Embryol* 1983;168:21–40.
63. Marin-Padilla M. Early ontogenesis of the human cerebral cortex. In: Peter A, Jones EG, eds. *Cerebral cortex,* vol 7: *Development and maturation of the cerebral cortex.* New York: Plenum, 1988:1–34.
64. Barkovich AJ, Gressens P, Evrard P. Formation, maturation, and disorders of brain neocortex. *AJNR* 1992;13:423–446.
65. Suzuki M, Choi BH. Repair and reconstruction of the cortical plate following closed cryogenic injury to the neonatal rat cerebrum. *Acta Neuropathol* 1991;82:93–101.
66. Aicardi J. The agyria-pachygyria complex: a spectrum of cortical malformations. *Brain Dev* 1991;13:1–8.
67. Warkany J, Lemire RJ, Cohen MM Jr. *Mental retardation and congenital malformations of the central nervous system.* Chicago: Yearbook, 1981.
68. Dobyns WB. The neurogenetics of lissencephaly. *Neurol Clin* 1989;7:89–105.
69. Dobyns W, Elias E, Newlin A, Pagon R, Ledbetter D. Causal heterogeneity in isolated lissencephaly. *Neurology* 1992;42:1375–1388.
70. Dobyns WB, Stratton RF, Greenberg F. Syndromes with lissencephaly. I: Miller-Dieker and Norman-Roberts syndromes and isolated lissencephaly. *Am J Med Genet* 1984;18:509–526.
71. Barkovich AJ, Koch TK, Carrol CL. The spectrum of lissencephaly: report of ten cases analyzed by magnetic resonance imaging. *Ann Neurol* 1991;30:139–146.
72. Dobyns WB, Kirkpatrick JB, Hittner HM, Roberts RM, Kretzer FL. Syndromes with lissencephaly. 2: Walker-Warburg and cere-

bral ocular muscular syndromes and a new syndrome with type 2 lissencephaly. *Am J Med Genet* 1985;22:157–195.

73. Garcia CA, Dunn D, Trevor R. The lissencephaly syndrome in siblings. *Arch Neurol* 1978;35:608–611.

74. Stewart RM, Richman DP, Caviness VS Jr. Lissencephaly and pachygyria: An architectonic and topographical analysis. *Acta Neuropathol* 1975;31:1–12.

75. Sarnat H. Role of the human fetal ependyma. *Pediatr Neurol* 1992;8:163–178.

76. Sarnat HB, Darwish HZ, Barth PG, et al. Ependymal abnormalities in lissencephaly/pachygyria. *J Neuropathol Exp Neurol* 1993; 52:525–541.

77. Barkovich AJ, Chuang SH, Norman D. MR of neuronal migration anomalies. *AJNR* 1987;8:1009–1017.

78. Zimmerman RA, Bilaniuk LT, Grossman RI. Computed tomography in migration disorders of human brain development. *Neuroradiology* 1983;25:257–263.

79. Williams RS, Swisher CN, Jennings M, Ambler M, Caviness VS Jr. Cerebroocular dysgenesis "Walker-Warburg" syndrome: neuropathologic and etiologic analysis. *Neurology* 1984;34:1531–1541.

80. Barth PG. Disorders of neuronal migration. *Can J Neurol Sci* 1987;14:1–16.

81. Rhodes RE, Hatten HP Jr, Ellington KS. Walker-Warburg syndrome. *AJNR* 1992;13:123–126.

82. Santavuori P, Somer H, Sainio K, et al. Muscle-eye-brain disease. *Brain Dev* 1989;11:147–153.

83. Takada K, Becker LE, Takashima S. Walker-Warburg syndrome with skeletal muscle involvement: a report of three patients. *Pediatr Neurosci* 1987;13:202–209.

84. Takada K, Nakamura H, Takashima S. Cortical dysplasia in Fukuyama congenital muscular dystrophy: a Golgi and angioarchitectonic analysis. *Acta Neuropathol* 1988;76:170–178.

85. Yoshioka M, Kuroki S, Kondo T. Ocular manifestations in Fukuyama type congenital muscular dystrophy. *Brain Dev* 1990;12: 423–426.

86. Yoshioka M, Saiwai S, Kuroki S, Nigami H. MR imaging of the brain in Fukuyama-type congenital muscular dystrophy. *AJNR* 1991;12:63–66.

87. Fukuyama Y, Kawazura M, Haruna H. A peculiar form of congenital muscular dystrophy. Report of fifteen cases. *Paediatr Universit (Tokyo)* 1960;4:5–8.

88. Fukuyama Y, Osawa M, Suzuki H. Congenital progressive muscular dystrophy of the Fukuyama type—clinical, genetic, and pathological considerations. *Brain Dev* 1981;3:1–29.

89. Yoshioka M, Kuroki S, Nigami H, Kawai T, Nakamura H. Clinical variation within sibships in Fukuyama-type congenital muscular dystrophy. *Brain Dev* 1992;14:334–337.

90. Leyten QH, Gabreels FJM, Renier WO, ter Laak HJ, Sengers RCA, Mullaart RA. Congenital muscular dystrophy. *J Pediatr* 1989;115:214–221.

91. Leyten QH, Renkawek K, Renier WO, et al. Neuropathological findings in muscle-eye-brain disease: neuropathological delineation of MEB-D from congenital muscular dystrophy of the Fukuyama type. *Acta Neuropathol* 1991;83:55–60.

92. Topaloglu H, Yalaz K, Kale G, Ergin M. Congenital muscular dystrophy with cerebral involvement—report of a case of "occidental type cerebromuscular dystrophy"? *Neuropediatrics* 1990; 21:53–54.

93. Topaloglu H, Yalaz K, Renda Y, et al. Occidental type cerebromuscular dystrophy: a report of eleven cases. *J Neurol Neurosurg Psychiatr* 1991;54:226–229.

94. Robain O, Lyon G. Les microcéphalies familiales par malformation cérébrale. *Acta Neuropathol* 1972;26:96–109.

95. Evrard P, de Saint-Georges P, Kadhim HJ, Gadisseux J-F. Pathology of prenatal encephalopathies. In: French J, ed. *Child neurology and developmental disabilities.* Baltimore: Paul H. Brookes, 1989:153–176.

96. Parain D, Gadisseux JF, Henocq A, Tayot J, Evrard P. Diagnostic prénatal et étude d'une microcéphalia vera à 26 semaines de gestation. In: Szliwowski H, Bormans J, eds. *Progrès en Neurologie Pédiatrique.* Bruxelles: Prodim, 1985:235–236.

97. Jammes JL, Gilles FH. Telencephalic development: matrix volume and isocortex and allocortex surface areas. In: Gilles FH, Leviton A, Dooling EC, eds. *The developing human brain.* Boston: John Wright, 1983:87–93.

98. Evrard P, Gadisseux JF, Lyon G. Les malformations du système nerveux. In: Royer P, ed. *Naissance du cerveau.* Paris: Lafayette, 1982:49–74.

99. Barkovich AJ, Kjos BO. Non-lissencephalic cortical dysplasia: correlation of imaging findings with clinical deficits. *AJNR* 1992;13:95–103.

100. Barkovich AJ, Kjos BO. Gray matter heterotopias: MR characteristics and correlation with developmental and neurological manifestations. *Radiology* 1992;182:493–499.

101. Smith AS, Weinstein MA, Quencer RM, et al. Association of heterotopic gray matter with seizures: MR imaging. *Radiology* 1988;168:195–198.

102. Barkovich AJ, Jackson DE Jr., Boyer RS. Band heterotopias: a newly recognized neuronal migration anomaly. *Radiology* 1989; 171:455–458.

103. Livingston JH, Aicardi J. Unusual MRI appearance of diffuse subcortical heterotopia or "double cortex" in two children. *J Neurol Neurosurg Psychiatry* 1990;53:617–620.

104. Palmini A, Andermann F, Aicardi J, et al. Diffuse cortical dysplasia, or the "double cortex" syndrome: the clinical and epileptic spectrum in 10 patients. *Neurology* 1991;41:1656–1662.

105. Martin N, Debussche C, De Broucker T, Mompoint D, Marsault C, Nahum H. Gadolinium-DTPA enhanced MR imaging in tuberous sclerosis. *Neuroradiology* 1990;31:492–497.

106. Gomez MR. *Tuberous sclerosis,* 2nd ed. New York: Raven, 1988.

107. Inoue Y, Nakajima S, Fukuda P, et al. Magnetic resonance images of tuberous sclerosis: further observations and clinical correlations. *Neuroradiology* 1988;30:379–384.

108. Barkovich AJ. Phakomatoses. In: Barkovich AJ, ed. *Pediatric Neuroimaging.* New York: Raven, 1990:123–148.

109. Braffman BH, Bilaniuk LT, Naidich TP, et al. MR imaging of tuberous sclerosis: pathogenesis of this phakomatosis, use of gadopentate dimeglumine, and literature review. *Radiology* 1992;183:227–238.

110. Falconer J, Wada J, Martin W, Li D. PET, CT, and MRI imaging of neuronal migration anomalies in epileptic patients. *Can J Neurol Sci* 1990;17:35–39.

111. Miura K, Watanabe K, Maeda N, et al. MR imaging and positron emission tomography of band heterotopia. *Brain Dev* 1993;15: 288–290.

112. Morell F, Whisler W, Hoeppner T, et al. Electrophysiology of heterotopic gray matter in the "double cortex" syndrome. *Epilepsia* 1992;33[suppl. 3]:76.

113. Barkovich AJ, Kjos BO. Schizencephaly: correlation of clinical findings with MR characteristics. *AJNR* 1992;13:85–94.

114. Guerrini R, Dravet C, Raybaud C, et al. Epilepsy and focal gyral anomalies detected by MRI: electroclinico-morphological correlations and follow-up. *Dev Med Child Neurol* 1992;34:706.

115. Palmini A, Andermann F, Olivier A, et al. Focal neuronal migration disorders and intractable partial epilepsy: a study of 30 patients. *Ann Neurol* 1991;30:741–749.

116. Guerrini R, Dravet C, Raybaud C, et al. Neurological findings and seizure outcome in children with bilateral opercular macrogyric-like changes detected by MRI. *Dev Med Child Neurol* 1992;34:694.

117. Becker PS, Dixon AM, Troncoso JC. Bilateral opercular polymicrogyria. *Ann Neurol* 1989;25:90–92.

118. Kuzniecky R, Andermann F, Tampieri D, Melanson D, Olivier A, Leppik I. Bilateral central macrogyria: epilepsy, pseudobulbar palsy, and mental retardation—a recognizable neuronal migration disorder. *Ann Neurol* 1989;25:547–554.

119. Barkovich AJ. Abnormal vascular drainage in anomalies of neuronal migration. *AJNR* 1988;9:939–942.

120. Henkes K, Hosten N, Cordes M, Neumann K, Hansen M-L. Increased rCBF in gray matter heterotopias detected by SPECT using ^{99m}Tc hexamethylpropylenamine oxime. *Neuroradiology* 1991;33:310–312.

121. Chugani HT, Shields WD, Shewmon DA, Olson DM, Phelps ME, Peacock WJ. Infantile spasms: PET identifies focal cortical dys-

genesis in cryptogenic cases for surgical treatment. *Ann Neurol* 1990;27:406–413.

122. Otsubo H, Chuang SH, Hwang PA, Gilday D, Hoffman HJ. Neuroimaging for investigation of seizures in children. *Pediatr Neurosurg* 1992;18:105–116.

123. Yakovlev PI, Wadsworth RC. Schizencephalies. A study of the congenital clefts in the cerebral mantle. 1. Clefts with fused lips. *J Neuropathol Exp Neurol* 1946;5:116–130.

124. Yakovlev PI, Wadsworth RC. Schizencephalies. A study of the congenital clefts in the cerebral mantle. 2. Clefts with hydrocephalus and lips separated. *J Neuropathol Exp Neurol* 1946;5:169–206.

125. Barkovich AJ, Norman D. MR of schizencephaly. *AJNR* 1988;9:297–302.

126. Aniskiewicz AS, Frumkin NL, Brady DE, Moore JB, Pera A. Magnetic resonance imaging and neurobehavioral correlates in schizencephaly. *Arch Neurol* 1990;47:911–916.

127. Miller GM, Stears JC, Guggenheim MA, Wilkening GN. Schizencephaly: a clinical and CT study. *Neurology* 1984;34:997–1001.

128. Chuang SH, Fitz CR, Chilton SJ, Harwood-Nash DC, Donoghue V. *Schizencephaly: spectrum of CT findings in association with septo-optic dysplasia.* Presented at Annual Meeting of the Radiological Society of North America. Washington, DC, 1984.

129. Barkovich AJ, Fram EK, Norman D. Septo-optic dysplasia: MR imaging. *Radiology* 1989;171:189–192.

130. Fitz CR, Harwood-Nash DC, Boldt DW. The radiographic features of unilateral megalencephaly. *Neuroradiology* 1978;15:145–148.

131. Barkovich AJ, Chuang SH. Unilateral megalencephaly: correlation of MR imaging and pathologic characteristics. *AJNR* 1990;11:523–531.

132. Kalifa CL, Chiron C, Sellier N, et al. Hemimegalencephaly: MR imaging in five children. *Radiology* 1987;165:29–33.

133. Townsend JJ, Nielsen SL, Malamud N. Unilateral megalencephaly: hamartoma or neoplasm? *Neurology* 1975;25:448–453.

134. Manz HJ, Phillips TM, Rowden G, McCullough DC. Unilateral megalencephaly, cerebral cortical dysplasia, neuronal hypertrophy, and heterotopia: cytomorphometric, fluorometric cytochemical, and biochemical analyses. *Acta Neuropathol (Berl)* 1979;45:97–103.

135. Sarwar M, Schafer M. Brain malformations in linear nevus sebaceous syndrome: an MR study. *J Comput Assist Tomogr* 1988;12:338–340.

136. Hager BC, Dyme IZ, Guertin SR, Tyler RJ, Tryciecky EW, Fratkin JD. Linear nevus sebaceous syndrome: megalencephaly and heterotopic gray matter. *Pediatr Neurol* 1991;7:45–49.

137. Peserico A, Battistella PA, Bertoli P, Drigo P. Unilateral hypomelanosis of Ito with hemimegalencephaly. *Acta Paediatr Scand* 1988;77:446–447.

138. Cusmai R, Curatolo P, Mangano S, Cheminal R, Echenne B. Hemimegalencephaly and neurofibromatosis. *Neuropediatrics* 1990;21:179–182.

139. King M, Stephenson J, Ziervogel M, Doyle D, Galbraith S. Hemimegalencephaly—a case for hemispherectomy? *Neuropediatrics* 1985;16:46–55.

140. Müller F, O'Rahilly R. Mediobasal prosencephalic defects, including holoprosencephaly and cyclopia, in relation to the development of the human forebrain. *Am J Anat* 1989;185:391–414.

141. Leech RW, Shuman RM. Holoprosencephaly and related midline cerebral anomalies: a review. *J Child Neurol* 1986;1:3–18.

142. Müller F, O'Rahilly R. The development of the human brain, including the longitudinal zoning in the diencephalon at stage 15. *Anat Embryol* 1988;179:55–71.

143. Probst FP. *The prosencephalies: morphology, neuroradiological appearances and differential diagnosis.* Berlin: Springer-Verlag, 1979.

144. Fitz CR. Holoprosencephaly and related entities. *Neuroradiology* 1983;25:225–238.

145. DeMyer W. Holoprosencephaly. In: Vinker PI, Bruyn JW, eds. *Handbook of clinical neurology.* Amsterdam: North-Holland, 1977:431–478.

146. DeMyer W. Holoprosencephaly (cyclopia-arhinencephaly). In:

Myrianthopoulos N, ed. *Malformations.* New York: Elsevier, 1987:225–244.

147. Cohen MM, Jirasek JE, Guzman RT, Gorlin RJ, Peterson MQ. Holoprosencephaly and facial dysmorphia: nosology, etiology, and pathogenesis. *Birth Defects* 1971;7:125–135.

148. Filly RA, Chinn DH, Callen PW. Alobar holoprosencephaly: ultrasonic prenatal diagnosis. *Radiology* 1984;151:455–459.

149. Nyberg DA, Mack LA, Bronstein A, Hirsch J, Pagan RO. Holoprosencephaly: prenatal sonographic diagnosis. *AJNR* 1987;8:871–878.

150. De Morsier G. Etudes sur les dysraphies cranio-encéphaliques. III. Agénésie du septum lucidum avec malformation du tractus optique. La dysplasie septo-optique. *Schweiz Arch Neurol Neurochir Psychiatr* 1956;77:267–292.

151. Stanhope R, Preece MA, Brook CGD. Hypoplastic optic nerves and pituitary dysfunction: a spectrum of anatomical and endocrine abnormalities. *Arch Dis Child* 1984;59:111–114.

152. Skarf B, Hoyt CS. Optic nerve hypoplasia in children: association with anomalies of the endocrine and CNS. *Arch Ophthalmol* 1984;102:62–67.

153. Izenberg N, Rosenblum M, Parks JS. The endocrine spectrum of septo-optic dysplasia. *Clin Pediatr* 1984;23:632–636.

154. Hoyt WF, Kaplan SL, Grumbach MM, Glaser T. Septo-optic dysplasia and pituitary dwarfism (letter). *Lancet* 1970;1:893–894.

155. Arslanian SA, Rouzfus WE, Foley TP Jr, Becker DJ. Hormonal, metabolic, and neuroradiologic abnormalities associated with septo-optic dysplasia. *Acta Endocrinol* 1984;107:282–288.

156. Brodsky MC, Glasier CM. Optic nerve hypoplasia: clinical significance of associated central nervous system abnormalities on magnetic resonance imaging. *Arch Ophthalmol* 1993;111:66–74.

157. Ouvrier R, Billson F. Optic nerve hypoplasia: a review. *J Child Neurol* 1986;1:181–188.

158. Shuman RM, Leech RW. Optic nerve hypoplasia: one part of a spectrum. *J Child Neurol* 1986;1:180.

159. Wilson DM, Enzmann DR, Hintz RL, Rosenfeld G. CT findings in septo-optic dysplasia: discordance between clinical and radiological findings. *Neuroradiology* 1984;26:279–283.

160. Barkovich AJ, Norman D. Absence of septum pellucidum: a useful sign in the diagnosis of congenital brain malformations. *AJNR* 1988;9:1107–1114.

161. Brodsky MC. Septo-optic dysplasia: a reappraisal. *Semin Ophthalmol* 1991;6:227–232.

162. Chiari H. Über Veränderungen des Kleinhirns infolge von Hydrocephalie des Grosshirns. *Deutsch Medizinische Wocherschrift* 1891;17:1172–1175.

163. Barkovich AJ, Wippold FJ, Sherman JL, Citrin CM. Significance of cerebellar tonsillar ectopia on MR. *AJNR* 1986;7:795–799.

164. Mikulis DJ, Diaz O, Egglin TK, Sanchez R. Variance of the position of the cerebellar tonsils with age: preliminary report. *Radiology* 1992;183:725–728.

165. Elster AD, Chen MYM. Chiari I malformations: clinical and radiologic reappraisal. *Radiology* 1992;183:347–353.

166. Vu BT, Mikulis DJ, Armstrong D, Pron G. *Normal position of the cerebellar tonsils in relation to the foramen magnum in children.* Presented at American Society of Neuroradiology, 31st Annual Meeting. Vancouver, BC, Canada, 1993:170.

167. Appleby A, Foster JB, Hankinson J, Hudgson P. The diagnosis and management of the Chiari anomalies in adult life. *Brain* 1969;91:131–140.

168. Banerji NR, Millar JHD. Chiari malformations presenting in adult life. *Brain* 1974;97:157–168.

169. Francis PM, Beals S, Rekate HL, Pittman HW, Manwaring K, Reiff J. Chronic tonsillar herniation and Crouzon's syndrome. *Pediatr Neurosurg* 1992;18:202–206.

170. Chumas PD, Armstrong DC, Drake JM, et al. Tonsillar herniation: the rule rather than the exception after lumboperitoneal shunting in the pediatric population. *J Neurosurg* 1993;78:568–573.

171. Hoffman HJ, Tucker WS. Cephalocranial disproportion. A complication of the treatment of hydrocephalus in children. *Childs Brain* 1976;2:167–176.

172. Naidich TP, McLone DG, Fulling KH. The Chiari II malforma-

tion: Part IV. The hindbrain deformity. *Neuroradiology* 1983;25: 179–197.

173. Vandertop WP, Asai A, Hoffman HJ, et al. Surgical decompression for symptomatic Chiari II malformation in neonates with myelomeningocele. *J Neurosurg* 1992;77:541–544.

174. McLone DG, Knepper PA. The cause of Chiari II malformation: a unified theory. *Pediatr Neurosci* 1989;15:1–12.

175. Naidich TP, Pudlowski RM, Naidich JB. Computed tomographic signs of the Chiari II malformation, Part II: Midbrain and cerebellum. *Radiology* 1980;134:391–398.

176. Naidich TP, Pudlowski RM, Naidich JB, Gornish M, Rodriguez FJ. Computed tomographic signs of the Chiari II malformation, Part I: Skull and dural partitions. *Radiology* 1980;134:64–71.

177. Naidich TP, Pudlowski RM, Naidich JB. Computed tomographic signs of the Chiari II malformation, Part III: Ventricles and cisterns. *Radiology* 1980;134:657–663.

178. Wolpert SM, Anderson M, Scott RM, Kwan ES, Runge VM. The Chiari II malformation: MR imaging evaluation. *AJNR* 1987;8: 783–791.

179. Friede RL. *Developmental neuropathology,* 2nd ed. Berlin: Springer-Verlag, 1989.

180. Caviness VS Jr, Rakic P. Mechanisms of cortical development: a view from mutations in mice. *Ann Rev Neurosci* 1978;1:297–326.

181. Gould BB, Rakic P. The total number, time of origin and kinetics of proliferation of neurons comprising the deep cerebellar nuclei in the Rhesus monkey. *Exp Brain Res* 1981;44:195–206.

182. Rakic P, Sidman RL. Histogenesis of cortical layers in human cerebellum, particularly the lamina dessicans. *J Comp Neurol* 1970;139:473–500.

183. Larroche J-C. Malformations of the nervous system. In: Adams J, Corsellis J, Duchen L, eds. *Greenfield's neuropathology,* 4th ed. New York: Wiley, 1984:385–450.

184. Lemire RJ, Loeser JD, Leech RW, Alvord EC. *Normal and abnormal development of the human nervous system.* Hagarstown, MD: Harper & Row, 1975.

185. Bonnevie K, Brodal A. Hereditary hydrocephalus in the house mouse. IV. The development of cerebellar anomalies during fetal life with notes on the normal development of the mouse cerebellum. *Lkr Norske Vidensk Akad Oslo 1 Matj-nat KI* 1946;4:4–60.

186. Hart MN, Malamud N, Ellis WG. The Dandy-Walker syndrome: a clinicopathological study based on 28 cases. *Neurology* 1972;22: 771–780.

187. Raimondi AJ, Sato K, Shimoji T. *The Dandy-Walker syndrome.* Basel: Karger, 1984.

188. Bindal AK, Storrs BB, McLone DG. Management of the Dandy-Walker syndrome. *Pediatr Neurosci* 1990–91;16:163–169.

189. Osenbach RK, Menezes AH. Diagnosis and management of the Dandy-Walker malformation: 30 years of experience. *Pediatr Neurosurg* 1992;18:179–189.

190. Maria BL, Zinreich SJ, Carson BC, Rosenbaum AE, Freeman JM. Dandy-Walker syndrome revisited. *Pediatr Neurosci* 1987; 13:45–51.

191. Golden JA, Rorke LB, Bruce DA. Dandy-Walker syndrome and associated anomalies. *Pediatr Neurosci* 1987;13.

192. Masdeu JC, Dobben GD, Azar-Kia B. Dandy-Walker syndrome studied by computed tomography and pneumoencephalography. *Radiology* 1983;147:109–114.

193. Macchi G, Bentivoglio M. Agenesis or hypoplasia of cerebellar structures. In: Myrianthopoulos N, ed. *Malformations.* New York: Elsevier, 1987:175–196.

194. Barkovich AJ, Kjos BO, Norman D, Edwards MSB. Revised classification of posterior fossa cysts and cyst-like malformations based on results of multiplanar MR imaging. *AJNR* 1989;10: 977–988.

195. Joubert M, Eisenring JJ, Robb JP, Andermann F. Familial agenesis of the cerebellar vermis. A syndrome of episodic hyperpnea, abnormal eye movements, ataxia, and retardation. *Neurology* 1969;19:813–825.

196. King MD, Dudgeon J, Stephenson JBP. Joubert's syndrome with retinal dysplasia: neonatal tachypnea as the clue to a genetic brain-eye malformation. *Arch Dis Child* 1984;59:709–718.

197. Kendall B, Kingsley D, Lambert SR, Taylor D, Finn P. Joubert syndrome: a clinical-radiological study. *Neuroradiology* 1990;31: 502–506.

198. Bolthauser E, Herdon M, Dumermuth G, Isler W. Joubert syndrome: clinical and polygraphic observations in a further case. *Neuropediatrics* 1981;12:181–191.

199. Obersteiner H. Ein Kleinhirn ohne Wurm. *Arb Neurol Inst (Wien)* 1914;21:124–136.

200. Truwit CL, Barkovich AJ, Shanahan R, Maroldo TV. MR imaging of rhombencephalosyanpsis: report of three cases and review of the literature. *AJNR* 1991;12:957–965.

201. Lhermitte J, Duclos P. Sur un ganglioneurone diffus du cortex du cervelet. *Bull Assoc Fr Étude Cancer* 1920;9:99–107.

202. Milbouw G, Born JD, Martin D, et al. Clinical and radiological aspects of dysplastic gangliocytoma (Lhermitte-Duclos disease): report of two cases and review of the literature. *Neurosurgery* 1988;22:124–128.

203. Roski RA, Roessmann U, Spetzler RF, Kaufman B, Nulsen FE. Clinical and pathological study of dysplastic gangliocytoma. *J Neurosurg* 1981;55:318–321.

204. Reeder RF, Saunders RL, Roberts DW, Fratkin JD, Cromwell LD. MRI in the diagnosis and treatment of Lhermitte-Duclos disease (dysplastic gangliocytoma of the cerebellum) *Neurosurgery* 1988;23:240–245.

205. Smith RR, Grossman RI, Goldberg H, et al. MR imaging of Lhermitte-Duclos disease: a case report. *AJNR* 1989;10:187–189.

206. Trandafir T, Lipot C, Froicu P. On a possible neuronal ridge origin of the adenohypophysis. *Endocrinologie* 1990;28:67–72.

207. Müller F, O'Rahilly R. The human brain at stage 16, including the initial evagination of the neurohypophysis. *Anat Embryol* 1989;179:551–569.

208. Ikeda H, Suzuki J, Sasano N, et al. The development and morphogenesis of the human pituitary gland. *Anat Embryol* 1988; 178:327–336.

209. Tagliavini F, Pilleri G. Mammillo-hypophyseal duplication (diplo-mammillo-hypophysis). *Acta Neuropathol* 1986;69:38–44.

210. Styne DM. Neurologic manifestations of endocrine diseases. In: Berg BO, ed. *Neurologic aspects of pediatrics.* Boston: Butterworth-Heinemann, 1992:439–466.

211. Kelly WM, Kucharczyk W, Kucharczyk J, et al. Posterior pituitary ectopia: and MR feature of pituitary dwarfism. *AJNR* 1988;9:453–460.

212. Kuriowa T, Okabe Y, Hasuo K, Yasumori K, Mizushima A, Masuda K. MR imaging of pituitary dwarfism. *AJNR* 1991;12:161–164.

213. Abrahams JJ, Trefelner E, Boulware SD. Idiopathic growth hormone deficiency; MR findings in 35 patients. *AJNR* 1991;12: 155–160.

214. Kallman F, Schoenfeld W, Barrera S. The genetic aspects of primary eunuchoidism. *Am J Ment Defic* 1944;48:203–236.

215. Schwanzel-Fukuda M, Bick D, Pfaff DW. Luteinizing hormone-releasing hormone (LHRL)–expressing cells do not migrate normally in an inherited hypogonadal (Kallmann) syndrome. *Mol Brain Res* 1989;6:311–326.

216. Schwanzel-Fukuda M, Abraham S, Crossin KL, Edelman GM, Pfaff DW. Immunocytochemical demonstration of neural cell adhesion molecule (NCAM) along the migration route of luteinizing hormone releasing hormone (LHRH) neurons in mice. *J Comp Neurol* 1992;321:1–18.

217. Valverde F, Heredia M, Santacana M. Characterization of neuronal cell varieties migrating from the olfactory epithelium during prenatal development in the rat. Immunocytochemical study using antibodies against olfactory marker protein and luteinizing hormone-releasing hormone. *Dev Brain Res* 1993;71:209–220.

218. Franco B, Guioli S, Pragliola A, et al. A gene deleted in Kallmann's syndrome shares homology with neural cell adhesion and axonal pathfinding molecules. *Nature* 1991;353:529–536.

219. Van Dop C, Burstein S, Conte FA, Grumbach MM. Isolated gonadotropin deficiency in boys: clinical characteristics and growth. *J Pediatr* 1987;111:684–692.

220. Truwit CL, Barkovich AJ, Grumbach MM. MR imaging of Kall-

mann syndrome: a disorder of the olfactory and genital systems caused by faulty neuronal migration. *AJNR* 1993;14:427–438.

221. Klingmüller D, Dewes W, Krahe T, Brecht G, Schweikert H-U. MR imaging of the brain in patients with anosmia and hypothalamic hypogonadism (Kallmann's syndrome). *J Clin Endocrin Metab* 1987;65:581–584.

222. Mazzola HK. Congenital malformations in the frontonasal area: their pathogenesis and classification. *Clin Plastic Surg* 1976;3: 573–609.

223. Kawamoto HK Jr. The kaleidoscopic world of rare craniofacial clefts: order out of chaos (Tessier classification). *Clin Plastic Surg* 1976;3:529–572.

224. Cohen MM. Craniosynostosis update 1987. *Am J Med Genet* 1988;4[suppl]:99–148.

225. Beighton P. *Inherited disorders of the skeleton.* Edinburgh: Churchill-Livingstone, 1988.

226. Bixler D, Ward RE. Craniosynostosis. In: Myrianthopoulos NC, ed. *Malformations.* In: Vinken P, Bruyn G, Klawans H, eds. *Handbook of clinical neurology.* New York: Elsevier, 1987:113–128.

227. Cohen MM Jr, Kreiborg S. The central nervous system in the Apert syndrome. *Am J Med Genet* 1992;35:36–45.

228. Taravath S, Tonsgard JH. Cerebral malformations in Carpenter syndrome. *Pediatr Neurol* 1993;9:230–234.

229. Murovic JA, Posnick JC, Drake JM, Humphreys RP, Hoffman HJ, Hendrick EB. Hydrocephalus in Apert syndrome: a retrospective review. *Pediatr Neurosurg* 1993;19:151–155.

230. Schinzel A. *Catalogue of unbalanced chromosome alterations in man.* Berlin: Walter de Gruyter, 1984.

231. Kumar AJ, Naidich TP, Stetten G, et al. Chromosomal disorders: background and neuroradiology. *Am J Neurorad* 1992;13:577–593.

232. Tamraz JC, Retmore MO, Iba-zizen MT, Lejeurn J, Cabanis EA. Contributions of MRI to the knowledge of CNS malformations related to chromosomal aberrations. *Human Genet* 1987;76: 265–273.

233. Martich V, Ben-Ami T, Yousefzadeh DK, Roizen NJ. Hypoplastic posterior arch of C-1 in children with Down syndrome: a double jeopardy. *Radiology* 1992;183:125–128.

234. Peuschel SM, Scola FH. Atlantoaxial instability in individuals with Down syndrome: epidemiologic, radiographic and clinical studies. *Pediatrics* 1987;80:555–560.

235. El-Khoury GY, Clark CR, Dietz FR, Harre RG, Tozzi JE, Kathol MH. Posterior atlantooccipital subluxation in Down syndrome. *Radiology* 1986;159:507–509.

236. Martel W, Tishler JM. Observations on the spine in mongoloidism. *AJR* 1966;97:630–638.

237. Menezes AH, Ryken TC. Craniovertebral abnormalities in Down's syndrome. *Pediatr Neurosurg* 1992;18:24–33.

238. Coria F, Quintana F, Villalba A, et al. Craniocervical abnormalities in Down syndrome. *Dev Med Child Neurol* 1983;25:252–254.

239. Inagaki M, Ando Y, Mito T, et al. Comparison of brain imaging and neuropathology in cases of trisomy 18 and 13. *Neuroradiology* 1987;29:474–479.

240. Golden J, Schoene W. Central nervous system malformations in Trisomy 9. *J Neuropathol Exp Neurol* 1993;52:71–77.

CHAPTER 6

The Phakomatoses

The phakomatoses are congenital malformations affecting mainly structures of ectodermal origin (i.e., the nervous system, the skin, the retina, and the globe and its contents); visceral organs are also involved, but in general to a lesser extent. Classically, four diseases are included in this group: Von Recklinghausen's neurofibromatosis, tuberous sclerosis (Bourneville's disease), retinocerebellar angiomatosis (Von Hippel-Lindau disease), and encephalotrigeminal angiomatosis (Sturge-Weber disease). Recently, several other hereditary diseases have been classified under the heading of phakomatoses; this chapter will include discussions of ataxia–telangiectasia, neurocutaneous melanosis, and the basal cell nevus syndrome because their neurologic and neuroradiologic manifestations are quite prominent.

NEUROFIBROMATOSIS TYPE I

Neurofibromatosis type I (NF1) is one of the most common autosomal dominant CNS disorders. It affects approximately one of every 3,000–5,000 people in the general population (1). Even after establishing the genetic distinction between NF1 and NF2, the argument continues to be made that NF1 is not a single disease (2,3). In fact, seven separate forms of NF1 have been described (2,3). The proposed subgroups of NF1 are not discussed here, as these are primarily variants on a cen-

TABLE 6.1. *Criteria for diagnosis of type I neurofibromatosis*

The diagnosis of NF1 requires two or more of the following:

1. Six or more café au lait spots over 5 mm in greatest diameter (over 15 mm in postpubertal individuals)
2. Two or more neurofibromas of any type or plexiform neurofibroma
3. Freckling in the axillary or inguinal areas
4. Optic glioma
5. Two or more Lisch nodules (pigmented hamartomas of the iris)
6. A distinctive osseous lesion, such as sphenoid dysplasia or thinning of long bone cortex
7. A first degree relative (parent, sibling, or offspring) with NF1

Adapted from ref. 41.

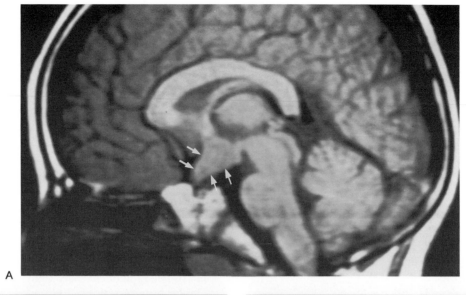

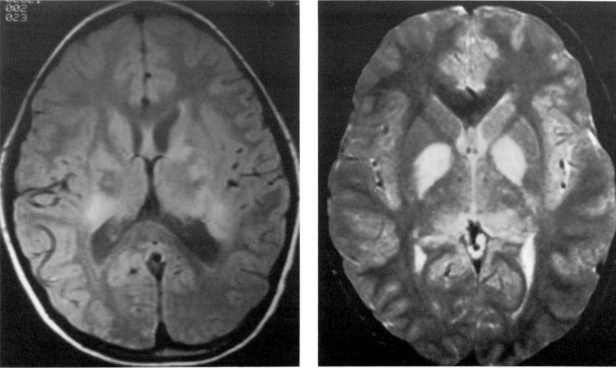

FIG. 6.1. Optic pathways glioma. **A:** Sagittal SE 600/20 image shows a mass (*arrows*) involving the optic chiasm, hypothalamus, and the anterior recesses of the third ventricle. **B:** Axial SE 2500/35 image at the level of the frontal horns shows high signal intensity extending to the level of the lateral geniculate bodies resulting from tumor involvement of the optic system. **C:** Axial SE 2500/70 image reveals high signal intensity in the globus pallidus bilaterally. These foci of high signal are believed to represent hamartomas.

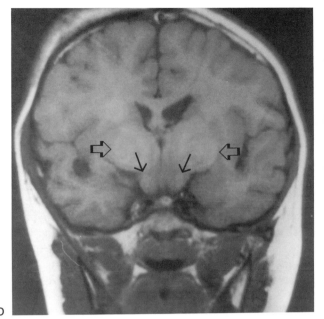

D

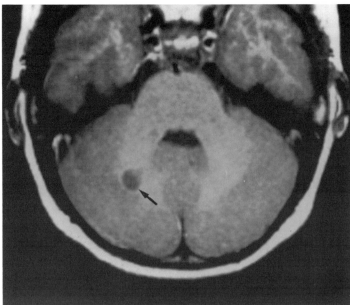

E

FIG. 6.1. (*Continued.*) D: Coronal SE 600/20 image shows these globus pallidus hamartomas (*open arrows*) to be slightly hyperintense. They also demonstrate a mild mass effect. The optic tracts are enlarged by tumor (*closed arrows*). E: This 1-cm focus of low signal intensity (*arrow*) in the right cerebellar white matter was an astrocytoma.

tral, well-defined set of clinical, pathologic, and radiologic manifestations.

NF1 is the disorder initially described by von Recklinghausen in 1882 (4). It is an autosomal dominant disease, the genetic locus of which is on the long arm of chromosome 17 (5). Diagnostic criteria of the disease are listed in Table 6.1.

Café au lait spots are the first manifestation of NF1 to develop, usually becoming evident during the first year of life. Freckling within the axilla will develop later in about two-thirds of patients (6–8). Cutaneous neurofibromas begin to appear around the onset of puberty and increase in number throughout life. Lisch nodules, which are best seen by slit lamp examination, begin to appear in childhood and are present in almost all affected adults (6–8). A number of other features are characteristic of this disease, the most important from the neuroimaging standpoint being gliomas of the optic pathway (and other intracranial astrocytomas), kyphoscoliosis, sphenoid wing dysplasia, vascular dysplasias, nerve sheath tumors, macrocephaly, seizures, and mental retardation (6–9).

Although the defining features occur in all NF1 patients, few of the other features are likely to be present in any particular patient. For example, one patient may have a normal vascular system and a normal intellect but have severe kyphoscoliosis and another may have a normal spine and normal mentation but severe hypertension from renal artery stenosis. The incidence of CNS manifestations in NF1 is about 15% (6,8).

Intracranial Manifestations

Optic Pathway Gliomas

The most common primary brain abnormality in NF1 is the optic pathway glioma (6,9,10). Optic gliomas can be isolated to a single optic nerve or can extend to both optic nerves, the chiasm and the optic tracts. Rarely, the tumor will extend beyond the lateral geniculate bodies into the optic radiations. Clinical studies indicate a poor prognosis for tumors that involve the optic chiasm or the optic tracts as compared to those restricted to the optic nerves (11,12). These tumors are most commonly of low histologic grade; in particular, those involving only the optic nerves are considered by some to be hamartomas rather than neoplasms. However, some can be highly malignant, demanding a very aggressive treatment approach (12). As discussed in Chapter 7, CT is an excellent method for evaluating tumors of the intraorbital optic nerves. The orbital fat provides intrinsic contrast against which to visualize these lesions. Enlargement of the optic nerve is usually fusiform, although occasionally the enlargement can be rather eccentric. Enlargement of the optic canals can be seen if bone windows are used. CT is less sensitive in assessing involvement of the optic chiasm. Unless the chiasm is very enlarged by gross tumor involvement, it is necessary to inject intrathecal water soluble contrast to visualize the chiasm adequately. In children, approximately 3 ml of nonionic contrast (concentration 150 mg of iodine per milliliter) is injected via lumbar puncture. The patient is tilted 45° head down (Trendelenburg) in the prone position for approximately 2 min, then transported to the CT scanner and imaged.

MR is the preferred imaging modality for evaluating the intracranial portion of the optic system. Assessment of the precise diameter of the intraorbital optic nerves may be hampered by chemical shift artifact resulting from the nerve's being adjacent to orbital fat. The use of a fat saturation pulse (13), however, will eliminate the chemical shift artifact and allow high-quality images to be obtained. The intracranial optic nerves, optic chiasm, optic tract, and optic radiations are all beautifully demonstrated with MR. Moreover, the use of MR eliminates exposure of the child's eyes to ionizing radiation. If CT is performed in children, 3-mm sections should be obtained in the axial plane; reformations can then be constructed in any desired plane. If MR is performed, short TR/TE axial and coronal sequences, using 3-mm slice thickness, should be obtained through the optic nerves and optic chiasm (Figs. 6.1–6.3). A routine brain scan should follow to look for involvement of the optic tracts and other areas of brain involvement. Long TR/TE images will show involvement of the optic tracts as high signal intensity extending along the tracts to the lateral geniculate bodies (Fig. 6.1). The short TR/TE images will show distortion of the normal architecture and enlargement of the optic nerves, chiasm, and/or tracts, depending upon the extent of involvement (Figs. 6.2, 6.3).

Other Gliomas

Astrocytomas are more common in NF1 than in the general population (6,9,10). These astrocytomas are most commonly juvenile pilocytic astrocytomas, but other low-grade (14) and higher-grade tumors also occur (15). Although the optic system is the most common portion of the CNS to be involved, the mesencephalic tectum (Fig. 6.4) is also often involved by neoplasia; other common locations for astrocytomas in patients with NF1 are the brain stem, and the cerebrum (Fig. 6.5) (9,10). Astrocytomas are discussed extensively in Chapter 7.

In a small but significant number of patients with NF1, hydrocephalus is present (16–18). The site of obstruction of CSF flow is usually the aqueduct of Sylvius;

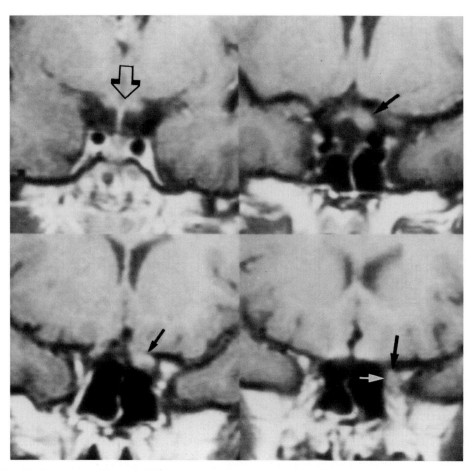

FIG. 6.2. Optic system glioma in NF1 patient. Coronal SE 600/15 images show enlargement of the intracranial left optic nerve (*closed arrows*) as it extends from the optic canal (*white arrow*) to the optic chiasm (*open arrow*).

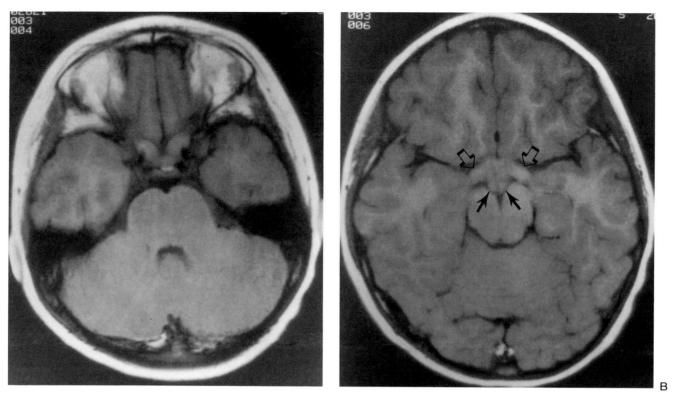

FIG. 6.3. Optic system glioma in NF1 patient. **A:** Axial SE 600/20 image shows enlargement of the intracranial segments of both optic nerves extending back to the level of the chiasm. **B:** Axial SE 600/20 image at a higher section shows enlargement of both optic tracts (*open arrows*) and extension of tumor into the interpeduncular cistern (*closed arrows*).

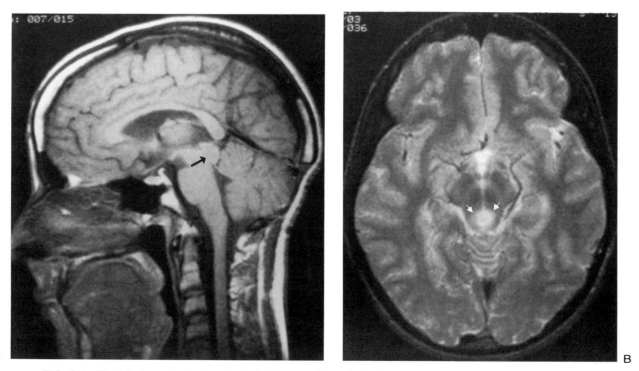

FIG. 6.4. Tectal glioma in NF1 patient. **A:** The quadrigeminal plate is bulbous and the aqueduct is occluded (*arrow*). A ventriculoperitoneal shunt was present (not shown). Note the posterior craniectomy defect from the biopsy of this lesion. **B:** Axial SE 2500/70 image reveals a large area of prolonged T2 relaxation in the region of the aqueduct and quadrigeminal plate (*arrows*).

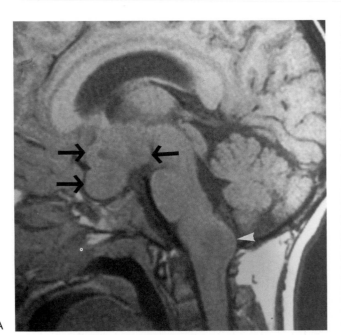

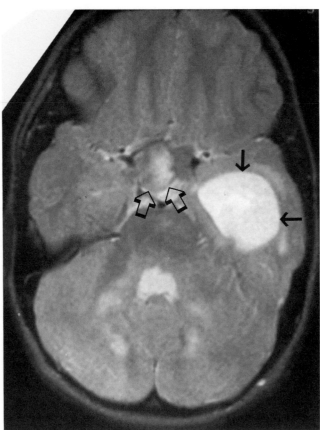

FIG. 6.5. NF1 patient with temporal lobe extension of optic chiasm/hypothalamic astrocytoma, brain stem astrocytoma, and hamartomas of the cerebellar white matter. **A:** Sagittal SE 600/20 image shows a large mass in the suprasellar cistern, optic chiasm, hypothalamus, and anterior third ventricle (*black arrows*). A second mass is seen in the medulla and cervical spinal cord with dorsal exophytic extension (*white arrow*). **B:** Axial SE 2800/70 image shows a large mixed-intensity astrocytoma filling the suprasellar cistern (*open arrows*) and a large high-intensity tumor within the left temporal lobe (*closed arrows*). The areas of high signal intensity in the pons and cerebellar white matter are common in NF1 and probably represent hamartomas.

this obstruction may result from benign aqueductal stenosis or gliomas of the tectum or tegmentum of the mesencephalon. The differentiation of these two causes of aqueductal stenosis is extremely difficult with CT (17). The tectal lesions usually do not show significant contrast enhancement when they are small, and therefore subtle calcifications or distortions of the posterior third ventricle and proximal aqueduct must be identified. The diagnosis of a tectal glioma is relatively simple using MR (Fig. 6.4). In contradistinction to benign aqueductal stenosis (in which the proximal aqueduct is dilated and the tectum displaced superiorly and thinned; see Chapter 8), gliomas enlarge the tectum and completely obliterate the aqueduct. Occasionally, the tectum may appear short and thick in aqueductal stenosis because of mass effect on the rostral aspect of the tectum by a dilated suprapineal recess (see Chapter 8). In these cases, the patient should be imaged after the infusion of IV contrast. An astrocytoma will often enhance, whereas a compressed tectum will not.

Vascular Dysplasia

Dysplasias of the cerebral vasculature can also occur in NF1. Most commonly, the dysplasia consists of intimal proliferation, with resultant stenosis or occlusion, in the carotid (common or internal), proximal middle cerebral, or anterior cerebral arteries; cerebral aneurysms are described as well, although less commonly (19). Many of the patients with vascular dysplasias are those who have been irradiated for optic nerve or optic chiasm gliomas, and presumably have a radiation arteritis. However, the known significant incidence of vascular dysplasia in other parts of the body and the presence of such vascular occlusions in a large number of patients without a history of irradiation make this vascular dysplasia a distinct clinical entity. Any child with NF1 who has seizures, mental retardation, paralysis, or severe headaches may have a vascular dysplasia, particularly in the absence of a brain tumor or hydrocephalus. Vascular dysplasia is difficult to detect with CT or MR, although occasionally one can

lier and is, in fact, a diencephalic structure that has been misnamed as a cranial nerve. The other cranial nerves are rarely, if ever, involved. When schwannomas occur in patients with NF1, the possibility of "overlap" syndromes (syndromes with characteristics of both NF1 and NF2) is often raised (20–22). Although patients with features of both NF1 and NF2 clearly exist, the true implications of the overlap in affected patients are unknown (22).

Bone Dysplasia

Other intracranial manifestations of NF1 include sphenoid wing dysplasia and dysplasia of the bone along the lambdoid suture. Only sphenoid dysplasia is of any clinical importance, as it allows herniation of the temporal lobes into the orbit (Fig. 6.8). The pulsations of the temporal lobe may be transmitted through the globe, thus being visible externally as pulsatile exophthalmos. The globe may be dysplastic or hypoplastic. Sphenoid wing dysplasia is often associated with plexiform neurofibromas in the orbit or periorbital regions (Fig. 6.8).

Plexiform Neurofibromas

Another cause of intracranial complications in NF1 is excessive growth of craniofacial plexiform neurofibromas. Plexiform neurofibromas are locally aggressive congenital lesions composed of tortuous cords of Schwann cells, neurons, and collagen in an unorganized intercellular matrix (9). They tend to progress along the nerve of origin (usually small, unidentified nerves) into the intracranial space, causing distortion and compression of the brain. Most commonly, growth occurs into the orbit where the neurofibromas act as masses, causing impaired ocular movements and exophthalmos.

On both MR and CT, plexiform neurofibromas appear as masses that most commonly arise in the region of the orbital apex or superior orbital fissure (Fig. 6.9), but they can occur anywhere in the body. They tend to be of low attenuation on CT and generally do not enhance after administration of intravenous contrast. On MR the masses are heterogeneous, displaying mostly low signal intensity as compared with brain on short TR/TE images and high signal intensity on long TR/TE images (Figs. 6.9–6.11) (23,24). Enhancement after administra-

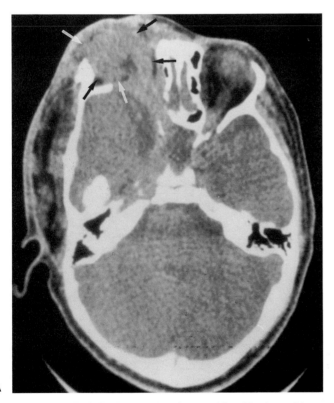
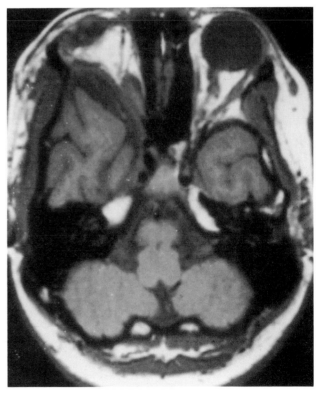

FIG. 6.8. Dysplasia of the sphenoid wing with associated plexiform neurofibroma. **A:** Axial CT shows absence of the greater wing of the right sphenoid bone. The large soft tissue mass (*arrows*) around the right orbit is a plexiform neurofibroma. **B:** Axial SE 600/15 image at a slightly lower level shows the anterior extension of the right temporal lobe with displacement of orbital contents.

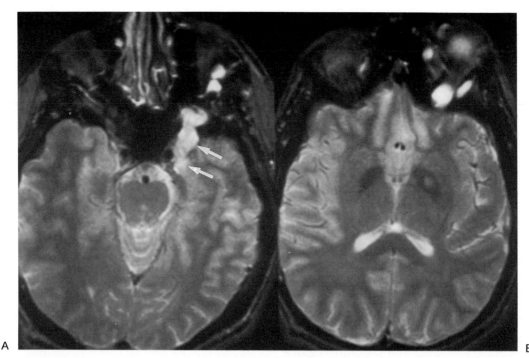

FIG. 6.9. Orbital plexiform neurofibroma. **A, B:** Axial SE 2800/70 images show nodular, round to ovoid areas of hyperintensity in the left orbit, representing a plexiform neurofibroma. Extension into the cavernous sinus (*arrows*) through a widened superior orbital fissure is seen.

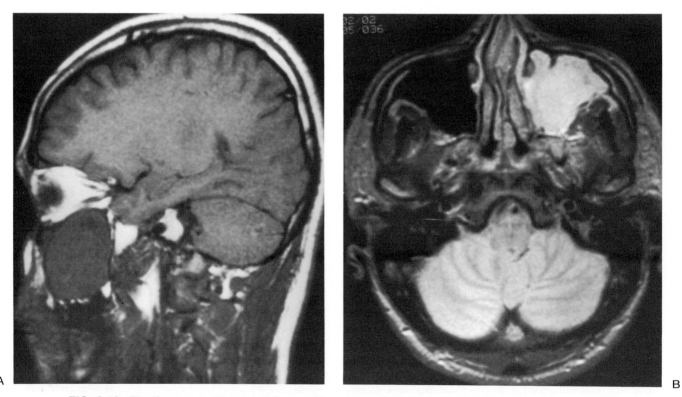

FIG. 6.10. Plexiform neurofibroma of the maxillary sinus. **A:** Sagittal SE 600/20 image in this patient with NF1 shows a large mass involving the left maxillary sinus. This mass is homogenous and shows a low signal intensity as compared to normal brain. **B:** Axial SE 2500/35 image shows the left maxillary plexiform neurofibroma to be hyperintense compared with white matter of the brain. Although these masses commonly grow out of the sinuses through foramina and fissures, this mass seems confined to the maxillary antrum.

tion of paramagnetic contrast is variable, although at least a portion of the tumor usually enhances. Careful evaluation of the images often reveals extension of orbital tumors into the cavernous sinus, nasopharynx, or pterygomaxillary fissure (Fig. 6.9).

Other Intracranial Lesions

MR imaging has disclosed the presence of characteristic foci of abnormal increased signal intensity in the pons, cerebellar white matter, internal capsule, and splenium of the corpus callosum on T2-weighted images in children with NF1 (Figs. 6.5, 6.11, 6.12) (25,26); the signal of these areas is normal on short TR/TE images. These lesions are characteristically multiple; they have no mass effect, do not elicit vasogenic edema, and do not enhance after intravenous administration of paramagnetic contrast. In the author's experience, they are seen in approximately 75% of patients with NF1 and in more than 90% of NF1 patients with optic gliomas. A recent

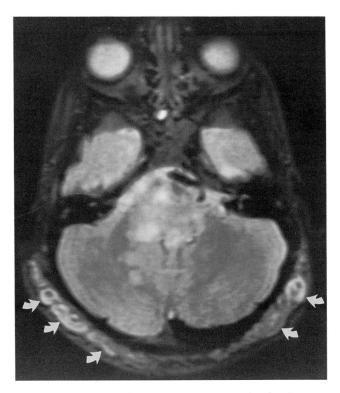

FIG. 6.11. Posterior fossa hamartomas and subcutaneous neurofibromas in an NF1 patient. Axial SE 2500/70 image reveals multiple foci of high signal intensity in the pons and cerebellar white matter. These foci are ill defined and have no mass effect. They could not be identified on short TR/TE images. All these factors suggest that these foci are hamartomas or areas of delayed myelination and not astrocytomas. Compare with Fig. 5.1E. The multiple subcutaneous heterogeneous nodular areas (*arrows*) of high signal intensity in the occipital region represent subcutaneous neurofibromas.

report (27) indicates that these lesions begin to appear at about age 3 years. They increase in number and size until the age of 10 or 12 years (Fig. 6.12); then they decrease in number and size. They are almost never seen in patients over the age of 20 years. A few of these regions have been biopsied; the histologic findings have been compatible with hamartomas or atypical glial cells, both of which are well-known pathologic findings in NF1 (9,28). Another possibility is that these are areas of disordered or dysplastic myelination because they initially develop normally and, after a period of growth (breakdown of the dysplastic myelin?), disappear (remyelinate?) on follow-up exams. In view of the frequency with which these lesions are seen, biopsy is not indicated as long as they occur in the characteristic locations (pons, midbrain, cerebellar white matter, internal capsule, splenium), are not seen on T1-weighted images, and lack associated mass effect, edema, and enhancement. However, it is recommended that the patients have a follow-up contrast-enhanced MR scan 6 months to a year after the first study to be sure that no enhancement or mass effect develops; a growing astrocytoma of the pons or cerebellum (which, when small, is indistinguishable from one of these lesions on noncontrast MR) will typically enhance or show mass effect on adjacent structures.

Foci of abnormal signal intensity are also seen in the globus pallidus of patients with NF1 (Figs. 6.1, 6.13). These foci differ from those in the pons and cerebellum in that they are slightly hyperintense on short TR/TE images (in addition to the hyperintensity on short TR images) and have some mild mass effect (26,29). These lesions are similar to those in the posterior fossa in that they do not enhance after administration of IV contrast. The characteristic lack of enhancement, location, bilaterality, and short T1 relaxation time help to differentiate these presumed hamartomas from astrocytomas.

Spine Manifestations

Scoliosis

Scoliosis is the most common skeletal abnormality reported in patients with NF1. In Holt's series, it was present in 32% of affected children; the incidence increases with age (30). The scoliosis is usually minimal or mild in degree but can be severe. It is most commonly the result of dysplasia of the of the vertebral bodies. Other vertebral manifestations of NF1 include hypoplasia of the pedicles, transverse processes, and spinous processes, scalloping of the posterior aspects of the vertebral bodies, and hyperplastic bone changes (30). It is not certain whether these bony anomalies result from a primary mesodermal dysplasia or are secondary to the effects of nerve sheath tumors. Plain film radiography is essential to demonstrate the scoliosis optimally. CT is the optimal modality

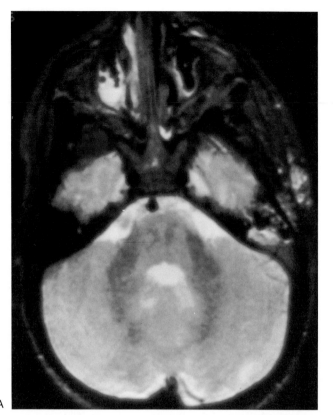
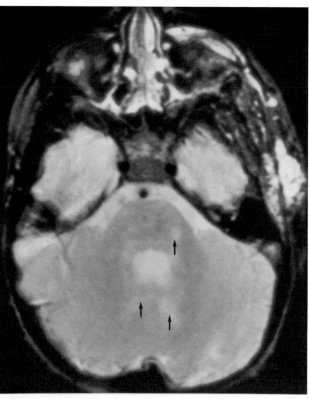

A   B

FIG. 6.12. Evolution of posterior fossa signal abnormalities in NF1. **A:** Axial SE 2500/70 image at age 2 years shows no white matter signal abnormalities. **B:** Follow-up scan 3 years later shows several new areas of T2 prolongation (*arrows*) in the pons and cerebellar white matter.

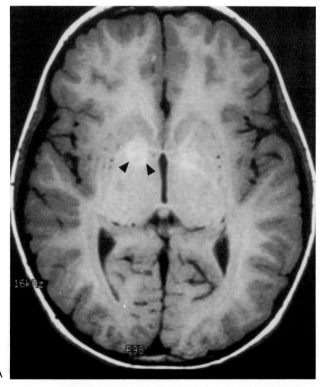
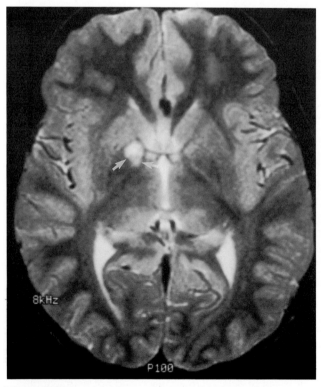

A   B

FIG. 6.13. Basal ganglia hamartoma in NF1. **A:** Axial SE 550/11 image shows a focus of T1 shortening (*arrowheads*) in the right globus pallidus. **B:** Axial SE 2800/70 image shows T2 prolongation of the lesion (*arrows*).

for demonstrating the changes of the individual vertebrae, as it shows superior bone detail. However, most of the bony changes are well visualized with high-quality MR studies.

When scoliosis is present, the question often arises as to whether it results from the dysplastic bone of neurofibromatosis or from an intrinsic spinal cord lesion such as a tethered cord, syringomyelia, or tumor. In the absence of any neurologic signs or symptoms, the incidence of an underlying spinal cord disorder is very low in patients with dextroscoliosis (convexity of the curvature to the right). However, patients with levoscoliosis—especially if it is rapidly progressive, associated with pain, or associated with neurologic deficits—have a significantly higher incidence of underlying spinal cord abnormalities (31). MR is the imaging modality of choice to examine such patients. Coronal sequences, followed by oblique sagittal and oblique axial images, are recommended to visualize the cord in these cases. The oblique sagittal and axial images should be obtained through each straight segment of spine, parallel and perpendicular, respectively, to the segment of spinal column (see discussion in Chapter 9). T1-weighted sequences should be obtained with a 3-mm slice thickness. If curved reformations are available on your MR, the scanner will allow you to define the curve of the scoliosis and will "straighten" the curve mathematically. Axial T1-weighted sequences through the L5–S1 level are recommended, in addition to the sagittal images, to assess the thickness of the filum accurately. If no lipoma or intrinsic spinal cord lesion (tumor or syringohydromyelia) is seen, the conus is at the normal (L2 or above) level, and the filum terminale measures 2 mm or less in diameter at the L5–S1 level, it is safe to assume that the scoliosis is a result of a bony dysplasia.

Nerve Sheath Tumors

Another major abnormality affecting the spine in NF1 is intra- or paraspinous neurofibroma (9,10). There has been a great deal of debate in the pathology literature as to whether the paraspinous tumors in NF1 are schwannomas or neurofibromas. Schwannomas are uncommon in NF1; conversely, neurofibromas are fairly distinctive features of von Recklinghausen's disease and rarely occur in any other setting. It is probably not possible to differentiate these tumor types by imaging; moreover, arguments as to the exact pathology and pathogenesis of these tumors continue (9,10). Neurofibromas are tumors of the nerve sheaths that also involve the nerves themselves. The cells of origin of these tumors are thought to be fibroblasts (10). Although isolated spinal neurofibromas can be seen in patients unaffected by NF1, patients with von Recklinghausen's disease can have neurofibromas of varying sizes at many levels throughout

the spinal canal (10,24). A recent study (32) has indicated that most nerve sheath tumors in NF1 are neurofibromas and that patients with NF1 typically have only a few (five or six) nerve sheath tumors. In contradistinction, patients with NF2 typically have many (more than 10) spinal nerve schwannomas (see the following section on NF2).

As they grow, the neurofibromas cause enlargement of the neural foramina by erosion of the bone. The neurofibromas have a characteristic appearance on both CT and MR. On CT, these lesions have low attenuation when compared to muscle; they widen the neural foramina by pressure erosion. If intrathecal contrast is introduced, the lesion (which can be intra- or extrathecal) may displace the spinal cord to the contralateral side of the canal. When bilateral neurofibromas are present at a single level, the cord can be compressed into a narrow, central band of tissue that is elongated in the anterior-posterior direction. Under these circumstances, the risk of damaging the cord during an attempted surgical decompression is very high. The MR appearance of neurofibromas is that of ovoid lesions that may be entirely within the spinal canal, causing canal enlargement, or may extend outward from the spinal canal through widened neural foramina (Figs. 6.14, 6.15) (24,32). Neurofibromas have a slightly greater signal intensity than skeletal muscle on T1-weighted sequences; on T2-weighted sequences, the periphery of the lesions tends to be of high

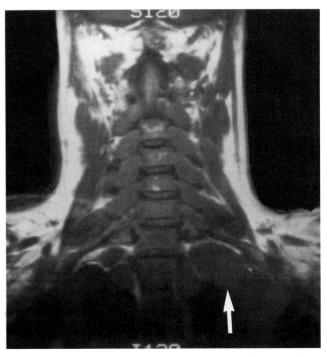

FIG. 6.14. Coronal SE 800/20 image in an NF1 patient reveals neurofibromas extending laterally from the neural foramina at every level. Also note the large neurofibroma at the apex of the left lung (*arrow*).

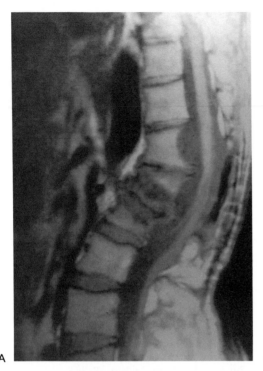
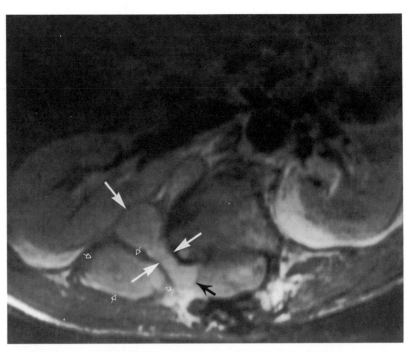

A   B

FIG. 6.15. Neurofibromas resulting in kyphosis. **A:** Focal kyphotic segment in patient with NF1. There is posterior scalloping of the vertebral body immediately above the kyphos. Posterior scalloping secondary to dural ectasia is a common bony change in the spine in NF1. A laminectomy has been performed in this patient. **B:** Axial SE 1000/20 image shows a neurofibroma extending through the neural foramen and on the right (*closed arrows*) and a second neurofibroma in the paraspinous muscles posterior to the foraminal mass (*open arrows*).

signal intensity with respect to muscle, whereas the center of the lesions is often of low signal intensity (24,32,33). The central area of decreased intensity is probably related to the known dense central core of collagen within these lesions (24,33). Collagen has a low mobile proton density and therefore gives a low signal intensity on T2-weighted images.

It is well established that malignant neurofibromas (neurofibrosarcomas) occur in NF1 (Fig. 6.16). It is not clear, however, whether these tumors result from malignant degeneration of preexisting tumors or whether they develop as malignancies *de novo* (9,10,34). Estimates of the frequency of these malignancies range from 3% to 13% (9,34). Since the lower numbers come from studies of children and the risk of malignancy is likely to increase with age, an incidence of 10% to 15% is likely. Neurofibrosarcomas usually present with localized motor deficits or pain and dysesthesias with or without evidence of a rapidly enlarging mass. On CT and MR, a neurofibrosarcoma cannot be differentiated from a benign neurofibroma or a schwannoma. The lesions tend to be large and relatively well circumscribed, and are uncommonly seen to invade adjacent structures. Increased internal heterogeneity may be seen; however, marked heterogeneity can be seen in benign tumors as well (23,35,36). Contrast enhancement is heterogeneous.

Those features that are most suggestive of malignant degeneration are a very large size and internal heterogeneity (24).

Meningoceles

Lateral meningoceles are diverticula of the thecal sac (most commonly at the thoracic level) that extend laterally through widened neural foramina. Some workers feel that the primary abnormality in affected patients is hypoplasia of the pedicles, which makes it possible for the dural sac to herniate laterally in response to spinal fluid pressure. Most authorities, however, feel that the meningoceles result from a primary dysplasia of the meninges (37), the same factor that results in scalloping of the posterior vertebral bodies. Weakness in the meninges allows the thecal sac to be focally stretched in response to CSF pulsations. The protrusions from the thecal sac slowly erode the bony elements of the neural foramina, allowing the meningoceles to form. The CT appearance of a lateral meningocele is that of a wide neural foramen with a CSF-attenuation dumbbell-shaped mass extending through it (Fig. 6.17). The corresponding vertebral body is usually markedly scalloped (38). The MR appearance of these lesions is similar in that the neural fo-

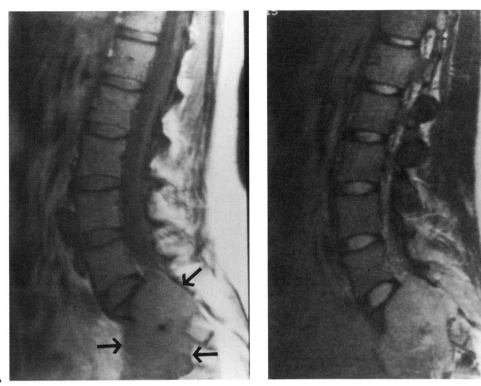

FIG. 6.16. Neurofibrosarcoma in NF1 patient. **A:** Sagittal SE 1000/20 shows a large mass involving the sacral spinal canal and eroding through the sacrum into the presacral space (*arrows*). The mass is largely homogeneous. **B:** SE 1000/70 image shows high signal intensity, similar to the intensity of intervertebral disk. It is not possible to confidently differentiate neurofibrosarcoma from a benign neurofibroma or schwannoma using CT or MR.

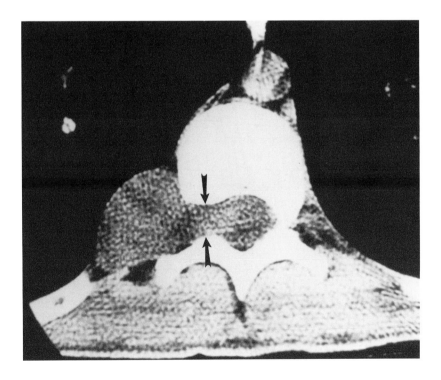

FIG. 6.17. Axial CT shows extension of a lateral thoracic meningocele into the paraspinous space. The meningocele, which is isodense with CSF, widens the neural foramen (*arrows*).

ramen is markedly widened and the spinal canal is enlarged as a result of scalloping of the posterior vertebral body at the level of the meningocele. The meningocele is isointense with CSF on T1- and T2-weighted images. These lesions can often be differentiated from neurofibromas by the absence of the central low-intensity focus on the T2-weighted images (24). Neurofibromas are of higher signal intensity than CSF on short TR/TE images.

NEUROFIBROMATOSIS TYPE II

NF2 has also been called neurofibromatosis with bilateral acoustic schwannomas. To be accurate, however, NF2 should not be considered a "form" of neurofibromatosis but rather a separate disease altogether. NF2 is associated with an abnormality of chromosome 22, verifying that it is a separate entity from von Recklinghausen's disease, which has a locus on chromosome 17 (5,39,40). NF2 is also autosomal dominant, but it is much less frequent than NF1, with an estimated incidence of one of every 50,000 people in the population (41). The major feature of NF2 is the presence in nearly all affected individuals of bilateral acoustic schwanno-

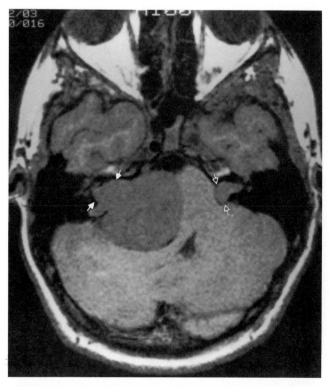

FIG. 6.18. Bilateral acoustic schwannomas in patient with NF2. Axial SE 600/20 image shows a large mass expanding the right internal auditory canal (*closed arrows*) and extending into the right cerebellopontine angle cistern. The brain stem is compressed and the fourth ventricle is compressed and pushed to the left of midline by this mass. A second, smaller tumor is seen in the left internal auditory canal and left cerebellopontine angle (*open arrows*).

TABLE 6.2. *Criteria for diagnosis of neurofibromatosis type II*

The criteria for diagnosis of neurofibromatosis type II are met by an individual who has:

1. Bilateral 8th nerve masses seen with CT or MR; or
2. A first-degree relative with NF2 and either
   a. A unilateral 8th nerve mass or
   b. Two of the following: neurofibroma, meningioma, glioma, schwannoma, or juvenile posterior subcapsular lenticular opacity

Adapted from ref. 41.

mas (Fig. 6.18). Other tumors of the central nervous system, particularly meningiomas, may be present as well. Cutaneous manifestations are much less frequent than in NF1. Less than half of affected patients will have café au lait spots, and, when present, the spots are pale and few in number (less than five). Cutaneous neurofibromas are minimal in size and number or absent (42). Lisch nodules are not present. NF2 has only recently been recognized as a distinct entity; earlier reports have therefore classified patients or families with NF2 with those having von Recklinghausen's disease. As a result of previous inaccurate classification, the exact manifestations of NF2 as compared to NF1 have not been clearly defined. The skeletal dysplasias, optic pathway gliomas, learning disabilities, and vascular dysplasias of NF1 are conspicuously absent in NF2. The established diagnostic criteria for NF2 are listed in Table 6.2.

Intracranial Manifestations

As a result of the absence of cutaneous and ocular manifestations, patients with NF2 may not develop any clinical manifestations of the disease until the second, third, or even fourth decade of life. Moreover, it may fall upon the radiologist to make the diagnosis of NF2 in affected patients. The characteristic intracranial abnormalities are schwannomas of the acoustic and other cranial nerves and meningiomas (often multiple, Figs. 6.19, 6.20). The imaging characteristics of schwannomas and meningiomas are described in Chapter 7. If bilateral acoustic tumors are present or a diagnosis of NF2 is suspected for other reasons, the imaging procedure of choice should be contrast-enhanced MR. Schwannomas and meningiomas both enhance brightly after the infusion of intravenous contrast. Multiple very small meningiomas and schwannomas that were not apparent on the precontrast scan are frequently identified on the postcontrast study (26) (Fig. 6.20).

An important point is that schwannomas and meningiomas are unusual tumors in children and young adults (under age 30 years). *If a meningioma or schwannoma is seen in a young patient, a contrast-enhanced MR scan should be obtained through the brain to look for other*

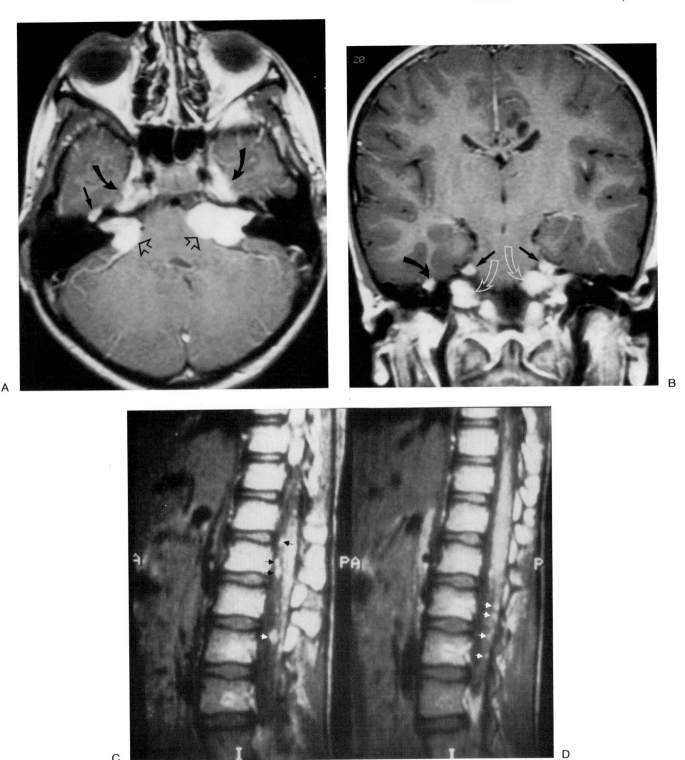

FIG. 6.19. NF2 with multiple schwannomas. **A:** Postcontrast axial SE 600/20 image of NF2 patient reveals bilateral acoustic schwannomas (*open arrows*) and a right facial schwannoma (*closed arrow*). Enlarged cavernous sinuses (*curved arrows*) suggest trigeminal schwannomas. **B:** Postcontrast coronal SE 600/20 image shows bilateral 5th nerve (*closed black arrows*), 8th nerve (curved white arrows) and right 7th nerve (*curved black arrow*) schwannomas. **C, D:** Postcontrast SE 600/20 image through the thoracolumbar spine shows multiple enhancing nerve root tumors (*arrows*), presumably schwannomas.

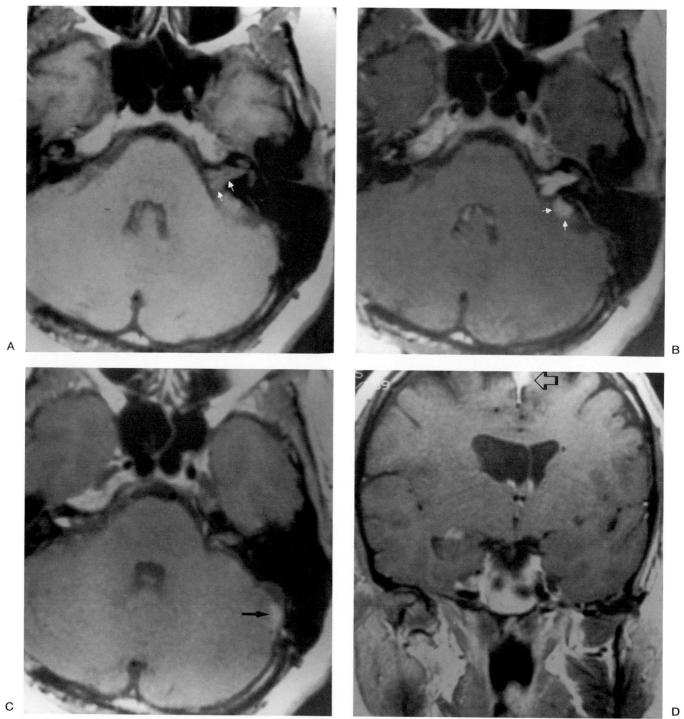

FIG. 6.20. NF2 with bilateral acoustic schwannomas and multiple meningiomas. The patient has had previous resection of a right-sided acoustic schwannoma. **A:** Noncontrast SE 600/20 image through the posterior fossa shows enlargement of the 7th and 8th nerve complex on the left (*arrows*). The patient has undergone a right occipital craniectomy. **B:** After infusion of IV contrast the left 7th and 8th nerve complex enhances. Moreover, a second, separate, enhancing focus is seen arising from the dura immediately posterior to the IAC (*arrows*). This proved to be a meningioma. **C:** Axial SE 600/20 image adjacent to B. A focus of enhancement is seen within the right internal auditory canal, suggestive of recurrent acoustic schwannoma. Additionally, another dural-based enhancing focus is seen on the left (*black arrow*); this proved to be another meningioma. **D:** Coronal SE 600/20 image reveals yet another unsuspected meningioma (*arrow*) arising from the falx.

asymptomatic schwannomas or meningiomas that may aid in establishing the diagnosis of NF2.

Spinal Manifestations

The characteristic spinal manifestations of NF2 are multiple paraspinal schwannomas and spinal cord ependymomas. Patients with NF2 more frequently develop symptoms of cord compression from the multiple nerve root tumors than do patients with NF1. Coronal imaging optimally shows the nerve root tumors and their relation to the spinal cord. Schwannomas may be intraspinal, may be extraspinal, or may involve both the intraspinal and extraspinal compartments, in addition to the intervening neural foramen. The tumors are isointense to neural tissue on short TR sequences, are hyperintense (usually) on long TR sequences, and enhance uniformly after intravenous administration of paramagnetic contrast. Axial images are helpful in evaluating any deformity of the cord and the relationship of the tumors to the cord (Fig. 6.21).

Intrinsic spinal cord tumors and syringohydromyelia occur with an increased incidence in NF2 (34). The most common intrinsic cord tumors are ependymomas. These can be solitary (most often involving the conus medullaris and filum terminale), or multiple, occurring at all levels of the neural axis. Contrast-enhanced MR is the imaging modality of choice. Without the administration of contrast, ependymomas of the spinal cord may be difficult to differentiate from multiloculated syringohydromyelia. Ependymomas and astrocytomas of the spinal cord are indistinguishable on CT and MR. However,

the presence of a centrally located, contrast-enhancing tumor with sharply marginated borders suggests the diagnosis of ependymoma. Further characteristics of intramedullary neoplasms are described in Chapter 10.

Meningiomas are common in the intraspinal as well as intracranial compartment in NF2 (34). As in patients without neurofibromatosis, spinal meningiomas are most common in the thoracic region. They are intradural, extramedullary masses that displace the spinal cord as they grow. These dural-based masses will sometimes cause pressure erosion of the adjacent bone. They can be identified as extramedullary, intradural masses on CT with intrathecal or IV contrast. MR is the preferred diagnostic modality. These lesions are usually isointense with cord on both short TR/TE and long TR/TE images. They will uniformly enhance after contrast infusion (32,43,44).

Syringohydromyelia has been described in association with neurofibromatosis. In the author's opinion, the syrinx is almost always a secondary phenomenon, resulting from either a primary tumor of the spinal cord or an intradural, extramedullary mass such as a meningioma or neurofibroma. The extramedullary masses cause syrinx formation by disturbing the normal CSF flow dynamics within the spinal canal (45,46). The syrinx will often disappear after removal of the tumor (46,47). The cause of the syrinx cavity resulting from primary spinal cord lesions is less clear. The syrinx most likely results from altered CSF dynamics in these patients as well; however, in some patients the syrinx may be caused by fluid secreted into the spinal cord and central canal by the tumor (48). If syringohydromyelia is seen in neurofibromatosis (either NF1 or NF2) and no extramedullary mass can be

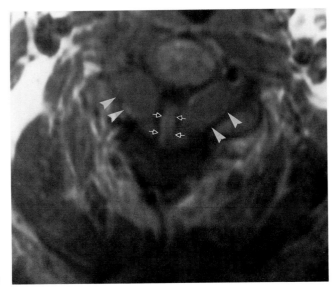

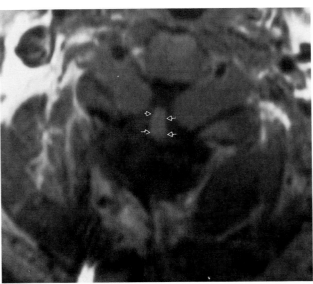

A

B

FIG. 6.21. Cervical paraspinal neurofibromas in NF2 patient. **A:** Neurofibromas are seen extending through and widening the neural foramina bilaterally (*arrowheads*). The spinal cord is compressed by the tumors into a narrow ribbon of tissue (*arrows*). **B:** At a slightly more caudal level, the tumors are located more laterally but the cord maintains its "ribbon" shape (*arrows*).

seen, a contrast-enhanced MR of the spinal cord should be performed in order to rule out an intramedullary lesion. Syringohydromyelia is discussed in more detail in Chapter 9.

OTHER FORMS OF NEUROFIBROMATOSIS

Although the previous sections have made the distinction of NF1 from NF2 seem clear, the reality is that some patients have a syndrome that appears to be an overlap between the two forms (20–22). For this reason, a third type, *NF3*, has been described, that combines some of the features of types I and II (2,3). The genetics of this group is not clear. Moreover, Riccardi has described several other forms of neurofibromatosis as well (2). *NF4* is a heterogeneous category representing a diversity of variant forms of neurofibromatosis. *NF5*, also known as segmental neurofibromatosis, involves only certain portions of the body. *NF6* patients have café au lait spots without neurofibromas. *NF7* is a late onset variety. Finally, an eighth category, *NF-NOS*, describes a number of forms of neurofibromatosis that do not fit into any of the preceding categories. It will be interesting to see how the categorization of these disorders evolves as we gain more experience with these diseases and more insight into their genetics.

TUBEROUS SCLEROSIS (BOURNEVILLE'S DISEASE)

Tuberous sclerosis is a familial disease that involves multiple organ systems. Classically, it has been characterized by the triad of mental retardation, epilepsy, and characteristic skin lesions known as adenoma sebaceum (49). Criteria for diagnosis of the disorder have recently been established and are listed in Table 6.3. The transmission of this disorder is thought to be autosomal dominant with low penetrance. The incidence is approximately one in 100,000 patients (49–51). No racial or sexual predilection has been detected. Tuberous sclerosis is postulated to result from an abnormality of the radial glial-neuronal unit in which the stem cells of all germ cell layers in certain portions of the germinal matrix are defective (52,53). As a consequence, dysplastic disorganized cells are present in the subependymal region, in the cortex, and along curvilinear pathways between them (52–54).

Myoclonic seizures that begin in infancy or early childhood are the presenting symptom of tuberous sclerosis in approximately 80% of patients. The seizures will often decrease in frequency as the patient gets older (55). The incidence of mental retardation ranges from 45% to 82%; most recent publications suggest that the lower number is more accurate (49,56). Among the retarded

TABLE 6.3. *Diagnostic criteria for tuberous sclerosis complex*

Primary features
Facial angiofibromas*
Multiple ungual fibromas*
Cortical tuber (histologically confirmed)
Subependymal nodule or giant cell astrocytoma (histologically confirmed)
Multiple calcified subependymal nodules protruding into the ventricle (radiographic evidence)
Multiple retinal astrocytomas*

Secondary features
Affected first-degree relative
Cardiac rhabdomyoma (histologic or radiographic confirmation)
Other retinal hamartoma or achromic patch*
Cerebral tubers (radiographic confirmation)
Noncalcified subependymal nodules (radiographic confirmation)
Shagreen patch*
Forehead plaque*
Pulmonary lymphangiomyomatosis (histologic confirmation)
Renal angiomyolipoma (radiographic or histologic confirmation)
Renal cysts (histologic confirmation)

Tertiary features
Hypomelanotic macules*
"Confetti" skin lesions*
Renal cysts (radiographic evidence)
Randomly distributed enamel pits in deciduous and/or permanent teeth
Hamartomatous rectal polyps (histologic confirmation)
Bone cysts (radiographic evidence)
Pulmonary lymphangiomyomatosis (radiographic evidence)
Cerebral white-matter "migration tracts" or heterotopia (radiographic evidence)
Gingival fibromas*
Hamartoma of other organs (histologic confirmation)
Infantile spasms

Definite TSC	Either one primary feature, two secondary features, or one secondary plus two tertiary features
Probable TSC	Either one secondary plus one tertiary feature, or three tertiary features
Suspect TSC	Either one secondary feature or two tertiary features

* Histologic confirmation is not required if the lesion is clinically obvious. TSC = tuberous sclerosis complex.

patients, approximately two-thirds will be moderately to severely retarded and one-third only mildly to moderately affected. Patients who manifest seizures before the age of 5 are more likely to have mental retardation than those who develop seizures at a later age (49,57).

Cutaneous Lesions

Although not radiologically apparent, cutaneous adenomas sebaceum are a major characteristic component of tuberous sclerosis and the imager should have a general knowledge of their characteristics. *Adenoma sebaceum* is the term used to describe a nodular rash of brownish red color that is disseminated over the face; the rash typically originates in the nasolabial folds and eventually spreads to cover the nose and the middle of the cheeks in the infraorbital region. These lesions, which are histologically classified as angiofibromas, appear between the ages of 1 and 5 years. Angiofibromas also occur in other areas of the body, most commonly the trunk, gingiva, and periungual regions. Depigmented nevi in the form of oval areas with irregular margins (ash-leaf spots) occur on the trunk and extremities and are as common as angiofibromas. In fact, depigmented nevi usually appear earlier than the adenoma sebaceum; as a result, they are frequently the cutaneous lesions that lead to a diagnosis of tuberous sclerosis in children with seizures (58). In light-skinned children, the depigmented nevi may be demonstrable only under an ultraviolet light. Café au lait spots are occasionally seen in patients with tuberous sclerosis, but their incidence is similar to that in the general population; their presence in isolation should not suggest a diagnosis of neurofibromatosis (59).

Ocular Lesions

Ocular findings are common in tuberous sclerosis. The most common of these is the retinal hamartoma, an astrocytic proliferation that is most commonly seen on or near the optic disc (49,51). Retinal hamartomas are usually present in both eyes and are often multiple (55). They originate as fairly flat, semitransparent, whitish lesions. Eventually, when they turn whitish gray or yellow and become nodular, they are said to resemble a clump of mulberries (60). When retinal hamartomas calcify, they can be seen on CT scan as small calcifications in the region of the optic nerve head (61). They have not been described on MR. The reader should be aware that, although they are most common in tuberous sclerosis (they are seen in over half the cases), retinal hamartomas can be seen occasionally in the other phakomatoses as well (61).

Brain Lesions

Subependymal Hamartomas

Several characteristic lesions occur in the brain in tuberous sclerosis. The most common of these are *subependymal hamartomas*, which differ histologically from the cortical hamartomas (tubers) and therefore behave differently on imaging studies. The subependymal nodules tend to be located along the ventricular surface of the caudate nucleus, most often on the lamina of the sulcus thalamostriatus immediately posterior to the fora-

men of Monro (51). Less commonly, the nodules may be detected along the frontal and temporal horns, the third ventricle or the fourth ventricle.

The imaging appearance of subependymal hamartomas changes with the age of the patient. They are rarely calcified in the first year of life; the number of calcifications typically increases with the age of the patient (56). Thus, they may be difficult to detect on CT scans of infants but become progressively easier to identify as they calcify (Fig. 6.22). On MR scans, subependymal hamartomas appear as irregular subependymal nodules that protrude into the adjacent ventricle. Their appearance changes as the signal of the surrounding white matter changes (54,62). In infants, who have unmyelinated white matter, the hamartomas are relatively hyperintense on short TR images and hypointense on long TR image (Fig. 6.23). As the brain myelinates, the subependymal nodules gradually become isointense with the white matter (Fig. 6.22). They are most easily visualized on T1-weighted images, where they contrast with low signal intensity of the CSF. Small nodules may not be apparent on long TR/TE spin echo images. Larger subependymal nodules manifest a variably low signal intensity on the long TR/TE images, depending upon the extent of calcification (54,63,64); T2*-weighted images are optimal for showing the calcification because of the magnetic susceptibility differences of calcium and brain. After intravenous administration of paramagnetic contrast, subependymal nodules show variable enhancement; some will enhance markedly, some mildly, and some not at all (Fig. 6.24) (54,65,66).

Giant Cell Tumors

Giant cell tumor is a term given to the enlarging subependymal nodules that are situated near the foramen of Monro. Anatomically, these tumors differ from the subependymal hamartomas by their size and their tendency to enlarge; their characteristic location and tendency toward enlargement usually result in a clinical presentation of hydrocephalus (54,67). Their incidence in tuberous sclerosis is approximately 5% to 10% (51,54, 56). Histologically, subependymal lesions in patients with tuberous sclerosis appear to span a continuum between subependymal hamartomas and giant cell tumors; although some lesions are clearly in one category or the other, many lesions have histologic characteristics of both (10,49).

On imaging studies, giant cell tumors are identified by their location near the foramen of Monro and the demonstration of tumor growth on serial studies. Neither signal intensity nor the presence or absence of enhancement is useful in making the distinction (54). If an enlarging, contrast-enhancing subependymal nodule is seen in the region of the foramen of Monro, it should be considered a giant cell tumor (Figs. 6.23A,B; 6.24A,B;

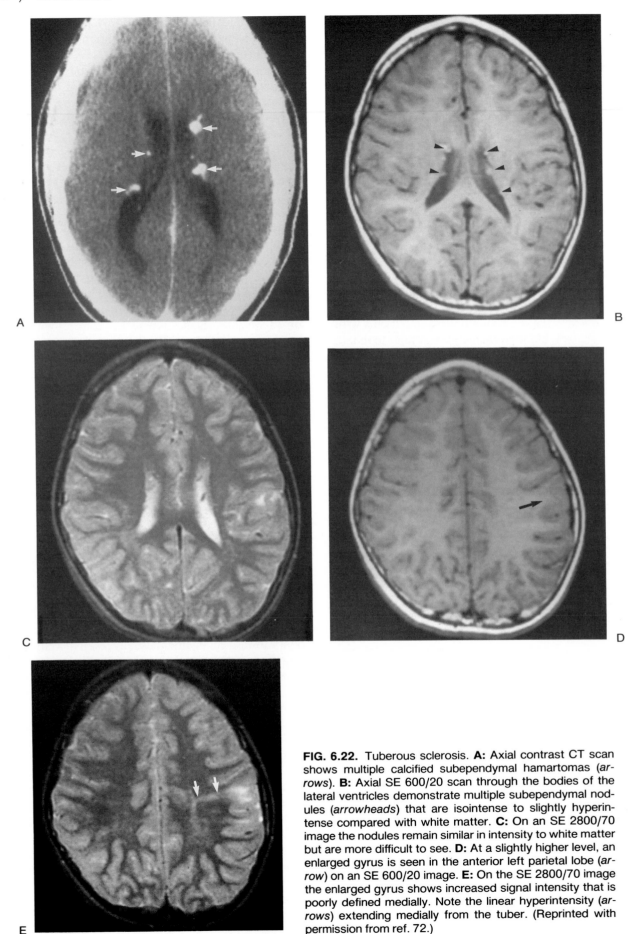

FIG. 6.22. Tuberous sclerosis. **A:** Axial contrast CT scan shows multiple calcified subependymal hamartomas (*arrows*). **B:** Axial SE 600/20 scan through the bodies of the lateral ventricles demonstrate multiple subependymal nodules (*arrowheads*) that are isointense to slightly hyperintense compared with white matter. **C:** On an SE 2800/70 image the nodules remain similar in intensity to white matter but are more difficult to see. **D:** At a slightly higher level, an enlarged gyrus is seen in the anterior left parietal lobe (*arrow*) on an SE 600/20 image. **E:** On the SE 2800/70 image the enlarged gyrus shows increased signal intensity that is poorly defined medially. Note the linear hyperintensity (*arrows*) extending medially from the tuber. (Reprinted with permission from ref. 72.)

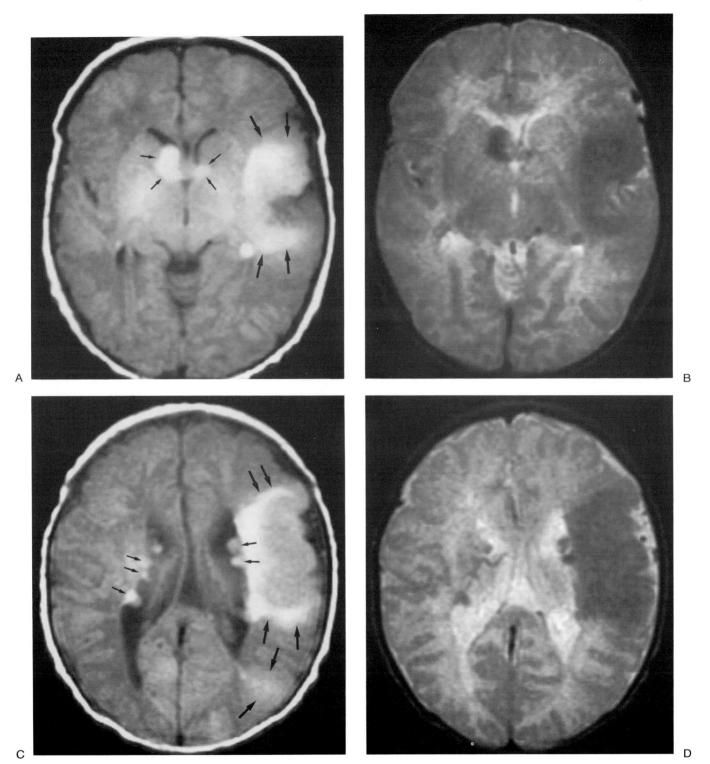

FIG. 6.23. Tuberous sclerosis in an infant. **A:** Axial SE 550/15 image shows hyperintense subependymal masses (*small arrows*), presumably giant cell tumors, at the foramina of Monro. A large cortical tuber (*large arrows*) is hyperintense compared to immature brain. **B:** Axial SE 3000/120 image shows that the lesions are hypointense to immature brain; they are similar to mature white matter in intensity. **C:** Axial SE 550/15 image 10 mm superior to (A) shows several hyperintense subependymal hamartomas (*small arrows*) and cortical tubers (*large arrows*) that are all hyperintense compared to immature brain. **D:** Axial SE 3000/120 at the same level as (C) shows the masses to be hypointense compared to immature brain. (C and D are reprinted with permission from ref. 72.)

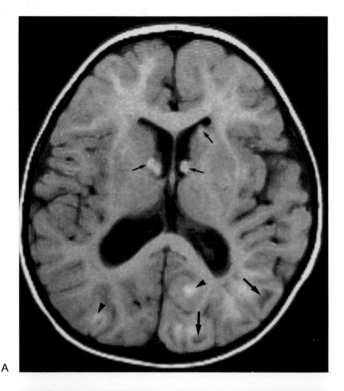

A

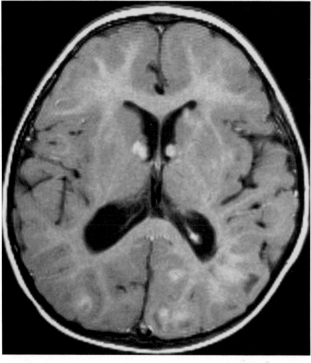

B

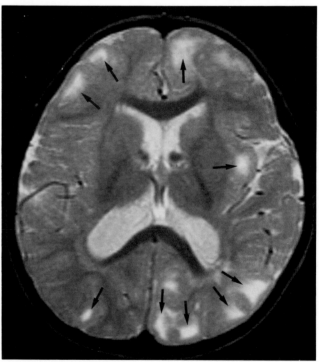

C

FIG. 6.24. Tuberous sclerosis. Variable enhancement of subependymal hamartomas. **A:** Axial SE 550/15 image shows several subependymal nodules (*small black arrows*) in the frontal horns; those at the level of the foramina of Monro are presumably giant cell tumors. Subcortical foci of high (secondary to calcification, *arrowheads*) and low (*large black arrows*) signal intensity represent cortical tubers. **B:** Postcontrast scan at same level as (A) shows some enhancement of the subependymal hamartomas but no enhancement of the cortical tubers. **C:** Axial SE 2800/70 image shows the subependymal hamartomas to be nearly isointense to mature white matter. Many more cortical tubers (*arrows*) are seen than on the T1-weighted images in (A) and (B).

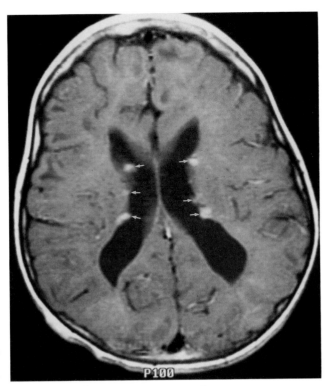
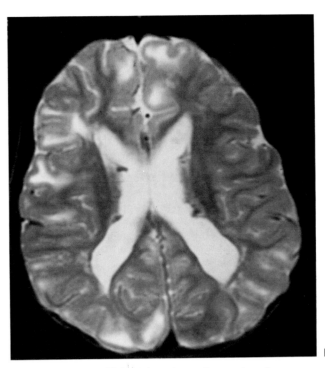

D

E

FIG. 6.24. (*Continued.*) **D:** Postcontrast T1-weighted image shows multiple enhancing subependymal hamartomas (*arrows*). **E:** Axial SE 2800/70 image at the same level as **D** shows that the subependymal hamartomas are harder to identify but the cortical tubers are more evident.

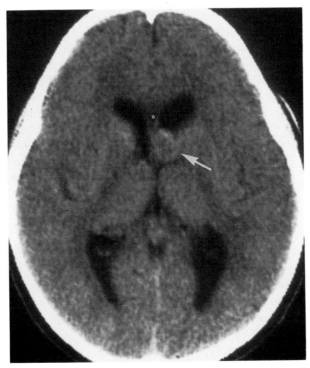
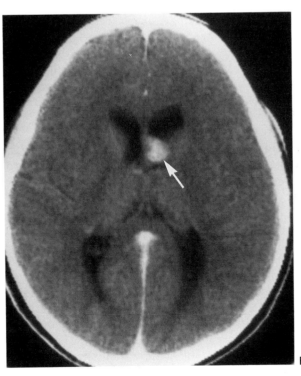

A

B

FIG. 6.25. Giant cell astrocytoma. **A:** Noncontrast CT shows a mass in the region of the left foramen of Monro in this patient with tuberous sclerosis (*arrow*). The left lateral ventricle is slightly enlarged, presumably as a result of partial obstruction of the foramen. **B:** After infusion of IV contrast, the intraventricular mass uniformly enhances (*arrow*). Giant cell astrocytomas characteristically enhance and occur at the foramen of Monro, whereas subependymal hamartomas do not enhance on CT and are nonenhancing or minimally enhancing on contrast-enhanced MR.

6.25). These tumors tend to grow into the ventricle and only rarely invade brain parenchyma. Occasionally, degeneration into higher-grade, or infiltrating, neoplasms can occur (67,68). Such degeneration should be suspected radiologically if the tumor is seen to invade the brain parenchyma or if rapid enlargement is seen. The treatment of benign giant cell tumors is controversial. Some surgeons believe that shunting of the obstructed lateral ventricle is sufficient unless local mass effect causes symptoms. Others believe that the tumor should be resected in order to cure the hydrocephalus and prevent possible degeneration into a higher-grade tumor. Rarely, giant cell tumors occur in patients with no other evidence of tuberous sclerosis (34). It has not been determined whether these neoplasms represent a forme fruste of tuberous sclerosis or a spontaneous tumor unrelated to the genetic abnormality that causes tuberous sclerosis.

Cortical "Tubers"

The *cortical hamartomas or "tubers"* are the most characteristic lesions of tuberous sclerosis pathologically. Macroscopically, they are smooth, whitish, slightly raised nodules that appear as enlarged, atypically shaped gyri; they may be round or polygonal. Histologically, they consist of bizarre giant cells, dense fibrillary gliosis, and diminished, disordered myelin sheaths (10,49,51). Any single patient may have as few as one to two or as many as 20–30 tubers (6,49,51). The proportion that calcify has not been reliably determined. The number of calcified cortical lesions seen on CT increases with age; by age 10, calcified cortical tubers are present in up to 50% of patients with tuberous sclerosis (56). The cortical calcifications may be gyriform, simulating the appearance of Sturge-Weber disease on CT (69).

In young patients (less than 1 year of age) cortical hamartomas appear on CT as lucencies within broadened cortical gyri (Fig. 6.26). The lucency diminishes with age, making the cortical hamartomas difficult to identify in older children and adults. In adults, this difficulty is exacerbated by beam hardening by the overlying calvarium, making identification of cortical tubers nearly impossible unless they are calcified (49). The MR appearance of cortical tubers also changes with age. In neonates, they appear as enlarged gyri that are hyperintense compared to the surrounding unmyelinated white matter on T1-weighted images and hypointense to white matter on T2-weighted images (Fig. 6.23). The appearance changes as the white matter myelinates; in older infants they appear as enlarged gyri with a low-intensity center on T1-weighted images and high signal intensity on T2-weighted images (Fig. 6.26). The lesions themselves seem predominantly subcortical, clearly separate from the overlying cortex (Figs. 6.22, 6.24, 6.26). The inner margins of the tubers are poorly defined on all im-

aging sequences. With increasing age, the tubers become isointense with white matter on the T1-weighted sequences; however, they remain hyperintense on the T2-weighted images (Fig. 6.22) (54,63,64,66). The signal characteristics probably result from the diminished myelin and dense gliosis within them. It is important to realize that the high signal intensity on the T2-weighted images does not imply malignant degeneration. In fact, neoplastic degeneration of cortical tubers is extremely rare. When cortical tubers calcify, they will often appear bright on T1-weighted images (Fig. 6.24), presumably because of T1 shortening caused by the crystals of calcium (70). Degenerated, calcified cortical tubers will sometimes enhance after contrast administration.

White Matter Lesions

Islets consisting of a grouping of neurons and glial cells are invariably present in the white matter of patients with tuberous sclerosis (10,51). Microscopically, the cells are often bizarre and gigantic, with characteristics of both neurons and glia; they are associated with areas of hypomyelination similar to those seen in the cortical tubers (10,51). Many of these clusters of heterotopic cells are microscopic and therefore do not appear on imaging studies. Those that are large enough to be seen have a variable appearance that depends upon the amount of calcification within them. On CT, these regions appear as low-attenuation, well-defined regions within the cerebral white matter that do not enhance after intravenous contrast infusion. When calcification occurs, it can involve part or all of the nodule. Partially calcified nodules will have a mixed attenuation, with one portion being of lower attenuation than the surrounding white matter and the other portion extremely high attenuation because of the calcification (49,56). On MR, these white matter islets have the same signal characteristics as cortical tubers (Figs. 6.22–6.24, 6.26). In older patients, they may be difficult to see on T1-weighted sequences; they can sometimes be identified as subtle, low-intensity regions. On the T2-weighted images, they appear as well-defined areas of high signal intensity (Fig. 6.22) (54,63,64,66). If the lesion is calcified, the calcification may appear as a low or high signal intensity on short TR images, depending upon the characteristics of the calcium crystals (70) (Fig. 6.24). As with cortical tubers, enhancement is only seen if the lesion has degenerated; under these conditions, calcification is usually present.

Occasionally, T2-weighted images will show linear or curvilinear regions of hyperintensity in the cerebral white matter, extending from subependymal hamartomas to cortical tubers (Fig. 6.22E) (54,71). These are believed to represent bands of unmyelinated, disordered cells along the pathway of the linear radial glial-neuronal unit (54,71,72). In theory, the primary brain abnormal-

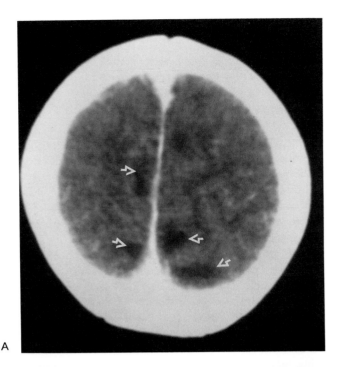

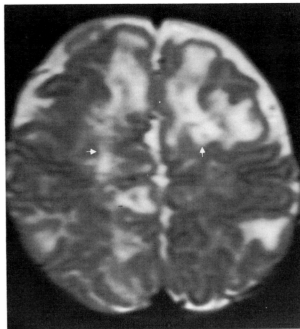

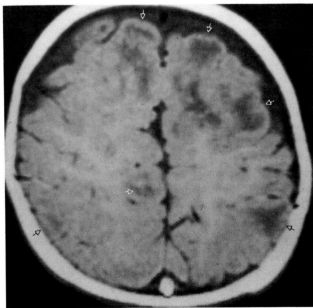

FIG. 6.26. Cortical tubers in an infant with tuberous sclerosis. **A:** Axial CT image shows multiple subcortical regions of low attenuation (*arrows*) in the cerebral hemispheres. Note that considerably fewer lesions are seen adjacent to the calvarium secondary to beam-hardening artifact. **B:** Axial SE 600/20 image reveals multiple cortical tubers (*open arrows*). In infants, these subcortical lesions appear as areas of low signal intensity on short TR/TE images with poorly defined medial borders. The involved gyri are enlarged. These lesions do not enhance after administration of IV contrast. **C:** Axial SE 2500/70 image at the same level in the same patient. The cortical tubers show a high signal intensity on long TR/TE images. Also notice areas of prolonged T2 relaxation in the white matter (*arrows*). These represent the so-called heterotopia of tuberous sclerosis that are histologically very similar to the cortical tubers.

ity in tuberous sclerosis is one of dysplastic stem cells in the germinal zone. The dysplastic stem cells give rise to dysplastic glia and neurons that fail to differentiate, migrate, and organize properly (53,72). The result is accumulations of disorganized collections of dysplastic cells in the subependymal and cortical regions, as well as along the curvilinear path between them.

Cerebellar Lesions

Cerebellar lesions have been described in tuberous sclerosis, but they are less common, occurring in approximately 10% of patients (54,56,57). The posterior fossa lesions are similar to those of the cerebral hemispheres, consisting of cortical tubers, heterotopic clusters in the white matter, and occasionally subependymal hamartomas (10,51,54). The hemispheric lesions are difficult to see by CT unless they are calcified, because of the severe beam hardening artifact that occurs in the posterior fossa. The CT and MR appearance of these cerebellar lesions is otherwise quite similar to the appearance of those in the cerebral hemispheres (54,56).

Non-CNS Lesions

Although brain, ocular, and cutaneous lesions are the hallmark of tuberous sclerosis, lesions also occur in the heart, kidneys, liver, lung, and spleen (49). Renal hamartomas occur in 40% to 80% of patients with tuberous sclerosis (51,73). Histologically, these lesions are *angiomyolipomas*; they often arise in young adulthood and enlarge slowly. They are usually asymptomatic, although hematuria, flank pain, or a palpable abdominal mass may be present. Malignant degeneration is rare. On ultrasound angiomyolipomas are well defined and highly echogenic. The CT and MR appearances are remarkable for the presence of fat. Benign *rhabdomyomas* of the heart are less common than the renal hamartomas but are important because they can present as a congenital cardiomyopathy (49,51). These tumors are always subendocardial and may be either circumscribed or diffuse. Because of their serious consequences, some authors feel that all patients with tuberous sclerosis should have screening echocardiography.

Pulmonary involvement is the next most common type of visceral abnormality in patients with tuberous sclerosis (49). The characteristic pulmonary lesion is called *lymphangioleiomyomytosis*. In this condition the lung parenchyma undergoes cystic changes with a myomatous proliferation of tissue and chronic fibrosis occurring in the septa between the cysts. Other types of visceral lesions include adenomas and lipomyomas of the liver, adenomas of the pancreas, and tumors of the spleen (49). Bone lesions consist of multiple dense lesions in the cra-

nium and cystic changes in the metacarpals and phalanges of the hands (10,49,51).

STURGE-WEBER DISEASE

Clinical Manifestations

Sturge-Weber disease, also known as encephalotrigeminal angiomatosis or meningofacial angiomatosis, is a congenital disorder that is marked by angiomatosis involving the face, the choroid of the eye, and the leptomeninges. The facial angioma, often referred to as a port wine vascular nevus, can involve part or all of the face. Other clinical components of this syndrome are seizures, hemiparesis, hemianopsia, and mental retardation. Although in most instances the condition appears sporadically, familial cases are reported. Both sexes are equally affected (74).

The facial nevus is composed of a plethora of thin-walled vessels that most closely resemble capillaries. It is present at birth—usually unilateral, although occasionally bilateral—and involves the middle portion of the face with no predilection for either side. The nevus does not change with advancing years. Rarely, Sturge-Weber syndrome has been reported without a facial nevus (75,76).

Patients with the Sturge-Weber syndrome generally develop normally until they begin to have focal or generalized seizures. Infantile spasms develop in approximately 90% of affected patients during the first year of life, followed by development of tonic, atonic, or myoclonic seizures (74,77). With time the seizures become progressively refractory to medication; they are accompanied by an increasing hemiparesis in about 30% of patients. Homonymous hemianopsia often accompanies the hemiparesis. The majority of affected patients are mentally retarded (74,77). Prognosis is poor when both cerebral hemispheres are involved or the majority of a single hemisphere is involved (77).

Brain Pathology

The major pathologic abnormality in Sturge-Weber disease is a meningeal angioma that is ordinarily confined to the pia mater. This pathologic process consists of multiple small venous channels that are matted together on the surface of the brain. The arteries are also abnormal, although involved to a lesser extent, and tend to undergo fibrosis. The combination of the facial and pial angiomatosis has been postulated to result from persistence of the architectonic features of the primordial sinusoidal vascular channels that are present between the fourth and eighth weeks of gestation (78,79). At that time the ectoderm, which is to form the skin of the upper part of the face, overlies that part of the neural tube destined to form the occipital and adjacent parts of the cerebrum. Normally, the superficial and deep portions of the vascular system become widely separated with the extensive subsequent growth of the cerebral hemispheres (78). According to Alexander, the persistence of primordial vessels may explain why facial nevi in the area of the ophthalmic division of the 5th nerve (in the frontal area) are associated with leptomeningeal angiomatosis in the occipital region, nevi in the region of the maxillary division are associated with angiomas in the parietal convexity, and nevi involving all three divisions are associated with angiomatosis of the entire convexity of the hemisphere, including the frontal lobe (74). Unfortunately, the correlation between the location of the facial nevus and the pial angioma is not absolute. For example, frontal angiomas can be present in association with maxillary nevi.

Cortical calcifications are another pathologic finding in Sturge-Weber syndrome. The calcifications occur exclusively in areas of the brain subjacent to the angioma. They begin in the subcortical white matter and later develop in the cortex, predominantly in cortical layers 2 and 3 (10,74). They are most frequently seen in the temporo-parieto-occipital region of the brain but can be located anywhere in the cerebrum (10,74,80). Cortical calcifications can be bilateral in up to 20% of patients (80). Although their cause is not confidently established, they are most likely the result of chronic ischemia that results from impaired venous drainage (23).

Imaging Manifestations in the Brain

Contrast-enhanced MR studies are the most accurate imaging studies for showing the extent of the pial angioma (81,82). Enhancement can sometimes be seen by CT if the patient is imaged in infancy, prior to the appearance of cortical calcifications (80); calcifications mask the enhancement. After intravenous administration of contrast, the angioma appears as an area of enhancement that seems to fill the subarachnoid space, covering the surfaces of the gyri and filling the cortical sulci (Figs. 6.27, 6.28). As demonstration of the extent of the angioma is critical in determining the patient's prognosis and the necessary extent of cortical resection, contrast-enhanced MR imaging should be performed in all patients for whom surgery for seizure control is planned (77,82).

The effects of the angioma (and the associated restricted cortical venous drainage) upon the underlying brain can also be assessed by imaging. As mentioned earlier, calcifications occur in the cerebral cortex underlying the pial angioma; they are the most frequent CT finding of Sturge-Weber disease (Fig. 6.29) (80,83). Calcifications most commonly occur unilaterally over the posterior portion of the hemisphere, although any portion of cerebral cortex may be involved. The calcification is

sometimes difficult to see on short TR spin echo MR imaging studies. It is more readily identified on long TR spin echo images and, especially, on gradient echo scans, which are more sensitive to the difference in magnetic susceptibility between normal brain and calcium (Fig. 6.27, 6.29). With the more sensitive techniques, a thin ribbon of low signal intensity will be seen in or subjacent to the cerebral cortex in the affected areas.

The choroid plexus is frequently enlarged in patients with Sturge-Weber disease, and abnormally prominent enhancement of the choroid may be seen ipsilateral to the angiomatous malformation (Figs. 6.27, 6.29) (84). On MR, the affected choroid plexuses are enlarged and are hyperintense to brain parenchyma on long TR images (84). This phenomenon is most commonly a result of hyperplasia of the choroid plexus, although angiomatous malformations of the choroid have been reported (79).

In the infant with Sturge-Weber syndrome, the white matter underlying the angioma may show accentuated T2 shortening compared to the remainder of the brain (Fig. 6.28) (85). Although it has been postulated that this finding represents accelerated myelination, the absence of early T1 shortening and the absence of any histologic evidence of accelerated myelination in affected patients makes it an unlikely cause of the signal change. Another more reasonable, but unproven, suggestion is that the T2 shortening is the result of increased deoxyhemoglobin in capillaries and veins. Presumably, the increased deoxyhemoglobin is the result of restricted superficial venous drainage, with consequent shunting of deoxygenated blood through the dilated deep medullary veins into the deep venous system (86).

The ipsilateral cerebral hemisphere is atrophic in most, but not all, patients with Sturge-Weber disease (Figs. 6.27, 6.29). As might be expected, atrophy is bilateral in those patients with bilateral angiomas (87). The white matter subjacent to the affected cerebral cortex appears as low density on CT scans and shows slight prolongation of T1 and T2 relaxation times on MR (80,88). These signal characteristics most likely represent gliosis in the ischemic underlying brain.

Cranial asymmetry often results from cerebral hemiatrophy. The ipsilateral calvarium is thickened and the ipsilateral paranasal sinuses and mastoid air cells are enlarged because of the lack of brain growth on the affected side. The thickened calvarium is seen on MR as a widening of the fat-filled high-intensity diploic space (Figs. 6.27, 6.29). Midline structures are often apparently displaced toward the side of the leptomeningeal angioma. Occasionally, an enlarged hemicranium may be seen on the side of the angioma. This paradoxical enlargement may be a result of subdural hematomas accumulating in the affected hemicranium secondary to the cerebral atrophy (89).

Occasionally, enlarged vessels are seen on CT and MR

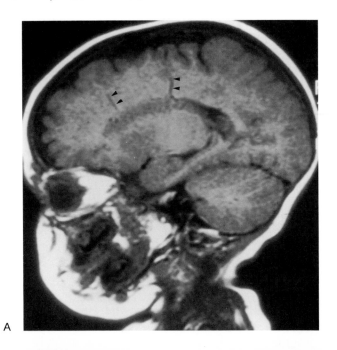

A

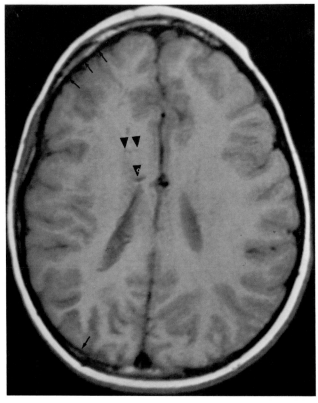

B

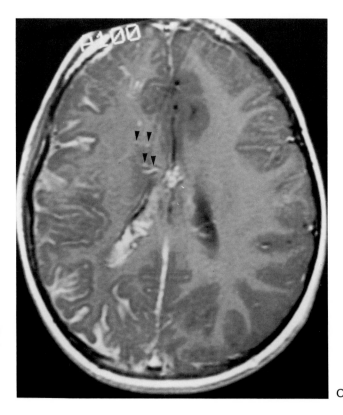

C

FIG. 6.27. Child with Sturge-Weber syndrome. **A:** Sagittal SE 500/15 image shows dilated periventricular veins (*arrowheads*). **B:** Axial SE 600/16 image shows thickening of the diploic space of the right hemicalvarium (*arrows*) compared to the left. A few enlarged periventricular vessels (*arrowheads*) are noted. **C:** Postcontrast T1-weighted image shows pial enhancement over the entire right hemisphere and enlargement of the right choroid plexus. The enlarged periventricular vessels (*arrowheads*) are enhancing, indicating that they are venous.

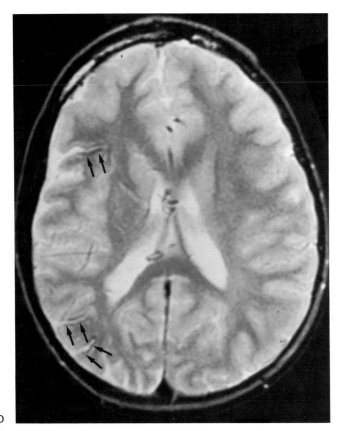
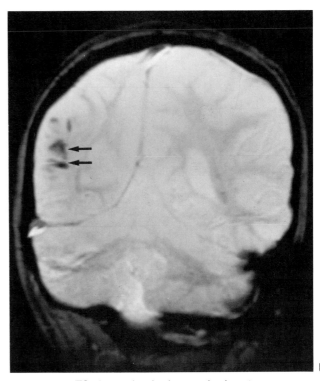

D

E

FIG. 6.27. *(Continued.)* **D:** Axial SE 2500/70 image shows some T2 shortening in the cerebral cortex *(arrows)*, suggesting calcification. **E:** Calcification *(arrows)* is much more obvious on this T2*-weighted gradient echo image.

studies in the subependymal and periventricular region of the brain (Figs. 6.27, 6.29). Although arteriovenous malformations may be seen in association with Sturge-Weber syndrome, the more likely cause for these enlarged deep hemispheric vessels is enlargement of the vessels of the deep venous system of the brain (86,90). When such enlargement occurs, it is a result of marked slowing of blood flow in, or possibly thrombosis of, the dysgenetic superficial venous system of the brain. The pial angiomatous malformation results in dysgenesis of, and diminished outflow through, the superficial venous system. Therefore, venous blood is shunted through the deep medullary veins and into the deep venous system of the brain (86,90). Such venous drainage should not be mistaken for arteriovenous malformations in which enlarged feeding arteries, as well as large veins, are present. The absence of superficial venous drainage in the region of the pial angioma was an important criterion in the diagnosis of Sturge-Weber disease prior to the advent of CT (86,90).

Positron emission tomography (PET) using ^{18}F-deoxyglucose has been used to study cerebral metabolism in patients with Sturge-Weber syndrome. In the early stages of the disease, the affected area is typically hypermetabolic. However, hypometabolism soon ensues (91).

Some authors have suggested that PET is useful in surgical planning when cortical resection is contemplated for treatment of intractable seizures and failure to attain developmental milestones (91). The value of PET, as compared to contrast-enhanced MR, has not been established.

Ocular Anomalies

Abnormalities of the globe are seen in about 30% of patients with Sturge-Weber disease (74,92). Pathologically, affected patients have angiomas of the choroid and sclera. They present with ocular pain or retro-orbital pain from glaucoma or with acute visual deterioration from retinal detachment. If the glaucoma begins *in utero,* the globe can enlarge as a result of the increased intraocular pressure. This condition is known as buphthalmos and is seen on CT and MR scans as a very large, somewhat elongated globe.

Extra-CNS Manifestations

Patients with Sturge-Weber syndrome do not typically have abnormalities of the thoracic or abdominal viscera.

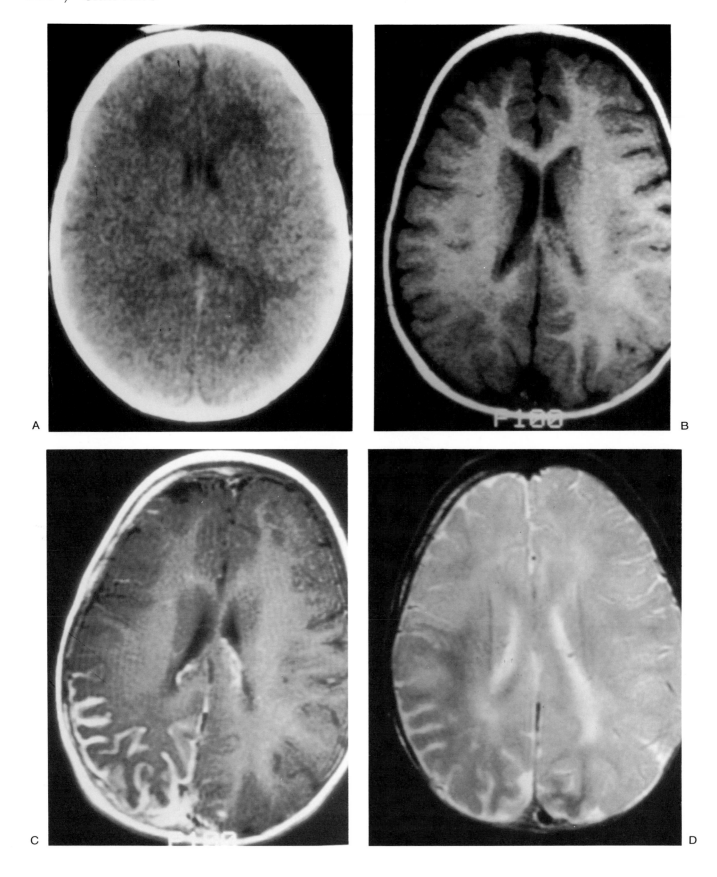

However, some patients will have angiomas of the viscera and extremities in conjunction with typical findings of Sturge-Weber syndrome (74,93,94). The angiomas can be localized or diffuse; they can be located in the intestine, kidneys, spleen, ovaries, thyroid gland, pancreas, or lungs (74). This combination of Sturge-Weber syndrome with involvement of the viscera and extremities is called Klippel-Trenaunay-Weber syndrome by some authors (23,95); others consider the entire complex to be a part of the Sturge-Weber syndrome (74,94).

VON HIPPEL-LINDAU DISEASE

Also known as CNS angiomatosis, von Hippel-Lindau disease is an autosomal dominant disorder with incomplete penetrance characterized by retinal angiomas, cerebellar and spinal cord hemangioblastomas, renal cell carcinomas, pheochromocytomas, angiomas of the liver and kidney, and cysts of the pancreas, kidney, liver, and epididymis (96,97). Both sexes are affected equally (98,99). The diagnosis is established if patients have more than one hemangioblastoma of the CNS, one hemangioblastoma with a visceral manifestation of the disease, or one manifestation of the disease and a known family history (99). The genetic abnormality, a defective tumor suppressor gene at chromosome 3p25-p26 has recently been identified (100); therefore, the disease may soon be diagnosed by molecular biological techniques, with potential for diagnosis *in utero*.

The initial symptoms of affected patients are usually the result of either the cerebellar or retinal tumors. Symptoms from the retinal angiomas usually antedate cerebellar complaints, but this order of events is by no means constant. The usual sequence of events is reactive retinal inflammation with exudate and hemorrhage, followed by retinal detachment, glaucoma, cataract, and uveitis. By the time the patient is seen because of decreasing visual acuity or eye pain, the secondary changes of retinal detachment may mask the underlying lesion. Headache, vertigo, and vomiting result from the cerebellar tumor and associated increased intracranial pressure, when present. Other cerebellar findings, such as dysdiadochokinesia, dysmetria, and Romberg's sign, are common (98). Uncommonly, patients may present with complaints of spinal cord dysfunction such as loss of sensation or impaired proprioception. It is rare, however, for patients to present with symptoms of spinal cord or

visceral lesions in this disease (99). Symptoms typically begin during the third or fourth decade of life; it is unusual for patients to present before the second half of the second decade (98,99).

Ocular Manifestations

Angiomas of the retina are observed in over half of affected patients; symptoms from these lesions are usually the earliest manifestation of the disease (99). Retinal angiomas are best demonstrated clinically, using indirect ophthalmoscopy and fluorescein angiography. The angiomas are multiple in up to two-thirds of patients and bilateral in up to 50% (98,99,101). Although CT and MR can detect the secondary retinal detachment, the retinal angiomas themselves are usually quite small and are rarely detected by imaging studies.

Brain and Spinal Cord Lesions

Cerebellar hemangioblastomas are present in more than half of patients with von Hippel-Lindau disease (98,99,101). They are the second most frequent source of initial symptoms and frequently recur after surgical resection. The most typical pathologic appearance is of a small, vascular tumor nodule in the wall of a large fluid-filled cyst within the cerebellar hemisphere (Fig 6.30). Between 20% and 40% of the tumors are solid (10). When the nodules of hemangioblastoma are large enough, they will show contrast enhancement on CT; however, when they are small, the tumor may be indistinguishable from a benign posterior fossa cyst, or in the absence of a cyst, they may not be detected at all (80,102). The MR appearance of the cystic lesions is that of sharply marginated cerebellar masses with prolongation of T1 and T2 relaxation time (103,104). If a solid nodule can be seen within the wall of the cyst, it will often have small tubular areas of flow void within it representing enlarged feeding and draining vessels (Fig. 6.30) (105). Solid hemangioblastomas appear as ill-defined solid cerebellar masses that are difficult to identify without the administration of paramagnetic contrast (Fig. 6.31) (103–105). In general, they show prolongation of both T1 and T2 relaxation times, although hemorrhage is occasionally present, resulting in high signal intensity on noncontrast T1-weighted images. MR contrast agents have increased sensitivity for detection of small lesions;

FIG. 6.28. Infant with Sturge-Weber syndrome. **A:** Axial CT image is normal. **B:** Axial SE 550/15 image shows a normal brain. **C:** Postcontrast T1-weighted image shows marked pial enhancement, representing the pial angioma, in the right parieto-occipital region and the left occipital lobe. **D:** Axial SE 2800/70 image shows T2 shortening in the white matter beneath the enhancing pia compared with the contralateral hemisphere.

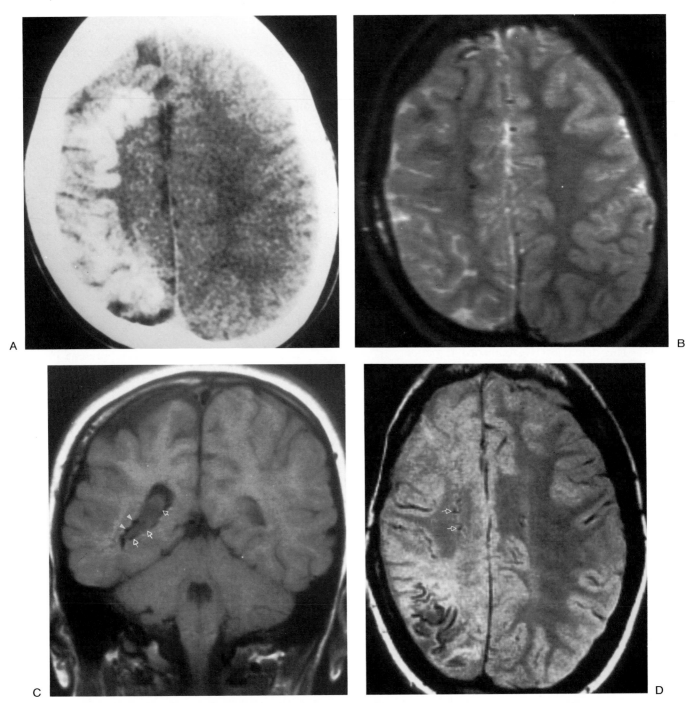

FIG. 6.29. Older child with Sturge-Weber syndrome. **A:** Axial noncontrast CT shows marked gyral calcification over most of the atrophic right cerebral hemisphere. When seen in conjunction with a port wine nevus, this finding is pathognomonic of Sturge-Weber disease. **B:** Axial SE 2500/70 image shows cortical atrophy and loss of underlying white matter. **C:** Coronal SE 600/20 image shows atrophy of the right hemisphere, prominent right choroid plexus (*arrows*), and dilated subependymal veins (*arrowheads*). The right side of the calvarium is thickened as a result of an enlarged diploic space. **D:** Axial SE 2800/30 image in a different patient shows atrophy of the right cerebral hemisphere, low signal intensity in the parieto-occipital cortex (as a result of cortical calcification), gliosis of the white matter, and dilated subependymal veins (*arrows*), as a result of shunting of cortical venous blood to the deep venous system.

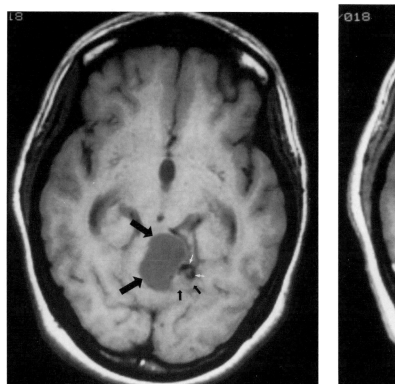
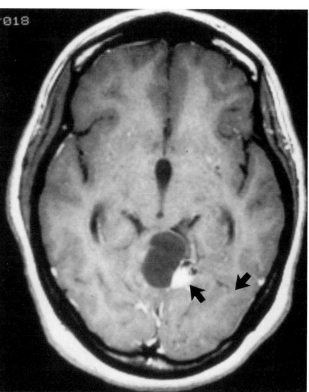

A   B

FIG. 6.30. Hemangioblastoma. **A:** Axial SE 600/20 image shows a cerebellar cyst (*large arrows*) with a mural nodule (*small black arrows*) containing a curvilinear flow void (*small white arrows*). **B:** Postcontrast image shows enhancement of the mural nodule (*arrows*).

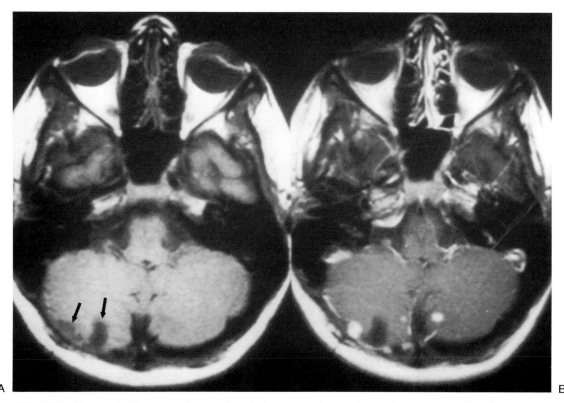

A   B

FIG. 6.31. Hemangioblastomas in von Hippel-Lindau syndrome. **A:** Axial noncontrast SE 600/16 image shows hypointensity (*arrows*) from prior surgery, but no evidence of recurrent tumor. **B:** Postcontrast scan shows multiple enhancing cerebellar tumors.

solid portions of tumor will enhance intensely (Figs. 6.31–6.33) (104). Angiography may still be performed to identify small tumor nodules within the wall of posterior fossa cysts and to identify other small hemangioblastomas that may be difficult to identify on imaging studies (80). The angiogram may also be of value if a surgical resection is required, as it will show the location and size of the arteries supplying the tumor. The angiographic appearance of the hemangioblastoma is highly characteristic, adding diagnostic specificity to a lesion that may be detected on CT/MR.

In the past, hemangioblastomas of the spinal cord were thought to be uncommon because of the rare clinical manifestations of spinal cord pathology in patients with von Hippel-Lindau disease. However, autopsy data suggest that these lesions may be more common than was previously suspected (10,98,99). Indeed, MR imaging demonstrates a considerably larger number and higher incidence of spinal cord hemangioblastomas than were previously felt to exist (103) (Fig. 6.32). Syringomyelia is present in the majority of patients with spinal cord hemangioblastoma; it is difficult to differentiate idiopathic syringomyelia from syringomyelia secondary to hemangioblastomas without the use of an MR contrast agent. Following intravenous administration of paramagnetic contrast, the tumor enhances markedly, facilitating the diagnosis (104,106). Another specific MR characteristic of spinal cord hemangioblastomas is the enlarged feeding and draining vessels that are manifest as serpiginous areas of flow void within the tumor (104,105).

Very rarely, hemangioblastomas may occur within the brain stem or the cerebral hemispheres (80,98,104). The radiographic appearance of these lesions is identical to that of the cerebellar or spinal cord hemangioblastomas. They may be cystic with a solid nodule or entirely solid; the solid portion shows curvilinear flow voids and marked contrast enhancement.

Visceral Manifestations of Von Hippel-Lindau Disease

Visceral lesions will be discussed briefly. The major visceral manifestation of this disease is the renal cell carcinoma, which occurs in up to 40% of patients. These tumors are frequently multicentric or bilateral (98). They occur later in life than most of the neurologic manifestations, with the average presentation during the fifth decade of life (99). Pheochromocytomas may be present in 10% to 15% of patients. Cysts occur in virtually all visceral organs, including the liver, omentum, mesentery, spleen, adrenal gland, and epididymis. Adenomas can occur in the liver and epididymis as well (99,102). Thus, affected patients must be evaluated with abdominal and pelvic imaging studies as well as neural axis imaging.

ATAXIA-TELANGIECTASIA

Clinical Manifestations

Ataxia-telangiectasia is an autosomal recessive disorder with an incidence of approximately one per 40,000 live births (107). The exact genetic abnormality is unknown; however, a high rate of spontaneous recombinations of DNA is found in affected patients, indicating that they may have defects in damage-sensitive cell cycle checkpoints. As a consequence, affected cells may replicate DNA or enter mitosis before repair of spontaneous DNA damage is complete (108). The disorder is characterized clinically by telangiectasias of the skin and eye, cerebellar ataxia, sinus and pulmonary infections, immunodeficiencies, and a propensity to develop malignancies (107,109,110). Affected patients usually present with cerebellar ataxia, which manifests itself when the child starts to walk. The ataxia is followed by a progressive neurologic deterioration. Eventually, the children are confined to a wheelchair and exhibit oculomotor abnormalities, dysarthric speech, choreoathetosis, endocrine abnormalities, and myoclonic jerks (107,109).

Characteristic skin changes (mucocutaneous telangiectasias) begin to appear between 3 and 6 years of age. They appear first on the bulbar conjunctiva and subsequently on the ears, face, neck, palate, dorsum of the hands, and antecubital and popliteal fossae. Other associated dermatologic changes can be seen as well (109,110). Recurrent bacterial and viral sinopulmonary infections occur in most patients, leading to bronchiectasis and pulmonary failure, the most common causes of death. Malignancies develop in 10% to 15% of affected patients (111). Lymphomas and leukemia predominate in younger patients, whereas epithelial malignancies occur much more frequently in adults (111,112).

Pathologic and Imaging Findings

The major neuropathologic finding in ataxia telangiectasia is degeneration of the cerebellar cortex. Neuronal degradation can be found in the vermis, the hemispheres, or both. The cause of this neuronal degeneration and atrophy has not been discovered; however, some authors have found associated cerebellar vascular anomalies, indicating a possible vascular etiology of the degenerative changes (109). Radiologically, the major abnormalities seen on both CT and MR are cerebellar cortical atrophy, manifested as diminished cerebellar size, dilatation of the fourth ventricle, and increased cerebellar folial prominence (80,113) (Fig. 6.34). More severe atrophy is associated with longer duration of the disease and more severe ataxia. Hemorrhage may occur as a result of rupture of parenchymal telangiectasias. Cerebral infarcts may result from emboli that are shunted through vascular malformations within the lungs.

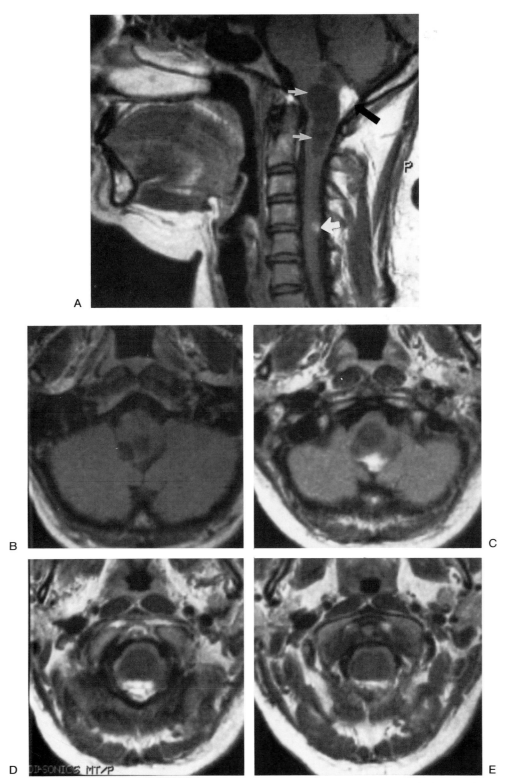

FIG. 6.32. Cervicomedullary and spinal cord hemangioblastomas in von Hippel-Lindau syndrome. **A:** Sagittal SE 500/25 image through the brain stem and spinal cord after IV contrast infusion. A cystic mass with an enhancing nodule is seen at the cervical-medullary junction with exophytic extension into the cisterna magna. A second lesion (*arrows*) is present at the C5-6 disk level dorsally. Both lesions were hemangioblastomas. The more caudal lesion was not clinically suspected. **B-E:** Axial images through the cervical-medullary junction shows the position of the mural nodule within the large cyst. The enhancing nodule can be well localized as a result of its marked contrast enhancement.

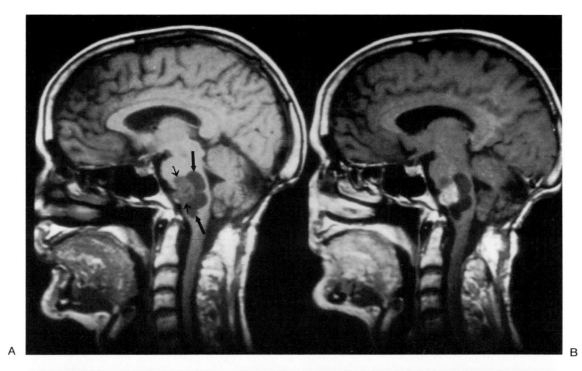

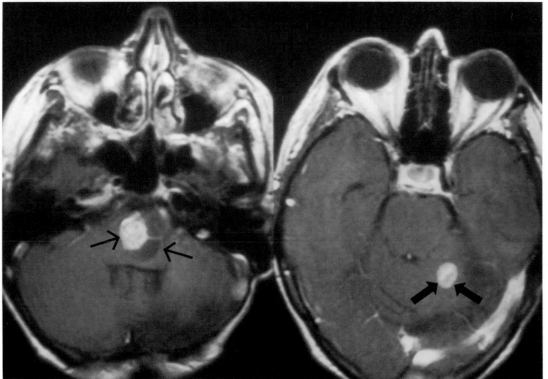

FIG. 6.33. Hemangioblastomas in von Hippel-Lindau syndrome. **A:** Sagittal SE 550/11 image shows a cystic mass (*large arrows*) with a mural nodule (*small arrows*) in the pons and medulla. The mural nodule contains curvilinear flow voids. The patient has had prior posterior fossa craniectomy for removal of cerebellar hemangioblastoma. **B:** After administration of paramagnetic contrast, the mural nodule enhances. **C:** Postcontrast axial image shows the enhancing pontomedullary tumor (*arrows*). **D:** Postcontrast axial image 15 mm superior to (C) shows a solid cerebellar hemangioblastoma (*arrows*).

When cerebellar atrophy is an isolated finding in a young child with cerebellar ataxia and progressive neurologic deterioration, the possible diagnosis of ataxia telangiectasia should be raised.

NEUROCUTANEOUS MELANOSIS

Clinical Criteria

Neurocutaneous melanosis was first described by Rokitansky, who reported a 14-year-old girl with a giant congenital melanocytic nevus and mental retardation who developed late-onset hydrocephalus (114). Since that initial report, nearly 100 cases have been reported. Giant congenital nevi are themselves a relatively rare birthmark, occurring in approximately one in 20,000–50,000 live births (115). Their cause is unknown, although they are thought to represent an error in morphogenesis of the embryonic neuroectoderm (115,116).

In 1972, Fox proposed the following criteria for diagnosing neurocutaneous melanosis: (1) unduly large or unusually numerous pigmented nevi in association with melanosis or melanoma of the pia-arachnoid; (2) no evidence of malignant change in any of the cutaneous lesions; and (3) no evidence of malignant melanoma in any organ apart from the meninges (115).

A revision of Fox's criteria has recently been proposed to define the population at risk more accurately (116): (1) large or multiple (three or more) congenital nevi in association with meningeal melanosis or CNS melanoma, where *large* is defined as a diameter equal to or greater than 20 cm in an adult, 9 cm on the scalp of an infant, or 6 cm on the body of an infant; (2) no evidence

of cutaneous melanoma, except in patients in whom the examined areas of the meningeal lesions are histologically benign; (3) no evidence of meningeal melanoma, except in patients in whom examined areas of the skin are histologically benign. Those cases with histologic confirmation are considered definite; all others are considered provisional diagnoses.

MR shows a high incidence of presence of foci of melanin in the brains of patients with giant cutaneous nevi. Thus, the incidence of neurocutaneous melanosis may be much higher than was previously suspected.

Pathologic Findings

Pathologists may find a substantial number of benign melanotic cells within the basilar meninges of normal patients at autopsy, as both melanocytes and the basilar pia-arachnoid derive from neural crest (117–119). Patients with NCM, however, have orders of magnitude more melanocytes, which may be distributed diffusely or demonstrate nodularity within the meninges (115,116). A number of potential explanations for the abnormal accumulation of melanocytes in the meninges have been proposed. These include (1) an abnormal migration of melanocyte precursors (120); (2) abnormal expression of melanin-producing genes within the leptomeningeal cells (121); or (3) a rapid proliferation of "normal" melanin-producing leptomeningeal cells. The abnormal melanin-producing cells are often present in the perivascular spaces along vessels that penetrate the brain from the basilar cisterns (115,116).

The anterior temporal lobes and cerebellum appear to be the most common locations for melanocytic accumu-

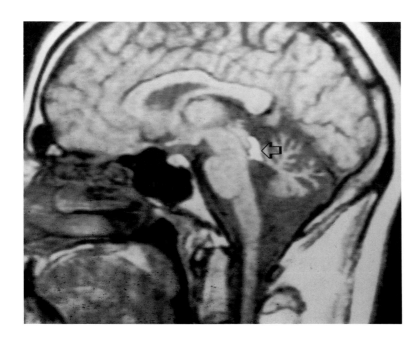

FIG. 6.34. Ataxia-telangiectasia. There is marked cerebellar atrophy. A posterior fossa hemorrhage is present (*arrow*), most likely resulting from rupture of a telangiectasia. (Courtesy Dr. K. Maravilla.)

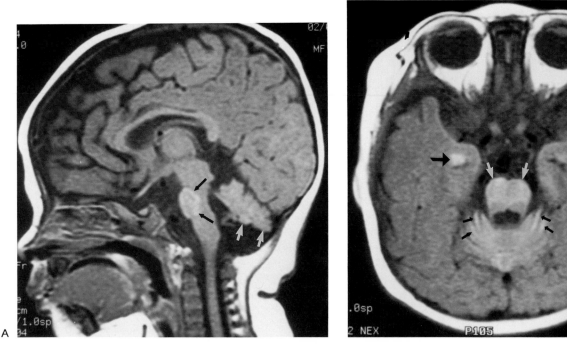

FIG. 6.35. Neurocutaneous melanosis. **A:** Sagittal SE 500/11 image shows hyperintensity in the basis pontis (*black arrows*) and cerebellar hypoplasia (*white arrows*). **B:** Axial SE 600/15 image shows hyperintense melanin deposits in the basis pontis (*white arrows*), right amygdala (*large black arrow*), and cerebellar folia (*small black arrows*).

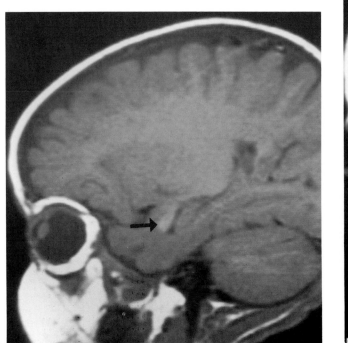

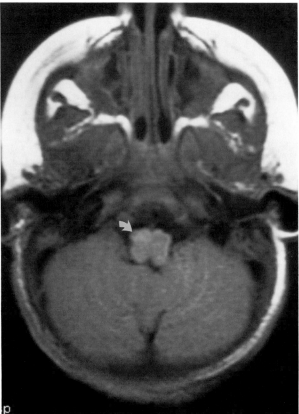

FIG. 6.36. Neurocutaneous melanosis. **A:** Parasagittal SE 600/15 image shows hyperintense focus of melanin (*arrow*) anterior to the temporal horn. **B:** Axial SE 600/16 image shows a focus of hyperintense melanin (*arrow*) in the right medullary pyramid.

lation in NCM (116,122–127). In the anterior temporal lobe, the amygdala seems particularly commonly affected (116,122,126–128). Other common locations include the thalami, cerebellum, and the base of the frontal lobe (116,122,128,129). It is likely that the melanocytes spread preferentially to these locations because of their close proximity to the basilar meninges.

Imaging Findings

CT scans in patients with neurocutaneous melanosis are normal unless a collection of melanocytes has converted into a melanoma. MR shows foci of T1, and sometimes T2, shortening in the brain parenchyma or meninges (Figs. 6.35, 6.36), signal characteristics that are compatible with deposits of melanin. The foci of abnormal signal are typically 3 cm or less in diameter; they are most commonly seen in the anterior temporal lobe, cerebellar nuclei, cerebellar white matter, and brain stem (Figs. 6.35, 6.36) (127,128,130). The T1 and T2 shortening is presumably the result of the presence of stable free radicals in melanin (identified by electron spin resonance studies (131,132)). The unpaired electrons in free radicals interact with water protons via an electron–proton/dipole–dipole interaction with subsequent shortening of both T1 and T2 relaxation times (133,134). Degeneration of the melanocytic accumulation into melanoma can only be determined by the identification of progressive growth of the lesion, by the presence of surrounding edema or mass effect, or by the presence of central necrosis (128). Some authors have identified abnormal meningeal enhancement on MR studies of patients with neurocutaneous melanosis (135), presumably resulting from the marked melanotic involvement of the meninges. However, this finding has not been confirmed in other studies, so the incidence of meningeal enhancement in affected patients is probably low. Other imaging findings in neurocutaneous melanosis include cerebellar (primarily vermian) hypoplasia (Fig. 6.35) (128,130), the Dandy-Walker malformation (129), and arachnoid cysts.

REFERENCES

1. Crowe FW, Schull WJ, et al. *A clinical, pathological, and genetic study of multiple neurofibromatosis.* Springfield, IL: Charles C Thomas, 1956.
2. Riccardi VM. Neurofibromatosis. *Neurol Clin* 1987;5:337–349.
3. Riccardi V. Neurofibromatosis: clinical heterogeneity. *Curr Probl Cancer* 1982;7:1–34.
4. Von Recklinghausen FD. Uber die multiplen Fibrome der Haut und ihre Beziehung zu den multiplen neuromen. In: Festschrift für Rudolf Virchow. Berlin: August Hirschwald, 1882.
5. Seizinger BR, Rouleau GA, Ozelins LJ, et al. Genetic linkage of von Recklinghausen neurofibromatosis to the nerve growth factor receptor gene. *Cell* 1987;49:589–594.
6. Berg BO. Neurocutaneous disorders. In: Berg BO, ed. *Neurologic manifestations of pediatrics.* Boston: Butterworth-Heinemann, 1992:485–498.
7. Berg BO. Current concepts of neurocutaneous disorders. *Brain Dev* 1991;13:9–20.
8. Huson SM, Harper PS, Compston DAS. Von Recklinghausen's neurofibromatosis: a clinical and population study in southeast Wales. *Brain* 1988;111:1355–1381.
9. Canale DJ, Bebin J. Von Recklinghausen disease of the nervous system. In: Vinken PJ, Bruyn GW, eds. *Handbook of clinical neurology: the phakomatoses.* Amsterdam: North-Holland, 1972:132–162.
10. DeRecondo J, Haguenau M. Neuropathologic survey of the phakomatoses and allied disorders. In: Vinken PJ, Bruyn GW, eds. *Handbook of clinical neurology: the phakomatoses.* Amsterdam: North-Holland, 1972:19–71.
11. Fletcher WA, Imes RK, Hoyt WF. Chiasmal gliomas: appearance and long-term changes demonstrated by computerized tomography. *J Neurosurg* 1986;65:154–159.
12. Alvord EC, Lufton S. Gliomas of the optic nerve or chiasm: outcome by patient's age, tumor site, and treatment. *J Neurosurg* 1988;68:85–98.
13. Simon JH, Szumowski J, Totterman S, et al. Fat suppression MR imaging of the orbit. *Am J Neurorad* 1988;9.
14. Parizel PM, Martin JJ, Van Vyre M, van den Hauwe L, De Schepper AM. Cerebral ganglioglioma and neurofibromatosis type 1. *Neuroradiology* 1991;33:357–359.
15. Hochstrasser H, Boltshauser E, Valavanis A. Brain tumors in children with Recklinghausen neurofibromatosis. *Neurofibromatosis* 1989;1:233–239.
16. Hosoda K, Kanazawa Y, Tanaka J, Tamaki N, Matsumoto S. Neurofibromatosis presenting with aqueductal stenosis due to a tumor of the aqueduct: case report. *Neurosurgery* 1986;19:1035–1037.
17. Pou-Serradell A, Ugarte-elola AC. Hydrocephalus in neurofibromatosis: contribution of MRI to its diagnosis. *Neurofibromatosis* 1989;2:218–226.
18. Afifi AK, Jacoby CG, Bell WE, Menezes AH. Aqueductal stenosis and neurofibromatosis: a rare association. *J Child Neurol* 1988;3:125–130.
19. Sobata E, Ohkuma H, Suzuki S. Cerebrovascular disorders associated with von Recklinghausen's neurofibromatosis. *Neurosurgery* 1988;22:544–549.
20. Sadeh M, Martinovits G, Goldhammer Y. Occurrence of both neurofibromatosis 1 and 2 in the same individual with a rapidly progressive course. *Neurology* 1989;39:282–283.
21. Michels VV, Whisnant JP, Garrity JA, Miller GM. Neurofibromatosis type 1 with bilateral acoustic neuromas. *Neurofibromatosis* 1989;2:213–217.
22. Is NF-1 always distinct from NF-2? (editorial). *Neurofibromatosis* 1989;2:193–194.
23. Smirniotopoulos JG, Murphy FM. The phakomatoses. *Am J Neuroradiol* 1992;13:725–736.
24. Burk DL, Brunberg JA, Kanal E, et al. Spinal and paraspinal neurofibromatosis: surface coil MR imaging at 1.5 T. *Radiology* 1987;162:797–801.
25. Brown EW, Riccardi VM, Mawad M, et al. MR imaging of optic pathways in patients with neurofibromatosis. *Am J Neuroradiol* 1987;8:1031–1035.
26. Aoki S, Barkovich AJ, Nishimura K, et al. Neurofibromatosis types 1 and 2: cranial MR findings. *Radiology* 1989;172:527–536.
27. Sevick RJ, Barkovich AJ, Edwards MSB, Koch T, Berg B, Lempert T. Evolution of white matter lesions in neurofibromatosis type 1: MR findings. *Am J Roentgenol* 1992;159:171–175.
28. Rubenstein LJ. The malformative central nervous system lesions in the central and peripheral forms of neurofibromatosis: a neuropathological study of 22 cases. In: Rubenstein AE, Bunge RP, Housman DE, eds. *Neurofibromatosis. Annals of the New York Academy of Sciences.* New York: New York Academy of Sciences, 1986:14–29.
29. Bognanno JR, Edwards MK, Lee TA, et al. Cranial MR imaging in neurofibromatosis. *Am J Neuroradiol* 1988;9:461–467.
30. Holt JF. Neuhauser lecture: neurofibromatosis in children. *Am J Roentengenol* 1978;130:615–639.
31. Barnes PD, Brody JD, Jaramillo D, Akbar JU, Emans JB. Atypi-

cal idiopathic scoliosis: MR imaging evaluation. *Radiology* 1993;186:247–253.

32. Halliday AL, Sobel RA, Martuza RL. Benign spinal nerve sheath tumors: their occurrence sporadically and in neurofibromatosis types 1 and 2. *J Neurosurg* 1991;74:248–253.

33. Suh J-S, Abenoza P, Galloway HR, Everson LI, Griffiths HJ. Peripheral (extracranial) nerve tumors: correlation of MR imaging and histologic findings. *Radiology* 1992;183:341–346.

34. Russell DS, Rubenstein LJ. Dysgenetic syndromes (phakomatoses) associated with tumors and hamartomas of the nervous system. In: Russell DS, Rubenstein LJ, eds. *Pathology of tumors of the nervous system*, 5th ed. Baltimore: Williams and Wilkins, 1989:766–784.

35. Kumar AJ, Kahadja FP, Martinez CR, et al. CT of extracranial nerve sheath tumors with pathological correlation. *J Comput Assist Tomogr* 1983;9:1037–1041.

36. Coleman BG, Arger PH, Dalinka MA, et al. CT of sarcomatous degeneration of neurofibromatosis. *Am J Roentengenol* 1983;140:383–387.

37. Miles J, Pennybacker J, Sheldon PH. Intrathoracic meningocele: its development and association with neurofibromatosis. *J Neurol Neurosurg Psychiatr* 1969;32:99–110.

38. Naidich TP, McLone DG, Harwood-Nash DC. Arachnoid cysts, paravertebral meningoceles, and perineural cysts. In: Newton TH, Potts DG, eds. *Computed tomography of the spine and spinal cord*. San Anselmo, CA: Clavedel, 1983:388–390.

39. Huson SM. The different forms of neurofibromatosis. *Br Med J* 1987;294:1113–1114.

40. Seizinger BR, Martuza RL, Gusella JF. Loss of genes on chromosome 22 in tumorogenesis of human acoustic neuroma. *Nature* 1986;322:664–667.

41. *Neurofibromatosis.* Presented at National Institutes of Health Consensus Development Conference. *Arch Neurol* 1988:575–578.

42. Serradell AP. Lésions centralées dans les neurofibromatoses: corrélations cliniques d'IRM et histopathologiques. *J Radiol* 1991;72:635–644.

43. Sze G, Abramson A, Krol G, et al. Gd-DTPA in the evaluation of intradural extramedullary spinal disease. *Am J Neuroradiol* 1989;9:153–163.

44. Valk J. Gd-DTPA in MR of spinal lesions. *Am J Neuroradiol* 1989;9:345–350.

45. Williams B. Progress in syringomyelia. *Neuro Res* 1986;8:130–145.

46. Sherman JL, Barkovich AJ, Citrin CM. The MR appearance of syringohydromyelia: new observations. *Am J Neuroradiol* 1986;7:985–995.

47. Castillo M, Quencer RM, Green BA, Montalvo BM. Syringomyelia as a consequence of compressive extramedullary lesions. *Am J Neuroradiol* 1987;8:973–978.

48. Nagahiro S, Matsukado Y, Kuratsu J, et al. Syringomyelia and syringobulbia associated with an ependymoma of the cauda equina involving the conus medullaris: case report. *Neurosurgery* 1986;18:357–360.

49. Gomez MR. *Tuberous sclerosis*, 2nd ed. New York: Raven, 1988.

50. Bender BL, Yunis EJ. The pathology of tuberous sclerosis. *Pathol Ann* 1982;17:339–382.

51. Donegani G, Grattarola FR, Wildi E. Tuberous sclerosis: Bourneville disease. In: Vinken PJ, Bruyn GW, eds. *Handbook of clinical neurology: the phakomatoses*. Amsterdam: North-Holland, 1972:

52. Seidenwurm DJ, Barkovich AJ. Understanding tuberous sclerosis. *Radiology* 1992;183:23–24.

53. Stefansson K, Wollmann RL, Huttenlocher PR. Lineages of cells in the central nervous system. In: Gomez MR, ed. *Tuberous sclerosis*, 2nd ed. New York: Raven, 1988:75–87.

54. Braffman BH, Bilaniuk LT, Naidich TP, et al. MR imaging of tuberous sclerosis: pathogenesis of this phakomatosis, use of gadopentate dimeglumine, and literature review. *Radiology* 1992;183:227–238.

55. Hanno R, Beck R. Tuberous sclerosis. *Neurol Clin* 1987;5:351–360.

56. Kingsley DPE, Kendall BE, Fitz CR. Tuberous sclerosis: a clinicoradiological evaluation of 110 cases with particular reference to atypical presentation. *Neuroradiology* 1986;28:171–190.

57. Lagos JC, Gomez MR. Tuberous sclerosis: reappraisal of a clinical entity. *Mayo Clin Proc* 1967;42:26–49.

58. Hurwitz S, Braverman IM. White spots in tuberous sclerosis. *J Pediatr* 1970;77:587–594.

59. Bell SD, MacDonald DM. The prevalence of café-au-lait patches in tuberous sclerosis. *Clin Exp Dermatol* 1985;10:562–565.

60. Nyboer JH, Robertson DM, Gomez MR. Retinal lesions in tuberous sclerosis. *Arch Opthalmol* 1976;94:1277–1280.

61. Hedges TR III, Pozzi-Mucelli R, Char DH, Newton TH. CT demonstration of ocular calcification: correlations with clinical and pathological findings. *Neuroradiology* 1982;23:15–21.

62. Christophe C, Bartholome J, Blum D, et al. Neonatal tuberous sclerosis. US, CT, and MR diagnosis of brain and cardiac lesions. *Pediatr Radiol* 1989;19:446–448.

63. Altman NR, Purser RK, Post MJD. Tuberous sclerosis: characteristics at CT and MR imaging. *Radiology* 1988;167:527–532.

64. Martin N, de Brouker T, Cambier J, Marsault C, Nahum H. MRI evaluation of tuberous sclerosis. *Neuroradiology* 1987;29:437–443.

65. Wippold FJ II, Baber WW, Gado M, Tobben PJ, Bartnicke BJ. Pre- and postcontrast MR studies in tuberous sclerosis. *J Comput Assist Tomogr* 1992;16:69–72.

66. Martin N, Debussche C, De Broucker T, Mompoint D, Marsault C, Nahum H. Gadolinium-DTPA enhanced MR imaging in tuberous sclerosis. *Neuroradiology* 1990;31:492–497.

67. Tsuchida T, Kamata K, Kwamata M, et al. Brain tumors in tuberous sclerosis. *Childs Brain* 1981;8:271–283.

68. Morimoto K, Mogami H. Sequential study of subependymal giant cell astrocytoma associated with tuberous sclerosis. *J Neurosurg* 1986;65:874–877.

69. Wilms G, van Wijck E, Demaerel PH, Smet M-H, Plets C, Brucher JM. Gyriform calcifications in tuberous sclerosis simulating the appearance of Sturge-Weber disease. *Am J Neuroradiol* 1992;13:295–297.

70. Henkelman MH, Watts JF, Kucharczyk W. High signal intensity in MR images of calcified brain tissue. *Radiology* 1991;179:199–206.

71. Inoue Y, Nakajima S, Fukuda P, et al. Magnetic resonance images of tuberous sclerosis: further observations and clinical correlations. *Neuroradiology* 1988;30:379–384.

72. Barkovich AJ, Gressens P, Evrard P. Formation, maturation, and disorders of brain neocortex. *Am J Neuroradiol* 1992;13:423–446.

73. Chonko AM, Weiss SM, Stein JH, et al. Renal involvement in tuberous sclerosis. *Am J Med* 1974;56:124–132.

74. Alexander GL. Sturge-Weber syndrome. In: Vinken PJ, Bruyn GW, eds. *Handbook of clinical neurology: the phakomatoses*. Amsterdam: North-Holland, 1972:223–240.

75. Roach ES. Diagnosis and management of neurocutaneous syndromes. *Semin Neurol* 1988;8:83–96.

76. Gorman MJ, Snead OC. Sturge-Weber syndrome without portwine nevus. *Pediatrics* 1977;60:785–786.

77. Pascual-Castroviejo I, Diaz-Gonzalez C, Garcia-Melian R, Gonzalez-Casado I, Muñoz-Hiraldo E. Sturge-Weber syndrome: study of 40 patients. *Pediatr Neurol* 1993;9:283–288.

78. Streeter GL. The developmental alterations in the vascular system of the brain of the human embryo. *Contrib Embryol Carneg Inst* 1918;8:5–38.

79. Wohlwill F, Yakovlev PI. Histopathology of meningo-facial angiomatosis (Weber disease): report of four cases. *J Neuropathol Exp Neurol* 1957;16:341–364.

80. Gardeur D, Palmieri A, Mashaly R. Cranial computed tomography in the phakomatoses. *Neuroradiology* 1983;25:293–304.

81. Sperner J, Schmauser I, Bittner R, et al. MR imaging findings in children with Sturge-Weber syndrome. *Neuropediatrics* 1990;21:146–152.

82. Benedikt RA, Brown DC, Walker R, Ghaed V, Mitchell M, Geyer CA. Sturge-Weber syndrome: cranial MR imaging with Gd-DTPA. *Am J Neuroradiol* 1993;14:409–415.

83. Coulam CM, Brown LR, Reese DF. Sturge-Weber syndrome. *Semin Roentgenol* 1976;11:55–59.

84. Stimac GK, Solomon MA, Newton TH. CT and MR of angiomatous malformations of the choroid plexus in patients with Sturge-Weber disease. *Am J Neuroradiol* 1986;7:623–627.

85. Jacoby CG, Yuh WTC, Afifi AK, Bell WE, Schelper RL, Sato Y. Accelerated myelination in early Sturge-Weber syndrome demonstrated by MR imaging. *J Comput Assist Tomogr* 1987;11:226-231.
86. Bentson JR, Wilson GH, Newton TH. Cerebral venous drainage pattern of the Sturge-Weber syndrome. *Radiology* 1971;102:111-118.
87. Kendall BE, Kingsley D. The value of CAT in craniocerebral malformations. *Br J Radiol* 1978;51:171-190.
88. Bilaniuk LT, Zimmerman RA, Hochman M, et al. MR of the Sturge-Weber syndrome. *Am J Neuroradiol* 1987;8:945-950.
89. Enzmann DR, Hayward RW, Norman D, Dunn RP. Cranial computed tomographic scan appearance of Sturge-Weber disease: unusual presentation. *Radiology* 1977;122:721-724.
90. Probst FP. Vascular morphology and angiographic flow patterns in Sturge-Weber angiomatosis: facts, thoughts and suggestions. *Neuroradiology* 1980;20:73-78.
91. Chugani HT, Mazziota JC, Phelps ME. Sturge-Weber syndrome: a study of cerebral glucose utilization with positron emission tomography. *J Pediatr* 1989;114:244-253.
92. Peterman AF, Hayles AB, Dockerty MB, Love JG. Encephalotrigeminal angiomatosis (Sturge-Weber Disease). *JAMA* 1958;167:2169-2176.
93. Williams DW III, Elster AD. Cranial CT and MR in Klippel-Trenaunay-Weber syndrome. *Am J Neuroradiol* 1992;13:291-294.
94. Venes JL, Linder S. Sturge-Weber-Dimitri syndrome. In: Edwards MSB, Hoffman HJ, eds. *Cerebral vascular disease in children and adolescents.* Baltimore: Williams and Wilkins, 1988:337-341.
95. Anlar B, Yalaz K, Erzen C. Klippel-Trenaunay-Weber syndrome: a case with cerebral and cerebellar atrophy. *Neuroradiology* 1988;30:360.
96. Von Hippel EV. Ueber eine sehr seltene Erkrankung der Netzhaut. *Albrecht von Graefes Archiv für Ophthalmologie* 1904;59:83-106.
97. Lindau A. Studien über Kleinhirncysten. Bau, Pathogenese und Beziehungen zur Angiomatosis retinae. *Acta Pathol Microbiol Scand* 1926;Suppl 1:1-128.
98. Grossman M, Melmon KL. Von Hippel-Lindau disease. In: Vinken PJ, Bruyn GW, eds. *Handbook of clinical neurology: the phakomatoses.* Amsterdam: North-Holland, 1972:241-259.
99. Horton WA, Wong V, Eldridge R. Von Hippel-Lindau disease. *Arch Int Med* 1976;136:769-777.
100. Latif F, Tory K, Gnarra J, et al. Identification of the von Hippel-Lindau disease tumor suppressor gene. *Science* 1993;260:1317-1320.
101. Huson SM, Harper PS, Hourihan MD, et al. Cerebellar hemangioblastoma and von Hippel-Lindau disease. *Brain* 1986;109:1297-1310.
102. Fill WL, Lamiell JM, Polk NO. The radiographic manifestations of von Hippel-Lindau disease. *Radiology* 1979;133:289-295.
103. Sato Y, Waziri M, Smith W, et al. Hippel-Lindau disease: MR imaging. *Radiology* 1988;166:241-246.
104. Ho VB, Smirniotopoulos JG, Murphy FM, Rushing EJ. Radiologic-pathologic correlation: hemangioblastoma. *Am J Neuroradiol* 1992;13:1343-1352.
105. Lee DR, Sanches J, Mark AS, Dillon WP, Norman D, Newton TH. Posterior fossa hemangioblastomas: MR imaging. *Radiology* 1989;171:463-468.
106. Bydder GM, Brown J, Niendorf HP, Young IR. Enhancement of cervical intraspinal tumors in MR imaging with IV Gd-DTPA. *J Comput Assist Tomogr* 1985;9:847-851.
107. Paller AS. Ataxia-Telangiectasia. *Neurol Clin* 1987;5:447-449.
108. Meyn MS. High spontaneous intrachromosomal recombination rates in ataxia-telangiectasia. *Science* 1993;260:1327-1330.
109. Sedgwick RP, Boder E. Ataxia-Telangiectasia. In: Vinken PJ, Bruyn GW, eds. *Handbook of clinical neurology: the phakomatosis.* Amsterdam: North-Holland, 1972:267-334.
110. Hosking G. Ataxia-telangiectasia. *Develop Med Child Neurol* 1982;24:77-80.
111. Frizzera G, Rosai J, Dehner LP, et al. Lymphoreticular disorders in primary immunodeficiencies: new findings based on up-to-date histologic classification of 35 cases. *Cancer* 1980;46:692-699.
112. Boder E. Ataxia-telangiectasia: an overview. In: Gatti RA, Swift M, eds. *Ataxia-telangiectasia: genetics, neuropathology, and immunology of a degenerative disease of childhood.* New York: Allen R Liss, 1985:1-63.
113. Sardanelli F, Pittiglio G, Mavilio N, et al. Sindrome di Louis-Bar, atassia-teleangiectasia: quadro clinica e tomografico MR in 4 casi. *Acta Neuroradiol* 1991;5:261-264.
114. Rokitansky J. Ein ausgezeichneter Fall von Pigment-Mal mit ausgebreiteter Pigmentierung der inneren Hirn- und Rüchenmarkshaute. *Allg Wien Med Z* 1861;6:113-116.
115. Fox H. Neurocutaneous melanosis. In: Vincken PJ, Bruyn GW, eds. *The phakomatoses.* New York: Elsevier, 1972:414-428.
116. Kadonaga JN, Frieden IJ. Neurocutaneous melanosis: definition and review of the literature. *Acad Dermatol* 1991;24:747-755.
117. Le Douarin N. *The neural crest.* Cambridge: Cambridge University Press, 1982.
118. O'Rahilly R, Muller F. The meninges in human development. *J Neuropathol Exp Neurol* 1986;45:588-608.
119. Yu H, Tsaur K, Chein C, et al. Neurocutaneous melanosis: electron microscopic comparison of the pigmented melanocytic nevi of skin and meningeal melanosis. *J Dermatol* 1985;12:267-276.
120. Stern CD, Artinger KB, Bronner-Fraser M. Tissue interactions affecting the migration and differentiation of neural crest cells in the chick embryo. *Development* 1991;113:207-216.
121. Kitamuira K, Takiguchi-Hayashi K, Sezaki M, Yamamoto H, Takeuchi T. Avian neural crest cells express a melanogenic trait during early migration from the neural tube: observations with the new monoclonal antibody, "MEBL-1." *Development* 1992;114:367-378.
122. Fox H, Emery JL, Goodbody RA, Yates PO. Neuro-cutaneous melanosis. *Arch Dis Child* 1964;39:508-516.
123. Fischer S. Primary perivascular cerebral, cerebellar and leptomeningeal melanoma. *Acta Psychiatr Scand* 1956;31:21-34.
124. Adeyanju M, Reyes MG, Junaid AT. Fatal pneumococcal infection in neurocutaneous melanosis. *J Child Neurol* 1988;3:293-294.
125. Lamas E, Diez Lobato R, Lotelo T, Ricoy JR, Castro S. Neurocutaneous melanosis: report of a case and review of the literature. *Acta Neurochir* 1977;36:93-105.
126. Thomas CS, Toone BK, Rose PE. Neurocutaneous melanosis and psychosis. *Am J Psychiatr* 1988;145:649-650.
127. Sebag G, Dubois J, Pfister P, Brunelle F, St-Rose C. Neurocutaneous melanosis and temporal lobe tumor in a child: MR study. *Am J Neuroradiol* 1991;12:699-700.
128. Barkovich AJ, Frieden I, Williams M. MR of neurocutaneous melanosis. *Am J Neuroradiol* (in press).
129. Kadonaga DJ, Barkovich AJ, Edwards MSB, Frieden IJ. Neurocutaneous melanosis in association with the Dandy-Walker malformation. *Pediatr Dermatol* 1992;9:37-43.
130. Ko S-F, Wang H-S, Lui T-N, Ng S-H, Ho Y-S, Tsai C-C. Neurocutaneous melanosis associated with inferior vermian hypoplasia: MR findings. *J Comput Assist Tomogr* 1993;17:691-695.
131. Sealy RC. Radicals in melanin biochemistry. *Methods Enzymol* 1984;105:479-483.
132. Jimbow K, Miyake Y, Homma K, et al. Characterization of melanogenesis and morphogenesis of melanosomes by physiochemical properties of melanin and melanosomes in malignant melanoma. *Cancer Res* 1984;44:1128-1134.
133. Burton DR, Forsen S, Karlstrom G, Dwek RA. Proton relaxation enhancement in biochemistry: a critical survey. *Prog NMR Spectroscopy* 1979;13:1-45.
134. Gomori JM, Grossman RI, Shields JA, Augsburger JJ, Joseph PM, DeSimeone D. Choroidal melanomas: correlation of NMR spectroscopy and MR imaging. *Radiology* 1986;158:443-445.
135. Rhodes RE, Riedman HS, Hatter HP Jr, Hockenberger B, Oakes WJ, Tomita T. Contrast-enhanced MR imaging of neurocutaneous melanosis. *Am J Neuroradiol* 1991;12:380-382.

CHAPTER **7**

Brain Tumors of Childhood

IDENTIFICATION OF BRAIN TUMORS IN PEDIATRIC PATIENTS

Brain tumors during childhood account for 15% to 20% of all primary brain tumors. CNS tumors are the second most common pediatric tumor, being exceeded only by leukemia (1,2). In most large series, posterior fossa tumors and supratentorial tumors occur with nearly equal frequency (3–6). However, supratentorial tumors are more common in the first 2–3 years of life, whereas infratentorial tumors predominate from ages 4 to 11 (3–10). Both locations develop tumors with equal frequency in children older than 10 years.

The symptoms of children with CNS tumors depend upon the age at the time of presentation. Infants present with increasing head circumference, nausea, vomiting, and lethargy (5). Children often have the same presenting symptoms and signs; in addition, they may complain of headache, seizures, or decreased visual acuity and develop focal neurologic signs, such as cranial nerve palsies, truncal and limb ataxia, and hemiparesis. Tumors developing in the region of the hypothalamus frequently produce endocrine dysfunction, such as diabetes insipidus, growth failure, or precocious puberty.

Masses are typically recognized on CT or MR on the basis of either density or signal intensity differences from normal brain, with mass effect causing distortion of normal brain structure, or the presence of abnormal enhancement after the intravenous administration of contrast. (In the normal central nervous system, contrast enhancement is only seen in the pituitary gland, pituitary stalk and its point of origin from the hypothalamus, pineal gland, and the choroid plexuses.) Almost all brain tumors are hypodense compared to normal brain on noncontrast CT images, hypointense to myelinated white matter on T1-weighted MR images, and hyperintense to myelinated white matter on T2-weighted MR images. Hemorrhage, necrosis, calcifications, and patterns and intensity of contrast enhancement vary among tumors of similar histologic class, and even more so among tumors of different cell type; these characteristics will be discussed more thoroughly later in the present chapter. All tumors exhibit mass effect. In the case of relatively slow-growing, peripheral tumors, the mass effect results in expansion or erosion of the cranial vault. In more rapidly growing, more central tumors, the effect is a displacement of structures. Displacement may result in herniation of brain tissue through or around rigid structures, such as the falx cerebri, tentorium cerebelli, or foramen magnum. Supratentorial masses typically cause herniation downward, through the tentorial incisura, whereas infratentorial masses cause upward tentorial herniation. Transtentorial herniation classically results in pressure on the midbrain, with secondary effects on eye movement and pupillary constriction (the "blown pupil"). Tentorial herniation may also result in compression of the posterior cerebral arteries between the midbrain and the tentorium, and consequent unilateral or bilateral infarction of the posterior cerebral artery distribution. Herniation of the cerebellar tonsils through the foramen magnum can occur with both supra- and infratentorial masses; tonsillar herniation, which is easily detected by MR, can lead to respiratory compromise.

If a mass is identified, it must be determined whether the lesion is intra- or extraparenchymal. In other words, does the mass arise from brain parenchyma or from extraparenchymal structures, such as meninges, choroid plexus, or the subarachnoid space? Extraparenchymal lesions typically displace, rather than invade, normal brain structures (Fig. 7.1); the brain may be displaced away from bone or dura, resulting in an enlarged cistern. Intraparenchymal masses tend to compress cisterns and sulci. A well-defined margin separates the extraparenchymal mass from the brain; usually, little or no edema surrounds the mass. Intraparenchymal masses often merge imperceptibly into the normal surrounding brain

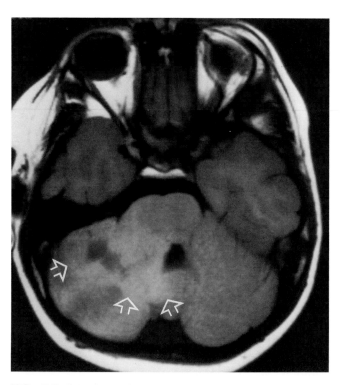

FIG. 7.2. Intraparenchymal tumor. Cerebellar glioma (arrows) blends imperceptibly into the surrounding brain. Mass effect compresses adjacent sulci.

(Fig 7.2) and may generate considerable edema. Other characteristics that are suggestive of an extraparenchymal origin are a relative paucity of mass effect for the size of the lesion, extension of the mass across the midline without involving a cerebral commissure, and relatively mild presenting symptoms. The reader should be aware, however, that the differentiation of intra- and extraparenchymal masses is not always easy. Intraparenchymal masses may be exophytic in nature, thereby enlarging the adjacent cistern, whereas extraparenchymal masses may invade the brain and elicit edema. Intraparenchymal masses may grow slowly and generate relatively little mass effect. However, the general rules outlined previously will allow determination of tumor origin in most cases.

Once the lesion is determined to be intraparenchymal, it must be determined whether the lesion is, in fact, a neoplasm. Infection and infarction can closely mimic the appearance of a neoplasm and must always be considered, at least momentarily, in the differential diagnosis. Cerebral abscesses (see Chapter 11) are intraparenchymal masses that are characterized by very rapid growth and by enhancing rims with a smooth inner margin; tumors typically grow more slowly and have more irregular enhancing rims. Infarctions are differentiated from tumors by location in a vascular distribution and involvement of both gray and white matter; tumors and infections typically originate in white matter or at the

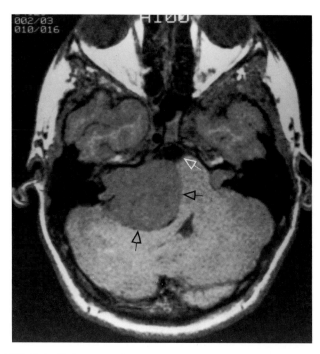

FIG. 7.1. Extraparenchymal tumor. Acoustic schwannomas in patient with neurofibromatosis type II. The tumors are sharply marginated (black arrows). The mass pushes brain away from the petrous bone, enlarging the cerebellopontine angle cistern (white arrow).

gray–white junction. However, some tumors are primarily cortical and have an imaging appearance that is identical to acute infarction. If differentiation is problematic based on imaging and clinical criteria, a follow-up study should be obtained before a biopsy. If the abnormality is an infarction, enhancement will develop within 5 days and mass effect will diminish by the end of the first week. Abscesses grow rapidly and the enhancing rim becomes better defined; tumors are unlikely to change during the 7-day period.

TECHNIQUES OF IMAGING PEDIATRIC BRAIN TUMORS

Although CT is probably the imaging method used most commonly for the initial diagnosis of intracranial neoplasms, MR is being used for preoperative evaluation with increasing frequency because the multiplanar imaging capability is extremely useful in determining the exact extent of the tumor and its relationship to surrounding normal structures. MR is particularly useful in the analysis of tumors of the posterior fossa, in which artifact from the surrounding bone hinders CT analysis. Moreover, MR is more sensitive than CT for the detection of tumor spread via the subarachnoid spaces, which is particularly common in pediatric tumors (11–13).

When CT is used as the method of radiologic evaluation, the patient should be scanned both with and without intravenous contrast in the axial plane. When the tumor originates in the posterior fossa, coronal images, either direct or reformatted, are often useful to evaluate the relationship of the tumor to the tentorium and the foramen magnum. Coronal images are particularly helpful in the evaluation of small lesions situated near dura or bone. Reformatted sagittal images may aid in evaluation of tumor of the midline structures, such as the third ventricle. The recommended contrast dose in these patients is 3 mg/kg of contrast (concentration 300 mg I_2/ml) up to a maximum dose of 120 ml. This is usually given in a single bolus immediately prior to the scan.

For MR evaluation, the standard sequence is sagittal T1-weighted images followed by axial T2-weighted spin echo or fast spin echo images (see Chapter 2 for more explicit imaging factors). Sequences should use a slice thickness of 5 mm or less and cover the entire brain. Supplemental T1-weighted images in either the coronal or axial plane can then be obtained through the tumor for better definition of its extent and relationship to surrounding normal structures. Postcontrast images should then be obtained in planes that are judged to be optimal from the precontrast studies. Generally, brain stem, suprasellar, and third- or fourth-ventricular masses are best imaged in the sagittal and coronal planes. Cerebral hemispheric masses are best imaged in the axial and coronal planes. Cerebellar hemispheric masses are best evaluated in the axial and coronal planes.

When paramagnetic contrast is used, it is administered in a dose of 0.1 mg/kg body weight, given as an intravenous bolus immediately prior to the study. It is important always to administer the contrast agent at the same time relative to scanning, as delays allow the contrast to diffuse farther in the extracellular space, resulting in larger regions of enhancement. Thus, variation in the time interval may result in a false interpretation of change in tumor size based on extent of enhancement. Flow compensation techniques (peripheral or cardiac gating, or gradient moment nulling) are useful when the tumor is in the posterior fossa, as spatial misregistration of the contrast-enhanced flowing blood will otherwise obscure vital areas. When imaging the spine for detection of drop metastases, sagittal 3 mm (or less) T1-weighted sections should be obtained prior to and following contrast administration. In the lumbar spine, fat saturation techniques are valuable in differentiating enhancing tumor from epidural fat (13).

CT is often more specific than MR for the prediction of tumor cell type. Small round cell tumors, such as germinomas and medulloblastomas, for example, are isodense or hyperdense compared with brain parenchyma prior to contrast administration, whereas astrocytomas of childhood are almost always hypodense. Therefore, suprasellar germinomas can be differentiated from suprasellar astrocytomas and medulloblastomas from cerebellar astrocytomas by CT. This differentiation is more difficult when using MR. The presence of calcifications, which can be a helpful factor in the characterization of craniopharyngiomas and teratomas, is more easily detected by CT than by MR. Other tumor characteristics, such as the presence of blood, are more readily detected by MR. The added anatomic information in terms of tumor extent and tumor spread provided by MR seems to more than compensate for the occasional reduction of preoperative histologic specificity (13).

In general, arteriography is not used for the evaluation of neoplasms unless a highly vascular lesion is suspected based on vascular flow voids seen on MR or in the unlikely situation that a vascular malformation cannot be ruled out by noninvasive studies. Arteriography may also be useful if noninvasive studies cannot clearly differentiate a dural-based lesion from a parenchymal lesion, a situation that usually arises in very large tumors. Because large tumors can parasitize blood flow, however, arteriography can be misleading, demonstrating dural vessels supplying intra-axial lesions or intracerebral vessels feeding extra-axial tumors.

Postoperative follow-up generally consists of both noncontrast and contrast-enhanced CT or MR scans in the immediate postoperative period (usually within 72 hours of surgery). Immediate evaluation by CT is especially indicated for any patient with delayed recovery from anesthesia or with a severe or unexpected postoperative neurologic defect. The timing of subsequent scans will depend on the child's clinical course and management protocol.

After the immediate postoperative period, the first imaging study should consist of both T1- and T2-weighted precontrast images and T1-weighted images after administration of contrast. The precontrast images are required to differentiate postoperative hemorrhage from residual enhancing tumor (14). Enhancement at the operative bed, usually in the form of a thin rim of enhancement, can be seen within 24 hours of tumor resection (15). The amount of enhancement at the tumor site increases rapidly during the postoperative period; thus, early imaging (in the first 72 hours) is important for assessing the extent of resection. Surgically induced enhancement at the operative margins progressively decreases on sequential exams after about 6 weeks and will generally disappear completely within 12 months (15). Meningeal and parenchymal enhancement are almost always seen on contrast-enhanced postoperative MR studies. Dural enhancement can be thin or thick but is usually smooth, is present over the cerebral convexities and along the tentorium, and may persist for 20 years or more (15,16). Nodular meningeal enhancement should raise suspicion for subarachnoid tumor spread.

One final important note concerns imaging of posterior fossa tumors. As mentioned earlier, misregistration of signal from flowing blood can cause artifacts, especially when the T1 relaxation time of the blood is decreased by intravenous administration of paramagnetic contrast. When looking for tumor recurrence or tumor spread in the postoperative patient, particularly in the posterior fossa, these artifacts are especially problematic. High doses of contrast may increase the magnitude of the artifact. Therefore, flow compensation techniques, through either gradient pulses or gating, are essential on postcontrast scans. A delay of 15–30 min after contrast administration may reduce the artifact, as the intravascular contrast will be reduced by redistribution; however, a price is paid in terms of increased imaging time.

POSTERIOR FOSSA TUMORS

Medulloblastomas (Primitive Neuroectodermal Tumor of the Posterior Fossa)

Medulloblastomas are highly malignant tumors composed of very primitive, undifferentiated small, round cells. These undifferentiated cells were given the name *medulloblast* by P. Bailey and Cushing in the early 1900s, hence the name *medulloblastoma* (17). Medulloblastomas are the most common posterior fossa tumor in children in most series, being slightly more common than the cerebellar astrocytoma. They comprise 15% to 20% of intracranial neoplasms in children and 30% to 40% of posterior fossa neoplasms in children (5,18,19). Males are affected two to four times as frequently as females. Approximately 40% of patients with medulloblastoma present within the first 5 years of life; 75% are seen in the first decade of life.

The duration of symptoms for patients with medulloblastoma is usually short; approximately half will have symptoms for less than 1 month prior to diagnosis. The most common symptoms are nausea, vomiting, and headaches. The high incidence of vomiting may be related to growth of the tumor in proximity to the area postrema, the emetic center of the brain, which is located near the inferior aspect of the fourth ventricle. In patients under a year of age, increasing head size is a frequent presenting symptom. In older children and adults, ataxia is the symptom that usually initiates medical attention. Rarely, paraparesis or symptoms referable to the cauda equina will result from tumor dissemination and necessitate medical evaluation (5,20).

Pathology

In contrast to adolescents and adults, in whom medulloblastomas are most often found in the cerebellar hemispheres, approximately two-thirds of medulloblastomas in children are located in the vermis. The tumor usually forms a well-defined vermian mass widening the space between the cerebellar tonsils. Anteriorly, it impinges upon the roof of the fourth ventricle and causes partial or complete obstruction to CSF flow. Posteriorly, it may project into the cisterna magna and extend downward to the level of the upper cervical cord (5,18). Occasionally, the tumor will extend laterally through the foramina of Luschka into the cerebellopontine angle cisterns. Invasion of the brain stem is seen in approximately one-third of patients, usually resulting from direct extension across the fourth ventricle (21). Invasion of the leptomeninges via dissemination along CSF pathways is frequent, with estimates as high as 100% of all cases (22–25). Intracranially, subarachnoid tumor spread is seen most prominently within the Sylvian fissures and at the base of the skull. Pathologically, subarachnoid tumor appears as small, grayish patches of tumor or as a continuous "frosting" of tumor on the pia. Retrograde spread through the aqueduct into the lateral and third ventricles can occur as well. From any of these sites, tumor may reinvade the cortex. Drop metastases to the spinal subarachnoid space and cauda equina are seen in approximately 40% of patients, most commonly at the thoracic and lumbosacral levels (22–25). Rarely, intramedullary metastases have been reported, presumably as a result of tumor dissemination into the central canal of the spinal cord. Systemic metastases are rare and have most commonly been seen at tumor recurrence. The skeleton is the most common site of involvement, followed by lymph nodes and lung (22).

Histologically, approximately half of these tumors are of the classic type, composed entirely of completely undifferentiated cells, whereas 25% are of the desmoplastic variety. Another 20% to 25% show glial or neuronal differentiation within the tumor, which may impart a poorer prognosis (26,27).

Imaging Studies

Classically, a typical medulloblastoma appears on CT as a well-defined, hyperdense tumor of the vermis (Fig. 7.3) or vermis and hemisphere. Isolated involvement of the hemisphere is rare and most commonly seen in adolescents and adults. As a result of their composition of small, round cells with a high nuclear-to-cytoplasmic ratio, medulloblastomas are almost always hyperdense or isodense, compared to surrounding brain, prior to the

administration of intravenous contrast. Mild to moderate edema surrounds the tumor in approximately 90% of patients. Hydrocephalus is present in approximately 95% of patients at the time of presentation. Enhancement, most commonly diffuse but sometimes patchy (3,28), is seen in greater than 90% of medulloblastomas.

Although the presence of cysts and calcifications was at one time thought to be unusual in medulloblastomas, recent series have revealed "atypical" features in 60% of CT studies, including calcification in up to 20% and cystic or necrotic, nonenhancing regions in close to 50% (Figs. 7.4, 7.5) (28,29). The presence of intratumoral hemorrhage is very uncommon. Although the presence of cystic, nonenhancing regions within the tumors may sway the radiologist toward the diagnosis of astrocytoma, it should be noted that the solid portions of astrocytomas are usually hypodense prior to the administration of IV contrast, whereas medulloblastomas are mostly isodense to hyperdense precontrast (Fig. 7.3A) (3). In the author's experience, the density of the tumor on the precontrast CT scan is the most reliable means of differentiating these tumors.

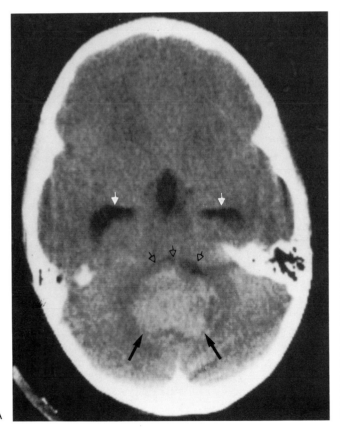

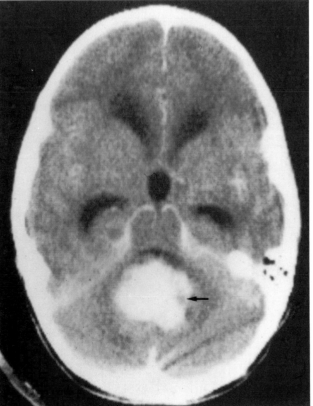

A

B

FIG. 7.3. Medulloblastoma. **A:** Noncontrast CT shows a high-density mass in the cerebellar vermis (*black arrows*) that is compressing the fourth ventricle (*open black arrows*). The dilated temporal horns (*white arrows*) show that hydrocephalus is present. **B:** After infusion of iodinated contrast, the tumor is seen to enhance markedly. A small lucent area on the left edge of the tumor (*arrow*) probably represents a focus of necrosis.

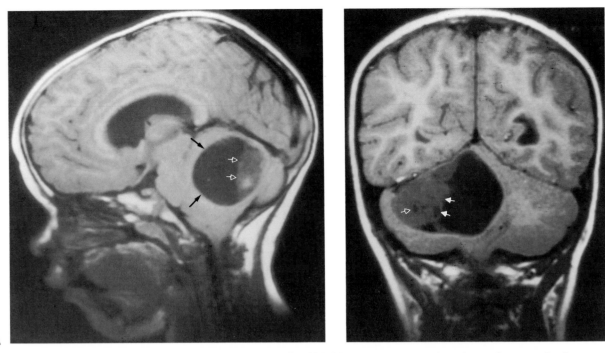

A

B

FIG. 7.4. Cystic medulloblastoma. **A:** Sagittal SE 600/20 image shows a largely cystic tumor in the cerebellar midline (*closed arrows*) with a solid portion located in the dorsal aspect of the cyst (*open arrows*). **B:** Coronal SE 600/20 image shows the dorsal solid portion of the tumor to be heterogeneous (*arrows*). This heterogeneity was previously thought to be uncommon in medulloblastomas but is increasingly being recognized.

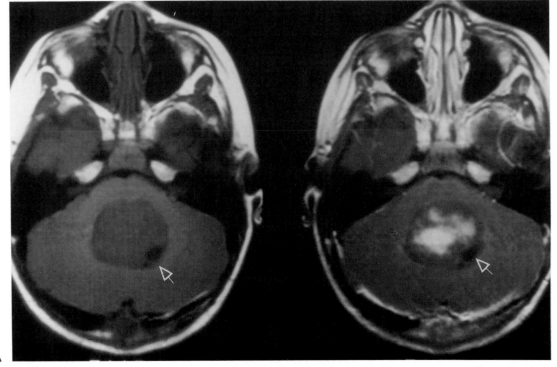

A

B

FIG. 7.5. Medulloblastoma. Unenhanced **(A)** and enhanced **(B)** T1-weighted images show a cystic component in the left posterolateral aspect of the tumor (*arrow*). The tumor incompletely enhances.

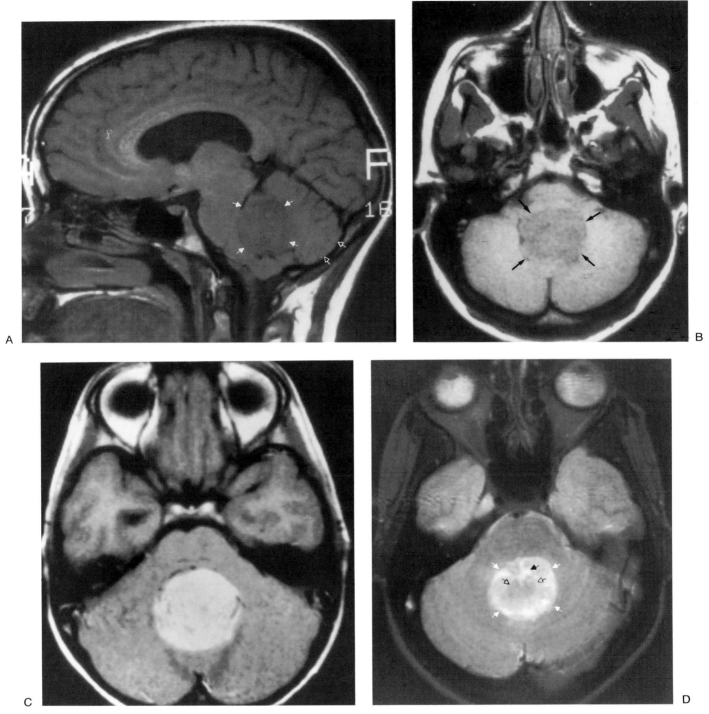

FIG. 7.6. Typical medulloblastoma. **A:** Sagittal SE 600/20 image shows a mass that is slightly lower in intensity than brain parenchyma sitting in the fourth ventricle (*arrows*). The cerebellar folia and fissures are somewhat poorly defined (*open arrows*). This is a common finding in medulloblastomas, probably because tumor spread has already occurred at the time of diagnosis. **B:** Axial SE 600/20 image shows the tumor mass sitting within the inferior fourth ventricle (*arrows*). **C:** Postcontrast axial SE 600/20 image shows uniform tumor enhancement. **D:** Axial SE 2000/80 image shows the tumor to be of slightly mixed signal intensity. The outer rim of high signal intensity most likely represents edema (*white arrows*). The mixed signal intensity central to the edema probably represents combinations of necrosis (high signal intensity; *closed black arrow*) and solid tumor (low signal intensity; *open black arrows*).

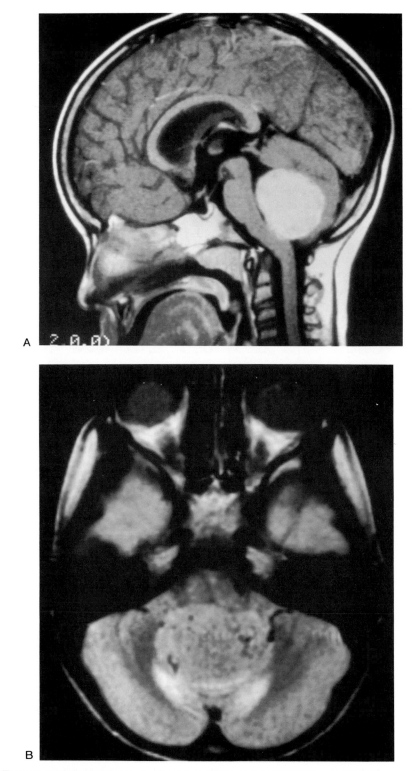

FIG. 7.7. Typical medulloblastoma. **A:** Contrast-enhanced sagittal T1-weighted image shows the uniformly enhancing tumor in the fourth ventricle. The aqueduct, third ventricle, and lateral ventricles are enlarged because of obstruction by the tumor. **B:** SE 2500/80 image show that the tumor is isointense with gray matter. The areas of hypointensity within the tumor were enlarged vessels.

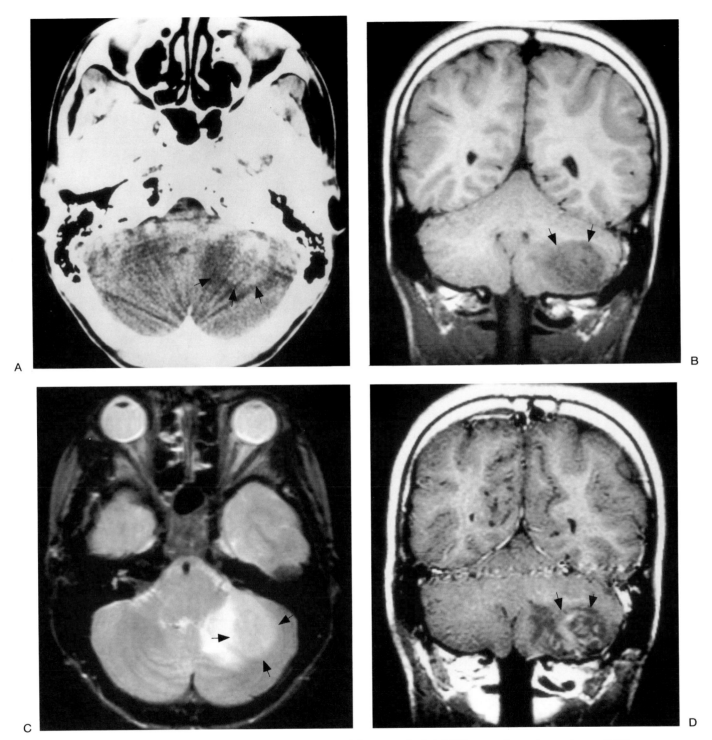

FIG. 7.8. Hemispheric medulloblastoma in an adolescent. **A:** Axial CT scan shows hyperdense mass (*arrows*) with surrounding edema in left cerebellar hemisphere. **B:** Coronal SE 616/15 image shows the mass (*arrows*) to be hypointense compared to surrounding brain. **C:** On axial SE 2500/80 image, the tumor (*arrows*) is isointense to gray matter and surrounded by hyperintense edema. **D:** Postcontrast SE 616/15 image shows heterogeneous enhancement of the tumor (*arrows*).

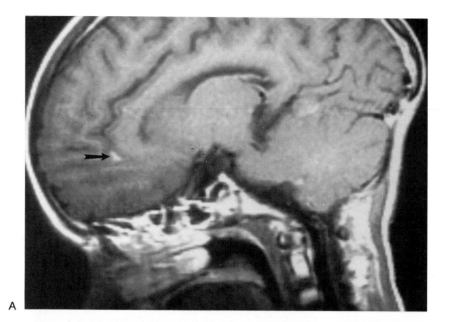

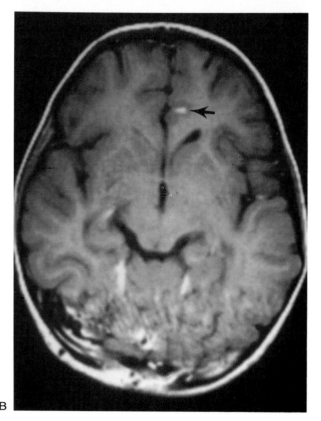

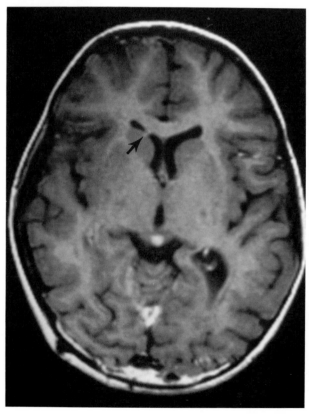

FIG. 7.9. Metastatic medulloblastoma. **A:** Sagittal SE 600/20 image after contrast enhancement shows high signal intensity in the frontal subarachnoid space (*arrow*). This high signal intensity represents enhancing metastatic tumor that has spread through the cerebrospinal fluid. **B:** Axial SE 600/20 image confirms the metastatic tumor spread (*arrow*). **C:** Axial SE 600/20 image 7.5 mm more cephalad shows a second metastatic focus in the right frontal horn (*arrow*).

The appearance of medulloblastoma on MR is variable and nonspecific. Tumor location and patient age are the most important factors in prospectively making the correct diagnosis. The most common appearance is of a hypointense mass compared with normal brain on short TR/TE images. The tumors are most commonly situated inferiorly within the vermis and can sometimes be seen originating from the inferior medullary velum (Figs. 7.6, 7.7). T2-weighted sequences typically reveal a heterogeneous hypo- or isointense (compared to gray matter) mass (Figs. 7.6, 7.7). The signal intensity presumably relates to the increased nuclear-to-cytoplasmic ratio of the tumor cells and, hence, to the reduced amount of free water within the tumor. Less free water results in a shortened T2 relaxation time and, hence, lower signal intensity on long TR, long TE images. The heterogeneity probably results from the aforementioned cysts and calcification (30). The enhancement pattern of the tumors after intravenous infusion of paramagnetic contrast is variable; enhancement may be uniform (Figs. 7.6, 7.7) or patchy (Fig. 7.5). Signal and enhancement characteristics of hemispheric medulloblastomas, seen in adolescents and adults, are similar to those of fourth-ventricular medulloblastomas seen in children (Fig. 7.8). One finding that has been helpful in identifying medulloblastomas on MR images has been to look at the distinctness of the cerebellar folia and fissures on the midline sagittal images. Because medulloblastomas spread so readily through the CSF, tumor coating the cerebellum often causes the fissures to appear effaced and the folia to appear blurred (Fig. 7.6A).

CSF spread of tumor is very poorly evaluated by MR without contrast. Therefore, paramagnetic contrast should be used in the evaluation of these patients both prior to and after resection of the tumor. The most common locations for intracranial metastases are the vermian cisterns, subependymal region of the lateral ventricles, and subfrontal region (Figs. 7.9–7.12). MR is, properly, replacing plain film and CT myelography to evaluate for the presence of drop metastases to the spinal cord or the cauda equina (11,12). On contrast-enhanced MR, drop metastases appear as brightly enhancing foci in the extramedullary, intradural, and, occasionally, intramedullary space (Figs. 7.9, 7.12). In the first few weeks after posterior fossa craniectomy, however, artifacts, presumably from spinal subdural collection and perhaps from "leakage" of contrast into the subarachnoid space, are common (31). *These artifacts can be very difficult to differentiate from CSF spread of tumor. These problems are best avoided by staging the tumor preoperatively with pre- and postcontrast scans of the brain and spine.*

Cerebellar Astrocytomas

Astrocytomas are the most common brain tumor in children, accounting for 40% to 50% of primary intra-

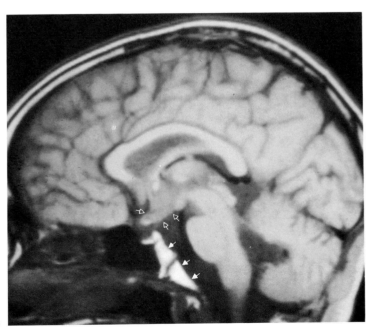
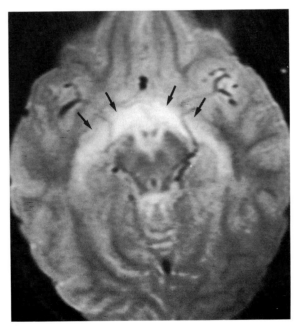

A   B

FIG. 7.10. Metastatic medulloblastoma. **A:** The patient has undergone a suboccipital craniectomy for tumor removal. The high signal intensity in the clivus (*closed white arrows*) is a result of fatty replacement secondary to radiation therapy. A soft tissue mass is seen in the anterior recesses of the third ventricle (*open white arrows*). **B:** Axial SE 2500/70 image shows high signal intensity from tumor extending posteriorly along the optic tracts (*arrows*).

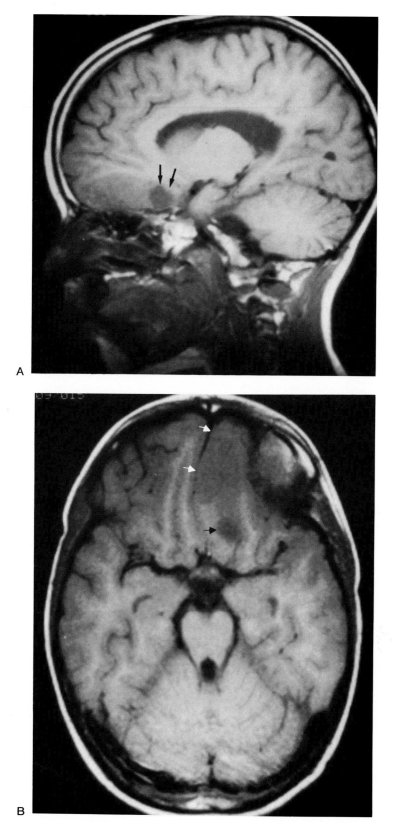

FIG. 7.11. Metastatic medulloblastoma. **A:** Parasagittal SE 600/20 image shows heterogeneous low signal intensity in the subfrontal region (*arrows*). **B:** Axial SE 600/20 shows diffuse low signal intensity in the region of the left gyrus rectus (*white arrows*), probably representing tumor and edema, and a cystic area (*black arrow*) that was necrotic tumor.

cranial neoplasms in this age group (3,5,6,18). Approximately 60% of astrocytomas in children are located in the posterior fossa, with 40% in the cerebellum and 20% in the brain stem. Astrocytomas have commonly been pathologically divided into four grades of malignancy, with the grade I lesions being the most benign and the grade IV lesions the most malignant (i.e., glioblastoma multiforme). At UCSF we use a different classification based on the degree of cellular anaplasia. Tumors are classified as astrocytoma, moderately anaplastic astrocytoma, highly anaplastic astrocytoma, or glioblastoma multiforme. Most cerebellar astrocytomas in children are of a specific histologic type, the juvenile pilocytic variety (JPA), which is considered a unique tumor and is generally separated from the classification listed earlier. JPAs are the most benign tumors of the CNS (19). Malignant astrocytomas of the cerebellum, even glioblastomas, however, can and do occur in children.

Juvenile pilocytic astrocytomas present with equal frequency in males and females. The peak incidence of these tumors is from birth to 9 years of age (32). Anaplastic astrocytomas (approximately 25% of pediatric cerebellar astrocytomas) are more common in older children, usually in the first half of the second decade (19,32). In general, patients with cerebellar astrocytomas, regardless of the histologic characteristics, present

with early morning headache and vomiting, which waxes and wanes over a period of months and finally becomes persistent and acute (5). Cerebellar signs, such as truncal ataxia or dysdiadochokinesia, will frequently localize the lesions to the cerebellum. Patients with cystic JPAs have an excellent prognosis, with a 25-year survival rate of nearly 90% (6). The 25% of patients with the solid cerebellar astrocytoma have a more guarded prognosis, with a 25-year survival rate of approximately 40% (6). With either variety, malignant transformation of benign cerebellar astrocytomas is exceedingly rare.

Pathology

Most cerebellar astrocytomas of childhood originate in the midline; they extend into the cerebellar hemispheres in approximately 30% of cases (18,19,33). Approximately 15% of these tumors involve only the cerebellar hemispheres. Cerebellar astrocytomas can be cystic, solid, or solid with a necrotic center (5,18,34). Most frequently, the cystic lesions have a tumor nodule found within the cyst wall; the remainder of the wall consists of nonneoplastic, compressed cerebellar tissue. Cystic astrocytomas with mural nodules account for approximately half of all cerebellar astrocytomas (3,5,18,34).

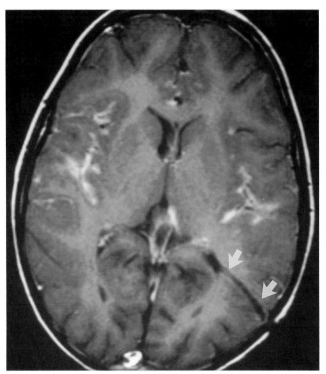
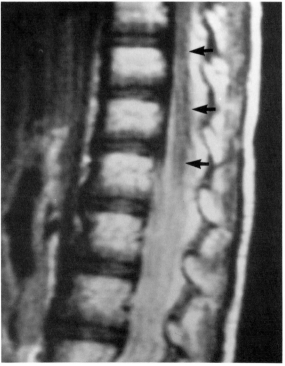

A

B

FIG. 7.12. Metastatic medulloblastoma. **A:** Axial SE 550/15 image shows enhancement in the subarachnoid space of the Sylvian fissures and callosal and cingulate sulci anteriorly. The curvilinear hypointensity (*arrows*) in the left temporo-occipital region is a shunt catheter. **B:** Postcontrast sagittal SE 500/15 image of the lumbar spine shows marked T1 shortening of the subarachnoid space, surrounding the spinal cord (*arrows*). The subarachnoid space was filled with tumor.

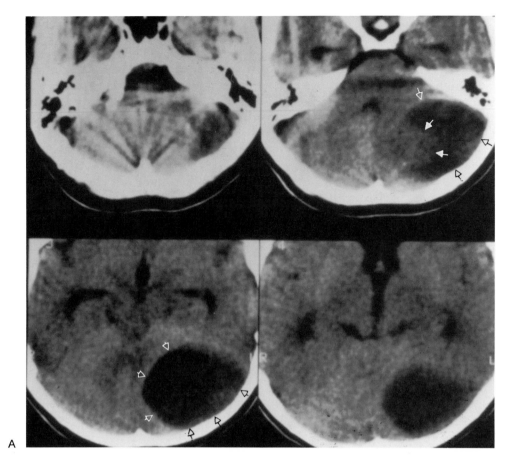

A

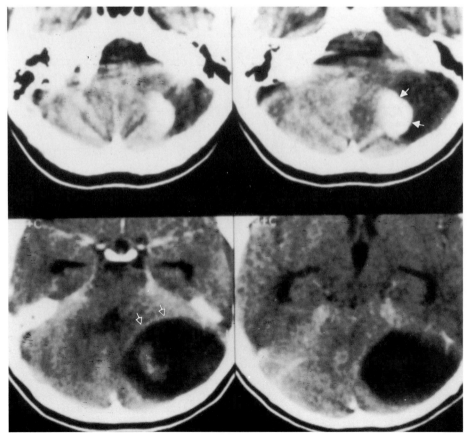

B

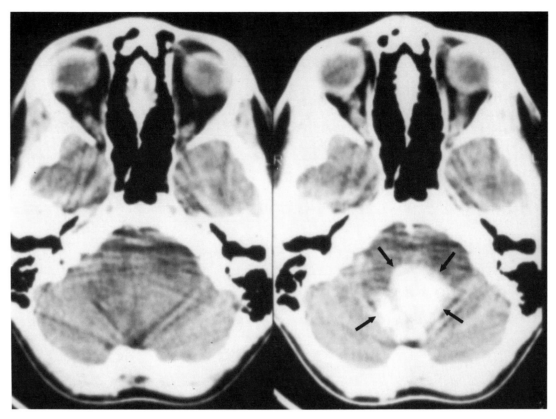

FIG. 7.14. Solid vermian astrocytoma. Noncontrast **(left)** and contrast-enhanced **(right)** CT scans through the cerebellum show an isodense vermian mass that completely obliterates the fourth ventricle. The mass is difficult to see on the noncontrast scan. After contrast administration, the tumor is seen to enhance uniformly (*arrows*).

Another 40% to 45% of cerebellar astrocytomas are composed of a rim of solid tumor with a cystlike, necrotic center. Necrosis of the tumor center is sometimes incomplete and on occasion results in a polycystic appearance (34). Nonnecrotic solid tumors are seen in less than 10%. The gross appearance does not correlate with histologic type (32).

Calcification is seen on histologic examination in 20% of cerebellar astrocytomas, most commonly in the solid variety. Tumoral hemorrhage is very rare. The tumor is usually large at the time of presentation, with an average diameter of more than 5 cm (18,19).

Pilocytic astrocytomas differ from most low-grade astrocytomas histologically in that the endothelial cells within the tumor have open tight junctions and fenes-

trations (35). The imaging implications of these "holes" in the vascular walls are a very profound enhancement of the tumors (see later).

Imaging Studies

Cerebellar astrocytomas are easily diagnosed by either CT or magnetic resonance. The typical appearance is that of a large vermian or hemispheric tumor that is predominantly cystic. The solid portion of the tumor is usually isodense or hypodense to normal brain tissue on noncontrast CT. Contrast enhancement is usually irregular, with half of the lesions showing mixed attenuation (3). In addition to the heterogeneities caused by cysts and

FIG. 7.13. Juvenile pilocytic astrocytoma of the cerebellum. **A:** Images from a noncontrast CT through the cerebellum. There is a cystic lesion involving the left cerebellar hemisphere (*open arrows*). A solid nodule of tumor that is of lower attenuation than surrounding cerebellum is located within the medial aspect of the cyst (*closed arrows*). **B:** After infusion of iodinated contrast, the nodule in the medial wall of the cyst is seen to enhance uniformly (*closed arrows*). The cyst wall does not enhance. The slight increased intensity seen in the ventral wall of the cyst (*open arrows*) results from compression of adjacent brain tissue.

tumor necrosis, heterogeneous enhancement is seen in the solid portion of the tumor; some degree of contrast enhancement is virtually always present (3). Tumors of pilocytic cytology show intense enhancement of their solid portions (36).

When the tumor is cystic with a mural nodule, the cyst is round or oval, whereas the mural nodule may be round, oval, or plaquelike. After infusion of IV contrast, the nodule shows an intense, homogeneous tumor blush (Fig. 7.13). The wall of the cyst may appear slightly hyperdense on CT because of the compressed cerebellar tissue, but it does not enhance; in these instances, pathology of the cyst wall almost never reveals tumor (6) (Fig. 7.13). When the cyst results from necrosis of a solid astrocytoma, it may be unilocular or multilocular. A well-defined mural nodule is not seen; instead, the entire circumference of the cyst is composed of tumor (3,6,37). Tumor enhancement surrounds the cyst and extends into the cerebellum, beyond the contour of the cyst. Solid tumors are usually round to oval, lobulated, and fairly well-defined masses that are iso- to hypointense precontrast and that show heterogeneous to homogeneous enhancement (Fig. 7.14). Rarely, no enhancement is discernible; nonenhancing tumors are essentially never of pilocytic histology.

The MR appearance of cerebellar astrocytomas is variable, depending upon the gross pathologic appearance. Solid and cystic components are identified, just as on CT. In general, solid portions appear as low-signal-intensity masses (although not as low as CSF) on T1-weighted sequences and as high-intensity masses (although not as high as CSF) on T2-weighted sequences (Figs. 7.15, 7.16). Solid portions of tumor will enhance with paramagnetic contrast in an identical fashion to their enhancement with iodinated contrast on CT. It is sometimes difficult to differentiate a solid from a cystic mass with noncontrast MR when the solid portion of the tumor is homogeneous. A tumor should not be called cystic merely because it demonstrates homogeneous low signal intensity on T1-weighted and homogeneous high signal intensity on T2-weighted images. Further evidence, such as wave forms from fluid pulsations or fluid–fluid levels should be sought to make this differentiation reliable.

Ependymomas

Ependymomas constitute 8% to 9% of primary CNS neoplasms in children and approximately 15% of poste-

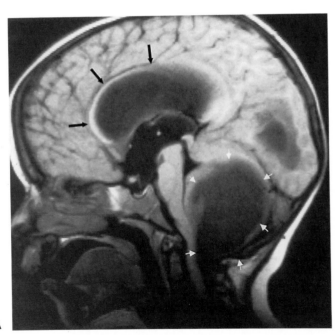

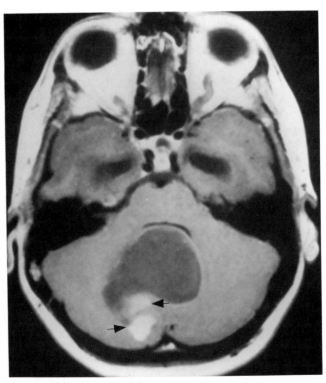

A   B

FIG. 7.15. Cystic juvenile pilocytic astrocytoma. **A:** Sagittal SE 500/40 image shows a large cystic mass involving the midline cerebellum (*white arrows*). Hydrocephalus is present, as indicated by the marked dilatation of the lateral and third ventricles and stretching of the corpus callosum (*black arrows*). **B:** Postcontrast SE 550/15 image through the posterior fossa in a different patient shows a large cystic mass occupying the vermis and extending into both cerebellar hemispheres. Enhancing mural nodules (*arrows*) are present posteriorly.

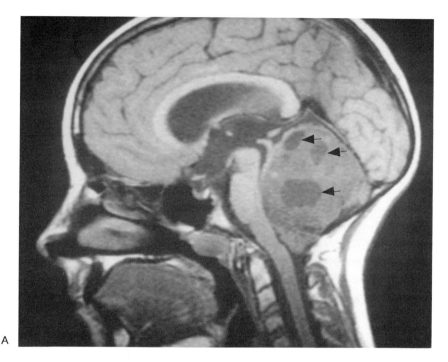

A

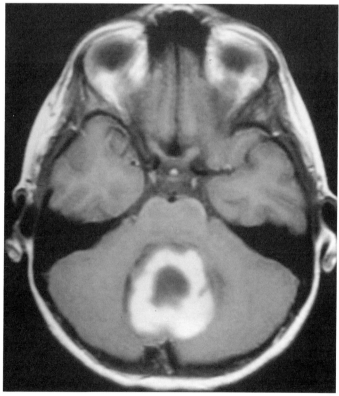

B

FIG. 7.16. Solid juvenile pilocytic astrocytoma with central necrosis. **A:** Sagittal SE 600/16 image shows large cerebellar mass with central foci of hypointensity (*arrows*). Obstructive hydrocephalus is present. **B:** Postcontrast scan shows that the solid portion of the tumor enhances uniformly, as characteristic of pilocytic astrocytomas. The central nonenhancing region is necrotic tumor.

rior fossa tumors in children. In childhood, intracranial ependymomas are more commonly infratentorial (70%) than supratentorial (30%). There is a slightly increased preponderance in males (38–40). Ependymomas of the posterior fossa have two age peaks, the first occurring between the ages of 1 and 5 years and the second in the mid-30s. Patients with ependymomas of the posterior fossa frequently present with a long clinical history. The delay in diagnosis probably results from the insidious onset of symptoms. The most common symptom is increased intracranial pressure (resulting from tumor obstructing the fourth ventricle), which develops in 90% of patients. Cerebellar signs, such as ataxia, are frequently present; motor and sensory deficits are uncommon (5,20).

Pathology

Ependymomas derive from differentiated ependymal cells that line the floor and roof of the fourth ventricle, extending into both lateral recesses and the foramina of Luschka. Additional ependymal cell rests are sometimes found far from ventricular linings, particularly in those areas where the ventricles are sharply angled, posterior to the occipital horns, and along the tela choroidia (19). Tumors may therefore originate either from the ependyma within the ventricles or from these ependymal cell rests.

Although most ependymomas are solid in nature, approximately 20% are very soft and deformable. Therefore, in contradistinction to most brain tumors (which grow as steadily enlarging masses), ependymomas can insinuate themselves through the subarachnoid spaces and around blood vessels and nerves, often surrounding and engulfing structures. Moreover, ependymomas tend to grow through the ventricular wall and become very adherent to surrounding brain. As a result of their adherence to surrounding brain and infiltrative growth pattern, ependymomas are quite difficult to cure; removal of the entire tumor is uncommon and the recurrence rate is high (5,20).

Ependymomas frequently grow out of the fourth ventricle and into surrounding cisterns and foramina. Approximately 15% extend into the cerebellopontine angles through the foramina of Luschka, and up to 60% grow through the foramina of Magendie into the cisterna magna, through the foramen magnum, and into the cervical spinal canal. Moreover, 30% to 40% of ependymomas invade the cerebellar parenchyma, permitting additional extension into the cerebellopontine angle. Occasionally, ependymomas of the cerebellopontine (C-P) angle can arise without evidence of tumor within the fourth ventricle or lateral recess, presumably originating from ependymal rests within the C-P angles (5,18,19).

Subarachnoid metastatic spread of benign ependymomas via cerebrospinal fluid is uncommon (approximately 10% to 12%) and correlates with histology (41).

When subarachnoid seeding is present, the presence of an anaplastic ependymoma or an ependymoblastoma should be suspected. Pathologically, calcification is seen in up to 50% of posterior fossa ependymomas; cysts are present in approximately 20% of patients (38).

Imaging Studies

The most characteristic appearance of a posterior fossa ependymoma on CT is that of an iso- to hyperdense fourth-ventricular mass with punctate calcifications, small cysts, and moderate enhancement with intravenous contrast (Fig. 7.17) (3,6). Extension of the tumor through the foramen of Luschka into the cerebellopontine angle or through the foramen magnum into the cervical spinal canal further supports the diagnosis of ependymoma.

On noncontrast CT, ependymomas are most commonly isodense with brain. Small lucencies are seen within the tumor in approximately 15% of cases, and nearly 50% will exhibit multifocal, small calcifications (Figs. 7.17, 7.18); large, clumplike calcifications are occasionally seen. Intratumoral hemorrhage can be seen in approximately 10% of patients. Infusion of IV contrast results in mild to moderate, heterogeneous enhancement of the solid portion of the tumor (3,40) (Figs. 7.17, 7.18).

Ependymomas may be heterogeneous on MR as well. T1-weighted images commonly reveal a slightly hypointense mass with respect to brain parenchyma with foci of marked hypointensity (Fig. 7.17). T2-weighted images reveal foci of high intensity (necrotic areas or cysts) and low intensity (calcifications or hemorrhage) within the tumor mass (Fig. 7.19). Fluid–fluid levels can sometimes be seen within the cysts. However, ependymomas may be homogeneous on all imaging sequences. The diagnosis of ependymoma is therefore difficult to make on the basis of signal characteristics. The most important imaging finding to identify ependymomas are extension of the tumor through the foramen of Magendie and the foramen magnum into the cervical canal dorsal to the cervical spinal cord (Figs. 7.17, 7.19). Similarly, extension of tumor through the foramen of Luschka (Fig. 7.19) into the cerebellopontine angle with insinuation around blood vessels and cranial nerves supports the diagnosis of ependymoma. The reader should note, however, that medulloblastomas can mimic this appearance. Astrocytomas involving the medulla frequently extend into the cervical spinal canal but are intramedullary (i.e., within the cord, not dorsal to it).

¹H MR Spectroscopy of Medulloblastomas, Cerebellar Astrocytomas, and Ependymomas

The literature contains little information about quantitation of spectra of pediatric brain tumors. However,

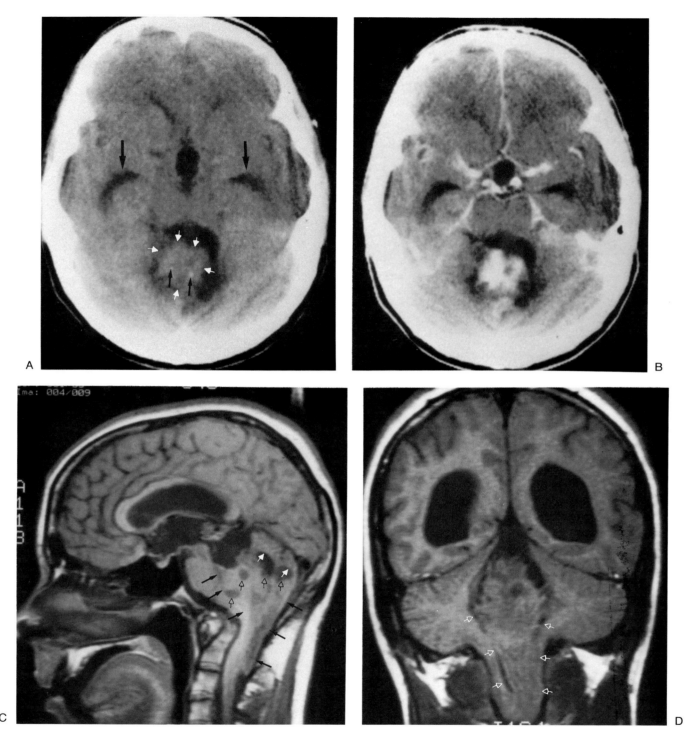

FIG. 7.17. Ependymoma. **A:** Noncontrast CT shows a mass within the fourth ventricle (*closed white arrows*). Punctate calcifications are seen within the mass (*small black arrows*). The temporal horns are dilated (*large black arrows*), confirming the presence of hydrocephalus. **B:** After infusion of iodinated contrast, the tumor heterogeneously enhances. **C:** Sagittal SE 600/20 image shows the tumor sitting within the fourth ventricle (*closed black arrows*) and extending down below the foramen magnum. Multiple cysts are seen within the tumor mass (*open black arrows*). The vermis is pushed superiorly by the mass (*white arrows*). **D:** The coronal SE 600/20 image shows the heterogeneous tumor extending inferiorly into the cervical spinal canal (*arrows*).

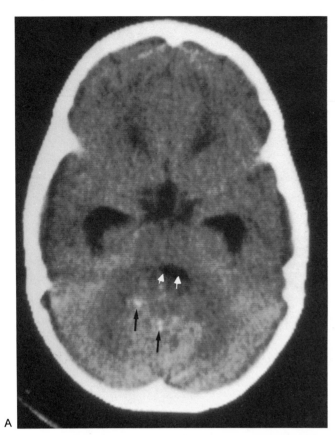 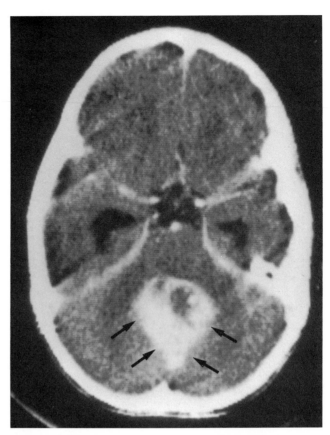

FIG. 7.18. Ependymoma. **A:** Axial noncontrast CT scan shows the heterogeneous tumor which is largely isodense with brain parenchyma compresses the fourth ventricle (*white arrows*). Multiple punctate calcifications are present (*black arrows*). **B:** After infusion of intravenous contrast, there is heterogeneous enhancement of the tumor (*arrows*).

some good, albeit preliminary, qualitative data have been reported on the spectra of pediatric cerebellar brain tumors (42). Proton spectra of normal cerebellum in the pediatric patient yields NAA/Cho > 1.7 and Cr/NAA > 1.1. Medulloblastomas usually yield NAA/Cho between 0 and 0.4, and Cr/NAA between 0 and 0.5. Low-grade astrocytomas and ependymomas typically have values between those of medulloblastomas and those of normal cerebellum. Therefore, proton MRS may be useful in prospectively differentiating medulloblastomas from astrocytomas and ependymomas (42).

Brain Stem Tumors

Brain stem gliomas constitute approximately 15% of all pediatric CNS tumors and account for 20% to 30% of infratentorial brain tumors. Males and females are affected with equal frequency. The peak incidence of these tumors is between 3 and 10 years of age, although they can be seen in infants as well as in adults (5,18,43). The advent of MR imaging has simplified the diagnosis of brain stem tumors; it has also given new information that has allowed the identification of subgroups with different therapeutic options and prognoses (43,44).

The classic presentation of a brain stem tumor is cranial nerve palsies, usually multiple, with pyramidal tract signs and cerebellar dysfunction (ataxia and nystagmus). Hydrocephalus and signs of increased intracranial pressure are uncommon. The prognosis for most patients is poor, with an overall 5-year survival rate of approximately 10% to 30%, despite therapy (5,43). Prognosis is dependent upon the location of the tumor, tumor size, and sharpness of tumor borders; therefore, the term *brain stem glioma* should probably be avoided and the tumor should be named for the part(s) of the brain stem involved. Pontine gliomas, which are usually poorly circumscribed and large, have extremely poor prognoses. However, more localized, smaller tumors, particularly those with cystic components and those originating in the midbrain and at the cervicomedullary junction, have much better prognoses, with 5-year survival rates as high as 73% (43,45–48).

Pathology

The most common site of origin of brain stem gliomas is the pons, followed by the midbrain and medulla. Pontine gliomas frequently extend inferiorly into the me-

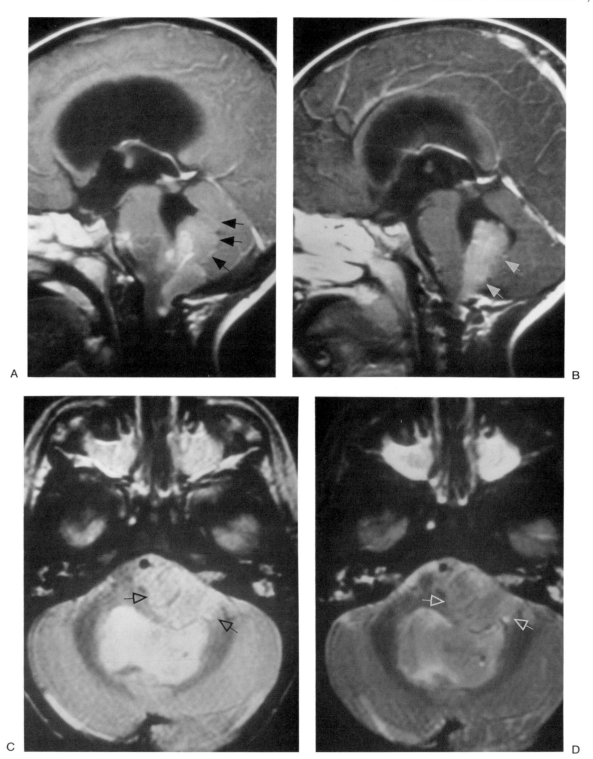

FIG. 7.19. Ependymoma with extension through foramen of Luschka. **A, B:** Postcontrast SE 650/29 images show a heterogeneously enhancing fourth ventricular mass (*arrows*) extending caudally through the foramen magnum. **C, D:** Axial SE 2800/30 (C) and 2800/80 (D) images show extension of the tumor through the left foramen of Luschka (*arrows*) into the cerebellopontine angle cistern and prepontine cistern.

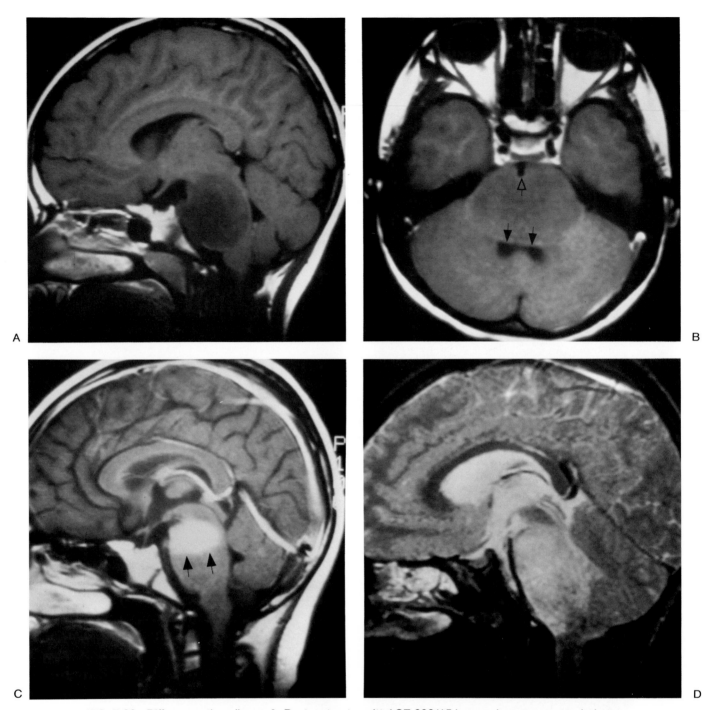

FIG. 7.20. Diffuse pontine glioma. **A:** Postcontrast sagittal SE 600/15 image shows an expanded pons with T1 prolongation involving more than 50% of the transverse diameter of the pons. The tumor does not enhance at all. **B:** Postcontrast axial SE 600/15 image shows the basilar artery (*open arrow*) engulfed by the mass. The anterior wall of the fourth ventricle (*closed arrows*) is flattened and posteriorly displaced by the tumor. **C:** After radiation therapy, the tumor has shrunken in size and the superior half of the tumor (*arrows*) shows enhancement. The development of enhancement after radiation is common in diffuse pontine gliomas and does not imply a change in tumor character. **D:** Sagittal FSE 4000/102 image. Sagittal T2-weighted images show the rostral and caudal extent of the tumor better than T1-weighted images.

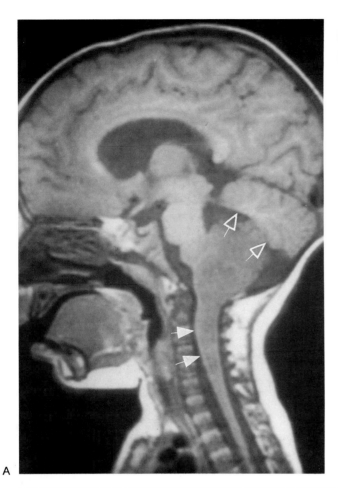

A

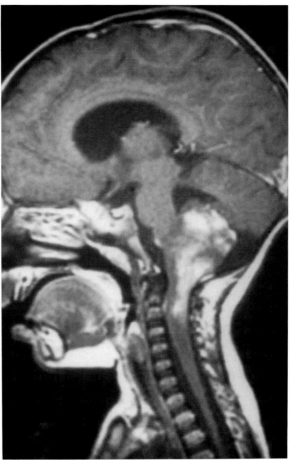

B

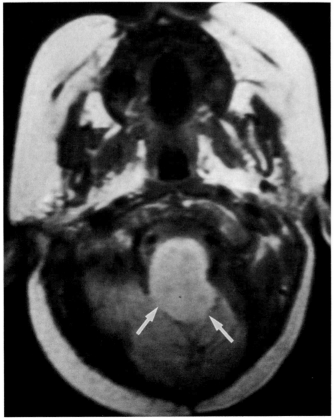

C

FIG. 7.21. Dorsally exophytic brain stem glioma extending into the cervical spinal cord. **A:** Sagittal SE 600/15 image shows a large tumor originating in the medulla and extending posteriorly between the cerebellar hemispheres. The cerebellum is pushed posteriorly and upward by the tumor mass (*open white arrows*). Caudal extension widens the cervical spinal cord (*closed white arrows*). **B:** Postcontrast sagittal SE 650/29 image shows heterogeneous enhancement of the mass. **C:** Axial SE 2500/30 image shows the medullary tumor (*arrows*) extending posteriorly between the cerebellar hemispheres.

dulla or posteriorly into the middle cerebellar peduncle and into the cerebellar hemisphere; they are usually diffuse and infiltrative. Gliomas of the midbrain frequently extend superiorly into the thalamus. As brain stem tumors enlarge, they cause diffuse expansion of the involved region. The surface is irregular and contains exophytic nodules that can grow into the cerebellopontine angle or prepontine cistern or can grow peripherally along the cranial nerves. Anterior growth frequently engulfs the basilar artery, which eventually lies within a deep groove bounded by tumor anteriorly and laterally (Fig. 7.20). Tumors of the cervicomedullary junction often grow dorsally into the cisterna magna, displacing the vermis (Fig. 7.21). Hemorrhage or cysts are present in approximately 25% of brain stem tumors, more commonly in focal tumors, and less commonly in diffuse pontine tumors (19,49).

Histologically, the tumor cells tend to infiltrate widely along the fiber tracts of the brain stem rather than to destroy them, so that one sees tumor cells intermingling intimately with neurons and nerve fibers (5,49). As a result of this characteristic, the appearance of the pons can return to normal after treatment with chemotherapy and irradiation of these tumors. Significant tumor recurrence is usually seen, however, within 18–24 months following radiation therapy (43,50).

In spite of the marked enlargement of the brain stem and frequent bulging of the brain stem into the fourth ventricle, hydrocephalus is uncommon in brain stem gliomas, except those involving the tectal plate. Tectal plate gliomas are discussed in the section on pineal region tumors.

Imaging Studies

On CT, brain stem gliomas almost always appear as an expanded area of medulla, pons, or midbrain that is hypodense to isodense prior to administration of IV contrast. Foci of hemorrhage are uncommon; when present, they are seen as localized areas of hyperdensity. Contrast enhancement is extremely variable; there may be homogeneous enhancement of parts of the tumor, heterogeneous enhancement of part of the tumor, heterogeneous enhancement of all of the tumor, or no enhancement of any of the tumor. The pattern of enhancement may change with time (3,6).

Expansion of the pons by the tumor will result in an increased sagittal dimension of the brain stem and posterior displacement of the fourth ventricle. In addition, the floor of the fourth ventricle may become flattened. When the tumor extends into the cerebellar peduncles, the lateral aspects of the fourth ventricle can be flattened, causing an apparent rotation of the ventricle. Exophytic extension of the tumor into the cerebellopontine angle can cause a paradoxical widening of the cerebellopontine

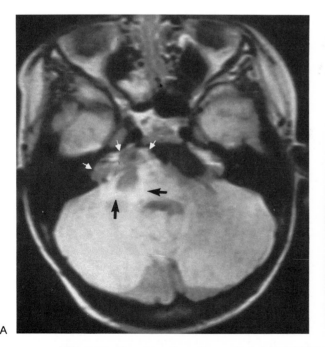
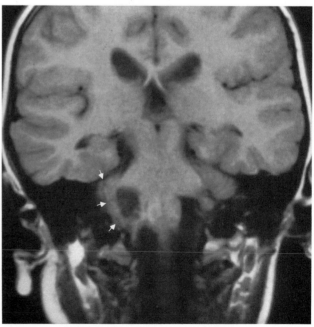

A

B

FIG. 7.22. Focal pontine glioma. **A:** Axial SE 2500/30 image shows a tumor, with local T2 prolongation (*black arrows*) arising in the lateral aspect of the pons and extending into the right cerebellopontine angle (*white arrows*). **B:** Coronal SE 600/20 image shows that the tumor is originating from the lateral pons and extending anterolaterally and inferiorly into the cistern (*arrows*).

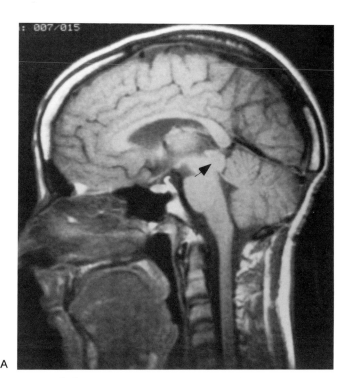
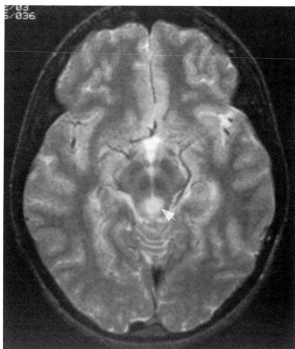

FIG. 7.23. Focal glioma of the quadrigeminal plate. **A:** Sagittal SE 600/20 image shows a tectal glioma (*arrow*) expanding the quadrigeminal plate. **B:** Axial SE 2800/80 image shows T2 prolongation (*arrow*) in the tectal region.

angle cistern on that side. Dorsal extension of the tumor through the vallecula into the cisterna magna can cause paradoxical anterior displacement of the fourth ventricle. When dorsal extension occurs, it is often difficult to differentiate the exophytic brain stem glioma from a cerebellar astrocytoma using axial images (3,6).

The use of MR greatly facilitates the diagnosis and exact localization of brain stem gliomas (Figs. 7.20–7.23). The characteristic MR appearance is of a mass expanding the brain stem and showing prolongation of T1 and T2 relaxation times with respect to normal brain. The appearance, therefore, is of a low-signal-intensity mass on T1-weighted images and a high-signal-intensity mass on T2-weighted images (Fig. 7.20).

Both diffuse and focal gliomas can show exophytic growth; the diagnosis of exophytic extension of tumor is easily diagnosed with MR (Figs. 7.20–7.22), aided by the multiplanar imaging capability. Diffuse pontine gliomas are almost always seen to engulf the basilar artery anteriorly (Fig. 7.20). Both diffuse and focal pontine gliomas can grow into the cerebellopontine angle cistern (Fig. 7.22). Medullary tumors that are exophytic posteriorly through the vallecula and are difficult to classify on axial images are easily diagnosed as brain stem tumors on sagittal images (Fig. 7.21). Focal tumors, whether in the medulla, pons, or midbrain, are usually of lower grade than other brain stem astrocytomas; therefore, some are amenable to surgical therapy. Because of their easy surgical

accessibility, dorsally exophytic medullary gliomas are particularly suited to surgical therapy (46,51,52). Focal tumors of the mesencephalic tectum (Fig. 7.23) are also usually of low grade, but because of the more difficult surgical access, they are treated more conservatively by most surgeons.

When using MR, it is most useful to categorize brain stem gliomas into groups, depending on the location of origin of the tumor and whether the tumor is focal or diffuse. Sagittal T2-weighted images (Fig. 7.20) should always be obtained to help the radiation oncologists determine the full extent of any tumor. *Diffuse neoplasms* tend to enlarge the affected area smoothly (Fig. 7.20) without focal areas of exophytic tumor. They are generally poorly marginated and involve more than 50% of the brain stem in the axial plane at the level of maximal involvement. Minimal or no contrast enhancement is seen initially, although enhancement is common after radiation therapy (Fig. 7.20C). Expansion of the brain stem by the tumor will result in an increased sagittal dimension of the brain stem and posterior displacement or flattening of the floor of the fourth ventricle. Extension into the cerebellar peduncles flattens the lateral aspects of the fourth ventricle, causing an apparent rotation of the ventricle. The basilar artery is often engulfed by anterior tumor extension. *Focal neoplasms* are generally well marginated and involve less than 50% of the brain stem in the axial plane (Figs. 7.21–7.23); these neoplasms appear to have a better prognosis (46,47). They often exhibit contrast enhancement in a homogeneous or heterogeneous fashion (Fig. 7.21). Focally exophytic components are common (Figs. 7.21, 7.22); dorsal extension of medullary gliomas through the vallecula into the cisterna magna were described earlier. Extension of the tumor into the cerebellopontine angle can cause a paradoxical widening of the cerebellopontine angle cistern on the affected side.

The major differential diagnoses of brain stem astrocytomas are encephalitis, resolving hematoma, vascular malformation, and tuberculoma. Because of its exquisite demonstration of blood and blood breakdown products, MR can differentiate brain stem astrocytomas from vascular malformations and subacute hemorrhage very easily. However, at this time, it is still not possible to differentiate an encephalitis or a tuberculoma definitively from a brain stem astrocytoma radiologically.

Schwannomas

Schwannomas are tumors derived of Schwann cells, which form the myelin sheaths around the axons of nerve roots. Schwannomas account for about 8% of primary tumors in the intracranial cavity; however, they are more frequent in adults and compose only 2% of posterior fossa tumors in children (5,18,53). When schwannomas are diagnosed in childhood, the possibility of type II neurofibromatosis (NF2, see Chapter 6) should be considered and an evaluation for other schwannomas and meningiomas should be carried out; they are rare in children outside the setting of NF2 (53). Schwannomas tend to occur at the sites of ganglia [i.e., at the transition from oligodendroglial cells to Schwann cells (54)]. For example, acoustic schwannomas tend to occur at Scarpa's ganglion, which lies within the internal acoustic canal or in the cerebellopontine angle. The location of the tumor often determines its presenting symptoms. Because schwannomas are tumors of the nerve sheath and not of the nerves themselves, patients present with neuropathy only if the schwannoma occurs within a bony canal. In such cases, outward growth of the tumor is restricted by bone; the neoplasm therefore grows centripetally into the nerve, causing compression of the nerve and, hence, a neuropathy (55). However, if the schwannoma occurs within the cranial cavity, symptoms will not occur until growth of the tumor compresses adjacent neural structures. The presenting signs and symptoms are those of brain stem compression or hydrocephalus from compression of the aqueduct or fourth ventricle. The most common nerve to be involved by a schwannoma is the 8th cranial nerve, followed by the 5th and 9th cranial nerves. Other intracranial schwannomas are extremely rare (54).

Imaging Studies

On noncontrast CT, schwannomas appear as hypo- to isodense masses that occasionally calcify. Central necrosis can occur in large lesions. After the infusion of intravenous contrast, the solid portion of the tumor typically shows homogeneous enhancement (54). When they occur within bony canals, schwannomas almost always enlarge the canals by pressure necrosis. For example, acoustic schwannomas normally enlarge the internal auditory canal, and facial schwannomas frequently enlarge the facial canal within the petrous bone.

On MR, schwannomas have prolonged T1 and T2 relaxation times (56–58). Large schwannomas often show heterogeneity with areas of high and low signal intensity on long TR sequences; the areas of T2 shortening are most likely caused by the by-products of intratumoral hemorrhage (Fig. 7.24), whereas the areas of long T2 are usually regions of cystic necrosis. Presentation with acute intratumoral hemorrhage is extremely rare. The enlarged cranial nerves coursing through enlarged neural foramina (i.e., the foramen ovale and foramen rotundum in trigeminal schwannomas and the internal auditory canal in acoustic schwannomas) and enlargement of adjacent CSF cisterns are easily demonstrated by MR. Administration of paramagnetic contrast results in enhancement of solid portions of the tumor (Fig. 7.25) (58). Several examples of schwannomas in the setting of NF2 are illustrated in Chapter 6.

Hemangioblastomas

Hemangioblastomas are relatively rare benign tumors of vascular origin, with an incidence ranging from 1% to 2.5% of intracranial neoplasms. Less than 20% of hemangioblastomas occur in children, with most being seen in young and middle-aged adults; the incidence in males exceeds that in females (5,18,19). Approximately 10% of hemangioblastomas occur in association with retinal angiomas, a condition known as von Hippel-Lindau disease (see Chapter 6). Patients with von Hippel-Lindau disease tend to have multiple hemangioblastomas of the CNS; multiple cysts or tumors involving the pancreas, liver, kidney, and lung; and rhabdomyomas of the heart. Patients with hemangioblastomas may present with erythrocythemia, thought to result from erythropoietin production by the tumor (5,18,19).

Pathology

Hemangioblastomas occur most commonly in the cerebellar hemisphere, especially the paramedian hemispheric area. Involvement of the spinal cord is not infrequent and is often accompanied by syringomyelia.

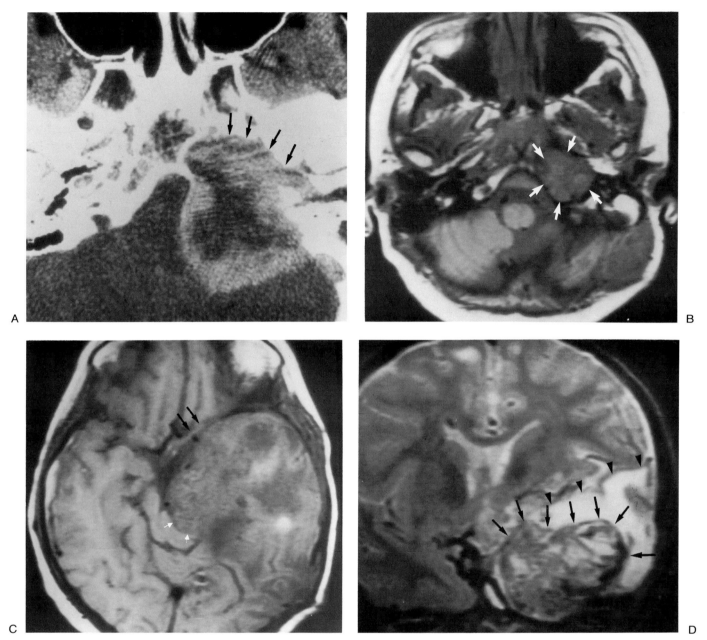

FIG. 7.24. Schwannoma of the fifth cranial nerve. **A:** Axial contrast-enhanced CT shows a large mass filling the cerebellopontine angle cistern, displacing the brain stem to the left, and eroding the skull base anteriorly (*arrows*). **B:** Axial SE 600/20 image shows tumor extension through the skull base in the region of the foramen ovale (*arrows*). **C:** Axial SE 600/20 at the level of the midbrain shows the tumor to be enormous at this level, invading the brain stem (*white arrows*) and displacing the optic tract (*black arrows*). Notice the marked heterogeneity of the tumor. Such heterogeneity is common in very large schwannomas. **D:** Coronal SE 2500/70 image shows the heterogeneous tumor (*black arrows*) surrounded by vasogenic edema (*arrowheads*).

Rarely, they may be located in the brain stem or the cerebral hemispheres. As they originate from the surface of the brain, a portion of the tumor is always connected to a pial surface. Hemangioblastomas are classically described as well-circumscribed, soft, cystic tumors with a mural nodule. However, solid hemangioblastomas are common, occurring in 30% to 40% of cases, particularly when the tumor is small. On gross inspection, the solid portion of the tumor may be intensely hemorrhagic. Calcification is not found in these lesions.

Imaging Studies

The CT appearance of hemangioblastomas is usually that of a cystic or solid posterior fossa lesion. When large enough, the solid portion of the tumor always enhances homogeneously and intensely after infusion of intravenous contrast. However, when the solid portion of the tumor is extremely small, it will not be seen on CT. Angiography will confirm the vascular component of the tumor and will detect small hemangioblastomas not seen on contrast CT. These very small lesions can usually be reliably detected on contrast-enhanced MR.

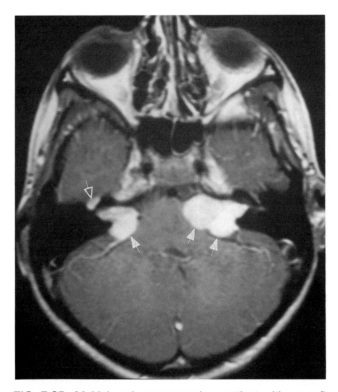

FIG. 7.25. Multiple schwannomas in a patient with neurofibromatosis type II. Post contrast SE 650/29 image shows bilateral enhancing acoustic schwannomas (*closed arrows*) and an enhancing facial nerve schwannoma (*open arrow*).

Multiple examples of MR images of hemangioblastomas are provided in Chapter 6, in the section on von Hippel-Lindau disease. The most common MR appearance is that of a cystic mass with a vascular mural nodule (59). The cyst may be hyperintense on T1-weighted images if hemorrhage has occurred recently. More commonly, cysts are hypointense on T1-weighted images and hyperintense on long TR/TE images (59,60). Moreover, on long TR images, a peripheral rim of hyperintensity may be seen as the result of surrounding edema. Solid portions of tumor enhance dramatically after intravenous infusion of paramagnetic contrast (61). When the mural nodule is small, it may be difficult to differentiate a hemangioblastoma from an arachnoid cyst. In such cases, contrast-enhanced MR should be obtained in at least two planes, as volume averaging may obscure a small region of enhancement in a single plane. If contrast-enhanced MR is not available, angiography is indicated to visualize the hypervascular nidus; many surgeons will order preoperative angiography on all suspected hemangioblastomas in order to know prospectively the location of the vascular pedicle. Preoperative embolization may serve to reduce blood loss and operative morbidity. When performed in at least two planes, contrast-enhanced MR imaging allows identification of very small tumor nodules, because they enhance intensely. In all patients with suspected or known von Hippel-Lindau disease, the spine should also be imaged, as affected patients have a surprisingly high incidence of spinal hemangioblastomas.

Embryonic Tumors (Epidermoids and Dermoids)

Presentation and Pathology

Dermoid and epidermoid tumors will be discussed in this section because they occur somewhat more frequently in the posterior fossa than in the supratentorial space or spine. Epidermoids develop from the ectoderm-derived epidermis, whereas dermoids arise not only from the epidermis but also from the subjacent dense connective tissue, the mesoderm-derived dermis. Both of these tumors are believed to arise from congenital rests of tissue that remain in the intracranial cavity as a result of incomplete separation of the neuroectoderm from the cutaneous ectoderm at the time of closure of the neural tube. Epidermoids are more common than dermoids (5,18,19).

The location of epidermoids shows a much greater variation than that of dermoids, as well as a greater tendency to deviate from the midline. The most frequent site is the cerebellopontine angle, followed by the pineal region, the suprasellar region, and the middle cranial fossa. Although epidermoids may present at any age, most are diagnosed in middle age with a peak incidence during the fifth decade. Epidermoids in the cerebellopontine angle tend to present with cranial neuropathies, whereas suprasellar epidermoids present with hydrocephalus, and middle cranial fossa epidermoids most frequently present with a chemical meningitis secondary to leakage of tumor contents into the subarachnoid space (5,18,19,62).

Dermoids are less common in the intracranial cavity than epidermoids but are more common in the spinal canal. In the intracranial cavity they are most frequently located in the posterior fossa, either within the vermis or in the fourth ventricle. In the spinal canal, most dermoids occur in the lumbosacral region, in either an extramedullary or an intramedullary location. Approximately 20% of dermoids are associated with dermal sinuses; those dermoids associated with dermal sinus tracts are most common in the spine, cerebellar vermis, and subfrontal regions. Symptoms from intraspinal dermoids usually arise in the first two decades of life, whereas intracranial dermoids present in the third decade. Symptoms may be the result of obstruction of the CSF pathways, of chemical meningitis from leakage of the contents of the cyst into the CSF, or (when associated with dermal sinus tracts) of infection and abscess formation within the tract or the dermoid itself (5,18,19,63).

Imaging Studies

CT scans show epidermoids as low-density, lobulated masses that occur in characteristic locations (Fig. 7.26). The density is often identical to that of CSF, making identification of these extra-axial lesions difficult. The introduction of water-soluble contrast into the subarachnoid space will demonstrate insinuation of the contrast into the interstices of the epidermoid, revealing its characteristic lobulated appearance (Fig. 7.26B). On MR, epidermoids appear as extra-axial masses with prolonged T1 and T2 relaxation times (Figs. 7.27, 7.28). Enhancement is not seen after infusion of intravenous contrast (Fig. 7.28). Occasionally, epidermoids have a short T1 (64); in this circumstance, they are difficult to differentiate from dermoids or lipomas. Differentiation can be made by the absence of chemical shift artifact associated with the short T1 of epidermoids; as epidermoids contain no fat, the short T1 derives from water protons. Alternatively, a fat saturation pulse can be applied; the high

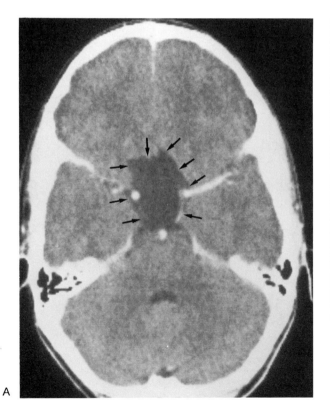

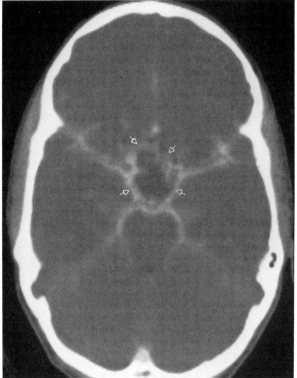

A   B

FIG. 7.26. Epidermoid tumor. **A:** Contrast-enhanced CT scan shows a low-attenuation, nonenhancing suprasellar mass (*arrows*). Note that the margins of the mass are somewhat irregular and lobulated. **B:** After introduction of intrathecal contrast, the contrast material can be seen to diffuse into the interstices of the mass, showing a characteristic lobulated appearance (*arrows*). This lobulated appearance is very characteristic of epidermoid tumors.

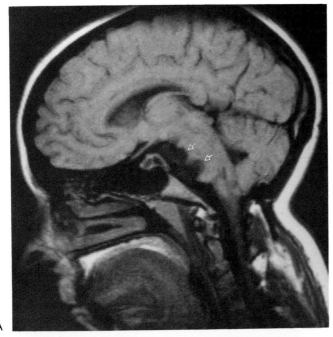

A

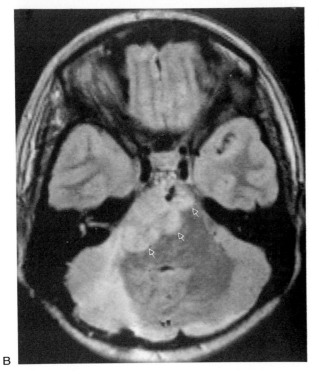

B

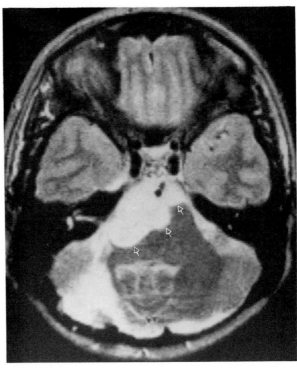

C

FIG. 7.27. Epidermoid. **A:** Sagittal SE 600/20 image shows lobulated indentations of the bases pontes (*arrows*). However, it is difficult to identify an actual mass within the prepontine cistern. Epidermoids are characteristically isointense with CSF. **B:** Axial SE 2500/30 image shows a lobulated mass in the prepontine cistern and cerebellopontine angle (*arrows*). The pons is displaced posteriorly and to the left. It is difficult to ascertain exactly where the mass ends and the adjacent cisterns begin. **C:** Axial SE 2500/70 at the same level as B. The tumor remains isointense with CSF (*arrows*).

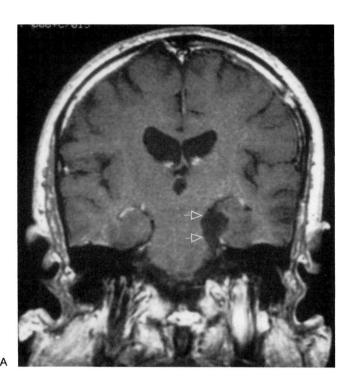
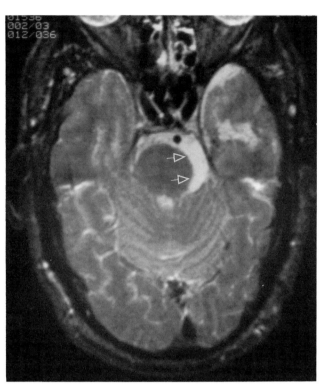

A

B

FIG. 7.28. Epidermoid. **A:** Postcontrast coronal SE 616/16 image shows an expanded left ambient cistern (*arrows*) with lateral displacement of the medial temporal lobe. No enhancement of the mass is present. **B:** Axial SE 2800/80 image shows the expanded cistern (*arrows*) with mild distortion of the adjacent pons.

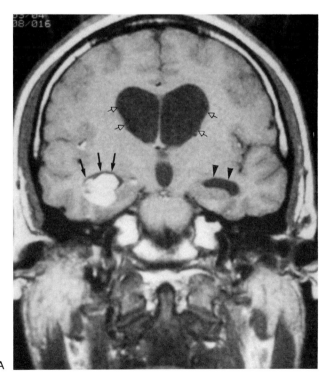
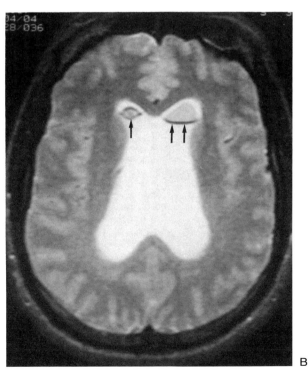

A

B

FIG. 7.29. Dermoid. **A:** Coronal SE 600/20 image shows a small mass of diminished T1 relaxation time within the right temporal lobe extending into the temporal horn of the right lateral ventricle (*closed arrows*). Note the dilatation of the left temporal horn (*arrowheads*) and the frontal horns (*open arrows*), indicative of hydrocephalus. **B:** Axial SE 2500/70 image shows fat floating within the frontal horns of lateral ventricles (*arrows*) as a result of rupture of the dermoid into the ventricular system. Note the chemical shift artifact manifested as the low signal intensity along the dorsal aspect of the dermoid in the left frontal horn.

signal from dermoids or lipomas will be saturated (disappear), but the high signal from epidermoids will remain unaffected. As with CT, however, most epidermoids have a signal intensity that is similar to CSF; difficulty therefore may arise in identifying the lesion and, once identified, in differentiating the epidermoid from an arachnoid cyst (see Chapter 8). Identification of a cisternal epidermoid is made by the enlargement of the occupied cisterns and the characteristic lobulated appearance of the mass (Figs. 7.27, 7.28) (65). Differentiation from arachnoid cysts is more difficult. A lobulated appearance and the presence of linear heterogeneities within the mass suggest that an epidermoid is present. Diffusion-weighted imaging can also be useful, as arachnoid cysts will have diffusion characteristics of a fluid (similar to CSF), whereas epidermoids will have diffusion characteristics of a solid (similar to brain tissue) (66). Alternatively, magnetization transfer techniques may be useful, as epidermoids will show significant transfer of magnetization from the solid matrix of the tumor to adjacent free water, but cysts show no magnetization transfer (67). Conspicuity is also improved by the use of heavily T1-weighted sequences, such as inversion recovery and three-dimensional gradient echo with gradient spoilers (SPGR, MP-RAGE).

The CT appearance of a dermoid is that of a fat-density, extra-axial mass that is usually located in the midline. As with epidermoids, enhancement is not seen after infusion of IV contrast unless the tumor is or has been infected (65). Whenever a midline dermoid or epidermoid tumor is encountered, the occipital and nasofrontal regions of the skull (when intracranial) or the posterior elements of the vertebra (when intraspinal) should be examined for defects that might indicate the presence of a dermal sinus tract. CT is more sensitive than MR for detection of the calvarial defect, although MR is more sensitive in detecting the tumor itself (68). Dermal sinuses result from a focal nondisjunction of neural ectoderm from cutaneous ectoderm and may be lined by fat (see Chapter 9). After infection, dermoid cysts have the typical appearance of an abscess with a uniform, contrast-enhancing rim surrounding them.

On MR, dermoids have shortened T1 and T2 relaxation times with associated chemical shift artifact, similar to lipomas (Figs. 7.29, 7.30) (for discussion of intracranial lipomas, see Chapter 5). However, dermoids are typically less lobulated than lipomas and will displace blood vessels and nerves; lipomas engulf vessels and nerves (see Chapter 5). Because affected patients often present with headaches from a chemical meningitis, inspection of the subarachnoid spaces and cerebral ventricles for fatty droplets should be performed. Occasionally, the dermoid contains a solid or cystic component (which will have a prolonged T1 and T2 compared with normal brain) or calcification [which has a variable signal on MR (69)].

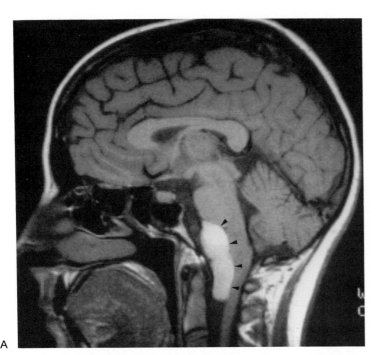

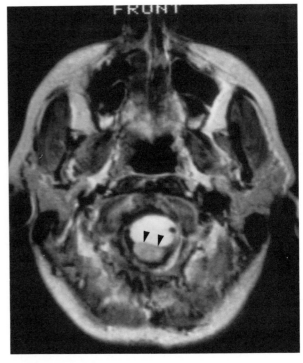

A   B

FIG. 7.30. Dermoid. A: Sagittal SE 600/20 image shows a slightly lobulated mass with diminished T1 relaxation time situated within the premedullary space and extending through the foramen magnum into the ventral spinal subarachnoid space (*arrowheads*). B: Axial SE 800/20 image at the C1 level shows the mass sitting ventral within the spinal canal, slightly compressing the spinal cord (*arrowheads*).

Teratomas

Intracranial teratomas are rare and account for only 0.5% of primary intracranial neoplasms. However, in children younger than 15 years old, they account for 2% of intracranial tumors. Moreover, teratomas represent a significant fraction of brain tumors that are diagnosed in infancy (see the section on tumors in first year of life at the end of this chapter). Intracranial teratomas are more common in males than females, as a result of the preponderance of pineal teratomas in males. The clinical presentation depends upon the location of the tumor. Hydrocephalus is common, as it is in other midline tumors (5,19).

Pathology

The pineal and parapineal regions are the most frequent sites of teratomas, followed by the third ventricular region (especially its floor) and the posterior fossa. Teratomas are less common in the spine than intracranially; they may occur at any spinal level and are associated with spina bifida occulta. Most teratomas are well circumscribed and benign, but some contain primitive elements and are highly malignant neoplasms that carry a poor prognosis. Some elaborate biochemical markers, such as alpha-fetoprotein and β-human chorionic gonadotropin, which can be measured in the CSF and serum. Grossly, teratomas are lobulated and variegated in appearance. The tumors tend to have both solid and cystic components and frequently contain calcification or bone. More malignant areas of tumor show less differentiation (5,19).

Imaging Studies

On both CT and MR, teratomas generally appear as heterogeneous lesions that are located in the midline. On CT, they can be reliably diagnosed if both fat and calcium are present; when fat and calcium are seen in association with a soft tissue intensity in a midline lesion, the diagnosis of teratoma should be suggested (Fig. 7.31A). Similarly, on MR, the presence of fat and soft tissue intensity together with punctate foci of low signal intensity (suggestive of calcium) in a midline mass should raise the suspicion of teratoma (Fig. 7.31B,C). The author has seen several patients, however, in whom teratomas were of homogeneous soft tissue intensity on both CT and MR. Teratomas with a homogeneous imaging appearance are commonly malignant and are indistinguishable from many other types of intrinsic brain tumors by imaging methods. The degree of contrast enhancement is variable. The lack of contrast enhancement suggests a low-grade tumor; however, the presence of enhancement does not assure that the tumor is malignant. Further examples of teratomas will be shown in the section on germ cell tumors and in the section on tumors in the first year of life.

Miscellaneous Tumors of the Posterior Fossa and Skull Base

Other tumors that occur in the posterior fossa in children are extremely rare. Although *meningiomas* do occur in children, they are unusual and are most frequently found in the supratentorial space in association with type II neurofibromatosis (see Chapter 6 and the section later in this chapter).

Chordomas are exceedingly rare in children and only a few dozen cases are described in the literature. In contrast to adult chordomas, which are most common in the sacral region, childhood chordomas are most common in the skull base and upper cervical vertebrae; the most common location is at the sphenoid–occipital synchondrosis (70). The behavior of these tumors in children is similar to that in adults (71). Chordomas are benign, slowly growing, locally infiltrative tumors that arise from notochordal remnants. Clivus chordomas usually produce marked destruction of the sphenoid bone, commonly extending into the sphenoid sinuses, nasopharynx, and, occasionally, ethmoid region. Patients with chordomas most frequently present with cranial neuropathies resulting from extension of tumor into the cranial neural foramina. On imaging studies, destruction of the clivus by the tumor mass is readily apparent (72) (Figs. 7.32, 7.33). When tumor extends into the nasopharynx, it is often difficult to differentiate from a primary nasopharyngeal tumor extending into the clivus. The presence of spicules of bone within a minimally enhancing tumor on CT should suggest the diagnosis of chordoma. The MR appearance of chordoma is that of a large intraosseous mass extending into the prepontine cistern, sphenoid sinuses, middle cranial fossa, or nasopharynx. Considerable posterior displacement of the brain stem may be present when the tumor is large (Figs. 7.32, 7.33). Typical chordomas have prolonged T1 and T2 relaxation values, whereas chondroid chordomas [which have a significantly better prognosis (73)] have less T2 prolongation. Enhancement is variable, ranging from minimal (Fig 7.32) to marked; in the author's experience, chordomas of childhood rarely enhance. No known correlation exists between degree of enhancement and tumor grade or prognosis.

Very rarely, *chondrosarcomas* arise from the skull base in children. Chondrosarcomas are malignant cartilaginous tumors that may arise *de novo* or from sarcomatous changes in benign cartilaginous tumors, such as chondromas or chondroblastomas. They are rarely seen in the pediatric age group, the mean age of presentation being

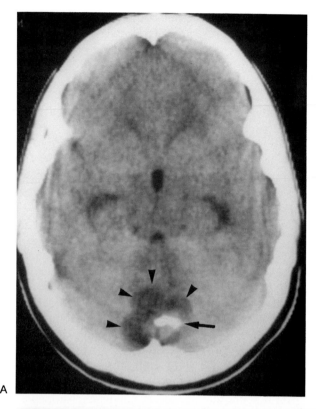

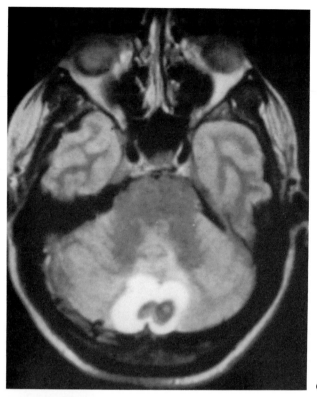

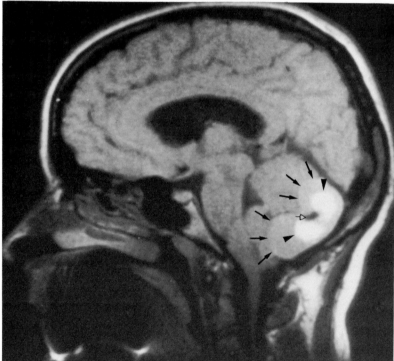

FIG. 7.31. Teratoma. **A:** Noncontrast axial CT shows a dorsal posterior fossa midline mass that has a heterogeneous appearance (*arrowheads*). A large focus of calcification is seen within the mass (*arrow*). Hydrocephalus is present, as manifested by the enlarged temporal horns. **B:** Sagittal SE 600/20 image shows the teratoma to be of mixed signal intensity. Fatty components are of very high signal intensity (*arrowheads*), soft tissue components are of soft tissue intensity (*closed arrows*), and the calcification is of very low intensity (*open arrow*). **C:** Axial SE 2500/30 image shows that the solid portion of the tumor is now of high signal intensity, whereas the fatty and calcified portions are now of low signal intensity.

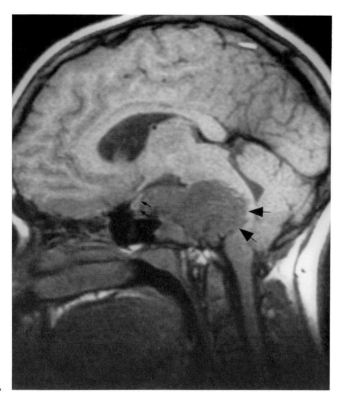

A

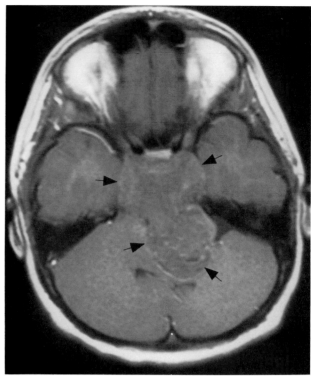

B

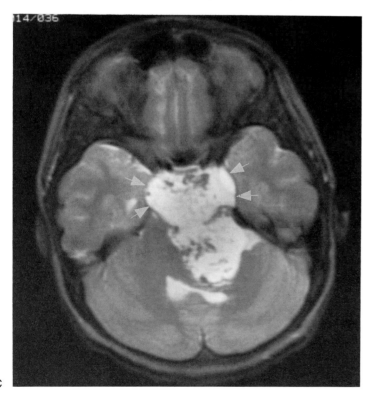

C

FIG. 7.32. Clivus chordoma. **A:** Sagittal SE 600/20 image shows a large mass (*large arrows*) pushing the pons posteriorly and pushing the pituitary gland (*small arrows*) anteriorly. The displacement of the pituitary implies an origin within the clivus. **B:** Postcontrast SE 600/15 image shows a nearly complete lack of enhancement of the tumor (*arrows*). **C:** Axial SE 2500/70 image shows lateral displacement of both temporal lobes (*arrows*) and posterolateral displacement of the pons by the hyperintense mass.

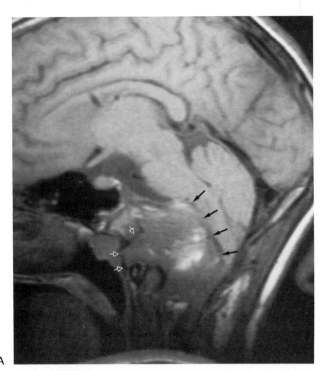
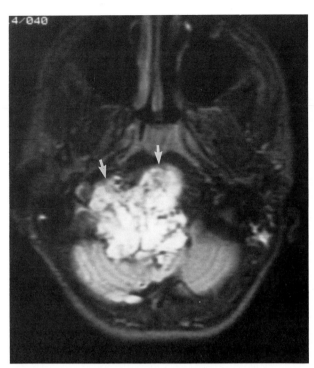

FIG. 7.33. Clivus chordoma. **A:** Sagittal SE 600/20 image shows a large mass that has arisen from and destroyed most of the basiocciput (*white arrows*). The brain stem is pushed dorsally and compressed by the mass (*black arrows*). **B:** Axial SE 2500/70 image shows prolonged T2 relaxation time within the tumor. In addition, note the extensive invasion and destruction of the skull base by this large, heterogeneous tumor (*arrows*).

in the third decade (62,74). Patients typically present with headache, sinus symptoms, proptosis, or cranial neuropathies. The most common locations are the petro-occipital, spheno-occipital, and sphenoethmoidal synchondroses, presumably arising from cartilaginous rests. Extension into the cavernous sinus, sella turcica, sphenoid sinus, or parapharyngeal space is common (75). On imaging studies, chondrosarcomas are heterogeneous (59% on MR, 44% on CT) secondary to mineralization and prominent fibrocartilagenous elements. The nonosseous elements have long T1 and T2 relaxation times and enhance markedly, but heterogeneously, after intravenous contrast administration. As the tumors often lie adjacent to fat in the marrow, infratemporal fossa, and deep facial regions, the use of fat saturation pulses is helpful on postcontrast studies. These tumors are nearly impossible to differentiate confidently from chordomas on imaging studies, as the appearance is essentially identical (Fig. 7.34).

Langerhans' cell histiocytosis (histiocytosis X) is a disorder of the reticuloendothelial system that rarely involves the CNS (76). When signs or symptoms are referable to the skull or nervous system, patients typically present with diabetes insipidus from involvement of the pituitary stalk (see section on sellar and suprasellar masses). However, patients may present with tender, palpable skull masses, with proptosis, or with evidence of

cerebral or cerebellar dysfunction (62,76,77). The most common imaging finding is that of a well-defined mass involving the calvarium or skull base. CT shows a sharply circumscribed skull lesion, most commonly involving the temporal bone, that enhances uniformly after administration of contrast (Fig. 7.35). MR shows the bone lesions as sharply defined soft tissue masses that have signal intensity comparable to skeletal muscle and enhance markedly after IV administration of paramagnetic contrast (Fig. 7.36) (78). Rarely, Langerhans' cell histiocytosis can affect regions of the brain other than the hypothalamus (76,79). Patients may present with acute neurologic deficit or with progressive neurologic deficits of insidious onset. Early cerebellar and long tract signs and symptoms may progress to profound neurologic dysfunction with or without intellectual deficits (76–78,80). Findings in the brain on imaging studies are variable. Affected patients may show diffuse regions of prolonged T1 and T2 relaxation time, of unknown nature, in the brain stem and corpus medullare of the cerebellum (Fig. 7.37). Some patients have punctate lesions scattered throughout the cerebrum, brain stem, and cerebellum. These punctate lesions, presumably composed of Langerhans' cells, enhance markedly after intravenous infusion of contrast (Fig. 7.38) (76–78,80). A few patients have extraparenchymal, dural-based, or intraventricular xanthofibromas that are characterized by significant en-

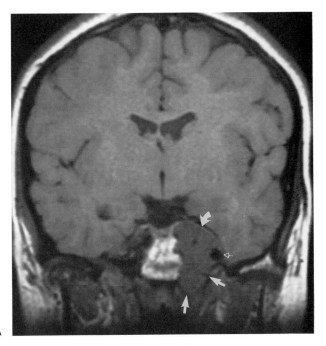

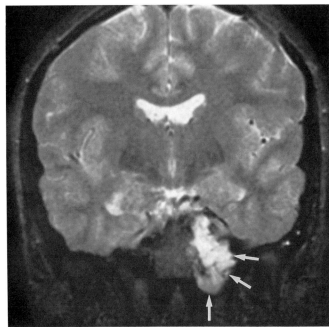

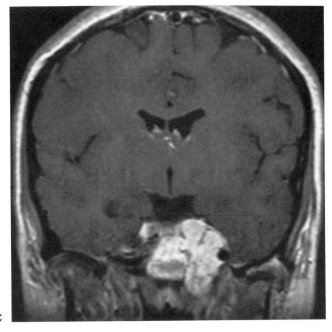

FIG. 7.34. Chondrosarcoma of the skull base in a child. **A:** Coronal SE 600/20 image shows a mass arising from the clivus and extending laterally. The curved arrow shows the dura displaced laterally by the tumor mass. The open arrow shows the carotid artery displaced far laterally. The straight white arrows show the inferior extent of the tumor. **B:** Coronal SE 2800/70 image shows that the tumor has prolonged T2 relaxation time (*arrows*). **C:** After infusion of paramagnetic contrast, the tumor becomes isointense with the bone marrow of the clivus.

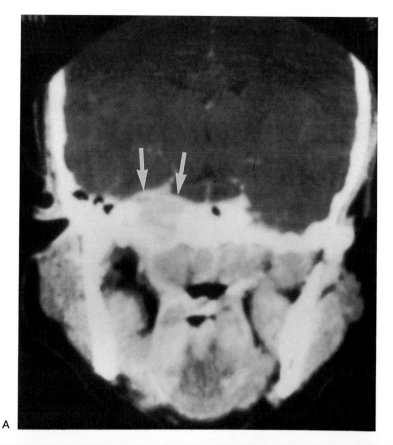

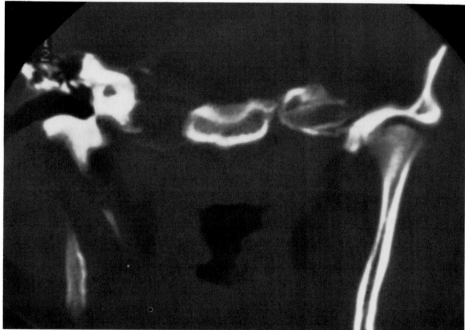

FIG. 7.35. Langerhans' cell histiocytosis of the skull base. **A:** Coronal contrast-enhanced CT scan shows an enhancing mass (*arrows*) at the petrous apex. **B:** Bone windows show a sharply demarcated defect in the petrous apex without any remaining bone.

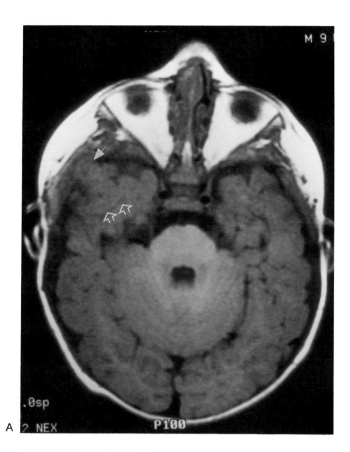

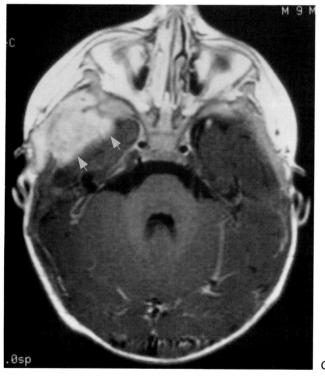

FIG. 7.36. Langerhans' cell histiocytosis of the skull base. **A:** Axial SE 600/16 image shows a mass (*open arrows*) eroding through the anterolateral wall of the right middle cranial fossa (*closed arrow*). **B:** Axial SE 2800/80 image better defines the mass (*arrows*), which has a hypointense rim. **C:** After administration of contrast, the mass (*arrows*) uniformly enhances.

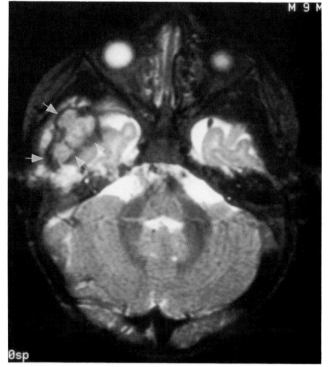

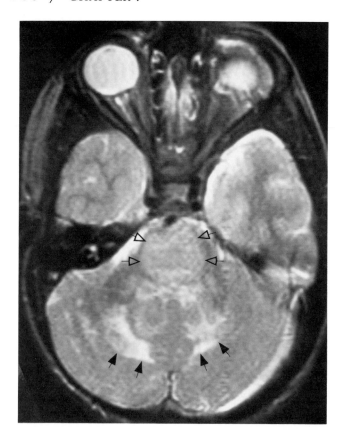

FIG. 7.37. Langerhans' cell histiocytosis involving the pons and cerebellar white matter. Axial SE 2800/80 image shows T2 prolongation in the central pons (*open arrows*) and in the white matter of the cerebellar hemispheres (*closed arrows*). These are the most common sites of parenchymal involvement.

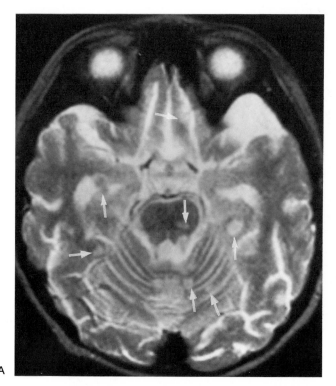

A

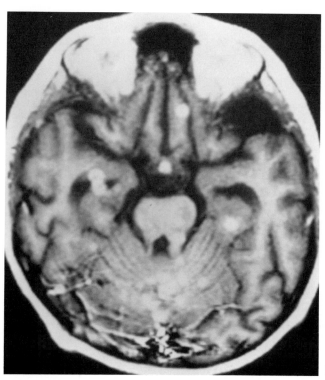

B

FIG. 7.38. Parenchymal involvement in Langerhans' cell histiocytosis. **A:** Axial SE 2800/80 image shows multiple parenchymal lesions of intermediate intensity (*arrows*) throughout the cerebrum and cerebellum. **B:** After administration of contrast, the lesions enhance uniformly.

hancement after contrast administration and marked hypointensity on T2-weighted images.

Although *neuroblastoma* most commonly presents with proptosis or a scalp mass secondary to metastasis to the orbital wall or calvarium (discussed later in this chapter), the tumor can originate in the upper cervical or skull base portions of the sympathetic chain. These primary neuroblastomas present as homogeneous, uniformly enhancing extraparenchymal masses in the cerebellomedullary or cerebellopontine angles. An extracranial, as well as intracranial, component will often be present, giving a clue to the correct diagnosis. Neuroblastoma primary to other parts of the body (abdomen, pelvis, or chest) may present with cranial neuropathy as a result of metastasis to the skull base (Fig. 7.39). The tumor appears as an enhancing, infiltrative mass that elevates the periosteum from the bone. Identification of a mass or of periosteal elevation is important in making the diagnosis of metastatic tumor to the skull base, as the normal infant's skull base contains hematopoietic marrow and enhances (81). As a result, enhancement of marrow in an infant or young child with neuroblastoma is not sufficient to establish a diagnosis of metastatic disease. Metastatic Ewing's sarcoma and leukemia can also involve the skull base; when imaged in isolation, metastatic neuroblastoma to the skull base cannot be differentiated from them.

SUPRATENTORIAL TUMORS

As previously stated, supratentorial tumors are more common than infratentorial tumors in patients less than 2 years and older than 10 years of age.

Tumors of the Cerebral Hemispheres

Hemispheric Astrocytomas

Astrocytomas of the cerebral hemispheres constitute approximately 30% of supratentorial brain tumors in children. Males and females are essentially equally affected, although most series show a slight male predominance. All pediatric age groups are affected, although there is a slight peak at 7–8 years of age. The presenting symptoms depend upon tumor location. Seizures, focal neurologic deficits, and symptoms of increased intracranial pressure are the most common presenting symptoms (the symptoms of increased intracranial pressure include headache, vomiting, and altered sensorium) (5,19,82–84).

Pathology

Grossly, hemispheric astrocytomas are similar to cerebellar astrocytomas; they can be solid, solid with a ne-

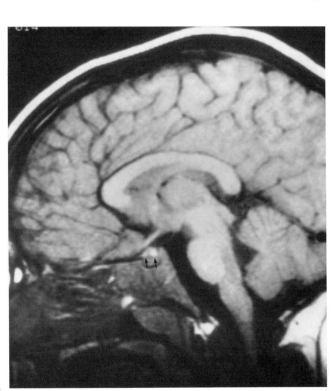

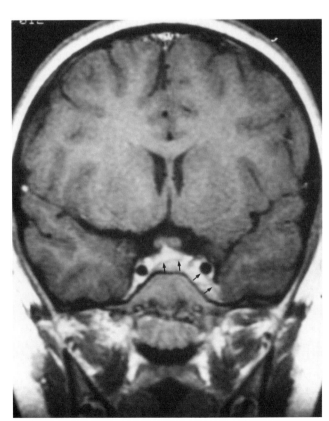

A   B

FIG. 7.39. Metastatic neuroblastoma to skull base. **A:** Sagittal SE 600/15 image shows elevation of the pituitary gland (*arrows*) by a mass that is isointense to the basisphenoid bone. **B:** Postcontrast coronal SE 600/29 image shows elevation of the periosteum (*arrows*) from the sphenoid bone by the tumor.

crotic center, or cystic with a mural nodule. Most have a low histologic grade, although glioblastoma multiforme does occur in childhood and has a better prognosis than in adults (85,86). Juvenile pilocytic astrocytomas are less common in the cerebral hemispheres than in the cerebellum, and therefore the overall prognosis of supratentorial astrocytomas is somewhat lower. There is no characteristic location for the tumors, although they tend to occur deep within the hemispheres, frequently involve the basal ganglia or thalamus, and may affect more than one lobe of the brain (5,19,82,84,87). They are often very large at the time of presentation.

Imaging Studies

CT of the brain reveals considerable variation in tumor appearance. The solid portion of the tumor tends to be iso- to hypodense prior to intravenous contrast administration. After infusion of contrast, the solid portion may enhance completely, partially, or not at all. The tumor can be completely solid, solid with a central area of necrosis, or cystic with an enhancing mural nodule. When cysts are large, it is often difficult to determine whether they are intraparenchymal or extraparenchymal. Therefore, it is important to administer contrast to the affected patients. The presence of an enhancing mural nodule (Fig. 7.40) makes the diagnosis of cystic astrocytoma likely. It is not possible radiographically to differentiate benign from malignant astrocytomas of the cerebrum. In general, malignant tumors tend to be larger and occur in younger children, but this difference is not significant enough to help determine pathology in individual cases (88). Occasionally, hemorrhage is seen in high-grade supratentorial astrocytomas (3).

On MR, astrocytomas typically appear as large, medially located hemispheric masses that have prolonged T1 and T2 relaxation values when compared with normal brain (Figs. 7.41, 7.42). Although typically found deep within the hemisphere, they can occur in the centrum ovale or in the cortex. It is difficult to differentiate a cystic from a solid tumor solely on a noncontrast MR. The presence of wave forms from pulsations of fluid within the tumor or the presence of a fluid–fluid level will confirm the presence of a cyst. In general, low-grade astrocytomas are homogeneous, free of hemorrhage, well circumscribed, and associated with only mild surrounding edema, whereas higher-grade tumors show heterogeneity, resulting from areas of necrosis or hemorrhage, and generate more extensive vasogenic edema (89) (Fig. 7.43). These characteristics are not absolute, however; low-grade tumors can have some high-grade characteristics and vice versa. Enhancement patterns after paramagnetic contrast infusion are similar to those seen on CT after infusion of iodinated contrast (Fig. 7.42). No characteristic features have been described that allow one to differentiate pediatric astrocytomas confidently

from ependymomas or oligodendrogliomas on the basis of MR features.

Giant Cell Tumors

The name *giant cell tumor* is given to a mass that is characteristically associated with tuberous sclerosis; when discovered, giant cell tumors should motivate a search for this condition, although the tumor may occasionally be found in other settings. Giant cell astrocytomas occur in 5% to 15% of patients with tuberous sclerosis (90). Males and females are equally affected. The tumor may be diagnosed at any age, but peak occurrence is between 5 and 10 years of age. The clinical presentation is almost always that of hydrocephalus. Rarely, the tumors can undergo malignant degeneration and invade surrounding brain (5,19,90,91).

Pathology

Giant cell tumors usually arise from the wall of the lateral ventricle near the foramina of Monro and produce hydrocephalus because of obstruction at the foramen. They are believed to arise from the subependymal hamartomas that are part of the tuberous sclerosis complex (see Chapter 6); in fact, the tumors bear histologic similarity to the subependymal hamartomas. Giant cell astrocytomas tend to be sharply defined and homogeneous on pathologic examination. Focal calcification is common. Although usually histologically benign, some show evidence of anaplasia (19,90).

Imaging Studies

The CT and MR findings of tuberous sclerosis are described in Chapter 6. The characteristic CT appearance of the giant cell astrocytoma is that of a hypo- to isodense, well-demarcated, rounded lesion in the region of the foramen of Monro, usually producing hydrocephalus (Fig. 7.44). Other subependymal masses, both calcified and noncalcified, are usually present. After the infusion of IV contrast, giant cell astrocytomas always uniformly enhance (3,92). Examination with MR also reveals a well-circumscribed, rounded mass in the region of the foramen of Monro, often extending into the frontal horn or body of the lateral ventricle, that is hypointense to isointense with brain tissue on T1-weighted sequences and hyperintense on T2-weighted sequences (Fig. 7.45) (91,93–95). Multiple smaller subependymal nodules are almost always present. Moreover, on MR one typically sees multiple cortical hamartomas that are identified by enlargement of the involved sulcus, variable signal intensity on T1-weighted sequences and high signal intensity on T2-weighted sequences (see Chapter 6 and Fig. 7.45). Infusion of Gd-DTPA results in uniform enhancement

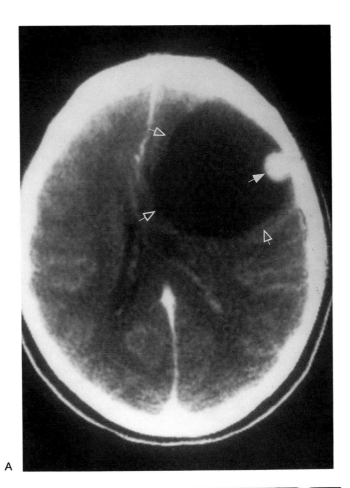

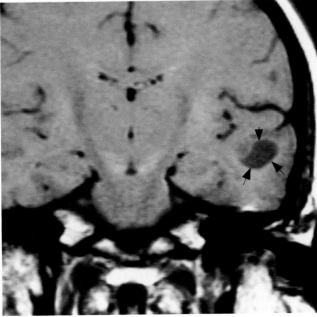

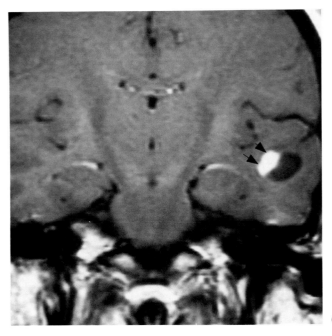

FIG. 7.40. Cystic astrocytomas. **A:** Postcontrast CT shows a large cyst (*open arrows*) with an enhancing mural nodule (*closed arrow*). When cysts are this large, it is difficult to determine whether they are intra- or extraparenchymal. Therefore, contrast should be administered to all patients with intracranial "cysts" to rule out the presence of an enhancing mural nodule. **B:** Noncontrast coronal SE 500/11 image shows a small cyst (*arrows*) in the temporal lobe. **C:** Postcontrast SE 500/11 image shows enhancement of a mural nodule (*arrows*) within the cyst.

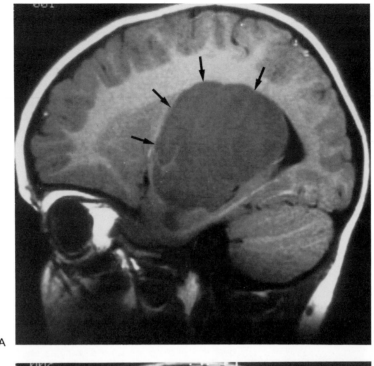

A

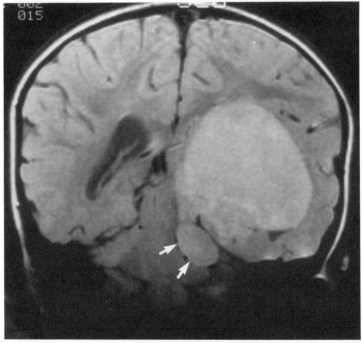

B

FIG. 7.41. Pilocytic astrocytoma. **A:** Parasagittal SE 600/20 image shows a large mass involving the left thalamus and extending into the left lateral ventricle (*arrows*). The mass appears largely homogeneous on this sequence. **B:** Coronal SE 2500/20 image shows the mass to have a prolonged T2 relaxation time. The mass extends across the tentorial incisura into the posterior fossa and is seen to compress the cerebellum slightly (*arrows*).

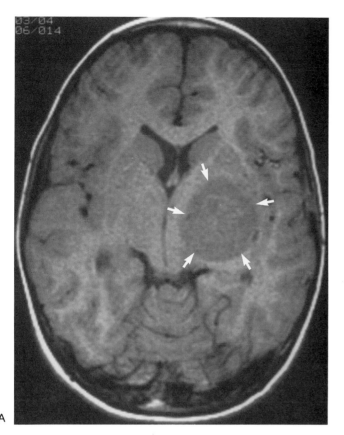

A

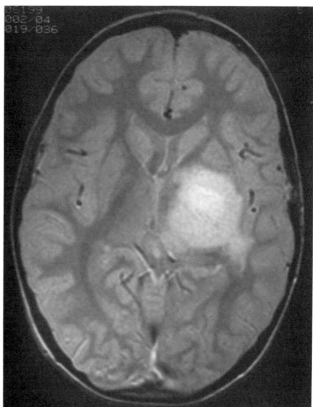

B

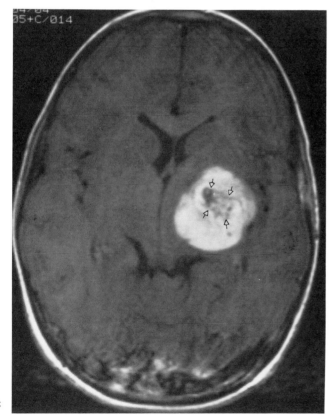

C

FIG. 7.42. Pilocytic astrocytoma. **A:** Axial SE 600/20 image shows a mass that is isointense with gray matter located in the left thalamic region (*arrows*). **B:** Axial SE 2800/30 image shows the mass to have a prolonged T2 relaxation time. **C:** After infusion of paramagnetic contrast, the tumor is seen to enhance brightly. A central area of heterogeneity is present (*arrows*) that was not appreciated on the precontrast study.

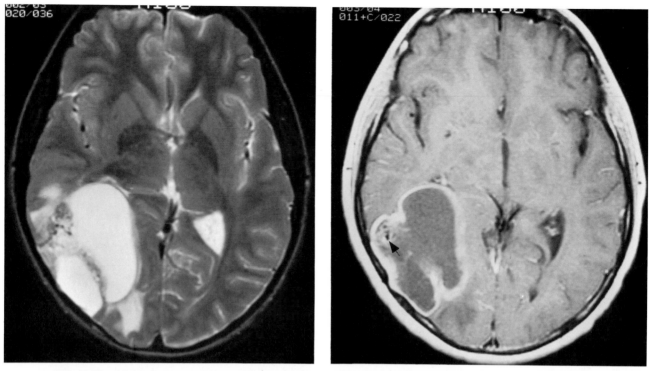

A

B

FIG. 7.43. Glioblastoma multiforme. **A:** Axial SE 2800/80 image shows a heterogeneous, partially cystic mass in the right temporo-occipital region with moderate peritumoral edema and significant mass effect upon adjacent structures. **B:** Postcontrast axial SE 616/15 image shows moderate rim enhancement and focal hypointensity in the right anterior portion (*arrow*) probably representing flow voids from feeding vessels.

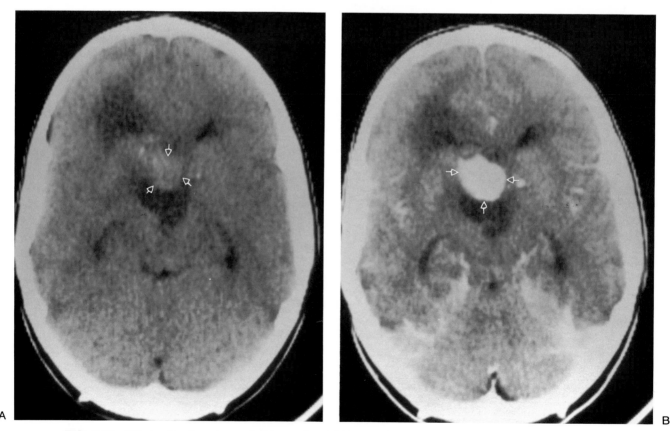

A

B

FIG. 7.44. Giant cell astrocytoma. **A:** Noncontrast CT scan through the level of the foramen of Monro shows a mass originating from the foramen of Monro (*arrows*) that is essentially isodense with brain. There is moderate vasogenic edema surrounding the mass. **B:** After infusion of iodinated contrast, the mass uniformly enhances (*arrows*).

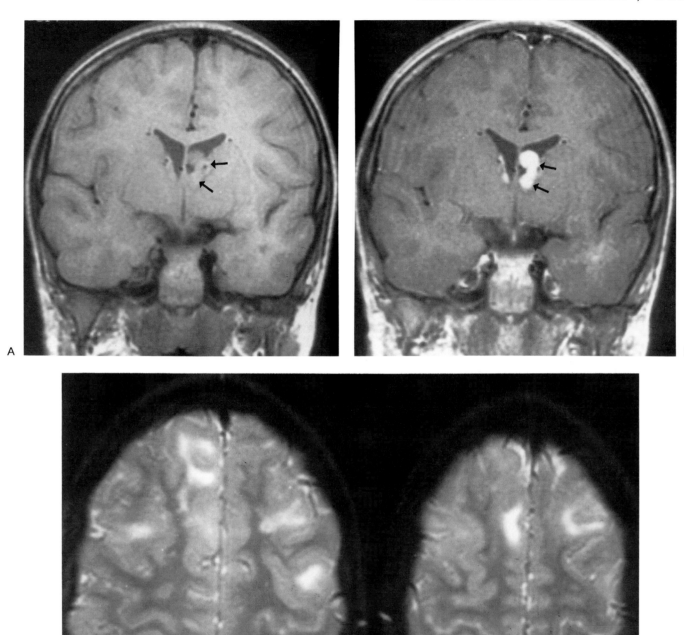

FIG. 7.45. Giant cell astrocytoma. **A:** Coronal SE 800/20 image shows a mass in the region of the left foramen of Monro (*arrows*) and extending into the frontal horn of the left lateral ventricle. **B:** After infusion of paramagnetic contrast, the mass is seen to enhance uniformly (*arrows*). **C:** Axial SE 2800/70 images near the vertex show multiple subcortical areas of prolonged T2 relaxation, compatible with the cortical tubers that are characteristic of tuberous sclerosis.

of the giant cell tumor (Fig. 7.45B) (91,94). As stated in Chapter 6, giant cell tumors are characterized by progressive but slow growth. If rapid growth or invasion of cerebral parenchyma is seen in a lesion originating in the region of the foramen of Monro, it should raise suspicion of anaplasia.

Gangliogliomas and Ganglioneuromas

Gangliogliomas and ganglioneuromas are tumors in which nerve cells and glial cells, usually astrocytes, participate in the neoplastic process; in this sense, they differ from most primary CNS neoplasms in which only the glial cells show neoplasia. Gangliogliomas and ganglioneuromas (also called gangliocytomas) are uncommon tumors, constituting approximately 3% of brain tumors in children and approximately 6% of supratentorial pediatric brain tumors. Both sexes are equally affected. Although presentation occurs most often during the second decade of life, it is not uncommon for patients with these tumors to present in adulthood. The clinical history of these slow-growing neoplasms is usually one of a protracted history of focal findings. When the motor cortex or temporal lobe is affected, the history tends to be one of long-standing focal epilepsy. Complete tumor removal generally alleviates the seizures (96). When the region of the third ventricle and hypothalamus is affected, symptoms tend to reflect hypothalamic dysfunction, resulting in obesity, diabetes insipidus, or bulimia. These tumors should not be confused with dysplastic cerebellar gangliocytomas (Lhermitte-Duclos syndrome), a congenital malformation described in Chapter 5 (5,97–100).

Pathology

Gangliogliomas and ganglioneuromas occur mainly in the cerebral hemispheres; the temporal lobes are most commonly affected, followed by the frontal lobe, parietal lobe, occipital lobe, third ventricle, and hypothalamus. The cerebellum, brain stem, and spinal cord can also be affected. The tumors tend to be small, firm, and well defined; foci of calcification and cysts are frequent. The differentiation between ganglioglioma and ganglioneuroma is histologic; if glial elements predominate, the lesion is called a ganglioglioma, and when neuronal elements predominate, the term *ganglioneuroma* (or *gangliocytoma*) is used. They are really two ends of the spectrum, however, and different components can predominate in different areas of the same lesion. It is therefore unrealistic to draw a rigid distinction between these tumor types, and they should be considered as a single entity (19,96,97,101). Temporal lobe gangliogliomas can be seen in association with, and are suspected to cause, mesial temporal sclerosis (102).

Imaging Studies

The CT appearance is that of a low-density, well-circumscribed lesion, typically located within the periphery of the hemisphere, with essentially no mass effect (Fig. 7.46). Solid portions of the tumor can be isodense or hypodense; when hypodense, care should be taken not to assume that the hypodense area is a cyst. Calcification is seen in approximately 35% of gangliogliomas on CT. Contrast enhancement is variable; part or all of the solid portion of the tumor may enhance, or contrast enhancement may be completely absent. Occasionally, the tumor can be surrounded by low-density edema. When the tumor is peripherally located within the cerebrum, erosion of the adjacent inner table of the calvarium may occur (6,100,103). On MR, the ganglioglioma may appear well or poorly circumscribed. They may be solid, be cystic, or have the appearance of many small cysts (Fig. 7.47). Signal intensity on T1-weighted sequences is variable (and often mixed); T2-weighted sequences generally reveal a high signal intensity of the tumor. Regions of slightly shortened T1 relaxation, probably representing calcification, may be helpful in identifying these neoplasms (Fig. 7.47). As on CT, the peripheral location within the hemispheres and the erosion of the adjacent calvarium can be helpful in making the diagnosis of ganglioglioma (104). When located in the hypothalamic area, gangliogliomas are difficult to differentiate from hypothalamic astrocytomas. When located peripherally, differentiation from astrocytomas, oligodendrogliomas, and dysembryoplastic neuroepithelial tumors is difficult.

Supratentorial Ependymomas

Supratentorial ependymomas comprise between 20% and 40% of childhood ependymomas. They occur in males more commonly than in females with a peak incidence between the ages of 1 and 5 years. The presenting symptoms depend upon the location of the tumor. Signs of increased intracranial pressure and focal seizures are the most common reasons for presentation (5,40,84).

Pathology

Supratentorial ependymomas are identical histologically to their infratentorial counterpart. Small foci of calcification are seen in about one-half of cases; cystic areas are common, especially in the larger lesions. These tumors are usually large at the time of presentation, probably because they are most commonly located in the frontal lobe, where they usually abut the wall of the frontal horn. They occur less frequently in the parietal and temporoparietal regions. In contrast to infratentorial ependymomas, the supratentorial variety is uncom-

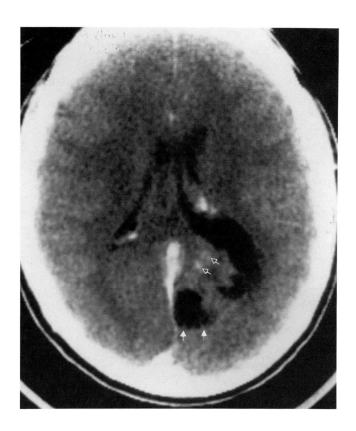

FIG. 7.46. Ganglioglioma. Axial contrast-enhanced CT scan shows a lesion of mixed signal intensity in the left occipital lobe near the visual cortex. Both calcifications (*open arrows*) and a low-intensity area (*closed arrows*) are present. Areas of low attenuation in gangliogliomas are not necessarily cystic.

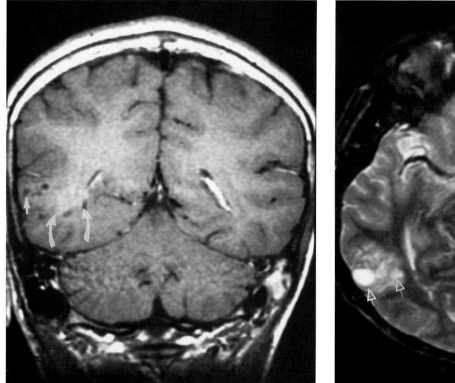

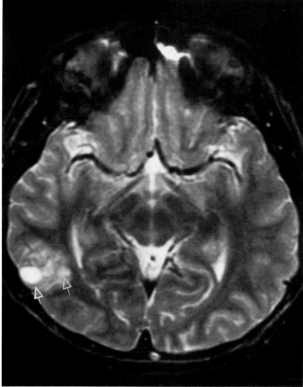

FIG. 7.47. Ganglioglioma. **A:** Coronal SE 616/15 image shows a small cyst (*small straight arrow*) in the right temporal cortex with hyperintensity (*curved arrows*) in the adjacent temporal white matter. **B:** Axial SE 2800/80 image shows the hyperintense tumor (*arrows*) in the right temporal cortex.

monly intraventricular; metastatic spread of tumor through the CSF is therefore uncommon (5,18,19).

Imaging Studies

As with the infratentorial ependymomas, those located supratentorially have an extremely variable appearance on both CT and MR. They tend to be isodense with normal brain on noncontrast CT scans; foci of calcification and cystic areas are frequently seen (Fig. 7.48). However, they may be hyperdense precontrast without calcification or cysts. After contrast administration the solid portion of the tumor enhances variably. As a rule, when one sees an isodense frontal or parietal juxtaventricular mass with foci of calcification and cysts that shows heterogeneous enhancement, the diagnosis of ependymoma should be entertained (6,40,105).

On MR, the major characteristic of the ependymoma is its heterogeneity. This heterogeneity results from the presence of intratumoral calcification, cysts, and, occasionally, hemorrhage, which combine to give a mixture of signal intensities with all imaging parameters (Fig. 7.49) (38). However, supratentorial ependymomas can appear homogeneous on MR (and thus be indistinguishable from low-grade astrocytomas) or ring enhancing with extensive edema indistinguishable from a high-grade astrocytoma or a primitive neuroectodermal tumor). When heterogeneity is seen in a midline tumor on MR, the first diagnosis considered should be teratoma. When heterogeneity is seen in a supratentorial tumor that is off the midline and extraventricular, both ependymomas and primitive neuroectodermal tumors should be considered likely diagnoses. When a markedly heterogeneous intraventricular tumor is seen, the diagnosis of a choroid plexus carcinoma should be suggested.

Primitive Neuroectodermal Tumor

Primitive neuroectodermal tumors (PNETs) were first conceptualized by Hart and Earl (106), who defined them as highly cellular tumors composed of more than 90% to 95% undifferentiated cells. Although foci of differentiation along glial or neuronal lines may be present within the tumor mass, the high percentage of undifferentiated cells set these tumors apart from other tumors. PNETs are histologically similar to medulloblastomas, pineoblastomas, and peripheral neuroblastomas. In fact, many neoplasms that were previously classified as primary cerebral neuroblastomas, primary cerebral medulloblastomas, ependymoblastomas, and undifferentiated small cell neoplasms of the brain are now considered by many to be PNETs, although some controversy exists regarding the classification of these neoplasms (19,107). PNETs are uncommon tumors, comprising less than 5% of supratentorial neoplasms in children. Although they have been described up to the age of 24 years, they are more commonly seen in children under the age of 5 years. No male or female predominance has emerged. Patients most frequently present with signs of increased intracranial pressure or seizures (108–110).

Pathology

PNETs most frequently occur in the deep cerebral white matter and are usually quite large at the time of presentation. Grossly, they have sharp margins, even though histologic examination shows spread of the tumor cells peripherally beyond the apparent tumor edge. Necrotic areas and foci of calcification are seen in about one-half of tumors. Seeding of tumor through the CSF pathways and metastases to the spinal cord, lungs, liver, and bone marrow have been reported (5,19,110).

Imaging Findings

The CT findings of PNETs are rather characteristic. On noncontrast CT, the solid portions of the tumor tend to be hyperdense when compared to normal brain, presumably because of the high nuclear-to-cytoplasmic ratio and the subsequent high electron density of the tumors. Cystic areas and foci of punctate calcifications are common, and hemorrhage is seen in approximately 10% (Fig. 7.50). After infusion of IV contrast, there is always some enhancement, which may be solid and homogeneous, heterogeneous, or ringlike, depending upon the size and number of associated cysts and necrotic foci (109,111,112).

The MR appearance of PNETs is that of a large, apparently well-marginated mass that can be located either in the cerebral hemisphere or in the lateral ventricle (Figs. 7.51, 7.52). As with ependymomas, the tumors are remarkable for their marked variability; appearance ranges from homogeneous to markedly heterogeneous to a rim of solid tumor surrounding central necrosis. Punctate calcifications may be inapparent or appear as foci of low signal intensity. The cystic areas are of low intensity on T1-weighted sequences and of very high intensity on T2-weighted sequences. When hemorrhage is present, it is of high signal intensity on the T1-weighted sequences and of mixed intensity on the T2-weighted sequences, depending upon the chemical state of the iron. Infusion of paramagnetic contrast results in enhancement similar to that seen on CT (113). When a large, sharply marginated mass is seen in a young child, the diagnosis of PNET should be suggested, particularly when the mass is markedly heterogeneous.

Rhabdoid Tumors

Malignant rhabdoid tumors are neoplasms of unknown histogenesis that were named because their light

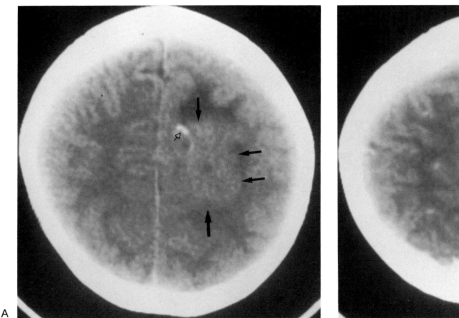
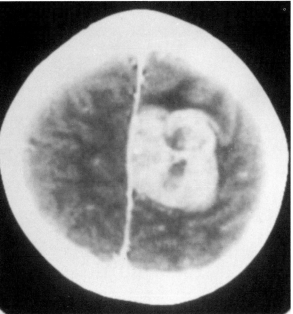

A

B

FIG. 7.48. Supratentorial ependymoma. **A:** Axial noncontrast CT scan shows a hemispheric mass (*arrows*) that is isodense with gray matter. A small focus of calcification (*open arrow*) is seen within the tumor mass. There is mild surrounding vasogenic edema. **B:** After infusion of iodinated contrast, there is heterogeneous contrast enhancement.

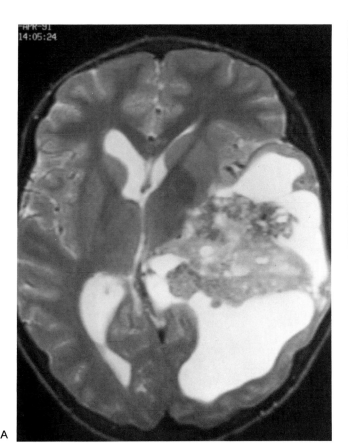
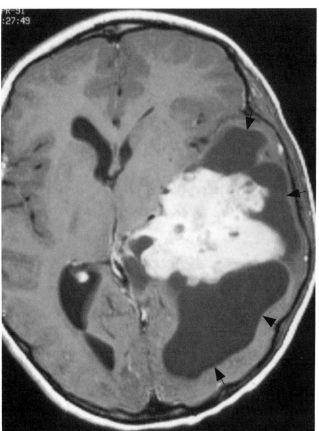

A

B

FIG. 7.49. Supratentorial ependymoma. **A:** Axial SE 2800/80 image shows a heterogeneous cystic and solid mass in the left temporal lobe. **B:** Postcontrast axial SE 650/15 image shows the solid portion of the tumor to enhance heterogeneously. The cysts (*arrows*) are hyperintense compared to ventricles and are therefore tumor cysts.

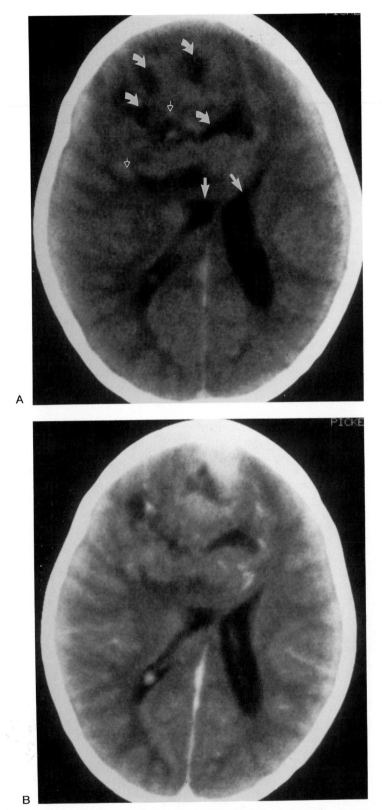

FIG. 7.50. Primitive neuroectodermal tumors. **A:** Noncontrast CT scan shows a large heterogeneous mass principally in the right frontal lobe that is extending across the midline and posteriorly displacing the lateral ventricles (*closed white arrows*). Foci of necrosis (*curved arrows*) and hemorrhage (*open white arrows*) are seen within the mass. **B:** After administration of iodinated contrast, there is moderate heterogeneous enhancement of the tumor.

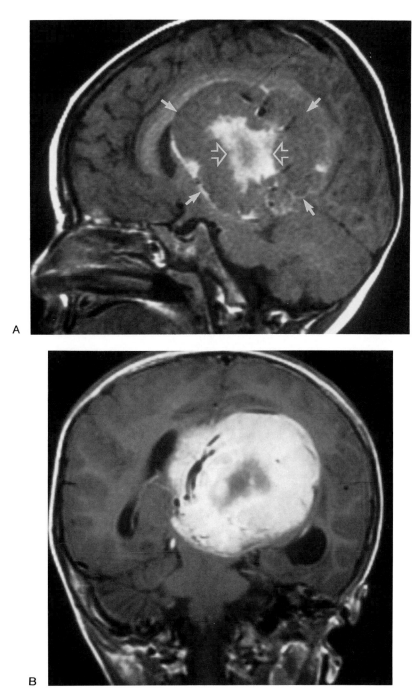

FIG. 7.51. Primitive neuroectodermal tumor. **A:** Parasagittal SE 600/20 image shows a large thalamic and intraventricular PNET (*closed arrows*) with a hemorrhagic center (*open arrows*). **B:** Coronal SE 600/ 20 image after infusion of paramagnetic contrast shows enhancement of the solid portion of the tumor.

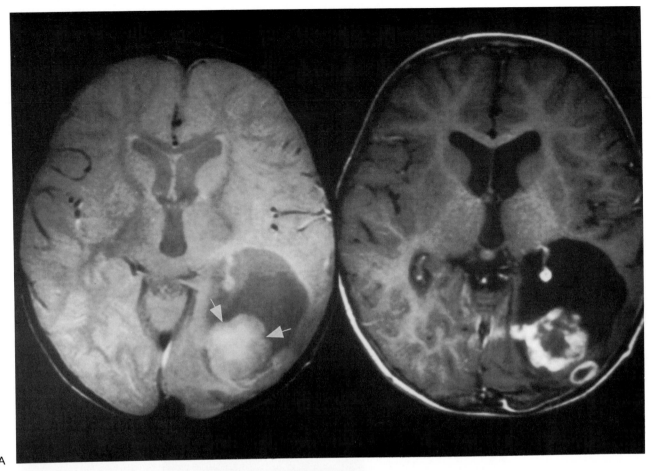

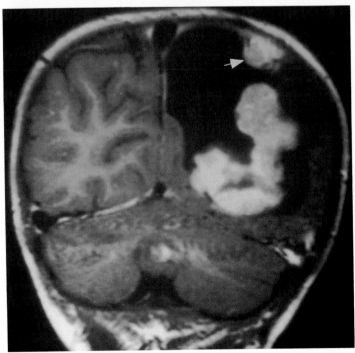

FIG. 7.52. Intraventricular primitive neuroectodermal tumor. **A:** Axial SE 2800/30 image shows the tumor (*arrows*) in the enlarged left occipital horn. The tumor is isointense to gray matter peripherally with a hyperintense center. **B:** Postcontrast axial image shows heterogeneous enhancement of the mass. **C:** Postcontrast coronal image shows the marked enlargement of the occipital horn more clearly. In addition, spread of the tumor to the superior wall of the ventricle (*arrow*) is appreciated.

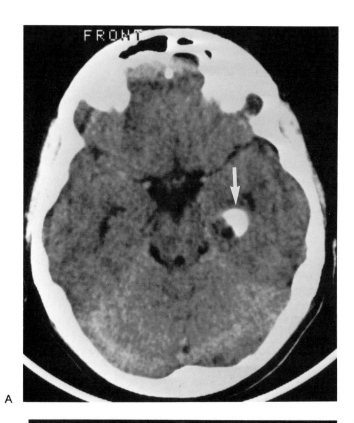

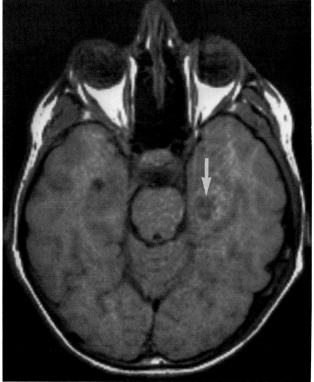

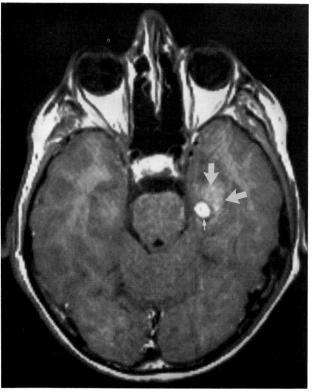

FIG. 7.53. Oligodendroglioma. **A:** Noncontrast CT shows a heavily calcified mass in the left temporal lobe with a medial hypodense component (arrow). **B:** Axial SE 480/20 shows the mass (*arrow*) to be heterogeneous. Artifact is misregistration from ocular motion. **C:** Postcontrast SE 480/20 shows marked enhancement of part of the tumor (*small arrow*). Less marked enhancement is seen anteriorly (*large arrows*) in tissue that, at surgery, was also found to be tumor.

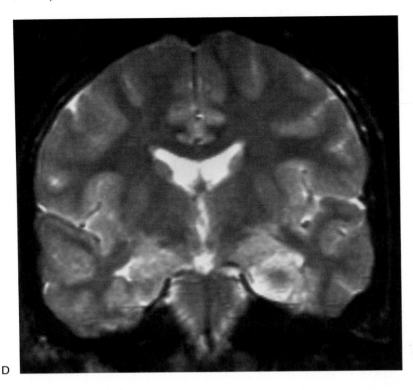

FIG. 7.53. (*Continued.*) **D:** Coronal SE 2000/80 image shows the tumor to be heterogeneous. (This case courtesy of Dr. Del Giudice, Napoli.)

D

microscopic appearance resembles that of rhabdomyo-sarcoma. Rhabdoid tumors rarely arise in the brain, being primarily malignant neoplasms of the kidney (114,115). Most reported cases of cerebral rhabdoid tumors have presented in the first decade of life with lethargy, vomiting, and visual disturbances. Prognosis is dismal, with survival of less than 1 year in most cases.

Pathologically, the tumors are solid with regions of necrosis. Histologic features include round to ovoid cells with eccentric nuclei and prominent nucleoli, abundant eosinophilic cytoplasm, and cytoplasmic hyaline inclusions.

On imaging studies, the tumors are usually large (averaging 5 cm in diameter) at the time of patient presentation. The masses are typically solid with areas of necrosis; the solid regions are iso- to hyperdense to gray matter on CT and isointense to gray matter on MR. The solid portions enhance heterogeneously after infusion of intravenous contrast (114,115).

Oligodendroglioma

Although they constitute 5% to 7% of brain tumors in the general population, oligodendrogliomas are rare in children. Little clinical information is available on their incidence or presentation in children. In general, oligodendrogliomas are hemispheric lesions that most commonly occur in the frontal lobes and are frequently calcified. They grow slowly and usually present with seizures (18,19). The CT appearance of oligodendrogliomas in children is that of hypo- to isodensity prior to

contrast infusion. Contrast enhancement is variable. Calcification and cysts (Fig. 7.53) are present in approximately 50%. Because the lesions are slow-growing, when they are located in the periphery of the brain, erosion of the adjacent inner table of the skull can be seen (3). The MR appearance of these lesions is completely nonspecific, with prolongation of T1 and T2 relaxation times. Regions of calcification may be hyperintense on T1-weighted images (Fig. 7.53). Solid portions of the tumor typically enhance moderately after administration of paramagnetic contrast. When they occur in the frontal lobes and are associated with calcification, cysts, and limited or absent contrast enhancement, a diagnosis of oligodendroglioma may be raised because these features would separate the tumor from most astrocytomas. When located in the temporal lobe, they are indistinguishable from gangliogliomas.

Dysembryoplastic Neuroepithelial Tumor

Dysembryoplastic neuroepithelial tumors (DNETs) are benign masses of the cerebral cortex that nearly always present as partial complex seizure disorders in children or young adults; other neurologic signs or symptoms are rarely present (116). Pathologically, more than 60% of DNETs are found in the temporal lobe, ~30% occur in the frontal lobe, and the rest are scattered through the parietal and occipital lobes. Cerebellar DNETs have not been described, although there is no reason to believe they do not exist (116,117). The tumors are solid but often have cystic or microcystic compo-

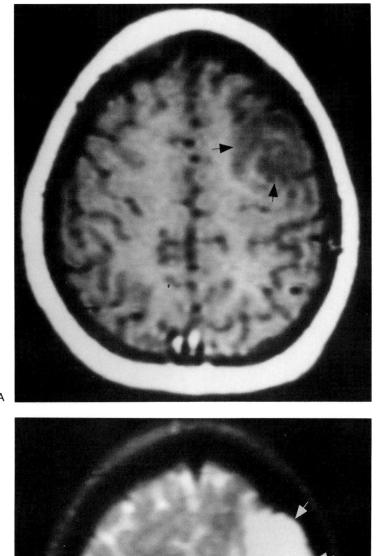

A

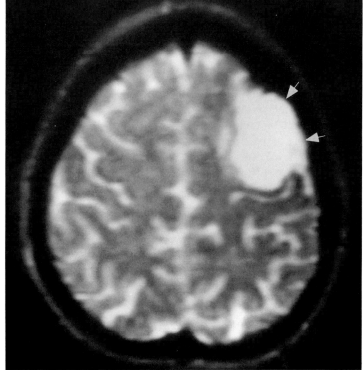

B

FIG. 7.54. Dysembryoplastic neuroepithelial tumor. **A:** Postcontrast axial SE 600/20 image shows a nonenhancing mass (*arrows*) in the left frontal lobe. **B:** Axial SE 2500/80 image shows scalloping of the inner table of the calvarium (*arrows*), indicating a slow-growing, superficial mass.

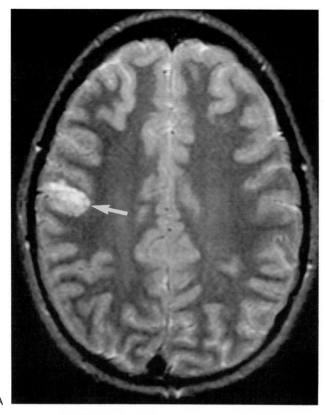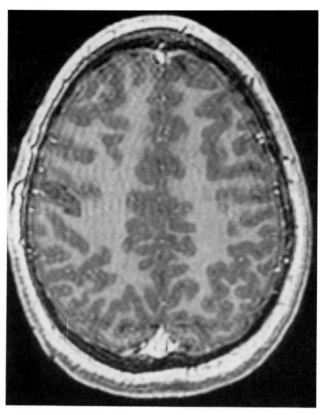

A   B

FIG. 7.55. Dysembryoplastic neuroepithelial tumor. **A:** Axial SE 2800/70 image shows multiple microcysts in affected right frontal gyrus (*arrow*). **B:** Postcontrast SPGR 45/7/35° image shows the multiple
microcysts without enhancement of the affected gyrus.

nents. Some are associated with cortical dysplasia, indicating a developmental defect during the second trimester *in utero*. Many tumors that, in the past, were
histologically classified as gangliogliomas or mixed oli-
goastrocytomas would probably be characterized as
DNETs if reviewed today. Imaging studies show nonenhancing cortical masses that are hypodense compared to
white matter on CT and have long T1 and T2 relaxation
characteristics compared to gray matter on MR (Fig.
7.54). If cystic or microcystic components are present,
they will appear as sharply defined areas of very long T1
and T2 relaxation (Fig. 7.55). Calcification may be present (116,117). Because the lesions are primarily cortical,
and therefore superficial, convexity DNETs may erode
the inner table of the skull (Fig. 7.54).

Meningioangiomatosis

Meningioangiomatosis is a disorder that involves the
cerebral cortex and, often, the overlying leptomeninges
(18). These rare, benign, hamartomatous lesions are
most commonly seen in association with type I neurofibromatosis, but they may be found as an isolated lesion.
Patients may present with seizures, headaches, or dizzi-

ness (118), but the majority of cases are found incidentally (119). The cause is unknown.

Pathology

Grossly, characteristic findings are cortical meningo-
vascular fibroblastic proliferation and leptomeningeal
calcification (119). Histologically, the disorder is characterized by a transcortical lesion composed of fascicles of
vascular fibromeninges. The fascicles contain central
capillaries. Adjacent cortex may contain neurofibrillary
tangles or hyalinization (119).

Imaging

On CT, meningioangiomatosis appears as a peripheral
mass that is hypodense prior to contrast administration
(Fig. 7.56A) (118,120), eliciting mild to moderate edema
in the adjacent white matter. No significant mass effect
is noted. MR scans show heterogeneous masses that are
iso- to hypointense compared with gray matter on T1-
weighted images and hypointense with a hyperintense
periphery on T2-weighted images (Fig. 7.56B) (118,

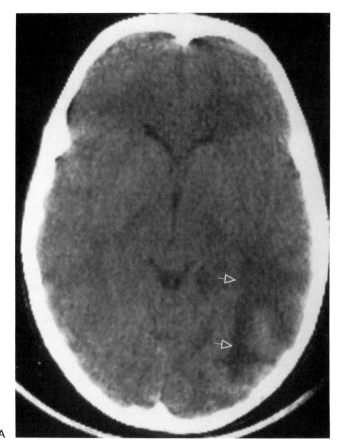
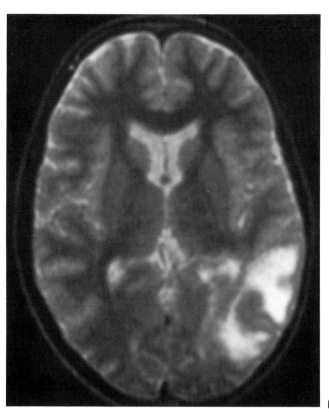

A

B

FIG. 7.56. Meningioangiomatosis. **A:** Noncontrast CT scan shows a region of hypodensity (*arrows*) in the left temporoparietal region. **B:** SE 2000/80 image shows a heterogeneous mass with central hypointensity and surrounding hyperintensity.

120,121). The single reported case of a postcontrast MR scan showed heterogeneous enhancement (120).

Sellar and Suprasellar Tumors

A Systematic Approach to Tumors of the Hypothalamus and Pituitary

Suprasellar masses can be differentiated to some degree before even looking at the neuroimaging study. It is important to recognize that some clinical signs and symptoms indicate hypothalamic involvement, whereas others indicate pituitary involvement. Knowledge of the characteristic modes of clinical presentation is important if the proper site is to be optimally imaged. Moreover, many tumor types present with specific clinical signs and symptoms. The most common presenting syndromes of hypothalamic and pituitary lesions and the lesions that most commonly cause them are listed in Table 7.1.

Chiasmatic/Hypothalamic Astrocytomas and Gliomas of the Optic Nerve

Gliomas originating in the optic chiasm often enlarge and involve the hypothalamus; similarly, astrocytomas

arising in the hypothalamus often grow inferiorly to involve the chiasm. Because the primary site of origin cannot be determined in many cases, we shall discuss these two lesions together. Astrocytomas of the optic chiasm and hypothalamus make up 10% to 15% of supratentorial tumors in children. Males and females are equally affected. The usual age at presentation is from 2 to 4 years, in contrast to gliomas that involve only the optic nerve, which present slightly later (6 years). The most common symptom is diminished visual acuity, which is noted in almost 50% of patients. The most common sign is optic atrophy. Large tumors produce hydrocephalus secondary to extension into the anterior third ventricle and obstruction at the level of the foramina of Monro. The combination of emaciation, pallor, alertness, and hyperactivity (the *diencephalic syndrome*) is seen in up to 20% of affected patients less than 3 years of age (5,18,19).

Pathology

Depending upon the series, 20% to 50% of patients with astrocytomas of the optic chiasm/hypothalamus have clinical evidence or a positive family history of neu-

TABLE 7.1. *Common presentations of hypothalamic and pituitary lesions*

Hypopituitarism
  Craniopharyngioma
  Kallman syndrome (see Chapter 5)
  Septo-optic dysplasia (see Chapter 5)
  Idiopathic

Diabetes insipidus
  Histiocytosis X
  Germ cell tumors
  Craniopharyngiomas
  Tuberculosis (see Chaper 11)

Precocious puberty (boys before age 9 years, girls before age 8 years)
  Hamartoma of the tuber cinereum
  Hypothalamic glioma
  Choriocarcinoma
  Teratoma
  Increased intracranial pressure
  Hydrocephalus
  Head trauma

Delayed puberty (boys after age 14 years, girls after age 13 years)
  Hypothalamic tumor
  Histiocytosis X
  Kallman syndrome (see Chapter 5)

Amenorrhea
  Pituitary adenoma
  Rathke's pouch cyst

rofibromatosis type I (NF1). In NF1 patients, the tumor usually begins in the intraorbital segment of the optic nerve and extends centrifugally toward the eye or centripetally toward the brain. The affected nerve expands in a fusiform fashion. Tumors originating within the optic nerve grow extremely slowly and are histologically similar to the juvenile pilocytic astrocytomas that occur in the cerebellum; malignant change is extremely rare in these tumors (122,123). However, tumors originating from the optic chiasm and the hypothalamus behave differently; they often are invasive and, on histologic examination, are identical to astrocytomas located throughout the cerebral hemispheres (5,124). It is noteworthy that, in adults, gliomas of the optic nerve and chiasm are usually highly malignant and aggressive, often proving fatal in less than 1 year.

Imaging Studies

The ready availability of fat suppression techniques on modern MR scanners (125) has made MR imaging the procedure of choice for evaluating tumors of the optic nerves and chiasm. CT displays the intraorbital portion of the nerve, contrasted by orbital fat, very nicely; however, the intracranial portions of the optic nerves and the chiasm are poorly seen by CT unless subarachnoid contrast is administered. When fat suppression techniques are used, MR imaging shows all portions of the optic nerves, the optic chiasm, the optic tracts, the hypothalamus, and the third ventricle. Moreover, MR allows the structures to be viewed in any plane; the coronal and sagittal planes are especially useful for evaluating tumors in the sellar and suprasellar regions.

CT remains adequate for evaluation of the intraorbital portions of the optic nerves. The enlargement of the optic nerve by tumor can be smooth and fusiform but is more commonly lobulated. The use of bone windows often reveals enlargement of the optic canals (Fig. 7.57) as a result of pressure erosion from the enlarged nerves. When the mass involves the intracranial optic nerves, optic chiasm, optic tracts, or hypothalamus, it almost always appears as a low-density, lobulated suprasellar mass prior to the administration of IV contrast. The tumors that grow along the optic nerves in patients with NF1 have a unique appearance in that the nerves have a characteristic downward kinking a few millimeters behind the globe, possibly as a result of nerve elongation (126). Hemorrhage, calcification, and cyst formation are very unusual in tumors of the optic nerves prior to radiation therapy. After intravenous contrast enhancement, the mass enhances heterogeneously and to a variable degree. When the tumor is very large, the enhancement can often be seen extending posteriorly from the mass along the optic tracts to the region of the lateral geniculate bodies (127,128).

MR imaging is optimal for showing the relationship of the mass to the chiasm, hypothalamus, and infundibulum. Moreover, when fat saturation and paramagnetic contrast agents are used, the intraorbital and intracanalicular portions of the nerve are demonstrated well (Figs. 7.58, 7.59). When tumor is primarily restricted to tubular enlargement of the optic nerves and chiasm, the tumor typically appears homogeneous; precontrast and enhancement are variable after intravenous administration of paramagnetic contrast (Fig. 7.59).

Astrocytomas of the optic chiasm and hypothalamus are almost always hypointense on T1-weighted sequences and hyperintense on T2-weighted sequences (Figs. 7.60, 7.61). When they are large and bulky, tumors of the chiasm and hypothalamus are typically heterogeneous, with large cystic and solid components; the solid portions typically enhance markedly after contrast administration (Fig. 7.61) (129). Although sagittal images best demonstrate the enlarged optic chiasm and hypothalamus, the coronal plane is optimal for visualization of tumor invasion of the cerebral hemispheres and identification of tumor in the optic canals, intracranial optic nerves, optic chiasm, and optic tracts. A small indentation in the superior surface of the tumor mass (Figs. 7.60,

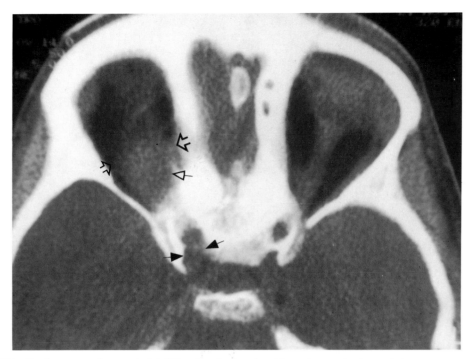

FIG. 7.57. Optic nerve glioma. Axial CT using bone algorithm shows the large left optic nerve tumor (*open black arrows*) and an expanded left optic canal (*closed black arrows*).

7.61) is often present, made by the anterior cerebral artery, which is often stretched over the top of the mass. A high signal intensity will often be seen extending from the optic chiasm to the lateral geniculate bodies on T2-weighted images. This finding may represent extension of tumor or edema within the optic tracts (126,130).

Craniopharyngiomas

Craniopharyngiomas are tumors that arise from remnants of the craniopharyngeal duct; they may occur anywhere along the stalk from the hypothalamus to the pituitary gland. They account for 3% of all intracranial tumors, 15% of supratentorial tumors, and 50% of suprasellar tumors in children. Although the incidence of craniopharyngiomas peaks between 10 and 14 years of age, a second peak occurs in the fourth to the sixth decade of life. Males are more commonly affected than females. Symptoms vary with the location of the tumor and the age of the patient at presentation. In general, symptoms consist of headaches, visual field defects secondary to compression of the optic chiasm and tracts, anterior pituitary dysfunction (growth failure) resulting from compression of the anterior pituitary and the hypothalamic–pituitary portal system, and hypothalamic dysfunction (usually manifest as diabetes insipidus) (5,129,131,132).

Pathology

Craniopharyngiomas may be either largely cystic, partly solid and partly cystic, or entirely solid. They vary greatly in size; small tumors present as solid or partly cystic nodules in the tuber cinereum, infundibulum, or sella, whereas large tumors are primarily cystic, often extending upward into the third ventricle or posteriorly and inferiorly to the level of the pons. When the tumor extends into the pituitary fossa, it is often of hour-glass shape; in such tumors, both the dorsum and tuberculum sellae are eroded. Although usually the tumors appear grossly well defined, they may invade the surrounding brain and are frequently surrounded by considerable gliosis. Foci of calcification and, on occasion, even frank bone formation may be present. The cyst fluid may be either straw-colored or a brownish, motor-oil-like substance that is rich in cholesterol crystals (5,19,129).

Surgeons divide craniopharyngiomas into three groups based on their location: sellar, prechiasmatic, and retrochiasmatic (131,132). *Sellar* craniopharyngiomas are usually small; they may invade the pituitary gland but usually do not distort the optic nerves, chiasm, or anterior cerebral arteries. *Prechiasmatic* craniopharyngiomas grow anteriorly between the optic nerves, displacing the chiasm posteriorly and elevating the anterior cerebral arteries; they rarely compress the third ventricle. *Retrochiasmatic* craniopharyngiomas can push the chi-

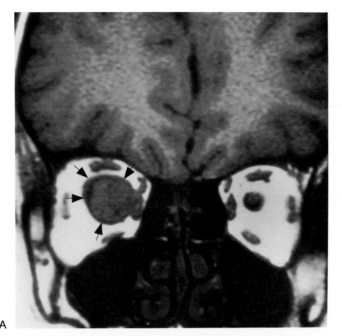

A

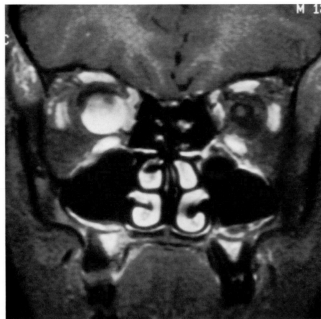

B

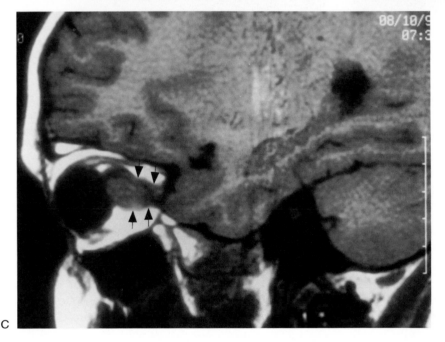

C

FIG. 7.58. Optic nerve glioma restricted to orbit. **A:** Coronal SE 550/15 image shows the markedly enlarged right optic nerve (*arrows*). **B:** Postcontrast fat suppressed coronal SE shows marked enhancement of the mass. Fat saturation is essential in performance of contrast enhanced studies of the orbits or head and neck. **C:** Sagittal SE 550/15 image shows ropelike enlargement (*arrows*) of the intraorbital optic nerve.

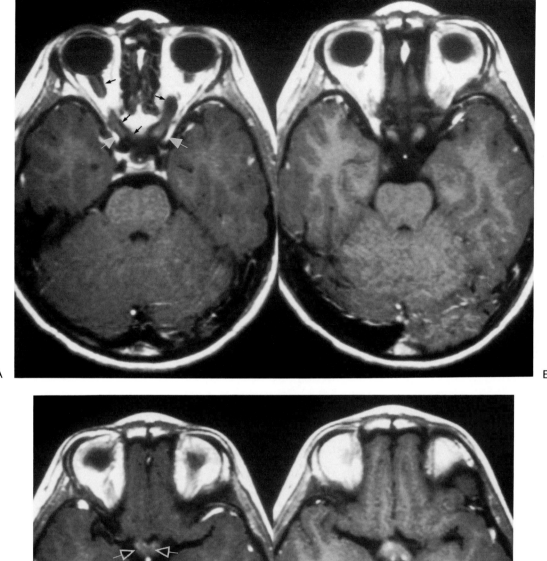

FIG. 7.59. Bilateral optic gliomas with intracranial extension to optic chiasm. **A–D:** Bilateral enlarged intraorbital optic nerves (*small black arrows*) can be seen extending through the optic canals (*closed white arrows*) and to the chiasm (*open white arrows*). Minimal enhancement of the nerves and chiasm is present.

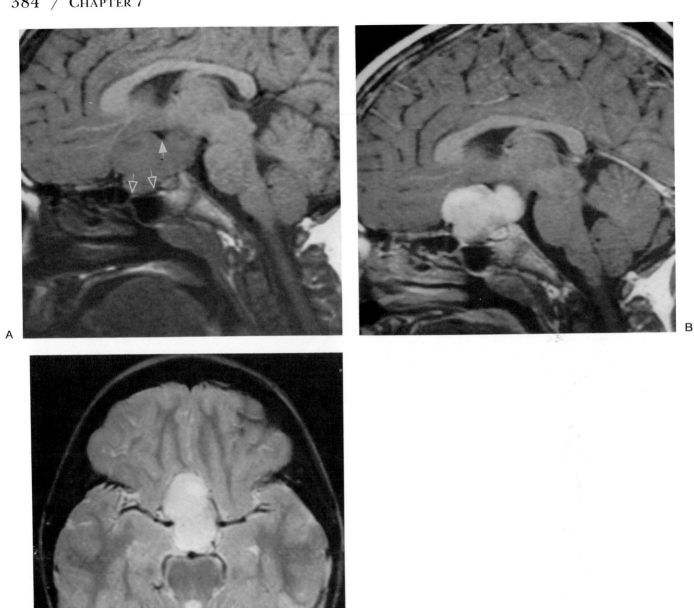

FIG. 7.60. Chiasmatic/hypothalamic glioma. **A:** Sagittal SE 600/20 image shows a lobulated suprasellar mass that erodes the posterior planum sphenoidale and tuberculum sella (*open arrows*). Indentation of the superior surface of the mass (*closed arrow*) by the anterior cerebral artery is characteristic. **B:** After administration of paramagnetic contrast, the tumor enhances uniformly. **C:** Axial SE 2500/70 image shows the tumor to be hyperintense.

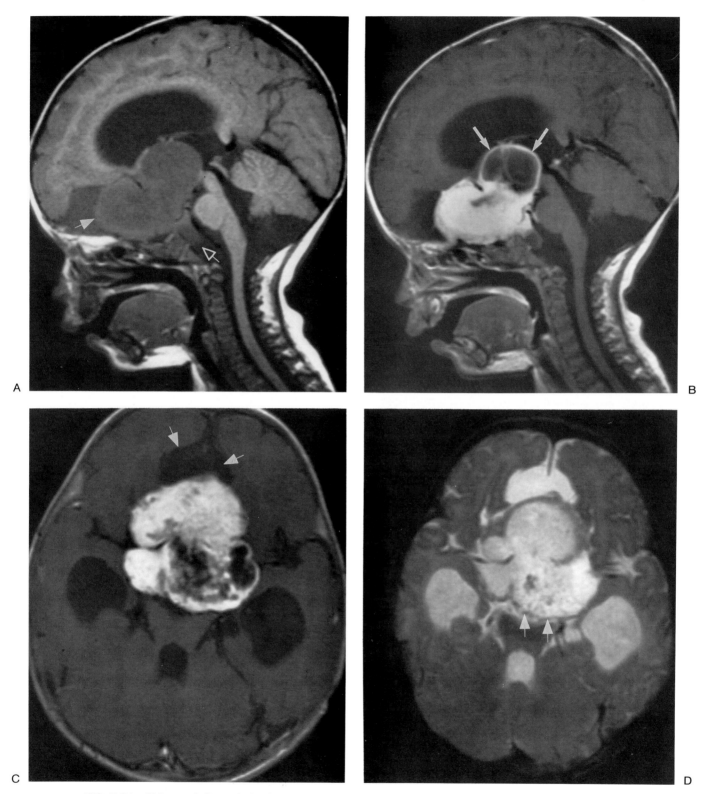

FIG. 7.61. Chiasmatic/hypothalamic glioma. **A:** Sagittal SE 600/20 image shows a large mass involving the suprasellar region, the anterior two-thirds of the third ventricle, anteroinferior interhemispheric fissure (*closed arrow*), and the prepontine cistern (*open arrow*). Significant hydrocephalus results from obstruction of the foramina of Monro. The optic chiasm cannot be discerned as a separate structure. **B:** After infusion of paramagnetic contrast, heterogeneous enhancement is observed. The superior portion of the tumor (*arrows*) is a large cyst. **C:** Postcontrast SE 650/29 image shows heterogeneous enhancement of the mass. The dilated anterior interhemispheric fissure (*arrows*) was the result of a cyst with nonenhancing walls extending anteriorly from the tumor. **D:** Axial SE 2800/70 image shows the tumor extending into the interpeduncular cistern (*arrows*) and splaying the cerebral peduncles. The tumor has a prolonged T2 relaxation time.

asm forward against the tuberculum sellae, fill the third ventricle, and extend into the prepontine cistern.

Imaging Studies

The CT appearance of craniopharyngiomas is characteristic (3,133). They are most frequently suprasellar in location; 90% have a cystic component and 90% are at least partially calcified. The calcification may be a thin, circumferential rim (usually around the cyst) or chunks of calcium within the solid portion of the tumor. Moreover, 90% of craniopharyngiomas enhance after the intravenous administration of iodinated contrast. Therefore, a cystic, contrast-enhancing suprasellar lesion with calcification is almost certainly a craniopharyngioma (Figs. 7.62, 7.63). If any two of these components are present, craniopharyngioma is a likely diagnosis. (Epi)-dermoid tumors can have the CT density of a cyst with foci of calcification, but (epi)dermoids, as stated earlier, do not enhance with IV contrast. Because craniopharyngiomas are often small, and the solid portion is generally isodense with brain, small tumors are sometimes difficult to identify on CT.

Craniopharyngiomas are also characteristic on MR studies, typically appearing as multilobular, multicystic masses extending upward from the region of the diaphragma sella (Figs. 7.63–7.66). The cystic areas may be high or low signal intensity with respect to brain tissue on T1-weighted sequences; the short T1 relaxation times, when present, are the result of very high protein content (134). Although both the cystic and solid components tend to be of high signal intensity on T2-weighted sequences, the cystic areas tend to be of higher signal intensity than the solid components (Fig. 7.64) (129,135). The solid portions of the tumor enhance heterogeneously after administration of paramagnetic contrast (Fig. 7.65); the thin walls of the cyst nearly always enhance (Figs. 7.64, 7.66) (129). Occasionally, craniopharyngiomas are entirely solid (Fig. 7.67); the solid tumors have an appearance and enhancement characteristics that are identical to the solid portion of more typical tumors. Rathke's cleft cysts are the only other lesions that originate in this area and have a high signal intensity on T1-weighted sequences. Since Rathke's cleft cysts tend to be small, intrasellar lesions that are approached trans-sphenoidally, the differentiation between an intrasellar craniopharyngioma and a Rathke's cleft cyst is entirely academic. When the cyst(s) of a craniopharyngioma is dark on T1-weighted images, differentiation from suprasellar astrocytoma may be difficult. The presence of calcification, heterogeneity of the solid portion of the tumor, enhancement of cyst walls, and enlargement of the sella turcica by extension of the tumor into the sella all suggest the diagnosis of craniopharyngioma.

It is important to realize that craniopharyngiomas extend into the middle cranial fossa, anterior cranial fossa, or posterior fossa (prepontine cistern) in about 25% of affected patients (Fig. 7.66) (136). This pattern of tumor extension should therefore suggest a diagnosis of craniopharyngioma. Very rarely, craniopharyngiomas can arise primarily in the third ventricle or in the optic chiasm (137). The characteristic lobulated, multicystic appearance and the inherent T1 shortening, if present, should aid in this diagnosis.

Hypothalamic Hamartomas (Hamartomas of the Tuber Cinereum)

Hypothalamic hamartomas are rare congenital malformations that are composed of normal neuronal tissue, located in the region of the mamillary bodies or tuber cinereum of the hypothalamus. Males are affected more commonly than females. The most common presenting symptom is isosexual precocious puberty, which usually manifests itself prior to the age of 2 years. The diagnosis, however, is frequently not made until 1 or 2 years later. Other symptoms associated with hypothalamic hamartomas include seizures [typically of the gelastic type ("laughing seizures") and more common when tumor diameter is more than 10 mm (138)], neurodevelopmental delay, and hyperactivity. Affected patients are commonly large for their chronological age (139,140). Although therapy is primarily medical, evidence has recently been presented that surgical removal of these tumors is curative (141).

Pathology

Hypothalamic hamartomas are well-defined, round to oval masses that usually project from the base of the brain into the suprasellar or interpeduncular cistern. They are usually attached to the tuber cinereum or the mamillary bodies by a thin stalk. Rarely, they can occur within the hypothalamus itself and no stalk is present. Histologically, hypothalamic hamartomas are composed of a heterotopic collection of large and small neurons, astrocytes, and oligodendroglial cells in proportion to normal neural tissue. They closely resemble the histologic pattern of the tuber cinereum. Calcification is rare, and hemorrhage is not described in these lesions (19,139,140).

Imaging Findings

On CT, hypothalamic hamartomas appear as rounded masses that are isodense with brain tissue; they sit within the suprasellar and interpeduncular cisterns. They are homogeneous and sharply marginated by the surrounding CSF. Enhancement does not occur after intravenous infusion of iodinated contrast (139,140,142). Rarely, cystic components can extend into the adjacent temporal fossa; under these circumstances, the solid, nonenhancing tumor may be difficult to identify prior to shunting of the cyst.

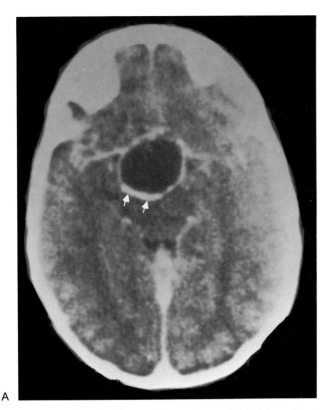
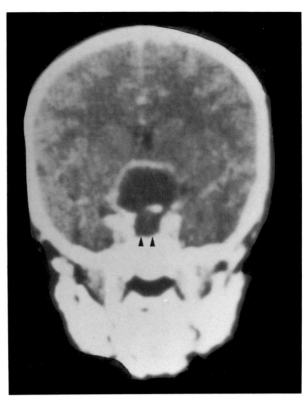

A

B

FIG. 7.62. Craniopharyngioma. **A:** Axial contrast-enhanced CT scan shows a low-density suprasellar mass with calcification of the posterior perimeter of the mass (*arrows*). There is a rim of enhancement around the low attenuation center. **B:** Coronal scan shows the low attenuation mass extending inferiorly into the sella (*arrow heads*). A rim of contrast enhancement is seen superiorly.

The MR appearance of hypothalamic hamartomas is typically that of a well-defined, round to ovoid mass within (Fig. 7.68), or suspended from (Fig. 7.69), the tuber cinereum or mamillary bodies. The hamartomas are isointense with brain on short TR/TE sequences and isointense to slightly hyperintense on long TR/TE sequences (143). They range in size from a few millimeters to 3 or 4 cm in diameter (139). No enhancement is seen after intravenous administration of paramagnetic contrast (143). The diagnosis is made by the characteristic location, isointensity to normal brain, and lack of enhancement (144–146).

Langerhans' Cell Histiocytosis (Histiocytosis X)

Langerhans' cell histiocytosis (LCH) was discussed briefly in the posterior fossa tumors section of this chapter, pertaining to its involvement of the brain stem, cerebellum, skull base, and calvarium. In this section, we consider involvement of the pituitary stalk, the most common intracranial manifestation of the disorder. Diabetes insipidus develops when more than 80% of neurons in the paraventricular and supraoptic nuclei of the hypothalamus are destroyed (147). It is present in 5% of patients with Langerhans' cell histiocytosis at the time of

diagnosis, but in up to one-third of affected patients on follow-up examinations (148).

When the pituitary stalk and hypothalamus are involved by LCH, the stalk is thickened (149). The thickening is difficult to see on CT without the use of intravenous contrast, especially if images are obtained only in the axial plane. When images are obtained in the coronal plane, both the thickening and the enhancement of the infundibulum can be appreciated (Fig. 7.70). MR is the imaging modality of choice, as the thickening and enhancement can be appreciated in both the sagittal and coronal planes (150). The thickened pituitary stalk enhances markedly after intravenous infusion of paramagnetic contrast. Prior to the onset of diabetes insipidus, the posterior pituitary retains its normal short T1 relaxation time. After the onset of diabetes insipidus, the high signal in the posterior pituitary on T1-weighted images is not present (151).

Pediatric Pituitary Tumors

Tumors of the pituitary gland are uncommon in children, with pediatric patients comprising only about 2% of those with pituitary adenomas (152,153). Those that do present in the pediatric age group typically present in

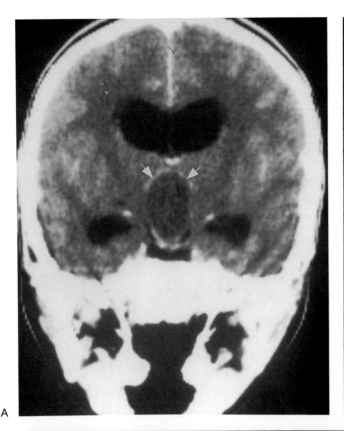

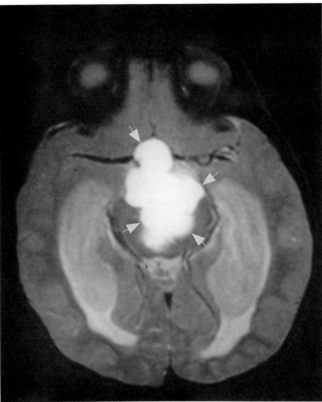

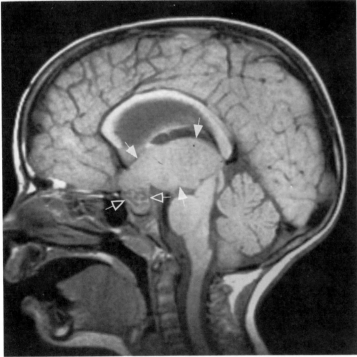

FIG. 7.63. Craniopharyngioma with extension into interpeduncular cistern. **A:** Coronal CT scan shows a suprasellar cyst with a thin rim (*arrows*) of enhancement or calcium. **B:** Sagittal SE 600/20 shows heterogeneous solid portion of tumor (*open arrows*) immediately superior to the pituitary gland and more hyperintense cystic portion (*closed arrows*) extending posteriorly into the interpeduncular cistern. Hydrocephalus is present secondary to obstruction of the foramina of Monro by the tumor. **C:** Axial SE 2500/70 image shows the hyperintense tumor (*arrows*) extending into the interpeduncular cistern. The irregular margin of the tumor with the cerebral peduncles does not necessarily imply invasion by the tumor.

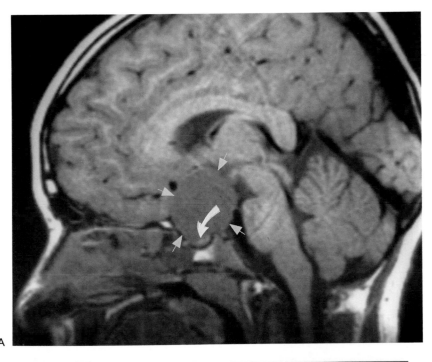

A

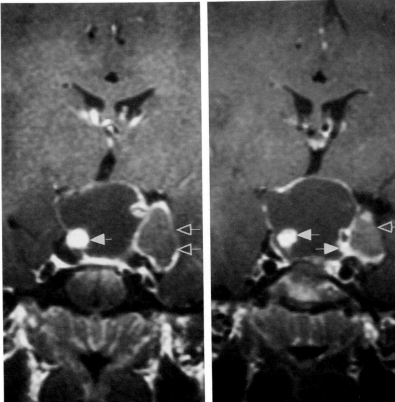

B,C

FIG. 7.64. Multicystic craniopharyngioma. **A:** Sagittal SE 600/15 image shows a mass (*straight arrows*) expanding the sella, compressing the pituitary gland (*curved arrow*), and superiorly displacing the floor of the third ventricle. **B, C:** Postcontrast coronal SE 650/29 images show the smaller cyst (*open arrows*) to be hyperintense compared to the larger cyst. Both cysts show thin rims of enhancement. The solid portions of the tumor (*closed arrows*) show greater enhancement. See **D** and **E** on following page.

adolescents (153). The most common hormonally active pituitary adenomas in the pediatric age group are prolactin-secreting adenomas (typically resulting in delayed menarche), ACTH-secreting adenomas (resulting in Cushing's disease), and growth hormone–secreting ad-

enomas (resulting in gigantism). About 25% of pediatric pituitary adenomas are nonfunctioning (131,153). In contrast to adults, pituitary tumors in children are more commonly macroadenomas than microadenomas. This fact may reflect a lack of symptoms in boys and premen-

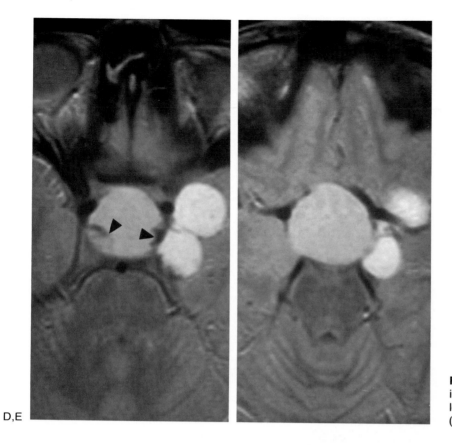

D,E

FIG. 7.64. (*Continued.*) **D, E:** Axial SE 2800/20 image shows differing intensity of the cysts and lower intensity of the solid tumor portions (*arrows*).

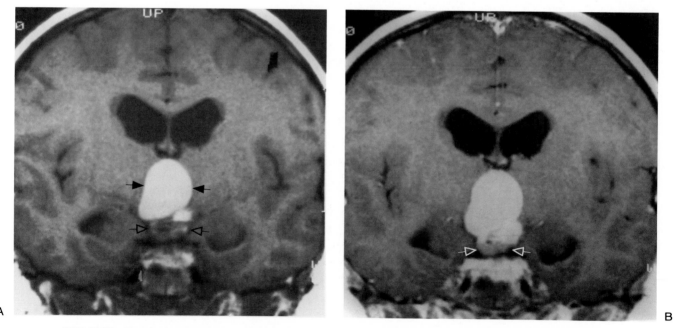

A

B

FIG. 7.65. Craniopharyngioma. **A:** Coronal SE 600/20 image shows tumor with heterogeneous hypointense solid portion (*open arrows*) and homogeneous hyperintense cystic portion (*solid arrows*). **B:** After contrast administration, the solid portion of the tumor enhances (*arrows*).

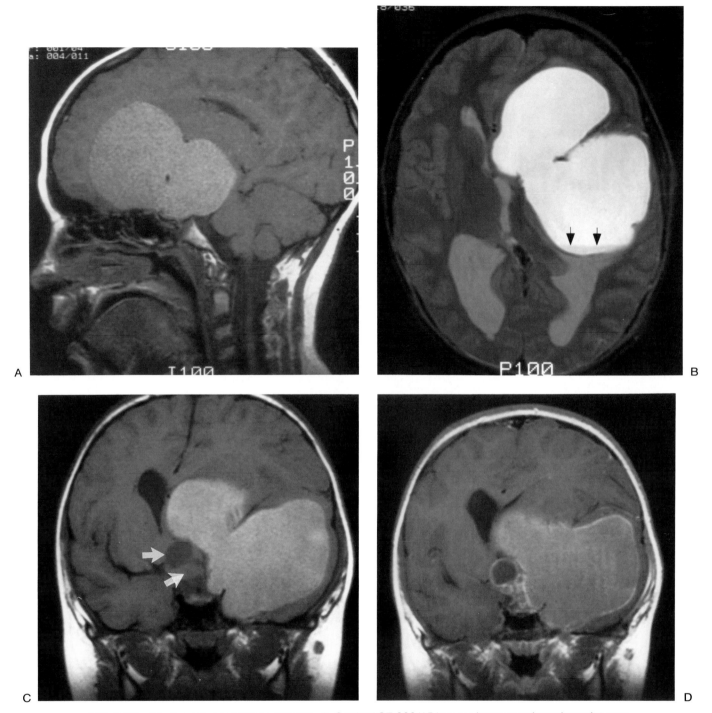

FIG. 7.66. Giant cystic craniopharyngioma. **A:** Sagittal SE 600/15 image shows very large hyperintense lobulated suprasellar mass. The sella turcica is enlarged beyond recognition. **B:** Axial SE 2800/70 image shows the lobulated cyst to be hyperintense compared to CSF. A fluid–fluid layer (*arrows*) is present. **C:** Coronal SE 650/20 image shows smaller cysts (*arrows*) that are hypointense compared with brain. The left temporal fossa is enlarged by the cyst. **D:** After administration of paramagnetic contrast, all the cysts show rim enhancement.

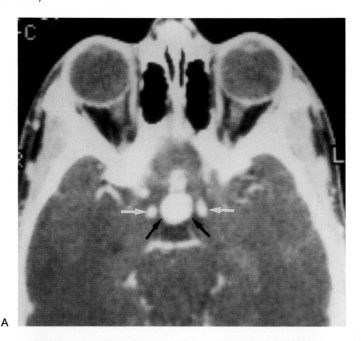

A

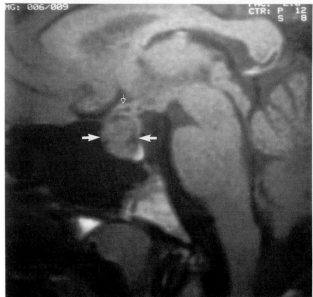

B

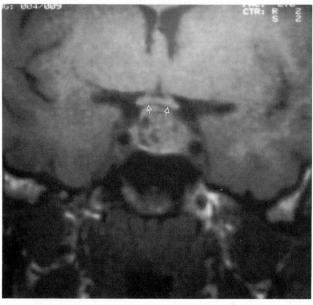

FIG. 7.67. Small intra- and suprasellar solid cranio-pharyngioma. **A:** Axial contrast-enhanced CT scan shows an enhancing mass in the suprasellar region (*black arrows*) situated between the two posterior clinoid processes (*white arrows*). **B:** Sagittal SE 600/20 image shows a heterogeneous mass within the sella and extending upward into the suprasellar region (*closed white arrows*). The optic chiasm (*open white arrow*) is slightly elevated by the mass. **C:** Coronal SE 600/20 image shows the mass sitting within the sella turcica and causing a slight upward displacement of the optic chiasm (*open arrows*).

C

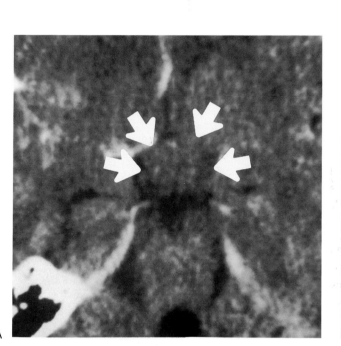

A

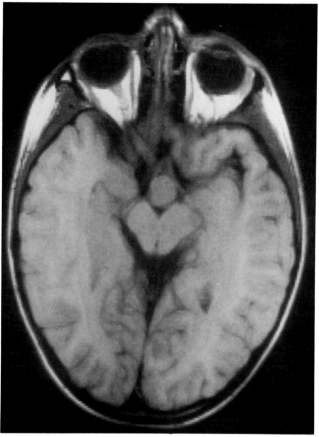

C

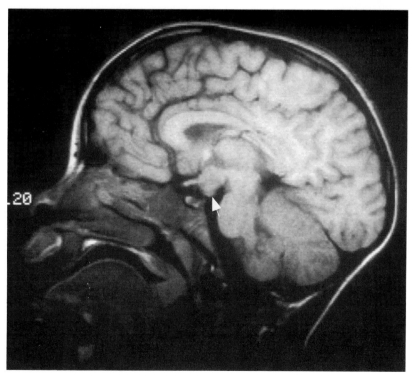

B

FIG. 7.68. Hypothalamic hamartoma within the floor of the third ventricle. **A:** Postcontrast CT scan shows soft tissue mass (*arrows*) filling suprasellar and interpeduncular cisterns. **B:** Sagittal SE 500/40 image shows soft tissue mass (*arrow*) in the floor of the third ventricle. **C:** Axial SE 500/40 image shows the mass sitting in the interpeduncular cistern.

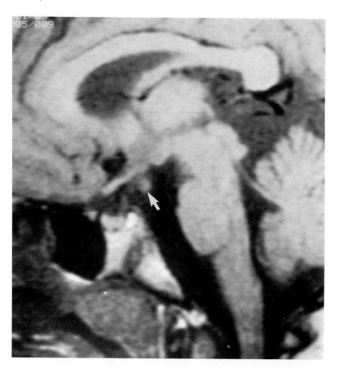

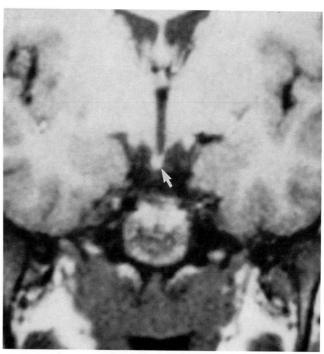

A   B

FIG. 7.69. Pedunculated hypothalamic hamartoma. **A:** Sagittal SE 600/20 image shows a small mass extending caudally from the tuber cinereum of the hypothalamus (arrow). **B:** Coronal SE 600/20 image shows this very small hypothalamic hamartoma (*arrow*) clearly outlined by CSF.

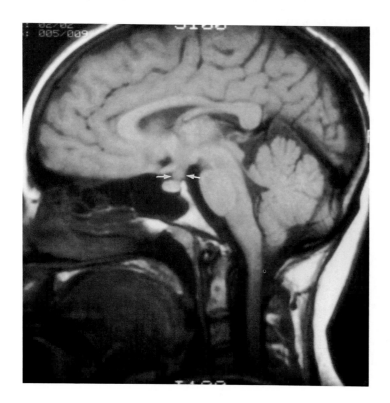

FIG. 7.70. Suprasellar histiocytosis X. Sagittal SE 550/15 image shows an enlarged infundibulum (*arrows*) and absence of the posterior pituitary gland (the "pituitary bright spot").

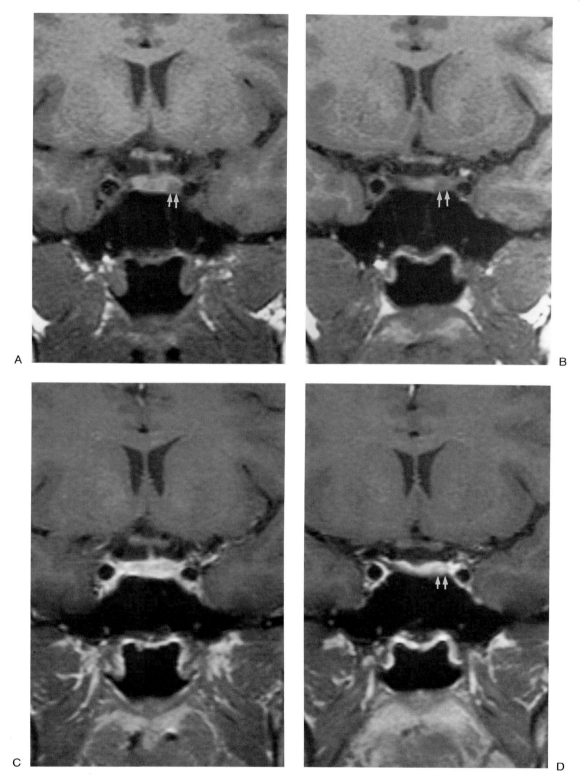

FIG. 7.71. Pituitary microadenoma. **A, B:** Coronal SE 600/15 images show a hypointense mass (*arrows*) in the left side of the pituitary gland. **C, D:** Postcontrast coronal SE 600/15 images show that the mass enhances slightly less than the pituitary gland (*arrows*).

archal girls with prolactin-secreting tumors. Large tumors may present with short stature, secondary to compromise of hypothalamic–pituitary function, or with visual disturbance if they extend into the suprasellar cistern (131,152,153).

The imaging appearance of pituitary adenomas in children is identical to that in adults. MR is the imaging modality of choice (154,155). Noncontrast thin section (3 mm or less) coronal and sagittal images should be acquired through the sellar and suprasellar regions. Microadenomas will appear as small (less than 1 cm) hypointense masses (Fig. 7.71) within the gland. Secondary signs include deviation of the pituitary stalk to the side opposite the tumor and upward convexity of the gland. Macroadenomas will expand the gland and, if the diaphragma sella is sufficiently large, will dumbbell into the suprasellar cistern, where the optic chiasm and infundibulum can be compressed. Lateral extension of the tumor can result in invasion of the cavernous sinuses (155). After intravenous contrast administration, microadenomas will typically remain hypointense compared to the enhancing gland on early images (154). However, if imaging is delayed, the adenoma will typically become isointense, or even hyperintense, compared with the surrounding normal gland (156). Therefore, the patient should be imaged as soon as possible after administration of contrast. Macroadenomas typically enhance uniformly and intensely (154). Caution must be exercised when examining the adolescent gland, as the hormonal changes during adolescence result in an enlargement of the gland, with upward convexity of the superior surface (see Chapter 2 and Fig. 2.18) (157). A focal lesion must be identified before an adenoma is diagnosed on the basis of the imaging study.

Rathke Cleft Cysts

Rathke cleft cysts are benign epithelium-lined cysts that contain mucoid material and arise primarily in the sella turcica. They are rare in children. Although often asymptomatic, they may produce symptoms by compression of the pituitary gland or suprasellar structures. They are thought to derive from remnants of Rathke's pouch, making them embryologically related to craniopharyngiomas (158). It is estimated that about two-thirds of children with symptomatic Rathke's cleft cysts present with manifestations of pituitary dysfunction, ranging from isolated hormonal deficiencies (typically growth hormone or prolactin) to generalized pituitary hypofunction. Visual disturbances are present in about half and headaches occur in about 30% (158).

CT scans typically show a round or lobulated intra- or suprasellar mass with attenuation values similar to CSF (159). MR shows round to ovoid, sharply defined mass that typically lies either between the anterior and posterior pituitary lobes or immediately anterior to the pituitary stalk (Fig. 7.72). The cyst has a variable signal intensity, ranging from iso- to hyperintense compared to CSF on T1-weighted images and from iso- to hypointense compared to CSF on T2-weighted images (160). No enhancement is seen after administration of paramagnetic contrast. Not uncommonly, the cyst is hyperintense compared to normal gland on precontrast MR images and hypointense compared to gland on postcon-

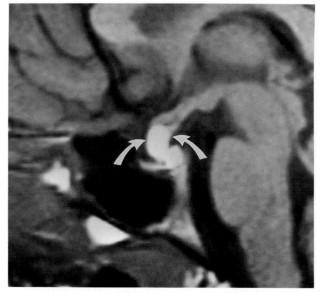
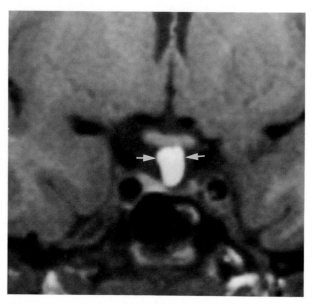

FIG. 7.72. Rathke cleft cyst. **A:** Sagittal SE 600/15 image shows an ovoid hyperintense mass (*arrows*) directly anterior to the infundibulum. **B:** Coronal SE 600/15 image shows the mass (*arrows*) situated between the pituitary gland and the optic chiasm.

trast images; when a sharply demarcated mass situated posterior to the anterior pituitary lobe has these signal characteristics, Rathke's cleft cyst should be strongly considered.

Suprasellar Arachnoid Cysts

Arachnoid cysts are discussed in Chapter 8.

Suprasellar Germ Cell Tumors

Germ cell tumors are discussed in the following section on tumors of the pineal region.

Pineal Region Masses

Germ Cell Tumors

Most tumors arising in the pineal region are germ cell tumors, a group of neoplasms that comprise about 3% to 8% of pediatric brain tumors (161,162). Of germ cell tumors, approximately 65% are germinomas (sometimes incorrectly referred to as atypical teratoma, pinealoma, or dysgerminoma), 26% are nongerminomatous (16% teratomas, 6% endodermal sinus tumors or embryonal cell carcinoma, and 4% choriocarcinomas), and 9% are mixed (162). Germ cell tumors are most common in the pineal region, but they can also occur in other areas of the brain, most commonly the suprasellar/hypothalamic region and the basal ganglia (161–163).

Germinomas

Germinomas are the most common neoplasm in the region of the pineal body, accounting for more than 50% of neoplasms in this area. Most germinomas occur in the second and third decades of life, with a peak incidence in the latter half of the second decade. They show approximately a 10:1 male predominance and most commonly present with hydrocephalus or the Parinaud syndrome (paralysis of upward gaze), resulting from compression of the aqueduct of Sylvius and mesencephalon, respectively. Approximately 35% of intracranial germinomas occur in the suprasellar region. Germinomas of the suprasellar region affect males and females equally and commonly present with symptoms indicative of hypothalamic involvement, such as diabetes insipidus, emaciation, or precocious puberty. It is of interest that patients with pineal germinomas frequently have symptoms indicative of hypothalamic involvement; these symptoms most likely result from spread of tumor through the CSF in the third ventricle to the infundibular recess with subsequent invasion of the hypothalamus. Some people, however, believe that the cause of these symptoms is multifocality of the tumor (5,19,161–164).

Less than 10% of intracranial germ cell tumors originate in the basal ganglia or thalamus. Affected patients show a male predominance and typically present with hemiparesis, mental status changes, or precocious puberty (165).

Pathology. Pineal germinomas usually are well-defined lesions restricted to the pineal gland; rarely, they occur in a parapineal location. Occasionally, adjacent structures, especially the quadrigeminal plate, are infiltrated by tumor. Suprasellar germinomas are round or lobulated masses occurring in the floor of the third ventricle, compressing and invading the optic chiasm and surrounding the pituitary stalk. They may extend upward into and infiltrate the walls of the third ventricle, mimicking an infiltrating glioma. Rarely, germinomas occur in the basal ganglia or thalamus. Metastatic spread occurs early and frequently via the CSF, often giving the involved surface of the brain a sugar-coated appearance (5,19,164,166–168).

Imaging Studies. The CT appearance of a germinoma is that of an iso- to hyperdense, well-marginated mass, typically occurring in either the pineal or suprasellar region. Occasionally, they originate in the deep gray matter of the brain. Uniform enhancement of the solid portions of the tumor is seen after intravenous infusion of contrast. Germinomas in the suprasellar and basal ganglia regions can be differentiated from astrocytomas by their high signal intensity relative to brain prior to contrast infusion (Fig. 7.73) (3,167–169). On MR, germinomas usually appear as well-marginated tumors, either round or lobulated, that demonstrate prolonged T1 and T2 relaxation times (Figs. 7.73, 7.74). Occasionally, a relatively short T2 relaxation time is present, resulting in a relatively low signal intensity mass on long TR/TE sequences (Fig. 7.74). The T2 shortening presumably results from the high nuclear-to-cytoplasmic ratio in these tumors with a resulting diminished free water content. When a relatively shortened T2 relaxation time is present in a suprasellar or pineal region tumor in an adolescent, the diagnosis of germinoma is suggested, although pineoblastomas can have the same appearance as pineal germinomas (170,171). Germinomas strongly enhance after infusion of paramagnetic contrast (Figs. 7.73–7.75), as do CSF-borne metastases to the brain (Fig. 7.75) and spine. In general, the differentiation of a suprasellar germinoma from a suprasellar astrocytoma is not possible using MR, although extension down the infundibulum may suggest germinoma (129). The differentiation is more easily made from the history; patients with suprasellar germinomas nearly always have diabetes insipidus at the time of presentation, whereas patients with suprasellar astrocytomas rarely develop diabetes insipidus until later in the course of the disease (129). Imaging is more helpful in differentiating suprasellar germinomas from craniopharyngiomas; germinomas rarely have cystic components and rarely calcify (129).

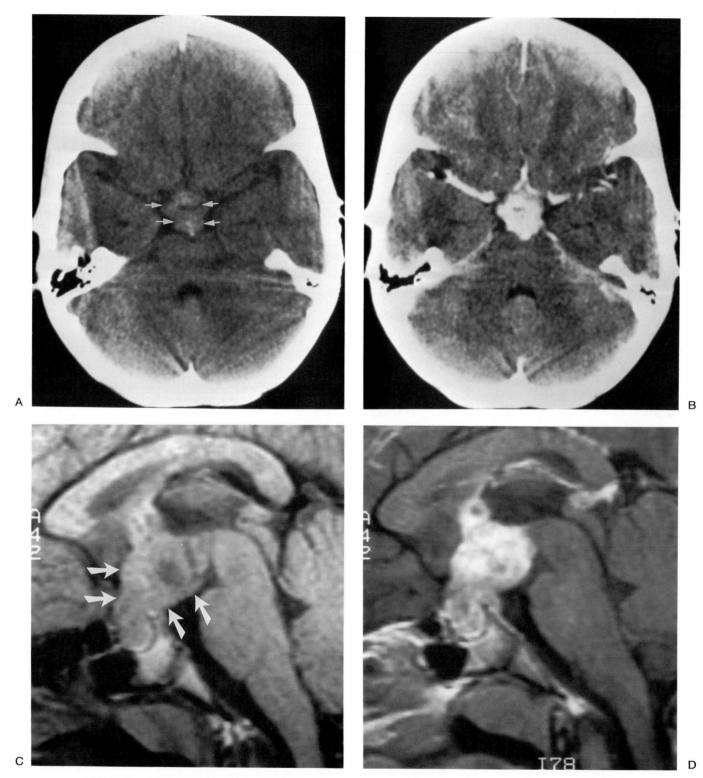

FIG. 7.73. Suprasellar germinoma. **A:** Axial noncontrast CT image shows the suprasellar mass (*arrows*) that is hyperdense compared to surrounding brain. Small, round cell tumors are typically hyperdense compared to normal brain. **B:** After administration of intravenous iodinated contrast, the germinoma uniformly enhances. **C:** Sagittal SE 600/20 image shows the mass (*arrows*) extending from the inferior third ventricle downward in to the sella turcica, filling the suprasellar cistern. **D:** Postcontrast sagittal image shows slightly heterogeneous enhancement of the tumor.

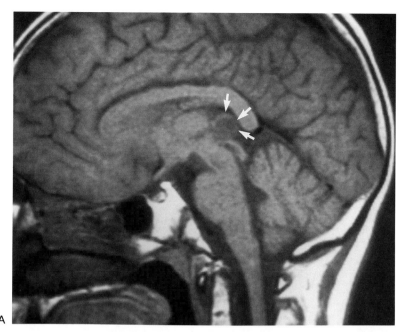

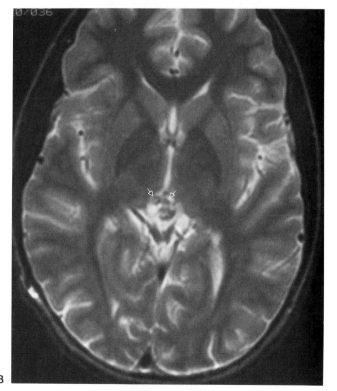

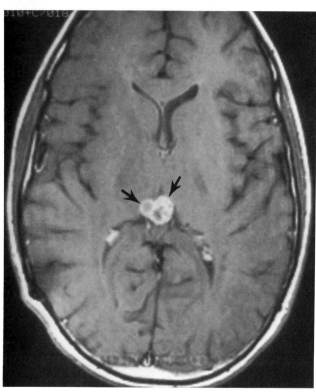

FIG. 7.74. Pineal germinoma. **A:** Sagittal SE 600/20 image shows a heterogeneous mass in the pineal region (*arrows*). **B:** Axial SE 2800/70 image shows the tumor mass to have a heterogeneous signal intensity with areas of short T2 relaxation time (*arrows*). **C:** After intravenous infusion of gadolinium-DTPA, there is marked contrast enhancement of the tumor (*arrows*).

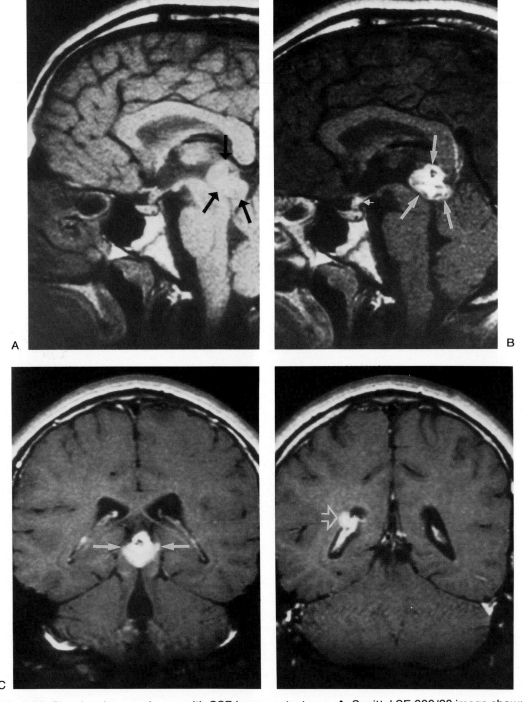

FIG. 7.75. Pineal region germinoma with CSF-borne metastases. **A:** Sagittal SE 600/20 image shows a large pineal region mass that has invaded the quadrigeminal plate (*arrows*). **B:** After intravenous infusion of paramagnetic contrast, heterogeneous enhancement of the pineal region mass is seen (*large white arrows*). In addition, a small focus of enhancement is seen in a thickened infundibulum (*small white arrow*). The patient had diabetes insipidus as a result of metastasis of tumor to the pituitary stalk. **C, D:** Coronal SE 800/20 images show the enhancing tumor mass in the pineal region (*closed arrows*) and a subependymal metastasis in the atrium of the right lateral ventricle (*open arrow*).

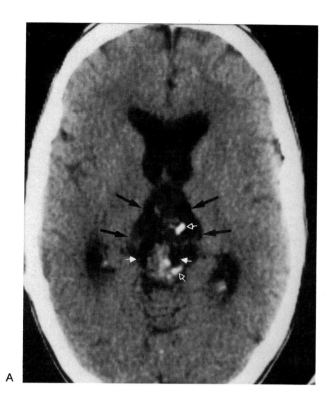

A

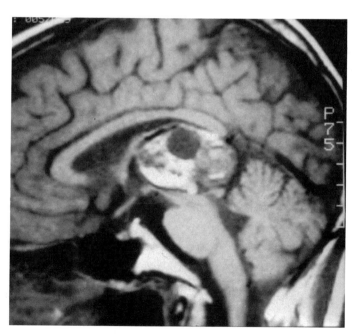

B

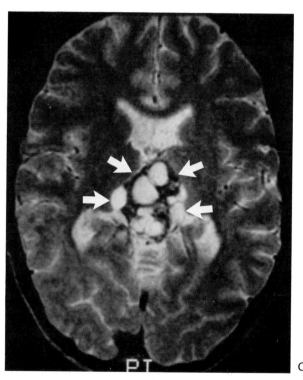

C

FIG. 7.76. Pineal region teratoma. **A:** Axial noncontrast CT scan shows a large mass in the pineal region and extending anteriorly into the third ventricle (*black arrows*). Foci of calcification (*open white arrows*) and fat (*closed white arrows*) are present as well. **B:** Sagittal SE 600/20 image shows the large heterogeneous tumor mass. The high-intensity regions represent fat. Calcification is not well seen on MR images. Note the extreme heterogeneity of the tumor. **C:** Axial SE 2800/70 image shows the markedly heterogeneous tumor with areas of high signal intensity, low signal intensity, and intermediate signal intensity occupying the pineal region and the third ventricle (*arrows*).

Teratomas

Although the pineal region is the most common site of intracranial teratomas, they may be situated in a parapineal region or in the suprasellar region. Pineal region teratomas are much less common than germinomas. As with germinomas, pineal teratomas occur almost exclusively in males; however, in contradistinction to germinomas, teratomas in the suprasellar location also have a marked male predominance. The peak incidence of presentation is in the second decade. Teratomas are similar to other germ cell tumors in that patients present with the Parinaud syndrome, hydrocephalus, and hypothalamic symptoms, the exact presentation being dependent upon tumor location (5,164,166,167).

Pathology. Teratomas are usually well-defined, extremely heterogeneous masses with a rounded or irregular, lobulated outline. Cystic areas and recognizable teratoma elements—such as cartilage, bone, hair, and fat—are common. In contrast to those in other parts of the brain, pineal region teratomas tend to be noninvasive (5,19).

Imaging Studies. As with teratomas in other parts of the brain and body, the hallmark of these tumors is their heterogeneity. On CT, they are distinguished by areas of fat and calcification in combination with cystic and solid areas (Fig. 7.76A). The MR appearance is also usually one of extreme heterogeneity (Fig. 7.76). The presence of fat, calcium, and soft tissue give a variegated appearance on T1- and T2-weighted images (Figs 7.76, 7.77) (129,171). Enhancement after infusion of intravenous contrast is not typically seen unless areas of malignant degeneration are present. An extremely heterogeneous mass in the pineal or suprasellar area should be strongly suggestive of a teratoma. The reader should be aware, however, that teratomas can be homogeneous on imaging studies. In such patients, the tumor is likely malignant and the diagnosis is unlikely to be made preoperatively.

Other Germ Cell Tumors

Choriocarcinoma, embryonal cell carcinoma, and *endodermal sinus tumors* are highly malignant germ cell tumors that occur in the pineal region. They generally present with either hydrocephalus and/or the Parinaud syndrome. Other than choriocarcinomas, these tumors do not have specific findings that allow them to be diagnosed radiographically. Choriocarcinomas are notoriously hemorrhagic; therefore, a hemorrhagic tumor in the pineal region (where most tumors have a very low

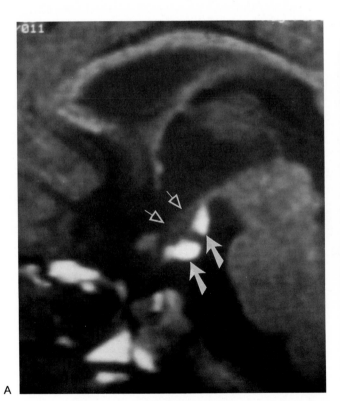
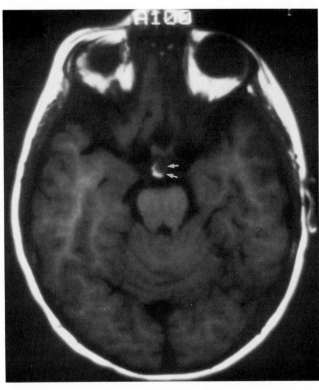

A   B

FIG. 7.77. Suprasellar teratoma. **A:** Sagittal SE 600/20 image shows a heterogeneous mass extending from the mamillary body to the infundibulum. Both fatty components (*solid arrows*) and nonfatty components (*open arrows*) are present. **B:** Axial SE 600/20 image shows the soft tissue mass (*arrows*) with a crescent of fat on the right side.

tendency to hemorrhage) is suggestive of a choriocarcinoma (164,167,171). Tumor markers, in particular placental alkaline phosphatase (PLAP), alpha-fetoprotein (AFP), and the beta subunit of human chorionic gonadotropin (β-HCG), are often secreted by germ cell tumors and can be assessed by serologic and CSF analyses. PLAP is secreted primarily by germinomas, β-HCG by choriocarcinomas, AFP by endodermal sinus tumors, and both AFP and β-HCG by embryonal cell carcinomas (172). Therefore, the specificity of preoperative diagnosis is aided by analysis of the tumor markers (172,173). An important concept is that approximately 10% of germ cell tumors contain more than one cell type; for example, there may be components of germinoma and embryonal cell carcinoma in the same tumor. Therefore, a needle aspiration of the tumor does not obtain adequate tissue to characterize the mass properly; open biopsy is necessary (173).

Pineal Parenchymal Tumors

Pineocytomas and pineoblastomas are both tumors that arise from pineal parenchymal cells. Both tumor types are considerably less common in children than pineal germ cell tumors. Pineocytomas are composed of relatively mature cells. They are usually circumscribed and noninvasive, are slowly growing, and may be found at any age; both sexes are equally affected. Because they are rare, the natural history of pineocytomas is not well defined (174). Some remain circumscribed and noninvasive; they are found after several years of clinical symptoms or disclosed at postmortem examination. Others metastasize extensively through the cerebrospinal fluid and behave more like the primitive tumor of this group, the pineoblastomas. Recent evidence indicates that pineocytomas in children are aggressive tumors that should be treated aggressively (175). Pineoblastomas are primitive, small round cell tumors that are highly cellular and resemble medulloblastomas histologically. They are highly malignant, demonstrating local invasion as well as distant spread through the cerebrospinal fluid. They may be found at any age but are more common in the pediatric age group (5,19).

Imaging Studies

Both pineocytomas and pineoblastomas are iso- to hyperdense on CT prior to contrast infusion (Fig. 7.78). In contrast to germinomas, which displace the calcified pineal gland, pineal parenchymal tumors usually contain areas of calcification within them; this is an important differentiating point (176). They are usually lobulated in appearance and show marked, uniform enhancement after the infusion of intravenous contrast (174,175,177,178). In this author's experience, pi-

neoblastomas more commonly have hypodense, nonenhancing foci within them and are larger and more irregular in shape at the time of presentation than pineocytomas or germinomas (Fig. 7.78). They frequently extend inferiorly into the posterior fossa and can invade the cerebellar vermis. Moreover, they can extend anteriorly into the third ventricle or laterally into the walls of the third ventricle. Pineocytomas tend to be smaller and much less invasive (3,167,169).

The MR appearance of pineal parenchymal tumors is nonspecific (171,179,180). They are usually iso- to hypointense on short TR/TE sequences and iso- to hyperintense on long TR/TE images (Fig. 7.78). *Pineocytomas* may be isointense with CSF on these sequences; they are differentiated from pineal cysts by the presence of trabeculae within the tumor mass and by diffuse enhancement after intravenous contrast administration (181). *Pineoblastomas* are usually larger and more lobulated than pineocytomas. Necrotic or cystic areas (hypointense on T1-weighted images and hyperintense on T2-weighted images) are commonly seen in larger tumors. The solid portions of the tumor enhance intensely after intravenous contrast administration (179,180). Very rarely, pineoblastomas can hemorrhage; the author has seen one such case. As with other pineal region tumors, pineoblastomas are known to metastasize frequently through the CSF; postcontrast scans of the entire neural axis are essential to detect and define subarachnoid tumor, which markedly enhances (182).

Dermoids and Epidermoids

Dermoids and epidermoids commonly occur in the pineal region. Their characteristics are described earlier in this chapter.

Pineal Region Gliomas

Gliomas, primarily astrocytomas, can also occur in the pineal region. Very rarely, these tumors develop from astrocytes within the pineal gland itself (183). Much more commonly, the tumors arise from adjacent brain parenchyma, such as the quadrigeminal plate, and grow into the pineal region secondarily (19,176). Patients typically present with headache secondary to hydrocephalus; they have few, if any, abnormalities on neurologic examination; thus, a significant delay often occurs between the onset of symptoms and the time of diagnosis (184). Histologically, most of the tumors in this region are pilocytic astrocytomas (184).

Imaging Studies

Imaging studies reveal a mass originating in the quadrigeminal plate, the medial temporal lobe, or the medial

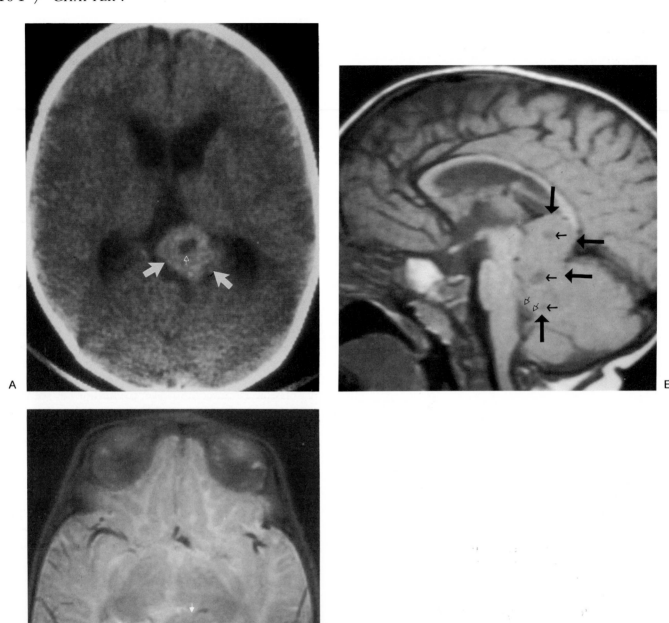

FIG. 7.78. Pineoblastoma. **A:** Noncontrast CT scan shows a mass in the pineal region (*arrows*). A small low attenuation center is seen within the mass (*open arrow*). Pineoblastomas are usually iso- to hyperintense with respect to brain on CT. **B:** Sagittal SE 600/20 image shows the mass extends from the pineal region well below the tentorial incisura into the posterior fossa (*large arrows*). There are multiple small cystic/necrotic areas within the tumor (*small arrows*). Note the inferior displacement of the fourth ventricle (*open arrows*). **C:** Axial SE 2000/80 image shows the solid portion of the tumor to be isointense with gray matter (*arrows*).

occipital lobe and growing into the pineal region (Fig. 7.79). If the tumor is very large at the time of the initial imaging study, the site of origin may become obscured; under these circumstances, differentiation of a primary pineal tumor from a parapineal tumor growing into the pineal region is impossible. The tumors are typically hypodense on CT and have long T1 and T2 relaxation times (hypointense on T1-weighted images and hyperintense on T2-weighted images) prior to contrast administration. After intravenous administration of contrast, the tumors typically enhance moderately to markedly (176,177,180).

Pineal Cysts

Small nonneoplastic cysts of the pineal gland are common, incidentally found in up to 40% of autopsies (185–187). Although many are too small to see on imaging studies, pineal cysts are, nonetheless, a frequent observation on MR studies of the brain, found in 1.5% to 4.3% of brain MR examinations (188–190). They are infrequently noted on CT scans, other than in retrospect, because they are isointense with CSF in the surrounding cisterns. On MR, they are most commonly appreciated on the sagittal images, where they appear as pineal masses that frequently cause a slight impression on the superior colliculi (Fig. 7.80A). An important factor in the differentiation of cysts from neoplasms is that cysts are rarely, if ever, associated with the Parinaud syndrome, and they are never the cause of hydrocephalus (190). In general, the MR appearance of pineal cysts is that of isointensity with CSF on T1-weighted images and slight hyperintensity with respect to CSF on T2-weighted images. The hyperintensity on the T2-weighted sequences is probably the result of loss of phase coherence of the protons in the moving CSF in the surrounding cisterns; the phase coherence of the protons within the cysts results in a higher relative signal intensity. Pineal cysts may very rarely hemorrhage; when hemorrhage is present, a high signal intensity is seen in the cyst on both short TR/TE and long TR/TE images and the cyst may enlarge, resulting in symptoms from local mass effect. After intravenous administration of paramagnetic contrast, the rim of normal pineal gland around the cyst typically enhances (Fig. 7.80B). The scan should not be delayed after contrast administration, as the cyst itself may enhance after prolonged delays, making differentiation from tumors impossible (191). The keys in making the diagnosis of pineal cyst by MR are the absence of clinical manifestations, the characteristic location, the isointensity with CSF on T1-weighted images, the absence of any internal structure within the lesion, and the presence of the typical rim of enhancement around the cyst.

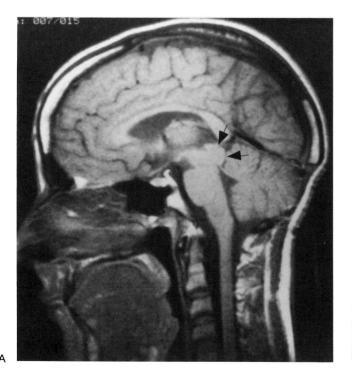
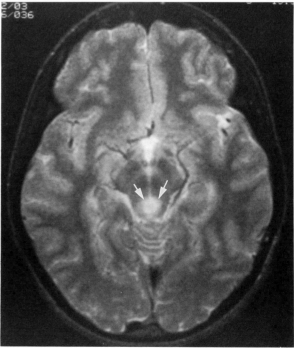

A

B

FIG. 7.79. Pineal region (quadrigeminal plate) astrocytoma. **A:** Sagittal SE 600/20 image shows enlargement of the quadrigeminal plate with extension of the mass (*arrows*) into the pineal region. **B:** Axial SE 2500/80 image shows the mass (*arrows*) to be hyperintense compared to surrounding brain tissue.

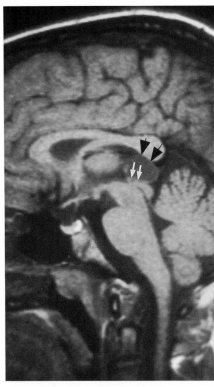
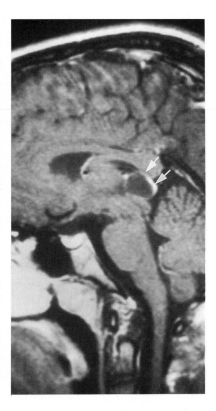

A,B

FIG. 7.80. Pineal cyst. **A:** Sagittal SE 600/ 20 image shows a homogeneous, sharply marginated ovoid mass in the pineal region (*large arrows*). The mass is isointense with CSF. Note that there is some distortion of the quadrigeminal plate (*small arrows*). In the absence of the Parinaud syndrome or hydrocephalus, such distortion should not cause alarm. These findings are classic for a pineal cyst. **B:** After administration of paramagnetic contrast, the rim of normal pineal gland around the cyst (*arrows*) enhances.

Extraparenchymal Tumors

Choroid Plexus Tumors

Choroid plexus papillomas and carcinomas are rare tumors that arise from the epithelium of the choroid plexus in both children and adults. They comprise approximately 5% of supratentorial tumors in children and less than 1% of all primary intracranial tumors. Choroid plexus tumors can occur at any age, but the majority are found in infants, or during the first 5 years of life. *Papillomas of the choroid plexus* are most often found in the first year of life; they are typically discovered because of the resultant severe hydrocephalus. *Choroid plexus carcinomas* make up 30% to 40% of choroid plexus tumors in children; they tend to present at a somewhat older age than papillomas, but usually within the first 5 years of life. The symptoms produced by carcinomas are more often neurologic deficits resulting from local brain involvement by tumor, rather than hydrocephalus. A marked male predominance has been noted for both papillomas and carcinomas (5,192–195).

Pathology

The most common site of origin of choroid plexus tumors in the pediatric age group is the lateral ventricle, the left side being more commonly involved than the right; tumors are rarely bilateral (192,194). The third and fourth ventricles are rarely involved in children, although the fourth ventricle is the most common site of origin of choroid plexus tumors in adults. Exceptionally, tumors may originate from choroid plexus in the cerebellopontine angle (196). Grossly, tumors of the choroid plexus are dark pink or red, globular masses with an irregular papillary surface resembling a cauliflower. They often cause considerable enlargement of the involved lateral ventricle. Papillomas tend to be well defined and quite separate from the surrounding brain. Small areas of hemorrhage may be present and multiple gritty foci of calcification are frequently found. Some choroid plexus papillomas show evidence of anaplasia and invasion of the adjacent brain. Anaplastic papillomas cannot be differentiated from carcinomas based on gross pathologic features; the distinction is based purely on characteristics of individual cells. Both aggressive papillomas and carcinomas show a marked propensity to metastasize through the CSF pathways, sometimes forming large subarachnoid masses (5,18,19).

Imaging Studies

The diagnosis of choroid plexus *papilloma* is easily made by CT. The tumor mass is isodense or mildly hyperdense to normal brain with occasional punctate foci of calcification. The most common location of the tumor is at the trigone, but papillomas may be located anywhere along the choroid plexus, including the frontal

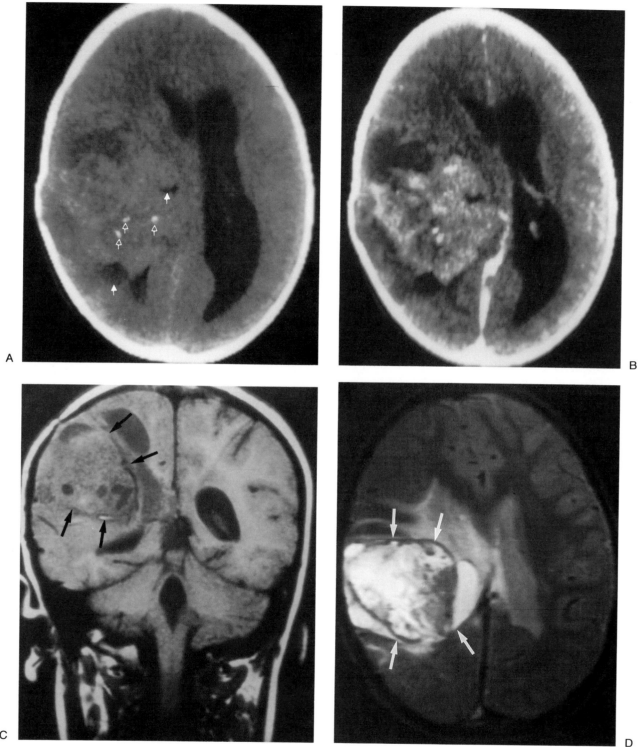

FIG. 7.81. Choroid plexus carcinoma. **A:** Axial noncontrast CT shows a large, high-attenuation mass involving the right lateral ventricle and the right cerebral hemisphere. Foci of calcification (*open arrows*) and cystic or necrotic areas (*closed arrows*) are seen within the tumor mass. **B:** After infusion of iodinated contrast, there is heterogeneous enhancement of the tumor mass. **C:** Recurrent tumor after surgery. Coronal SE 800/20 image shows a large heterogeneous tumor mass (*arrows*) underlying the craniotomy flap. **D:** Axial SE 2000/80 image shows the extremely heterogeneous tumor mass (*arrows*) with surrounding vasogenic edema.

horn and third ventricle. Homogeneous enhancement is seen after infusion of IV contrast. Although usually unilateral, bilateral papillomas have been reported (192). Occasionally, papillomas grow through the ependyma and into the surrounding white matter, inciting surrounding edema. These aggressive papillomas have a more irregular appearance more closely resembling a carcinoma; histologically, they show a higher degree of anaplasia than the less aggressive papillomas. Choroid plexus *carcinomas* tend to appear much more aggressive than papillomas. Carcinomas are irregular in contour, are of mixed density prior to contrast enhancement, and have a prominent but variable enhancement pattern. Cysts and hemorrhage are often present within the tumor. Carcinomas nearly always grow through the ventricular wall into the brain and incite vasogenic edema (Fig. 7.81) (3,6,192,195,197,198).

The MR appearance of choroid plexus *papilloma* is that of a lobulated intraventricular mass that tends to be homogeneous on both T1-weighted and T2-weighted sequences (Fig. 7.82). They are typically somewhat hypointense compared to gray matter on T2-weighted images, a characteristic that may aid in their preoperative diagnosis. Foci of hemorrhage or calcium are occasionally present. Uniform, intense enhancement follows intravenous administration of paramagnetic contrast (Figs. 7.82, 7.83) (194,197). Fourth ventricular papillomas may originate within or grow through the foramina

of Luschka, presenting as a cerebellopontine angle or cerebellomedullary angle mass (Fig. 7.83). Fourth ventricular papillomas are more common in adults than in children.

Choroid plexus *carcinomas* are heterogeneous in appearance and usually invade the surrounding brain through the ventricular wall, inciting vasogenic edema (Fig. 7.81). Carcinomas often have areas of high and low signal intensity on both T1- and T2-weighted images, resulting from hemorrhage and cyst formation. The frontal, occipital, or temporal horn of the affected lateral ventricle becomes encysted in more than 80% of patients (13,193). Choroid plexus papillomas are easily diagnosed on both CT and MR by their characteristic location and appearance. Carcinomas are more difficult to firmly diagnose pathologically because of their resemblance to primitive neuroectodermal tumors and ependymomas.

Meningiomas and Related Tumors

Intrinsic meningeal tumors in childhood are uncommon, comprising only 1% to 2% of primary brain tumors. In contrast to adults, in whom a female predominance exists, males and females seem to be equally affected in the pediatric age group. No definite age peak is noted within the pediatric population. The clinical pre-

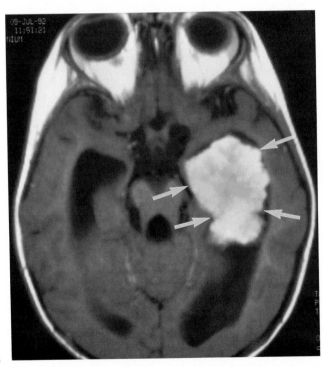
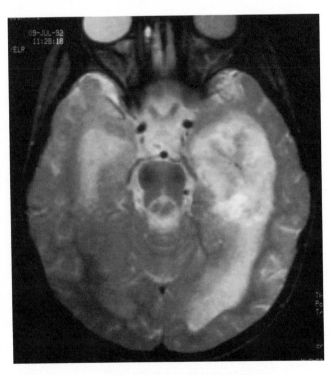

A

B

FIG. 7.82. Choroid plexus papilloma. **A:** Postcontrast axial SE 550/19 image shows a lobulated enhancing mass within the temporal horn of the left lateral ventricle (*arrows*). **B:** Axial SE 2500/70 image shows the heterogeneous mass to be relatively hypointense and filling the left anterior temporal horn. There is no surrounding vasogenic edema and no evidence of invasion of the cerebral parenchyma.

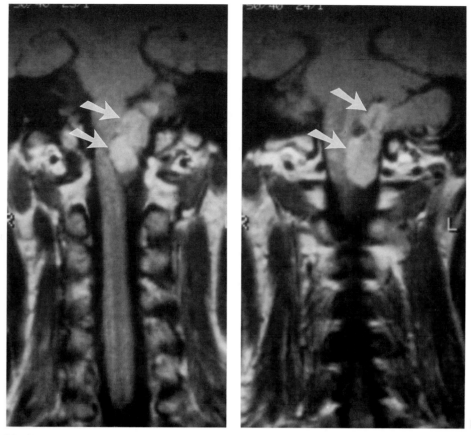

FIG. 7.83. Fourth ventricular choroid plexus papilloma extending through foramen of Luschka. **A, B:** Postcontrast coronal SE 650/40 images show the lobulated enhancing tumor (*arrows*) extending out the left foramen of Luschka into the cerebellomedullary angle cistern and into the cervical subarachnoid space.

sentation is variable and depends upon the site of the tumor (199–201). The presence of a meningioma in a child should raise suspicion for neurofibromatosis type II (see Chapter 6) and initiate a search for other meningiomas or schwannomas.

Pathology

Meningeal tumors of childhood include meningiomas (which are by far the most common), meningeal fibromas, meningeal sarcomas, and meningeal melanomas (200,202). In addition to their rarity, several features characterize meningeal tumors in children. They are often very large and are more frequently malignant than adult meningiomas; in several series more than 50% of pediatric meningiomas were malignant (5,19,199,201). For some reason, meningiomas in childhood sometimes originate in the Sylvian fissure and lack a dural attachment, a finding that may imply origin from heterotopic meningeal rests within the brain. Moreover, a higher percentage of meningiomas in the pediatric age group is intraventricular (199–201). In general, pediatric meningiomas have been found to show rapid growth, malignant changes, and poor outcome. A high mortality rate and

high incidence of sarcomatous degeneration have frequently been reported (19,199,201).

Imaging Studies

CT studies have revealed a heterogeneous appearance of these tumors. Associated hyperostosis is seen in approximately one-half of the patients, and half have intratumoral calcification. The tumors are iso- to hyperdense precontrast, and the solid portion of the tumor shows diffuse contrast enhancement (Fig. 7.84). Cystic and necrotic changes are more frequent in pediatric patients than in adults, possibly because of the larger size at the time of diagnosis. The presence of atypical CT features, such as hemorrhage, heterogeneous enhancement, cyst formation, or poorly defined margins, suggests a malignant tumor, such as meningeal sarcoma or meningeal PNET. Intraventricular meningiomas arise from the choroid plexuses and have the same signal characteristics as those originating in the dura (199,200,203).

On MR, pediatric meningiomas are generally large masses that arise from the dura, the choroid plexuses, or ectopic dural rests in the Sylvian fissures. Meningiomas typically have well-defined margins and are isointense to

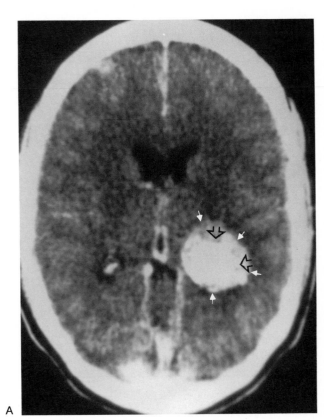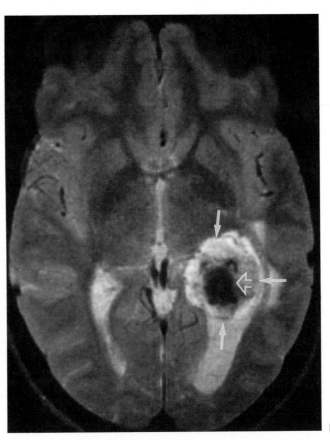

A   B

FIG. 7.84. Meningioma. **A:** Contrast-enhanced CT scan shows a mass within the atrium of the left lateral ventricle. The periphery (*white arrows*) is enhancing, whereas the central portion (*open black arrows*) is densely calcified. **B:** Axial SE 2500/70 image shows the meningioma (*closed white arrows*) in the atrium of the left lateral ventricle. The densely calcified center (*open arrow*) is of very low signal intensity.

gray matter on T1-weighted sequences and iso- to hyperintense to gray matter on T2-weighted sequences. Cystic and necrotic areas, if present, have prolonged T1 and T2 relaxation times compared to the solid portion of the tumor, which shows uniform enhancement after intravenous infusion of paramagnetic contrast. Densely calcified areas will be of very low intensity, whereas areas that are less densely calcified may appear iso- or hyperintense on noncontrast T1-weighted images (Fig. 7.84B). Arteriography can be helpful in affected patients, especially if a characteristic homogeneous tumor blush is seen along with vascular supply from meningeal vessels. The reader should keep in mind, however, that meningeal tumors can parasitize blood flow from intracerebral vessels and, thus, incorrectly suggest a primary intracerebral tumor. Similarly, intracerebral tumors can parasitize flow from meningeal vessels to mimic meningeal tumors.

Leukemia and Lymphoma

Metastases to the brain and meninges from systemic malignancies are rare in childhood. The exceptions to this rule are childhood leukemia and lymphoma. The most common finding in *leukemia* is enlargement of the ventricles and sulci. Although some have suggested that the brain atrophy was a result of radiotherapy and chemotherapy, Kretzschmar and colleagues (204) found that 31% of children with acute lymphocytic leukemia have enlarged ventricles before treatment, suggesting that these changes represent hydrocephalus, not atrophy, and are caused by the disease, not by the treatment. Although meningeal and parenchymal metastatic disease are occasionally seen, they are far less common than enlargement of the ventricles and sulci. On CT, only 5% of leukemic patients with CNS symptoms show contrast enhancement of the meninges (3). When lymphomas and leukemias do involve the brain, they appear on CT as areas of iso- to hyperdense signal prior to contrast enhancement. On MR, these masses tend to be slightly hypointense with respect to brain on short TR/TE sequences and iso- to slightly hyperintense on long TR/TE sequences. All lesions show diffuse and prominent enhancement, on both CT and MR, after infusion of IV contrast. There are no characteristic locations within the brain.

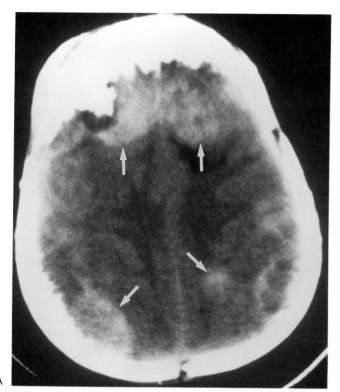

A

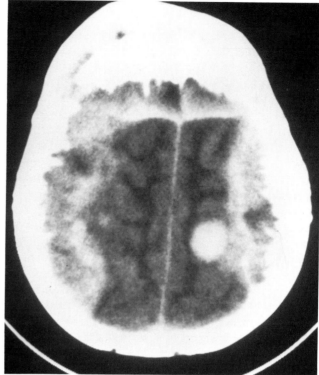

B

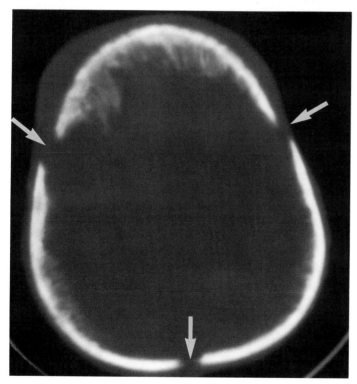

C

FIG. 7.85. Metastatic neuroblastoma to calvarium. **A:** Noncontrast CT scan shows multiple intracranial hyperdense masses (*arrows*), some of which appear to be intraparenchymal in origin. Bony spicules extend intracranially from the calvarium. **B:** After intravenous contrast infusion, the masses heterogeneously enhance. **C:** Bone windows show the characteristic bony spicules radiating centripetally from the calvarium. Also notice the splitting of the coronal and sagittal sutures (*arrows*), another characteristic finding in metastatic neuroblastoma.

Calvarial Tumors

Tumors arising from the calvarium were discussed in Chapter 5, under the Cephalocele section entitled "Fontanel Dermoids and Other Calvarial Masses of Childhood." *Neuroblastoma metastases* should also be mentioned in this section. Neuroblastomas are common tumors of childhood that can involve the central nervous system either by direct extension (primarily in the spine; see Chapter 10) or, more commonly, by blood-borne metastases. Neuroblastoma metastases rarely involve the brain; instead, they characteristically involve the orbit and calvarium. On CT, calvarial metastases from neuroblastoma show a characteristic appearance of a mass (or masses) growing inward from the bone with spicules of bone radiating centripetally within it (Fig. 7.85). Calvarial metastases can grow centripetally into the intracranial space and mimic intracranial masses. Coronal images will help to verify a dural or extradural origin of these lesions. On MR, the metastases appear as soft tissue intensity masses originating within the calvarium (Fig. 7.86). They enhance markedly, on both CT and MR, after administration of contrast. The elevated periosteum will enhance as well and may be a helpful sign in differentiating metastatic tumor from the normal hematopoietic marrow of childhood.

TUMORS OF THE HEAD AND NECK IN CHILDHOOD

Ocular Tumors

Retinoblastoma is the most common intraocular malignancy in childhood. It most often presents in early childhood with leukocoria, or "cat's eye reflex." Ten percent of retinoblastomas are inherited by an autosomal dominant mechanism; those that are hereditary are more commonly bilateral. In 2% to 5% of patients with bilateral retinoblastomas, a small cell tumor in the pineal region (pineoblastoma) will eventually develop, although the pineal tumor is rarely present at the time the ocular tumors present. When tumors are found in both globes and in the pineal region, the term *trilateral retinoblastoma* is applied. Overall, there is a 31% incidence of bilaterality and a 33% incidence of multifocality (205). Eighty percent of retinoblastomas occur in patients less than 2 years old. Subsequent neoplasms, most commonly soft tissue sarcomas, develop in 10% to 15% of affected patients.

The usual CT appearance is that of a calcified mass within the globe. The mass, which may be of any size, arises from the retina, but the borders may be ill defined, making the retinal origin unclear. Calcification is seen in 95% of these tumors and may be large, small, single, or multiple (Fig. 7.87A). Enhancement is usually seen after contrast administration. The tumor may extend through the sclera into the orbital lymphatics or through the optic nerve intracranially; both pathways of extension are well visualized by CT. Because the presence of calcification is the most important factor in the identification of these tumors, CT should be the primary imaging modality used in patients presenting with leukocoria, although retinoblastomas can be identified by MR (Fig. 7.87B) (205,206). The primary differential diagnosis is *Coats' disease*, which is a degenerative proliferative disease of the retina. In Coats' disease, secretions that are high in cholesterol content escape into the subretinal area, causing retinal detachment and hemorrhage (Fig. 7.88) (207). Coats' disease has an identical appearance on CT to larval granulomatosis (Fig. 7.89), caused by a *Toxocaris canii* infection (208). Both are differentiated from retinoblastoma by the absence of calcification on CT. Another anomaly that results in leukocoria, retinal detachment, and subretinal hemorrhage is the *persistent hyperplastic primary vitreous* (Figs. 7.90, 7.91). Differentiation from retinoblastoma is made by the absence of calcification and by the presence of a hypoplastic globe on the affected side (209). Occasionally, a persistent hyaloid canal can be seen, confirming the diagnosis (Fig. 7.90).

Retrobulbar Orbital Masses

Retrobulbar orbital masses in children include a wide range of pathologies, including vascular tumors (lymphangiomas, varices, and hemangiomas), rhabdomyosarcomas, neurofibromas, infections, cysts, dermoids, cephaloceles, gliomas, meningiomas, Langerhans' cell histiocytosis, leukemic infiltrates, and metastatic neuroblastoma (210–214). Dermoids and cephaloceles were discussed in Chapter 5. Infections are discussed in Chapter 11, and optic gliomas, meningiomas, and Langerhans' cell histiocytosis were discussed earlier in this chapter. The remaining pathologies will be discussed briefly.

Vascular Tumors

Orbital hemangiomas and lymphangiomas are best thought of as hamartomatous malformations that arise from an anlage of vascular mesenchyme that is capable of differentiating into both lymphatic vessels and blood vessels, as well as other mesenchymal tissues (215,216).

Capillary hemangiomas are the most common vascular mass to present in the orbit in children. These malformations, which have a female predominance, typically present at birth or shortly thereafter and show rapid growth during the first 6 months of life. They typically cease growth during the second year of life and then slowly involute over the subsequent 5–6 years (215,216). CT scans show a diffuse, usually poorly marginated mass that is typically retrobulbar. The mass may be outside

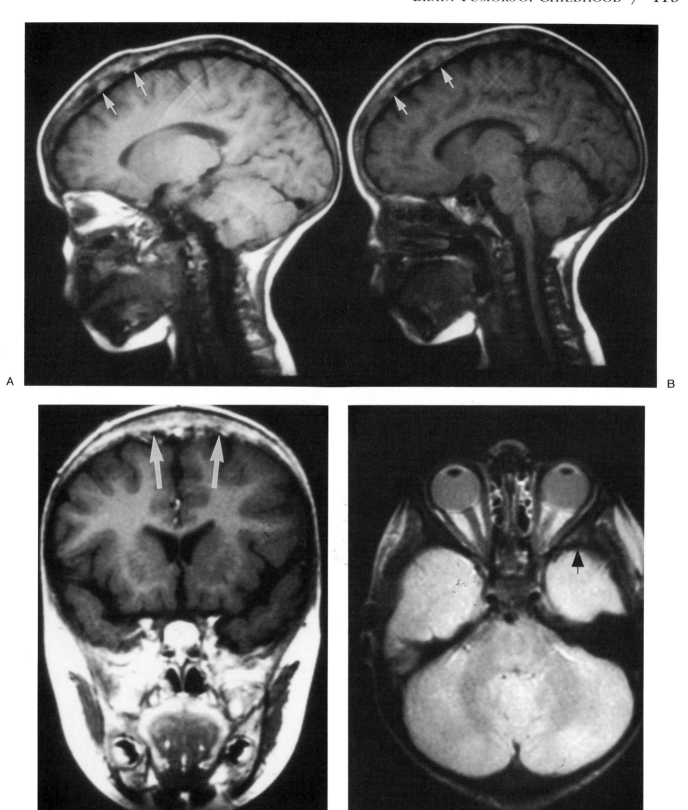

FIG. 7.86. Metastatic neuroblastoma to calvarium and orbital wall. **A, B:** Sagittal SE 600/20 images show thickened, heterogeneous calvarium (*arrows*). **C:** Postcontrast coronal SE 600/20 image shows marked enhancement (*arrows*) of the affected calvarium. **D:** Axial SE 2700/30 image shows expanded, hyperintense lateral orbital wall (*arrow*), secondary to presence of metastatic tumor.

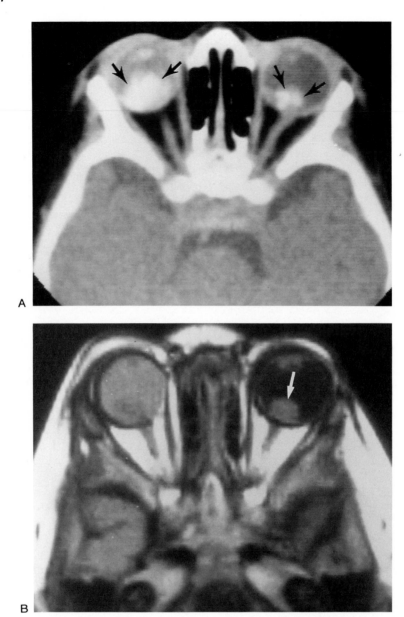

FIG. 7.87. Bilateral retinoblastomas. **A:** Axial noncontrast CT through the globes shows calcified masses arising from the retina bilaterally (*arrows*). There is no evidence of extension of tumor outside of the globes. The pineal region was spared in this patient. **B:** Axial SE 500/40 image shows the mass in the left globe extremely well (*arrow*). The mass in the right globe is not well seen because of high signal in the vitreous resulting from hemorrhage and proteinaceous exudate.

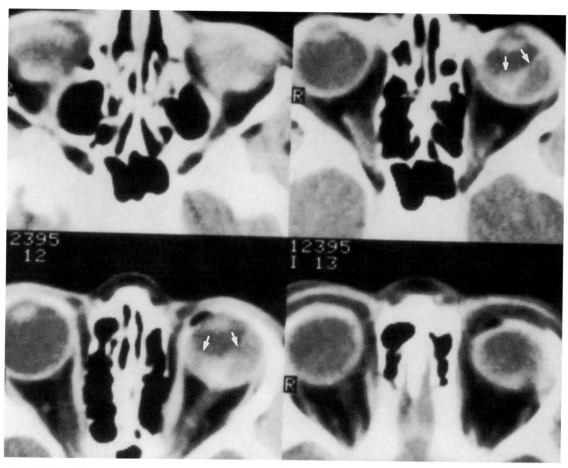

FIG. 7.88. Coats' disease. Axial CT images show crescentic hyperdensity (*arrows*) in the posterior left globe secondary to subretinal hemorrhage. The globe is of normal size and no calcification is present, suggesting the diagnosis of Coats' disease.

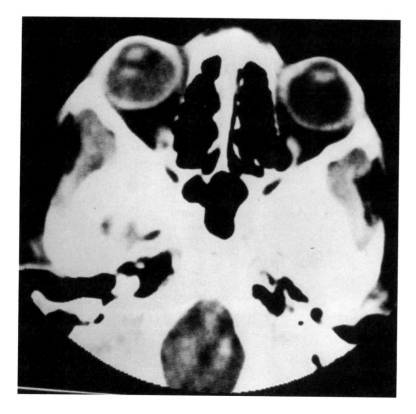

FIG. 7.89. Larval granulomatosis. Axial CT shows crescentic hyperdensity in the posterior right globe. The appearance is identical to that of Coats' disease (Fig. 7.88). (This case courtesy Dr. Sylvester Chuang, Toronto.)

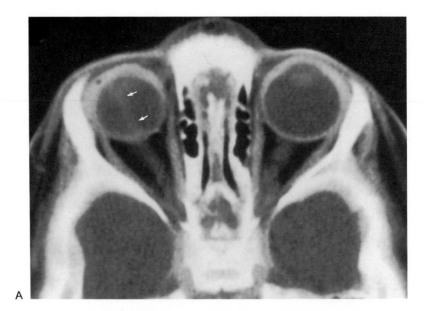

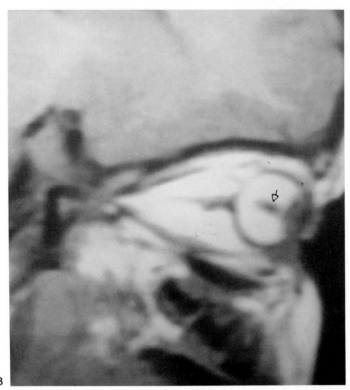

FIG. 7.90. Persistent hyperplastic primary vitreous. **A:** Axial CT through the globes shows a hypoplastic right globe. Moreover, a streaky density is seen extending toward the head of the optic nerve through the vitreous (*arrows*). This represents a persistent hyaloid canal and confirms the diagnosis of persistent hyperplastic primary vitreous. **B:** Sagittal SE 600/20 image shows the vitreous to contain hemorrhagic components. The hyaloid canal can be seen outlined by the hemorrhagic vitreous (*arrow*).

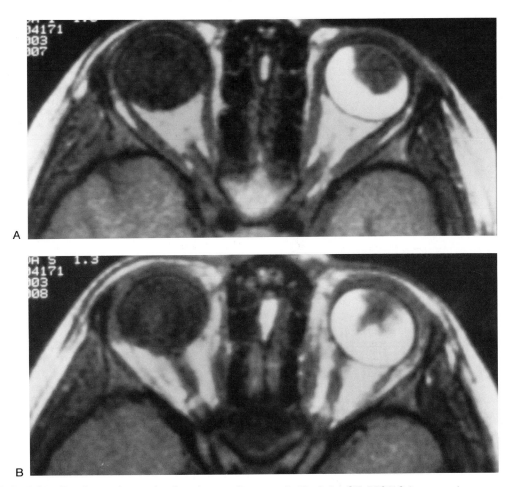

FIG. 7.91. Persistent hyperplastic primary vitreous. **A, B:** Axial SE 550/16 images show crescentic hemorrhage in the posterior left globe. The left globe is smaller than the right globe. The combination of microphthalmia and retinal detachment is strongly suggestive of PHPV.

the cone of extraocular muscles (extraconal), inside the muscle cone (intraconal), or both. Diffuse enhancement is seen after administration of iodinated contrast (Fig. 7.92). MR shows the tumor as slightly hyperintense compared to extraocular muscles and hypointense compared to fat on T1-weighted images. On T2-weighted images, capillary hemangiomas are hyperintense compared to muscle and hypointense compared to fat. Curvilinear flow voids, representing blood vessels, are typically present within the mass; this finding is useful in differentiating hemangiomas from more aggressive lesions, such as rhabdomyosarcomas. The affected orbit is often enlarged, probably as a result of the congenital nature of the lesion (216,217).

Most *lymphangiomas* present during childhood; they are the most common vascular mass of the orbit presenting between the ages of 1 and 15 years. Patients typically present with recurrent episodes of proptosis that result from recurrent hemorrhages within the mass. On CT, lymphangiomas are heterogeneous, poorly defined lesions that cross anatomic boundaries such as the conal

fascia and orbital septum (Fig. 7.93). Small focal calcifications, representing phleboliths, are occasionally seen. Areas of hyperdensity, representing acute hemorrhage, may be present, especially after recent exacerbation of proptosis. Enhancement is heterogeneous (210,217). On MR, lymphangiomas appear as lobulated masses containing septi that divide it into multiple cysts and lobules that have varying sizes and intensities on both T1- and T2-weighted images. The majority of the mass is typically hypointense to muscle on T1-weighted images and hyperintense to muscle on T2-weighted images (Fig. 7.94). The variations of intensity are the result of differing amounts of blood and protein in the cysts. Fluid–fluid levels may be present within the cysts (Fig. 7.94); if present, they are strongly suggestive of lymphangioma. Heterogeneous enhancement follows intravenous administration of paramagnetic contrast (216).

Cavernous hemangiomas uncommonly present in children, becoming symptomatic more commonly in young and middle-aged adults (215). They typically present with painless proptosis that remains unchanged

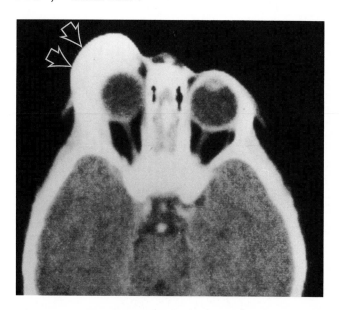

FIG. 7.92. Capillary hemangioma. Postcontrast axial CT shows a homogeneously enhancing mass (*arrows*) anterolateral to the globe. Capillary hemangiomas can be intraconal, extraconal, or both.

with Valsalva maneuvers, differentiating them from orbital varices, which enlarge during a Valsalva maneuver (215). On CT, cavernous hemangiomas appear as homogeneously enhancing round or ovoid masses that are usually intraconal and spare the orbital apex. Calcified phleboliths are frequently seen within the mass (217). On MR, cavernous hemangiomas appear as homogeneous, well-defined, round or ovoid, slightly lobulated masses that are usually intraconal (Fig. 7.95). They are isointense to the orbital muscles on T1-weighted images, hyperintense to the orbital muscles on T2-weighted images, and homogeneously enhance after intravenous infusion of paramagnetic contrast (216).

Orbital varices are venous malformations that occur in the retrobulbar region. They typically present in later childhood or adulthood with intermittent proptosis that is exacerbated by a Valsalva maneuver, bending over, or lying prone. On CT and MR, varices are identified by a curvilinear configuration, the presence of calcified phleboliths, intense enhancement after contrast administration, and an increase in size in the prone position or with a Valsalva maneuver. On occasion, images obtained in a

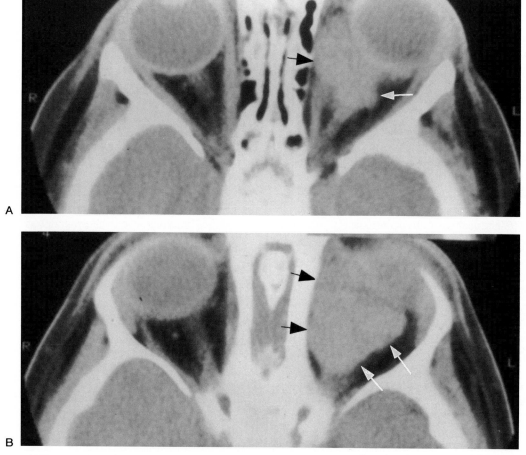

FIG. 7.93. Lymphangioma. **A, B:** Axial noncontrast CT images show an irregular, lobulated mass (*arrows*) in both the extra- and intraconal spaces of the left orbit, causing mild proptosis.

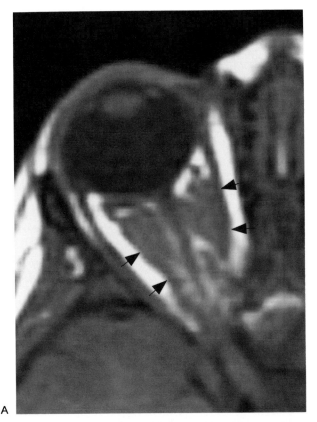

A

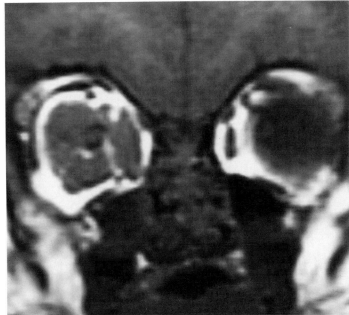

B

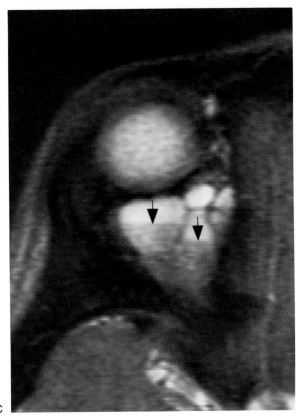

C

FIG. 7.94. Lymphangioma. **A:** Axial SE 450/11 image shows an irregular mass (*arrows*), primarily intraconal, in the right orbit. **B:** Coronal SE 500/11 image shows the mass as being difficult to separate from the orbital cone and optic nerve. **C:** Axial FSE 3000/ 102 image shows fluid–fluid levels (*arrows*) within the mass, strongly suggesting lymphangioma.

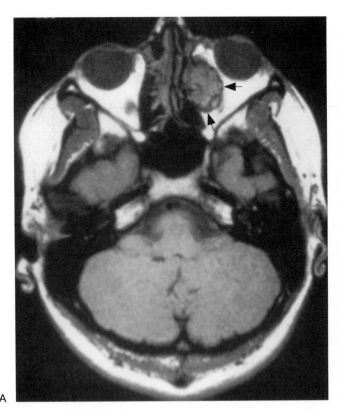
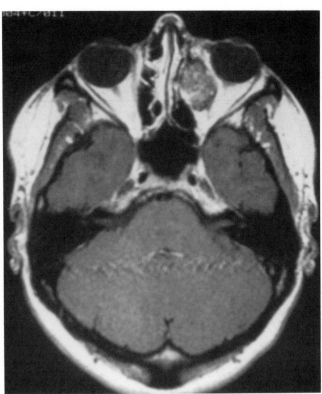

A

B

FIG. 7.95. Cavernous hemangioma. **A:** Axial SE 550/15 image shows a lobulated mass (*arrows*) in the medial left orbit. Cavernous hemangiomas can be intraconal, extraconal, or both. **B:** After infusion of paramagnetic contrast, heterogeneous enhancement is seen.

supine position without Valsalva may be normal; if the proper history is obtained, further scans should be obtained during the maneuvers. CT is probably a better study because of the shorter imaging times that allow scanning to be performed during a Valsalva maneuver (216,217).

Orbital Cysts

When retro-orbital cysts are seen in infants and children, the most common cause is a severe colobomatous malformation of the globe. *Ocular colobomas* are anomalies of the globe that result from a failure of the posterior midline of the globe (the choroidal fissure) to close properly, with consequent localized defects in the uvea, retina, and optic nerve (214,218). Colobomas are typically bilateral, constitute about 2% of congenital ocular anomalies, and are often associated with anomalies of the brain or other viscera. Most colobomas are too small to be detected by imaging. When detected, the most common configuration is that of the "morning glory anomaly," so named because of the funnel-shaped appearance of the posterior globe (Fig. 7.96) (218,219). Sometimes, the inner layer of the retina proliferates at the margins of the coloboma and protrudes outward to form a cyst. The cyst may be small with a normal-sized globe, moderate

in size with a slightly small globe, or large with a small, malformed globe (Figs. 7.97, 7.98). MR and CT are useful for making an accurate diagnosis and characterization of the cyst and for assessing the brain for other anomalies. Both the cyst and globe are isointense to normal vitreous on all imaging sequences. Contrast enhancement is not seen (214,218,219).

Orbital Neoplasms

Granulocytic Sarcoma (Chloroma)

Granulocytic sarcomas are solid tumors of immature granulocytes that develop in some patients with myelogenous or myelomonocytic leukemia (220). They most commonly occur in the skin, bones, sinuses, and orbits but rarely involve the central nervous system. Although granulocytic sarcomas arising in other areas usually develop during relapses in patients with known leukemia, those arising in the orbit may be the initial manifestation of leukemia (220,221). After testing, most affected patients are found to have simultaneous evidence of bone marrow or peripheral blood disease. Although most patients present with proptosis, some may have pain and chemosis, suggesting an inflammatory disorder. CT

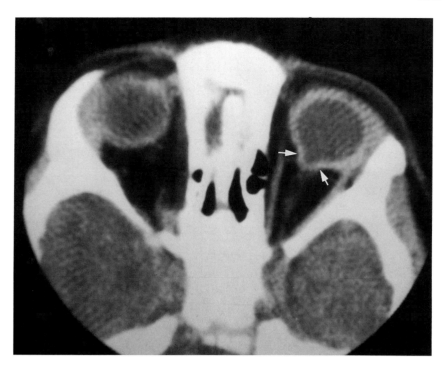

FIG. 7.96. Coloboma. Axial CT shows a midline protrusion (*arrows*) of the vitreous in the posterior globe. This appearance is quite specific for a coloboma.

shows poorly defined, homogeneous soft tissue masses that may be intra- or extraconal. The masses typically infiltrate the orbital fat and conform to orbital structures; bone erosion is very rare. These characteristics are typical of lymphocytic orbital infiltrates; however, lymphocytic orbital infiltrates other than granulocytic sarcomas are uncommon in children. About half are bilateral at the time of presentation; *bilaterality of orbital masses in children is uncommon, so this finding should arouse suspicion of a granulocytic sarcoma.* On MR, granulocytic sarcomas are hypointense compared to muscle on T1-weighted images and iso- to hyperintense compared to muscle on T2-weighted images (220,221). They enhance intensely after administration of intravenous contrast.

Metastatic Neuroblastoma

Metastatic neuroblastoma, although already mentioned twice in this chapter with regard to calvarial and skull base masses, must be discussed in this section as well, as it is the most common tumor to metastasize to the orbit in infants and young children (215). As many as 8% of patients with neuroblastoma present with orbital symptoms, and bilateral orbital lesions are noted in as many as 40% of patients with metastatic disease (215,216). Patients typically present with rapidly progressive proptosis. CT shows a soft tissue mass that typically arises from a partially destroyed superolateral orbital wall; the bone typically shows a permeated pattern or elevation of the periosteum secondary to rapid growth

of tumor (Fig. 7.99). MR shows focal or extensive soft tissue, often partially hemorrhagic, expanding the orbital wall and growing into the orbit. Nonhemorrhagic portions of tumor typically remain isointense to muscle on both T1- and T2-weighted images. The tumor enhances markedly after intravenous infusion of contrast.

Plexiform Neurofibroma

Plexiform neurofibromas are highly vascular, poorly defined, and diffusely infiltrative masses involving peripheral nerves and connective tissue that are only seen in the setting of neurofibromatosis type I (NF1; see Chapter 6). The tumor tends to grow centripetally along the nerve from the periphery toward the center. When they involve the orbit, plexiform neurofibromas present with proptosis, visual loss, and marked facial asymmetry (215). They appear on both CT and MR as serpiginous, irregular, poorly marginated masses that engulf normal orbital structures (Fig. 7.100). The involved orbit is often enlarged and the adjacent greater sphenoid wing is often dysplastic. The mass often extends through the superior orbital fissure into the cavernous sinus, which may also be expanded (Fig. 7.100B). On CT, the masses are isodense with the extraocular muscles. On MR, they are isointense with muscle on T1-weighted images and hyperintense compared with muscle on T2-weighted images. Contrast enhancement is variable (216,217). MR is the imaging study of choice because of the ability to analyze for cavernous sinus involvement without the use of

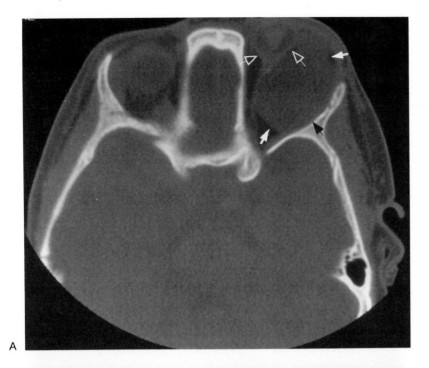

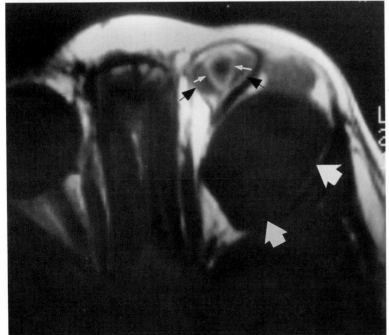

FIG. 7.97. Coloboma with cyst. **A:** Bone algorithm CT shows that the left orbit is enlarged. A small malformed globe (*open arrows*) is situated anteromedially, displaced by a large, lateral cyst (*closed arrows*). **B:** Axial SE 550/15 image obtained with a 3-cm surface coil shows the shrunken, malformed globe (*closed black arrows*) with lens (*small white arrows*) and posterolateral cyst (*large white arrows*).

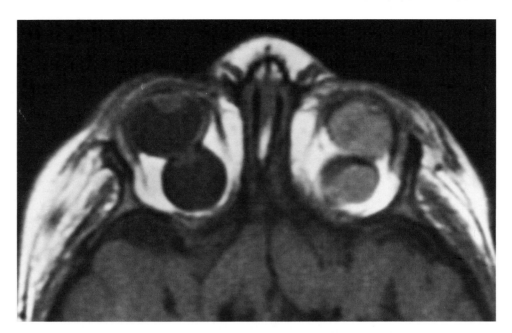

FIG. 7.98. Bilateral colobomas with cysts. Axial SE 500/11 image shows bilaterally small globes with cysts extending from the posterior midline of the globes. The left globe and colobomatous cyst are hyperintense secondary to subretinal hemorrhage. (This figure courtesy Dr. Sylvester Chuang, Toronto.)

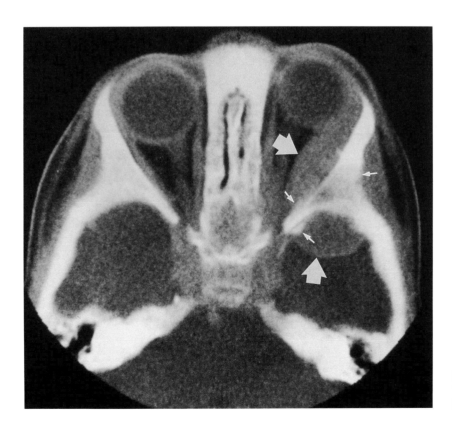

FIG. 7.99. Metastatic neuroblastoma to orbit. Axial CT shows a mass (*large arrows*) arising within the lateral wall of the orbit. Periosteal reaction (*small arrows*) is indicated by irregular thickening of the bone.

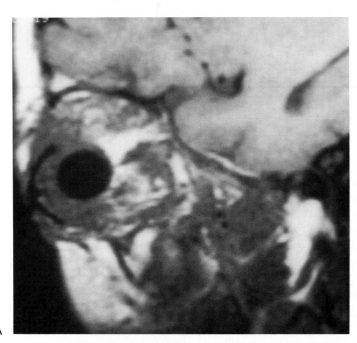

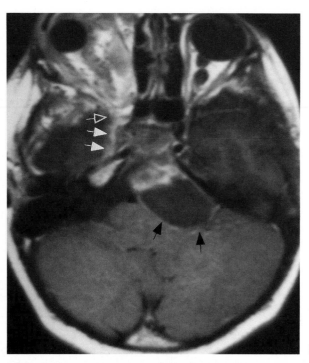

FIG. 7.100. Orbital plexiform neurofibroma. **A:** Parasagittal SE 500/15 image shows numerous irregular curvilinear streaks in the expanded right orbit of this patient with neurofibromatosis type I. **B:** Postcontrast axial image shows some enhancement of the curvilinear structures. Extension is seen through the enlarged superior orbital fissure (*open arrow*) into the cavernous sinus (*closed arrows*). This patient also had a parenchymal astrocytoma (*black arrows*).

contrast and the ability to analyze the brain for other manifestations of NF1. In the setting of NF1, no significant differential diagnosis exists.

Rhabdomyosarcomas

Rhabdomyosarcomas are discussed in the following section.

Masses of the Face and Neck

Rhabdomyosarcomas

Rhabdomyosarcomas are the third most common primary childhood malignancy of the head and neck, following intracranial brain tumors and retinoblastomas in frequency. They comprise 4% to 8% of all malignant tumors in children less than 15 years old. Forty percent of rhabdomyosarcomas arise in the head and neck, with the orbit and nasopharynx most commonly involved, followed by the paranasal sinuses and middle ear. Intracranial involvement usually results from extension of ex-

tracranial tumor into the cranial vault through fissures and foramina. However, very rarely, primary intracranial rhabdomyosarcomas do occur; they cannot be differentiated radiographically from other primary intra-axial brain tumors (222–224).

Clinically, it is useful to classify rhabdomyosarcomas of the head and neck by site of origin (225). Three major groups are identified: (1) parameningeal, (2) orbital, and (3) other head and neck locations. The parameningeal group—consisting of tumors originating in the middle ear, nasopharynx, paranasal sinuses, and nasal cavity—is of particular importance from the neuroimaging perspective. Tumors in these locations have the poorest prognosis because they commonly invade the skull or spread intracranially via skull base foramina. Orbital rhabdomyosarcomas can also spread intracranially, typically through the orbital fissures into the cavernous sinuses and middle cranial fossae.

On CT, rhabdomyosarcomas are usually isodense with brain prior to contrast enhancement; they uniformly enhance after the infusion of contrast (Fig. 7.101). If intracranial extension occurs, the foramen or fissure through which the extension has occurred is usu-

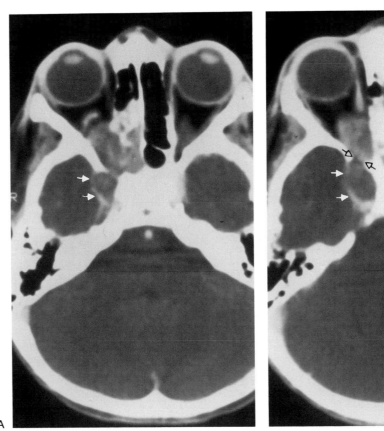

A   B

FIG. 7.101. Rhabdomyosarcoma. **A:** Contrast-enhanced CT through the mid-orbits shows a mass near the apex of the right orbit and extending into the posterior ethmoidal air cells. The mass extends through the superior orbital fissure into the cavernous sinus (*arrows*). **B:** Image 5 mm higher than A shows the mass filling and expanding the right cavernous sinus (*arrows*) and widening the superior orbital fissure (*open arrows*).

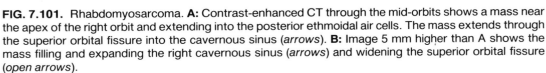

ally expanded. The extradural mass adjacent to the expanded foramen usually demonstrates a wide base against the inner table of the skull; meningeal enhancement indicates a poor prognosis (226). Usually, an extracranial or petrosal mass is also visible (222–224,227). The MR findings are usually those of a mass that is isointense to muscle on T1-weighted images and hyperintense to muscle on T2-weighted images (Figs. 7.102, 7.103). The tumors are often heterogeneous on T2-weighted images. Extension of tumor through a foramen or fissure is more easily visualized with MR due to the lack of beam-hardening artifact from the skull base; however, erosion or infiltration of the skull base without intracranial extension is difficult to appreciate on MR and better evaluated with CT. Administration of paramagnetic contrast results in uniform tumor enhancement, which aids in the localization of intracranial tumor (222,228). The identification and localization of extracranial tumor, however, is more difficult after contrast administration because the muscles of the neck enhance to become isointense with tumor and obscure fat planes; therefore, contrast-enhanced MR imaging should always include fat satura-

tion pulses (Fig. 7.104). Although the CT and MR findings are not specific, the diagnosis of rhabdomyosarcoma can be suggested from imaging studies because it is by far the most common primary extracranial tumor that invades the cranial vault in childhood. When available, MR is the imaging modality of choice for these tumors because the coronal and sagittal sections are extremely helpful in evaluating the invasion of the cavernous sinus and the extradural space. Moreover, MR better defines ports for irradiation because of its multiplanar capability.

Juvenile Angiofibromas

Juvenile angiofibromas are highly vascular, locally invasive, histologically benign tumors that arise in the sphenopalatine foramen, nasopharynx, or posterior nasal cavity of adolescent boys. Local spread into the sphenoid sinus, pterygopalatine fossa, infratemporal fossa, orbit, and middle cranial fossa is often seen by the time

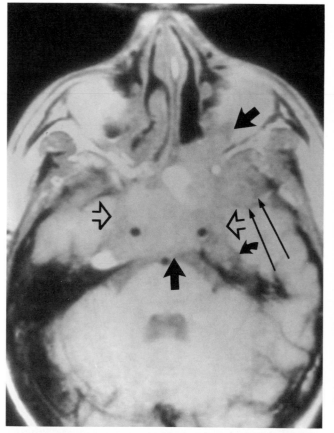

A

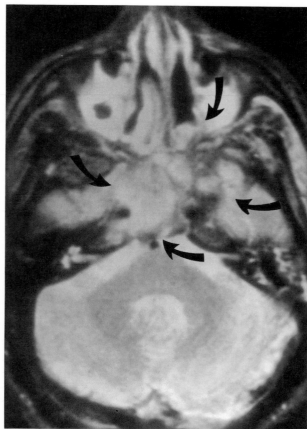

B

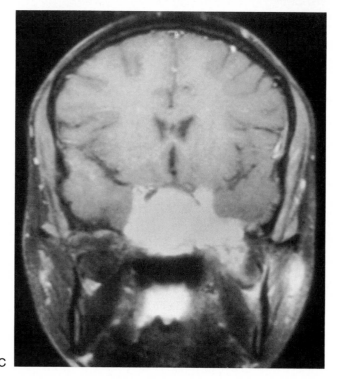

C

FIG. 7.102. Rhabdomyosarcoma. A: Axial SE 550/15 image shows a large mass in the clivus, laterally displacing the lateral walls of the cavernous sinuses (*open arrows*), extending into the prepontine cistern (*large closed arrow*), extending through the inferior orbital fissure into the left orbit (*small closed arrow*), filling the anterior aspect of the left middle cranial fossa (*long arrows*), and growing into the left petrous apex (*curved arrow*). **B:** Axial SE 2500/70 image shows the heterogeneous mass (*arrows*) to be hyperintense compared to skeletal muscle. **C:** Postcontrast SE 550/16 image shows homogeneous enhancement of the tumor.

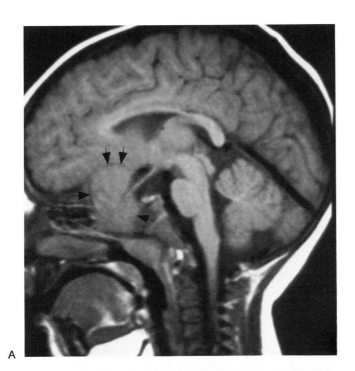

A

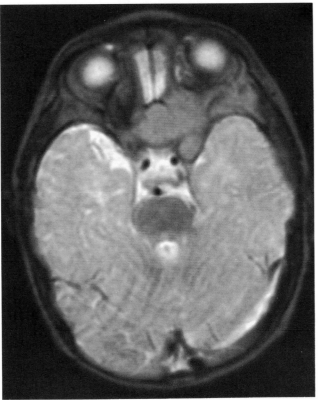

B

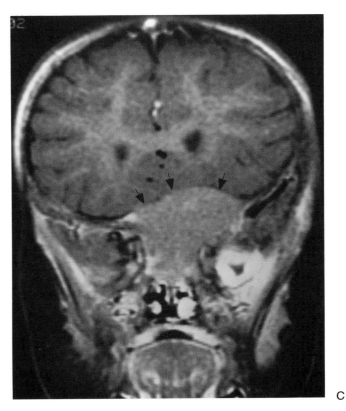

C

FIG. 7.103. Rhabdomyosarcoma. **A:** Sagittal SE 550/16 image shows a mass (*arrows*) growing upward from the nasal cavity through the sphenoid bone and into the inferior anterior cranial fossa. **B:** Axial SE 2500/70 image shows the mass to be in the sphenoid bone, enlarging the left anterior clinoid process. **C:** Postcontrast coronal SE 550/15 image shows moderate enhancement of the mass (*arrows*).

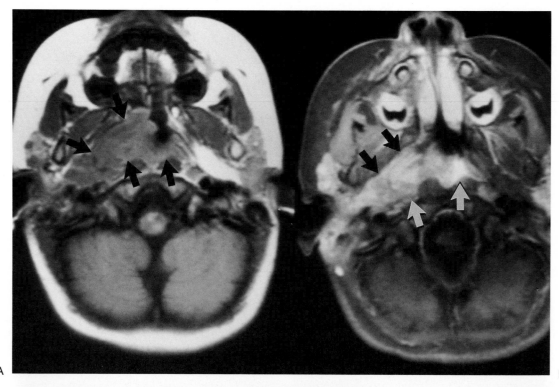

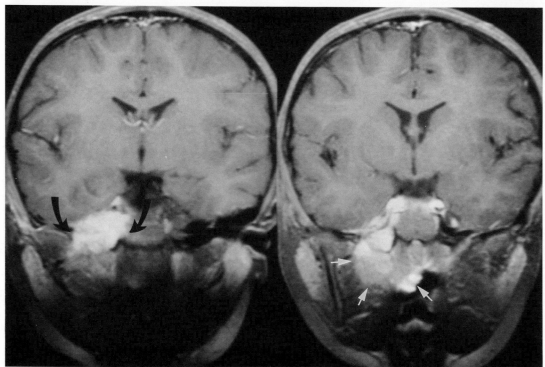

FIG. 7.104. Rhabdomyosarcoma. Value of fat suppression. **A:** Noncontrast SE 500/15 image shows a nasopharyngeal mass (*arrows*) compressing and laterally displacing the parapharyngeal fat stripe. **B:** Postcontrast fat-suppressed image 1 cm inferior to A shows the heterogeneously enhancing mass (*arrows*) distinctly separate from infratemporal and marrow fat. **C, D:** Postcontrast coronal fat suppressed images show enhancing nasopharyngeal tumor (*white arrows*) growing intracranially through a large hole (*curved black arrows*) in the skull base, presumably the expanded foramen ovale.

of presentation. Affected patients typically present with nasal obstruction, recurrent epistaxis, and, in severe cases, recurrent nosebleeds. In advanced cases, proptosis or cranial neuropathies may develop (222,229,230).

CT typically shows a sharply marginated, homogeneous soft tissue mass in the nasopharynx and pterygopalatine fossa, causing anterior bowing of the posterior wall of the maxillary sinus. Expansion through the roof of the nasopharynx into the sphenoid sinus is common. Homogeneous enhancement is seen after intravenous infusion of iodinated contrast (Fig. 7.105) (222,229,230). MR shows the mass to be hypo- to isointense compared with muscle on T1-weighted images and iso- to hyperintense compared with muscle on T2-weighted images (Fig. 7.106). Marked, uniform enhancement is seen after intravenous administration of paramagnetic contrast. Punctate and curvilinear regions of low signal intensity can be seen on both T1- and T2-weighted images, representing the prominent tumor vessels that are characteristic of these tumors; however, tumor vessels are not always seen by MR and their absence in a mass otherwise typical for juvenile angiofibroma does not negate the diagnosis (222,230). Treatment of choice is by intravascular techniques.

Melanotic Neuroectodermal Tumors of Infancy

Melanotic neuroectodermal tumors of infancy are tumors of mesodermal origin that typically involve the skull, dura, or face. Patients typically present with a mass and discoloration of adjacent skin. The tumors secrete high levels of vanillomandelic acid and homovanillic acid in the urine, which can be used to make a preoperative diagnosis and to identify tumor recurrence at an early stage. Local resection is often curative (231,232). CT shows a soft tissue mass that usually arises in the bones of the face. The bone can show expansion, hyperostosis, erosion, or osteogenesis; in some reported cases, all these characteristics have been present in the same patient in different areas of tumor. MR shows a soft tissue mass that is isointense to muscle on T1-weighted images and iso- to hyperintense to muscle on T2-weighted images. T1 shortening from melanin is not reported in most cases. Rarely, melanotic neuroectodermal tumors of infancy can originate intracranially, presumably from mesodermal elements within the stroma of the choroid plexus. These tumors are in no way distinguishable from the more common neoplasms that arise in those locations by radiologic criteria (231,232).

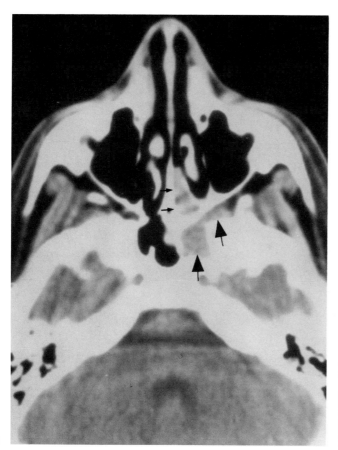

A

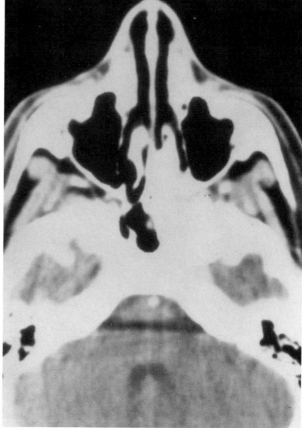

B

FIG. 7.105. Juvenile nasopharyngeal angiofibroma. **A, B:** Axial noncontrast (A) and postcontrast (B) CT images show an intensely enhancing mass (*arrows*) in the left nasal cavity extending into the sphenopalatine foramen.

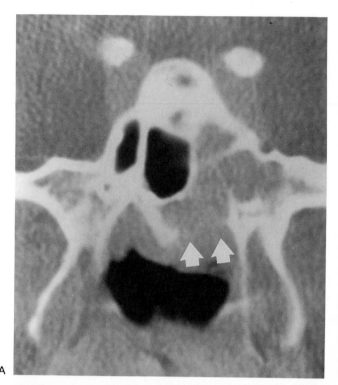

A

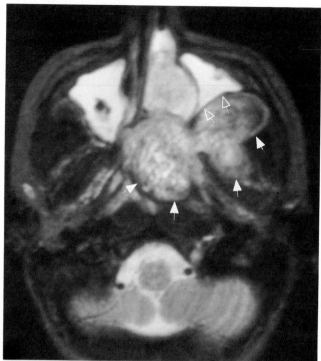

C

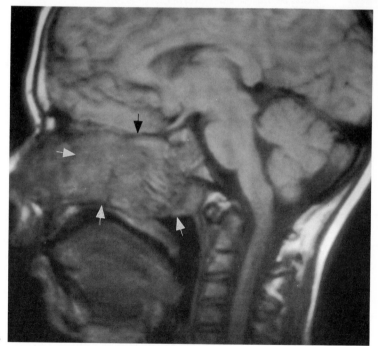

B

FIG. 7.106. Juvenile nasopharyngeal angiofibroma. **A:** Coronal noncontrast CT image (*bone window*) shows a mass (*arrows*) in the pterygopalatine region growing into the left sphenoid sinus. **B:** Sagittal SE 600/20 image shows a nasal mass (*arrows*) growing posteriorly into the sphenoid sinus and basisphenoid bone. **C:** Axial SE 2500/70 image shows the heterogeneous, hypointense mass (*closed white arrows*) in the nasal cavity, nasopharynx, and retromaxillary region. The posterior wall of the left maxillary sinus (*open white arrows*) is bowed anteriorly, a classic sign of juvenile nasopharyngeal angiofibromas.

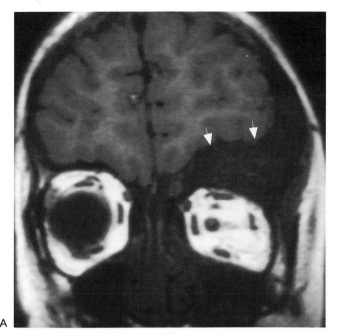

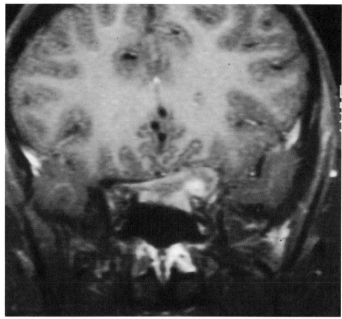

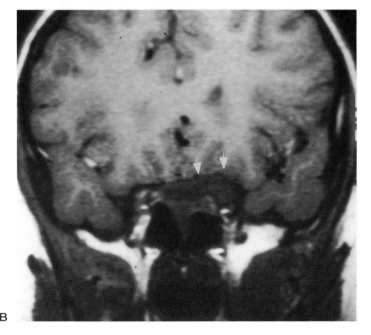

FIG. 7.107. Fibrous dysplasia of the orbitosphenoid region. **A:** Coronal SE 550/15 image shows expanded orbital roof (*arrows*). **B:** Coronal SE 550/15 image shows the left side of the sphenoid bone (*arrows*) to be enlarged. Compare with Fig. 7.103. **C:** After administration of paramagnetic contrast, the expanded sphenoid heterogeneously enhances, as is typical for fibrous dysplasia.

Fibrous Dysplasia of the Skull Base

Fibrous dysplasia is mentioned in this section only because it can mimic skull base and head-and-neck tumors, such as rhabdomyosarcomas and juvenile nasal angiofibromas on MR imaging (Fig. 7.107). Affected bone is expanded and will enhance dramatically. A noncontrast CT scan (Fig. 7.108) with bone algorithm will show the classic "ground glass" appearance of fibrous dysplasia, confirming the proper diagnosis.

TUMORS IN THE FIRST YEAR OF LIFE

The distribution of primary brain tumors in the first year of life is different from the distribution of the entire pediatric period. Although different groups report different incidences of tumors in infants (3,8–10, 233,234), certain definite trends emerge. Suprasellar lesions seem more common during the first year of life than during the pediatric years as a whole. Of these, the most common are suprasellar astrocytomas, which are usually grade II or grade III astrocytomas arising in the hypothalamus. Choroid plexus papillomas and carcinomas have a much higher relative incidence in the first year of life, representing 15% to 20% of all tumors in this age group. Medulloblastomas, although peaking in fre-

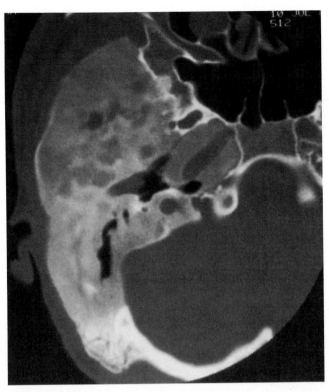

FIG. 7.108. CT of fibrous dysplasia of temporal bone. Axial bone algorithm CT image shows the temporal bone to be diffusely expanded, with a "ground glass" appearance.

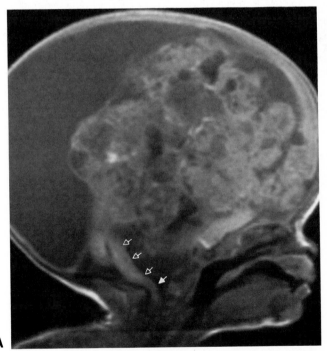

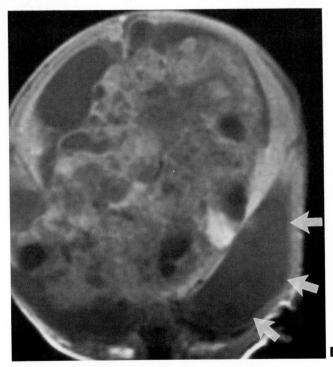

FIG. 7.109. Teratoma in a newborn. **A:** Sagittal SE 500/20 image shows an enormous, heterogeneous mass involving the frontal, temporal, and parietal lobes in this newborn infant. There is marked hydrocephalus. The brain stem is pushed posteriorly and inferiorly (*open arrows*) and is kinked at the cervicomedullary junction (*closed arrow*). **B:** Coronal SE 700/20 image shows markedly dilated temporal horns (*arrows*) in addition to the huge, extremely heterogeneous tumor occupying the majority of the intracranial space. (This case courtesy of Dr. T. Ito.)

quency toward the latter half of the first decade, frequently present during the first year of life and are considerably more common than other posterior fossa tumors in this age group. Posterior fossa ependymomas also seem relatively more common in younger children, whereas cerebellar and brain stem astrocytomas are uncommon. In some series, primitive neuroectodermal tumors appear frequently within the first year of life, with an incidence nearly equal to that of choroid plexus papillomas. In other series, teratomas are the most frequent brain tumor diagnosed in the first year of life. Teratomas are diagnosed most frequently in the first few months after birth (Fig. 7.109); their incidence of presentation drops off steadily thereafter.

Clinical presentation is different in patients in the first year of life as well (10,233). Focal neurologic deficits are almost always absent because of the relative immaturity of the central nervous system. Infants with infratentorial tumors tend to present with vomiting and increased sleepiness; increasing head size and developmental delays are noted in approximately one-half of affected patients. Among infants with supratentorial tumors, an increasing head size is seen in about one-half, vomiting and lethargy or irritability develop in approximately one-third, and seizures are seen in approximately 20%. Those infants with hypothalamic/chiasmal gliomas tend to present with decreased appetite, poor weight gain, and abnormal eye movements.

Treatment of very young children also differs from those in the older age group (10,233). The treatment of children under the age of 2 is compromised by the immaturity of the brain, the highly malignant nature of the neoplasms, the delay in diagnosis (because of a low index of suspicion and nonspecific clinical findings), the large bulk of tumor found at presentation, and the reduced radiation dose used in this age group. A reduced radiation dosage is necessary because of the immaturity of the brain and the high incidence of subsequent vasoocclusive disease that occurs when radiation is given to very young children. In general, a conservative approach is recommended in children with optic gliomas and low-grade supratentorial astrocytomas. Radiation is deferred until the child is 3–4 years old, when he or she can better tolerate its effects on the CNS. Presently, several centers are using postoperative chemotherapy with delayed radiation; early results have been encouraging and neurotoxicity has been low (235).

REFERENCES

1. Young JL, Heise HW, Silverberg E, et al. *Cancer incidence, survival and mortality for children under 15 years of age.* New York: American Cancer Society, 1978.
2. Tadmor R, Harwood-Nash DC, Scotti G, et al. Intracranial neoplasms in children: the effect of computed tomography on age distribution. *Radiology* 1982;145:371–373.
3. Fitz CR. Neoplastic diseases. In: Gonzales CF, Grossman CB, Masdeu JC, eds. *Head and spine imaging.* New York: Wiley, 1985:385–410.
4. Farwell JR, Dohrmann GJ, Flannery JT. Central nervous system tumors in children. *Cancer* 1977;40:3123–3132.
5. Amador LV. *Brain tumors in the young.* Springfield, IL: Charles C Thomas, 1983.
6. Naidich TP, Zimmerman RA. Primary brain tumors in children. *Semin Roentgenol* 1984;19:100–114.
7. Hooper R. Intracranial tumours in childhood. *Childs Brain* 1975;1:136–140.
8. Radkowski MA, Naidich TP, Tomita T, Byrd SE, McLone DG. Neonatal brain tumors: CT and MR findings. *J Comput Assist Tomogr* 1988;12:10–20.
9. Tadmor R, Harwood-Nash DCF, Savoiardo M. Brain tumors in the first two years of life: CT diagnosis. *Am J Neuroradiol* 1980;1:411–417.
10. Tomita T, McLone DG. Brain tumors during the first twenty-four months of life. *Neurosurgery* 1985;17:913–919.
11. Kramer E, Rafto S, Packer R, Zimmerman RA. Comparison of myelography with CT follow-up versus gadolinium MRI for subarachnoid metastatic disease in children. *Neurology* 1991;41:46–50.
12. Blews DE, Wang H, Kumar AJ, Robb PA, Phillips PC, Bryan RN. Intradural spinal metastases in pediatric patients with primary intracranial neoplasms: Gd-DTPA enhanced MR vs CT myelography. *J Comput Assist Tomogr* 1990;14:730–735.
13. Barkovich AJ. Neuroimaging of pediatric brain tumors. In: Berger MS, ed. *Pediatric neuro-oncology.* In: Winn HR, Mayberg MR, eds. *Neurosurgery clinics of North America.* Philadelphia: Saunders, 1992:739–770.
14. Dickman C, Rekate HL, Bird CR, Drayer BP, Medina M. Unenhanced and gadolinium-DTPA-enhanced MR imaging in postoperative evaluation of pediatric brain tumors. *J Neurosurg* 1989;71:49–53.
15. Elster AD, Dipersio DA. Cranial postoperative site: assessment with contrast-enhanced MR imaging. *Radiology* 1990;174:93–98.
16. Hudgins PA, Davis PC, Hoffman JC Jr. Gadopentetate dimeglumine enhanced MR imaging in children following surgery for brain tumor: spectrum of meningeal findings. *Am J Neuroradiol* 1991;12:301–308.
17. Bailey P, Cushing H. Medulloblastoma cerebelli. A common type of midcerebellar glioma of childhood. *Arch Neurol Psychiatry* 1925;14:192–224.
18. Rubenstein LJ. *Tumors of the central nervous system. Atlas of tumor pathology.* 2nd series, Fascicle 6. Washington, DC: Armed Forces Institute of Pathology, 1972.
19. Russell DS, Rubenstein LJ. *Pathology of tumors of the nervous system.* Baltimore: William and Wilkins, 1989.
20. Albright L. Posterior fossa tumors. In: Berger MS, ed. *Pediatric neuro-oncology. Neurosurgery clinics of North America.* Philadelphia: Saunders, 1992:881–891.
21. Park TS, Hoffman HJ, Hendrick EB, et al. Medulloblastoma: clinical presentation and management; experience at the Hospital for Sick Children. Toronto, 1950–1980. *J Neurosurg* 1983;58:543–552.
22. George RE, Laurent JP, McCluggage CW, Cheek WR. Spinal metastasis in primitive neuroectodermal tumors (medulloblastoma) of the posterior fossa: evaluation with CT myelography and correlation with patient age and tumor differentiation. *Pediatr Neurosci* 1986;12:157–160.
23. Stanley P, Senac MO Jr, Segall HD. Intraspinal seeding from intracranial tumors in children. *Am J Roentgenol* 1985;144:157–161.
24. Packer RJ, Siegel KR, Sutton LN, et al. Leptomeningeal dissemination of primary central nervous system tumors of childhood. *Ann Neurol* 1985;18:218–221.
25. Tomita T, McLone DG. Spontaneous seeding of medulloblastoma; results of CSF cytology and arachnoid biopsy from the cisterna magna. *Neurosurgery* 1983;12:265–267.
26. Farwell JR, Dohrmann GJ, Flannery JT. Medulloblastoma in childhood: an epidemiological study. *J Neurosurg* 1984;61:657–664.

27. Al-Mefty O, Jinkins JR, El-Senoussi M, et al. Medulloblastomas: a review of modern management with a report on 75 cases. *Surg Neurol* 1985;24:606–624.

28. Sandhu A, Kendall B. Computed tomography in management of medulloblastomas. *Neuroradiology* 1987;29:444–452.

29. Nelson MD, Diebler C, Forbes WSC. Pediatric medulloblastoma: atypical CT features at presentation in the SIOP II trial. *Neuroradiology* 1991;33:140–142.

30. Meyers SP, Kemp SS, Tarr RW. MR imaging features of medulloblastomas. *Am J Roentgenol* 1992;158:859–865.

31. Wiener MD, Boyko OB, Friedman HS, Hockenberger B, Oakes WJ. False positive spinal MR findings for subarachnoid spread of primary CNS tumor in postoperative pediatric patients. *Am J Neuroradiol* 1990;11:1100–1103.

32. Gjerris F, Klinken L. Long-term prognosis in children with benign cerebellar astrocytoma. *J Neurosurg* 1978;49:179–184.

33. Ringertz N, Nordenstam HJ. Cerebellar astrocytoma. *Neuropathol Exp Neurol* 1951;10:343–367.

34. Gol A, McKissock W. The cerebellar astrocytomas: a report on 98 verified cases. *J Neurosurg* 1959;16:287–296.

35. Sato K, Rorke LB. Vascular bundles and wickerworks in childhood brain tumors. *Pediatr Neurosci* 1989;15:105–110.

36. Lee YY, van Tassel P, Bruner JM, Moser RP, Share JC. Juvenile pilocytic astrocytomas: CT and MR characteristics. *Am J Roentgenol* 1989;152:1263–1270.

37. Zimmerman RA, Bilaniuk LT, Bruno L, et al. Computed tomography of cerebellar astrocytoma. *Am J Roentgenol* 1978;130:929–933.

38. Centano RS, Lee AA, Winter J, Barba D. Supratentorial ependymomas: neuroimaging and clinicopathological correlation. *J Neurosurg* 1986;64:209–215.

39. Pierre-Kahn A, Hirsch JF, Roux FX, et al. Intra-cranial ependymomas in childhood: survival and functional results of 47 cases. *Childs Brain* 1983;10:145–156.

40. Swartz JD, Zimmerman RA, Bilaniuk LT. Computed tomography of intracranial ependymomas. *Radiology* 1982;143:97–101.

41. Salazar M. A better understanding of CNS seeding and a brighter outlook for postoperatively irradiated patients with ependymoma. *Int J Radiat Oncol Biol Phys* 1983;9:1231–1235.

42. Wang Z, Zimmerman RA, Sutton L, Haselgrove J, Rorke L. Proton MR spectroscopy of pediatric cerebellum brain tumors. *Radiology* 1993;189(P):195.

43. Packer RJ, Nicholson HS, Vezina LG, Johnson DL. Brainstem Gliomas. In: Berger MS, eds. *Pediatric neuro-oncology. Neurosurgery clinics of North America.* Philadelphia: Saunders, 1992:863–879.

44. Grigsby PW, Thomas PR, Schwartz HG, Fineberg BB. Multivariant analysis of prognostic factors in pediatric and adult thalamic and brainstem tumors. *Int J Radiat Oncol* 1989;16:649–655.

45. Edwards MSB, Wara WM, Barkovich AJ. Focal brain-stem astrocytomas causing symptoms of involvement of the facial nucleus: long term survival in six pediatric cases. *J Neurosurg* 1994;80:20–25.

46. Epstein F, Wisoff JH. Intrinsic brain stem tumors of childhood: surgical indications. *J Neuro-oncol* 1988;6:309–317.

47. Barkovich AJ, Krischer J, Kun LE, et al. Brain stem gliomas: a classification system based on magnetic resonance imaging. *Pediatr Neurosci* 1990–1991;16:73–83.

48. Stroink AR, Hoffman HJ, Hendrick EB, Humphreys RP. Diagnosis and management of pediatric brainstem gliomas. *J Neurosurg* 1986;65:745–750.

49. Mantravardi RVP, Phatak R, Bellur S, et al. Brainstem glioma: an autopsy study of 25 cases. *Cancer* 1982;49:1294–1296.

50. Smith RR, Zimmerman RA, Packer RJ, et al. Pediatric brainstem glioma; post-radiation clinical and radiographic follow-up. *Neuroradiology* 1990;32:265–271.

51. Epstein F, Wisoff J. Intra-axial tumors of the cervico-medullary junction. *J Neurosurg* 1987;67:483–487.

52. Stroink AR, Hoffman HJ, Hendrick EB, Humphreys RP, Davidson G. Transependymal benign dorsally exophytic brain stem gliomas in childhood: diagnosis and treatment recommendations. *Neurosurgery* 1987;20:439–444.

53. Allcutt DA, Hoffman HJ, Isla A, et al. Acoustic schwannomas in children. *Neurosurgery* 1991;29:14–19.

54. Pinto RS, Kricheff II. Neuroradiology of intracranial neuromas. *Semin Roentgenol* 1984;14:44–52.

55. Latack JT, Gabrielson TD, Knake JE, et al. Facial nerve neuromas: radiologic evaluation. *Radiology* 1983;149:731–739.

56. Kingsley DPE, Brooks GB, Leung AWL, Johnson MA. Acoustic neuromas: evaluation by MR imaging. *Am J Neuroradiol* 1985;6:1–5.

57. Gentry LR, Jacoby CG, Turski PA, et al. Cerebellopontine angle-petromastoid mass lesions: comparative study of diagnosis with MR imaging and CT. *Radiology* 1987;162:513–520.

58. Curati WL, Graif M, Kingsley DPE, et al. Acoustic neuromas: Gd-DTPA enhancement in MR imaging. *Radiology* 1986;158:447–451.

59. Lee DR, Sanches J, Mark AS, Dillon WP, Norman D, Newton TH. Posterior fossa hemangioblastomas: MR imaging. *Radiology* 1989;171:463–468.

60. Sato Y, Waziri M, Smith W, et al. Hippel-Lindau disease: MR imaging. *Radiology* 1988;166:241–246.

61. Ho VB, Smirniotopoulos JG, Murphy FM, Rushing EJ. Radiologic-pathologic correlation: hemangioblastoma. *Am J Neuroradiol* 1992;13:1343–1352.

62. Shah MV, Haines SJ. Pediatric skull, skull base, and meningeal tumors. In: Berger MS, ed. *Pediatric neuro-oncology. Neurosurgical Clinics of North America.* Philadelphia: Saunders, 1992:893–924.

63. Maravilla KR. Intraventricular fat-fluid level secondary to rupture of an intracranial dermoid cyst. *Am J Roentgenol* 1977;128:500–501.

64. Horowitz BL, Chari MV, James R, Bryan RN. MR of intracranial epidermoid tumors: correlation of in vivo imaging with in vitro C13 spectroscopy. *Am J Neuroradiol* 1990;11:299–302.

65. Zimmerman RA, Bilaniuk LT, Dolinskas C. Cranial CT of epidermoid and congenital fatty tumors of maldevelopment origin. *CT* 1979;3:40–47.

66. Tsuruda JS, Chew WM, Moseley ME, Norman D. Diffusion-weighted MR imaging of the brain: value of differentiating between extraaxial cysts and epidermoid tumors. *Am J Neuroradiol* 1990;11:925–931.

67. Chew WM, Rowley HA, Barkovich AJ. Magnetization transfer contrast imaging in pediatric patients. *Radiology* 1992;185(P):281.

68. Barkovich AJ, Vandermarck P, Edwards MSB, Cogen PH. Congenital nasal masses: CT and MR imaging features in 16 cases. *Am J Neuroradiol* 1991;12:105–116.

69. Henkelman MH, Watts JF, Kucharczyk W. High signal intensity in MR images of calcified brain tissue. *Radiology* 1991;179:199–206.

70. Wold LE, Laws ER. Cranial chordomas in children and young adults. *J Neurosurg* 1983;59:1043–1047.

71. Handa J, Suzuki F, Nioka H, Koyama T. Clivus chordoma in childhood. *Surg Neurol* 1987;28:58–62.

72. Meyer JE, Oot RF, Lindfors KK. CT appearance of clival chordomas. *J Comput Assist Tomogr* 1986;10:34–38.

73. Sze G, Uichanco LS, Brant-Zawadzki MN, et al. Chordomas: MR imaging. *Radiology* 1988;166:187–191.

74. Voorhies SP, Sundaresan N. Tumors of the skull. In: Wilkins RH, Rengachary SS, eds. *Neurosurgery.* New York: McGraw-Hill, 1984:984–1009.

75. Meyers SP, Hirsch WL Jr, Curtin HD, Barnes L, Sekhar LN, Sen C. Chondrosarcomas of the skull base: MR imaging features. *Radiology* 1992;184:103–108.

76. Grois N, Barkovich AJ, Rosenau W, Ablin AR. Central nervous system disease associated with Langerhans' cell histiocytosis. *Am J Pediatr Hematol/Oncol* 1993;15:245–254.

77. Hayward J, Packer R, Finley J. Central nervous system and Langerhans' cell histiocytosis. *Med Pediatr Oncol* 1990;18:324–328.

78. Rosenfield NS, Abrahams J, Komp D. Brain MR in patients with Langerhans' cell histiocytosis: findings and enhancement with Gd-DTPA. *Pediatr Radiol* 1990;20:433–436.

79. Ragland RL, Moss DS, Duffis AW, et al. CT and MR findings in diffuse cerebral histiocytosis. *Am J Neuroradiol* 1991;12:525–526.

80. Thorphy MJ, Crosley CJ. Multifocal eosinophilic granuloma and the cerebellum. *Ann Neurol* 1980;8:454–457.

81. Applegate GR, Hirsch WL, Applegate LJ, Curtin HD. Variability in the enhancement of the normal central skull base in children. *Neuroradiology* 1992;34:217–221.

82. Palma L, Guidetti B. Cystic pilocytic astrocytomas of the cerebral hemispheres: surgical experience with 51 cases and long term results. *J Neurosurg* 1985;62:811–815.

83. Mercuri S, Russo A, Palma L. Hemispheric supratentorial astrocytomas in children. Long-term results in 29 cases. *J Neurosurg* 1981;55:170–173.

84. Berger MS, Keles GE, Geyer JR. Cerebral hemispheric tumors of childhood. In: Berger MS, ed. *Pediatric neuro-oncology. Neurosurgery clinics of North America.* Philadelphia: Saunders, 1992: 839–852.

85. Artico M, Cervoni L, Celli P, Salvati M, Palma L. Supratentorial glioblastoma in children: a series of 27 surgically treated cases. *Childs Nerv Syst* 1993;9:7–9.

86. Dropcho EJ, Wisoff JH, Walker RW, Allen JC. Supratentorial malignant gliomas in childhood: a review of fifty cases. *Ann Neurol* 1987;22:355–364.

87. Tomita T, McLone DG, Naidich TP. Mural tumors with cysts in the cerebral hemispheres of children. *Neurosurgery* 1986;19:998–1005.

88. Joyce P, Bentson J, Takahashi M, et al. The accuracy of predicting histologic grades of supratentorial astrocytomas on the basis of computerized tomography and cerebral angiography. *Neuroradiology* 1978;16:346–348.

89. Drayer BP, Johnson BP, Bird CR, Flom RA, Hodak JA. Magnetic resonance imaging and glioma. *BNI Quarterly* 1987;3:44–55.

90. Reagan TJ. Neuropathology. In: Gomez MR, eds. *Tuberous Sclerosis,* 2nd ed. New York: Raven, 1988:63–74.

91. Braffman BH, Bilaniuk LT, Naidich TP, et al. MR imaging of tuberous sclerosis: insights into the pathogenesis of this phakomatosis, comments on the role of gadopentate dimeglumine, and literature review. *Radiology* 1992;.

92. Gardeur D, Palmieri A, Mashaly R. Cranial computed tomography in the phakomatoses. *Neuroradiology* 1983;25:293–304.

93. Martin N, de Brouker T, Cambier J, Marsault C, Nahum H. MRI evaluation of tuberous sclerosis. *Neuroradiology* 1987;29:437–443.

94. Martin N, debussche C, de Broucker T, Mompoint D, Marsault C, Nahum H. Gadolinium-DTPA enhanced MR imaging in tuberous sclerosis. *Neuroradiology* 1990;31:492–497.

95. Altman NR, Purser RK, Post MJD. Tuberous sclerosis: characteristics at CT and MR imaging. *Radiology* 1988;167:527–532.

96. Mickle JP. Ganglioglioma in children: a review of 32 cases. *Pediatr Neurosurg* 1992;18:310–314.

97. Sutton LN, Packer RJ, Rorke LB, et al. Cerebral gangliogliomas during childhood. *Neurosurgery* 1983;13:124–128.

98. Johansson JH, Rekate HL, Roessmann U. Gangliomas: pathological and clinical correlation. *J Neurosurg* 1981;54:58–63.

99. Garrido E, Becker LF, Hoffman HJ, et al. Gangliomas in children: a clinicopathological study. *Childs Brain* 1978;4:339–346.

100. Tampieri D, Moumdjian R, Melanson D, Ethier R. Intracerebral gangliogliomas in patients with partial complex seizures: CT and MR imaging findings. *Am J Neuroradiol* 1991;12:749–755.

101. Mizuno J, Nishio S, Barrow DL, Davis PC, Tindall GT. Ganglioglioma of the cerebellum. *Neurosurgery* 1987;21:584–588.

102. Otsubo H, Hoffman HJ, Humphreys RP, et al. Evaluation, surgical approach and outcome of seizure patients with gangliogliomas. *Pediatr Neurosurg* 1990–91;16:208–212.

103. Smith NM, Carli MM, Hanieh A, Clark B, Bourne AJ, Byard RW. Gangliogliomas in childhood. *Childs Nerv Syst* 1992;8:258–262.

104. Demierre B, Stichnoth FA, Hori A, Spoerri O. Intracerebral ganglioma. *J Neurosurg* 1986;65:177–182.

105. Armington WG, Osborn AG, Cubberly DA, et al. Supratentorial ependymomas: CT appearance. *Radiology* 1985;157:367–372.

106. Hart MD, Earle KM. Primitive neuroectodermal tumors of the brain in children. *Cancer* 1973;3232:890–897.

107. Horton BC, Rubinstein LJ. Primary cerebral neuroblastoma: a clinicopathological study of 35 cases. *Brain* 1976;99:735–736.

108. Ashwal S, Hinshaw DB Jr, Bedros A. CNS primitive neuroectodermal tumors of childhood. *Med Pediatr Oncol* 1984;12:180–188.

109. Kingsley DPE, Harwood-Nash DCF. Radiological features of the neuroectodermal tumors of childhood. *Neuroradiology* 1984;26: 463–467.

110. Kosnik EJ, Bocsel CP, Bay J, et al. Primitive neuroectodermal tumors of the central nervous system in children. *J Neurosurg* 1978;48:741–746.

111. Altman N, Fitz CR, Chuang SH, Harwood-Nash DC, Cotter C, Armstrong D. Radiologic characteristics of primitive neuroectodermal tumors in children. *Am J Neuroradiol* 1985;6:15–18.

112. Chambers EF, Turski PA, Sobel D. Radiologic characteristics of primary cerebral neuroblastomas. *Radiology* 1981;139:101–104.

113. Davis P, Wichman RD, Takei Y, Hoffman JC Jr. Primary cerebral neuroblastoma: CT and MR findings in 12 cases. *Am J Neuroradiol* 1990;11:115–120.

114. Briner J, Bannwart F, Kleihues P, et al. Malignant small cell tumor of the brain with intermediate filaments: a case of a primary cerebral rhabdoid tumor. *Pediatr Pathol* 1985;3:117–118.

115. Hanna SL, Langston JW, Parham DM, Douglass EC. Primary malignant rhabdoid tumor of the brain: clinical, imaging, and pathologic findings. *Am J Neuroradiol* 1993;14:107–115.

116. Dumas-Duport C, Scheithauer BW, Chodkiewicz J-P, Laws ER Jr, Vedrenne C. Dysembryoplastic neuroepithelial tumor: a surgically curable tumor of young patients with intractable partial seizures. *Neurosurgery* 1988;23:545–556.

117. Koeller KK, Dillon WP. Dysembryoplastic neuroepithelial tumors: MR appearance. *Am J Neuroradiol* 1992;13:1319–1325.

118. Aizpuru RN, Quencer RM, Norenberg M, Altman N, Smirniotopoulos M. Meningioangiomatosis: clinical, radiologic, and histopathologic correlation. *Radiology* 1991;179:819–821.

119. Halper J, Scheithauer B, Okazaki H, et al. Meningio-angiomatosis: a report of six cases with special reference to the occurrence of neurofibrillary tangles. *J Neuropathol Exp Neurol* 1986;45:426–446.

120. Partington CR, Graves VB, Hegstrand LR. Meningioangiomatosis. *Am J Neuroradiol* 1991;12:549–552.

121. Kuzniecky R, Melanson D, Robitaille Y, Olivier A. Magnetic resonance imaging of meningio-angiomatosis. *Can J Neurol Sci* 1988;15:161–164.

122. DeRecondo J, Haguenau M. Neuropathologic survey of the phakomatoses and allied disorders. In: Vinken PJ, Bruyn GW, eds. *Handbook of clinical neurology: the phakomatoses.* Amsterdam: North-Holland, 1972:19–71.

123. Stern J, DiGiancinto GV, Housepian EM. Neurofibromatosis and optic glioma. Clinical and morphological correlations. *Neurosurgery* 1979;4:524–527.

124. Alvord EC, Lufton S. Gliomas of the optic nerve or chiasm: outcome by patient's age, tumor site, and treatment. *J Neurosurg* 1988;68:85–98.

125. Simon JH, Szumowski J, Totterman S, et al. Fat suppression MR imaging of the orbit. *Am J Neuroradiol* 1988;9.

126. Imes RK, Hoyt WF. MR imaging signs of optic nerve gliomas in neurofibromatosis 1. *Am J Ophthalmol* 1991;111:729–734.

127. Savoiardo M, Harwood-Nash DC, Tadmor R, Scotti G, Musgrave MA. Gliomas of the intracranial anterior optic pathways in children. *Radiology* 1981;138:601–610.

128. Fletcher WA, Imes RK, Hoyt WF. Chiasmal gliomas. Appearance and long term changes demonstrated by computed tomography. *J Neurosurg* 1986;65:154–159.

129. Kollias SS, Barkovich AJ, Edwards MSB. Magnetic resonance analysis of suprasellar tumors of childhood. *Pediatr Neurosurg* 1991–1992;17:284–303.

130. Brown EW, Riccardi VM, Mawad M, et al. MR imaging of optic pathways in patients with neurofibromatosis. *Am J Neuroradiol* 1987;8:1031–1035.

131. Rutka JT, Hoffman HJ, Drake JM, Humphreys RP. Suprasellar and sellar tumors in childhood and adolescence. In: Berger MS, ed. *Pediatric Neuro-oncology.* Philadelphia: Saunders, 1992:803–820.

132. Hoffman HJ, da Silva M, Humphreys RP, et al. Craniopharyngioma in children: fifteen years of management. *J Neurosurg* 1992;76:47–52.

133. Fitz CR, Wortzman G, Harwood-Nash DC. CT in craniopharyngiomas. *Radiology* 1978;127:687–691.

134. Ahmadi J, Destian S, Apuzzo MLJ, Segall HD, Zee C-S. Cystic

fluid in craniopharyngiomas: MR imaging and quantative analysis. *Radiology* 1992;182:783–785.

135. Pusey E, Kortman KE, Flannigan BD, et al. MR of craniopharyngiomas: tumor delineation and characterization. *Am J Neuroradiol* 1987;8:439–445.

136. Young SC, Zimmerman RA, Nowell MA, et al. Giant cystic craniopharyngiomas. *Neuroradiology* 1987;29:468–473.

137. Rush JL, Kusske JA, De Feo DR, et al. Intraventricular craniopharyngioma. *Neurology* 1975;25:1094–1096.

138. Mahachoklertwattana P, Kaplan S, Grumbach MM. The luteinizing hormone-releasing hormone-secreting hypothalamic hamartoma is really a congenital malformation: natural history. *J Clin Endocrinol Metab* 1993;77:118–124.

139. Diebler C, Ponsot G. Hamartomas of the tuber cinereum. *Neuroradiology* 1983;25:93–101.

140. Sato M, Ushio Y, Arita N, Mogami H. Hypothalamic hamartoma: report of two cases. *Neurosurgery* 1985;16:198–206.

141. Albright AL, Lee PA. Neurosurgical treatment of hypothalamic hamartomas causing precocious puberty. *J Neurosurg* 1993;78:77–82.

142. Lin S-R, Bryson MM, Goblen RP, Fitz CR, Lee Y-Y. Radiologic findings of hamartomas of the tuber cinereum and hypothalamus. *Radiology* 1978;127:697–703.

143. Boyko OB, Curnes JT, Oakes WJ, Burger PC. Hamartomas of the tuber cinereum: CT, MR, and pathologic findings. *Am J Neuroradiol* 1991;12:309–314.

144. Hahn FJ, Leibrock LG, Huseman CA, Makos MM. The MR appearance of hypothalamic hamartomas. *Neuroradiology* 1988;30:65–68.

145. Markin RS, Leibrock LG, Huseman CA, McComb RD. Hypothalamic hamartoma: a report of 2 cases. *Pediatr Neurosci* 1987;13:19–26.

146. Nishio S, Fujiwara S, Aiko Y, Takeshita I, Fukui M. Hypothalamic hamartoma: report of two cases. *J Neurosurg* 1989;70:640–645.

147. Felig P, Baxter JD, Broadus AJ, Frohman LA. Endocrinology and metabolism. In: Robertson GL, eds. *Posterior pituitary.* New York: McGraw-Hill, 1987:338–385.

148. Dunger D, Broadbent V, Yeoman E. The frequency and natural history of diabetes insipidus in children with Langerhan-cell histiocytosis. *N Engl J Med* 1989;321:.

149. Manelfe C, Louvet JP. CT in diabetes insipidus. *J Comput Assist Tomogr* 1979;3:309–316.

150. Tien R, Newton TH, McDermott MW, Dillon WP, Kucharczyk J. Thickened pituitary stalk on MR images in patients with diabetes insipidus and Langerhan-cell histiocytosis. *Am J Neuroradiol* 1990;11:703–708.

151. Maghnie M, Arico M, Villa A, Genovese E, Beluffi G, Severi F. MR of the hypothalamic–pituitary axis in Langerhans cell histiocytosis. *Am J Neuroradiol* 1992;13:1365–1371.

152. Haddad SF, Van Gilder JC, Menezes AH. Pediatric pituitary tumors. *Neurosurgery* 1991;29:509–514.

153. Laws ER, Sheithauer BW, Groover RV. Pituitary adenomas in childhood and adolescence. *Prog Exp Tumor Res* 1987;30:359–361.

154. Newton DR, Dillon WP, Norman D, et al. Gd–DTPA–enhanced MR imaging of pituitary adenomas. *Am J Neuroradiol* 1989;10:949–954.

155. Kucharczyk W, Davis DO, Kelly WM, Sze G, Norman D, Newton TH. Pituitary adenomas: high resolution MR imaging at 1.5 T. *Radiology* 1986;161:761–765.

156. Sakamoto Y, Takahashi M, Korogi Y, Bussaka H, Ushio Y. Normal and abnormal pituitary glands: gadopentate dimeglumine-enhanced MR imaging. *Radiology* 1991;178:441–445.

157. Elster AK, Chen MYM, Williams DW III, Key LL. Pituitary gland: MR imaging of physiologic hypertrophy in adolescence. *Radiology* 1990;174:681–685.

158. Voelker JL, Campbell RL, Muller J. Clinical, radiographic, and pathologic features of symptomatic Rathke's cleft cysts. *J Neurol Sci* 1991;74:535–544.

159. Okamoto S, Handa H, Yamashita J, Ishikawa M, Nagasawa S. CT in intra- and suprasellar epithelial cysts (symptomatic Rathke cleft cysts). *Am J Neuroradiol* 1985;6:515–519.

160. Kucharczyk W, Peck WW, Kelly WM, Norman D, Newton TH. Rathke cleft cysts: CT, MR imaging, and pathologic features. *Radiology* 1987;165:491–496.

161. Hoffman HJ, Otsubo H, Hendrick EB, et al. Intracranial germ-cell tumors in children. *J Neurosurg* 1991;74:545–551.

162. Felix I, Becker LE. Intracranial germ cell tumors in children: an immunohistochemical and electron microscopic study. *Pediatr Neurosci* 1990–1991;16:156–162.

163. Komatsu Y, Narushima K, Kobayashi E, et al. CT and MR of germinoma in the basal ganglia. *Am J Neuroradiol* 1989;10:S9–S11.

164. Shokry A, Janzer RC, von Hochstetter AR, et al. Primary intracranial germ cell tumors: a clinicopathological study of 14 cases. *J Neurosurg* 1985;62:826–830.

165. Yasue M, Tanaka H, Nakajima M, et al. Germ cell tumors of the basal ganglia and thalamus. *Pediatr Neurosurg* 1993;19:121–126.

166. Jennings MT, Gelman R, Hochberg F. Intracranial germ cell tumors: natural history and pathogenesis. *J Neurosurg* 1985;63:155–167.

167. Jooma R, Kendall BE. Diagnosis and management of pineal tumors. *J Neurosurg* 1983;58:654–665.

168. Soejima T, Takeshita I, Yamamoto H, Tlukamoto Y, Fukui M, Matsuoka S. CT of germinomas in basal ganglia and thalamus. *Neuroradiology* 1987;29:366–370.

169. Casenave P, Eresue J, Guibert-Tranier F, Piton J, Caille JM. Tumors of the pineal region: diagnostic problems. *J Neuroradiol* 1984;11:47–63.

170. Kilgore DP, Strother CM, Starshak RJ, Haughton VM. Pineal germinoma: MR imaging. *Radiology* 1986;158:435–438.

171. Tien RD, Barkovich AJ, Edwards MSB. MR imaging of pineal tumors. *Am J Neuroradiol* 1990;11:557–565.

172. Baumgartner JE, Edwards MSB. Pineal tumors. In: Berger MS, ed. *Pediatric neuro-oncology.* Philadelphia: Saunders, 1992:853–862.

173. Edwards MSB, Hudgins RJ, Wilson CB, Levin VA, Wara WM. Pineal region tumors in children. *J Neurosurg* 1988;68:689–697.

174. Vaquero J, Ramiro J, Martinez R, Coca S, Bravo G. Clinicopathological experience with pineocytomas: report of five surgically treated cases. *Neurosurgery* 1990;27:612–618.

175. D'Andrea AD, Packer RJ, Rorke LB, et al. Pineocytomas of childhood. A reappraisal of natural history and response to therapy. *Cancer* 1987;59:1353–7.

176. Zimmerman RA, Bilaniuk LT, Wood JH, Bruce DA, Schut L. CT of pineal, parapineal, and histologically related tumors. *Radiology* 1980;137:669–677.

177. Chang T, Teng MM, Guo WY, Sheng WC. CT of pineal tumors and intracranial germ–cell tumors. *Am J Neuroradiol* 1989;10:1039–44.

178. De Campo MP, Davis MD. The role of CT in the diagnosis and management of childhood pineal region tumours. *Australas Radiol* 1991;35:336–339.

179. Muller-Forell W, Schroth G, Egan PJ. MR imaging in tumors of the pineal region. *Neuroradiology* 1988;30:224–231.

180. Zee CS, Segall H, Apuzzo M, et al. MR imaging of pineal region neoplasms. *J Comput Assist Tomogr* 1991;15:56–63.

181. Nakagawa H, Iwasaki S, Kichikawa K, et al. MR imaging of pineocytoma: report of two cases. *Am J Neuroradiol* 1990;11:195–198.

182. Rippe D, Boyko OB, Friedman HS, et al. Gd-DTPA-enhanced MR imaging of leptomeningeal spread of primary intracranial CNS tumor in children. *Am J Neuroradiol* 1990;11:329–332.

183. Zang X, Nilaver G, Stein BM, Fetell MR, Duffy PE. Immunocytochemistry of pineal astrocytes: species differences and functional implications. *J Neuropathol Exp Neurol* 1985;44:486–495.

184. Boydston WR, Sanford RA, Muhlbauer MS, et al. Gliomas of the tectum and periaqueductal region of the mesencephalon. *Pediatr Neurosurg* 1991–92;17:234–238.

185. Megyeri L. Cystische Veränderungen des Corpus pinale. *Frankfurt Z Pathol* 1960;70:699–704.

186. Hasegawa A, Ohtsubo K, Mori W. Pineal gland in old age: quantitative and qualitative morphological study of 168 human autopsy cases. *Brain Res* 1987;409:343–349.

187. Cooper ER. The human pineal gland and pineal cysts. *J Anat* 1932;67:28–46.

188. Mamourian AC, Towfighi J. Pineal cysts: MR imaging. *Am J Neuroradiol* 1986;7:1081–1086.
189. Lee DH, Norman D, Newton TH. MR imaging of pineal cysts. *J Comput Assist Tomogr* 1987;11:586–590.
190. Golzarian J, Balériaux D, Bank WO, Matos C, Flament-Durand J. Pineal cyst: normal or pathological? *Neuroradiology* 1993;35:251–253.
191. Mamourian AC, Yarnell T. Enhancement of pineal cysts on MR images. *Am J Neuroradiol* 1991;12:773–774.
192. Tomita T, McLone DG, Flannery AM. Choroid plexus papillomas of neonates, infants, and children. *Pediatr Neurosci* 1988;14:23–30.
193. St. Clair SK, Humphreys RP, Pillay PK, Hoffman HJ, Blaser SI, Becker LE. Current management of choroid plexus carcinoma in children. *Pediatr Neurosurg* 1991–1992;17:225–233.
194. Ellenbogen RG, Winston KR, Kupsky WJ. Tumors of the choroid plexus in children. *Neurosurgery* 1989;25:327–335.
195. Boyd MD, Steinbok P. Choroid plexus tumors: problems in diagnosis and management. *J Neurosurg* 1987;66:800–805.
196. Martin N, Pierot L, Sterkers O, Mompoint D, Nahum H. Primary choroid plexus papilloma of the cerebellopontine angle: MR imaging. *Neuroradiology* 1990;31:541–543.
197. Coates TL, Hinshaw DB Jr, Peckman N, et al. Pediatric choroid plexus neoplasms: MR, CT, and pathologic correlations. *Radiology* 1989;173:81–88.
198. Kendall B, Rerder-Grosswasser I, Valentine A. Diagnosis of masses presenting within the ventricles on computed tomography. *Neuroradiology* 1983;25:11–22.
199. Drake JM, Hedrick EB, Becker LE, et al. Intracranial meningiomas in children. *Pediatr Neurosci* 1986;12:134–139.
200. Hope JKA, Armstrong DA, Babyn PS, et al. Primary meningeal tumors in children: correlation of clinical and CT findings with histologic type and prognosis. *Am J Neuroradiol* 1992;13:1353–1364.
201. Perilongo G, Sutton L, Goldwein JW, et al. Childhood meningiomas: experience in the modern era. *Pediatr Neurosurg* 1992;18:16–23.
202. Reyes-Mugica M, Chou P, Gonzalez-Crussi F, Tomita T. Fibroma of the meninges in a child: immunohistological and ultrastructural study. *J Neurosurg* 1992;76:143–147.
203. Sano K, Wakai S, Ochiai C. Characteristics of meningiomas in childhood. *Childs Brain* 1981;8:98–106.
204. Kretchmer K, Gutjahr P, Kutzner J. CT studies before and after CNS treatment for acute lymphocytic leukemia and malignant non-Hodgkins lymphoma in childhood. *Neuroradiology* 1980;20:173–180.
205. Price HI, Batnitzky S, Danzinger A, Karlin CA, Goldberg L. The neuroradiology of retinoblastoma. *Radiographics* 1982;2:7–23.
206. Hedges TR, Pozzi-Mucelli R, Char DH, Newton TH. CT demonstration of ocular calcifications: correlations with clinical and pathological findings. *Neuroradiology* 1982;23:15–21.
207. Sherman JL, McLean IW, Brallier DR. Coats' disease: CT–pathologic correlation in two cases. *Radiology* 1983;146:77–78.
208. Edwards MG, Pordell GR. Ocular toxocariasis studied by CT scanning. *Radiology* 1985;157:685–686.
209. Mafee MF, Goldberg MF, Valvassori GE, Capek V. CT in the evaluation of patients with persistent hyperplastic primary vitreous (PHPV). *Radiology* 1982;145:713–717.
210. Graeb DA, Rootman J, Robertson WD, Lapointe JS, Nugent RA, Hay EJ. Orbital lymphangiomas: clinical, radiologic and pathologic characteristics. *Radiology* 1990;175:417–421.
211. Hopper KD, Sherman JL, Boal DK, Eggli KD. CT and MR imaging of the pediatric orbit. *Radiographics* 1992;12:485–503.
212. Lallemand DP, Brasch RC, Char DH, Norman D. Orbital tumors in children. *Radiology* 1984;151:85–88.
213. Nugent RA, Lapointe JS, Rootman J, Robertson WD, Graeb DA. Orbital dermoids: features on CT. *Radiology* 1987;165:475–478.
214. Simmons JD, Lamasters D, Char DH. CT of ocular colobomas. *Am J Roentgenol* 1983;141:1223–1226.
215. Rootman J. *Diseases of the orbit.* Philadelphia: Lippincott, 1988.
216. Bilaniuk LT, Zimmerman RA, Newton TH. Magnetic resonance imaging: orbital pathology. In: Newton TH, Bilaniuk LT, eds. *Radiology of the eye and orbit.* Clavadel, 1990:5.1–5.84.
217. Char DH, Unsöld R, Sobel DF, Salvolini U, Newton TH. Computed tomography: ocular and orbital pathology. In: Newton TH, Bilaniuk LT, eds. *Radiology of the eye and orbit.* Clavadel, 1990:9.1–9.64.
218. Mafee M, Jampil LM, Langer BG, Tso M. CT of optic nerve colobomas, morning glory anomalies, and colobomatous cyst. *Radiol Clin North Am* 1987;25:693–699.
obomas, morning glory anomalies, and colobomatous cyst. *Radiol Clin North Am* 1987;25:693–699.
219. Bilaniuk LT, Farber M. Imaging of developmental anomalies of the eye and orbit. *Am J Neuroradiol* 1992;13:793–803.
220. Jakobiec FA. Granulocytic sarcoma. *Am J Neuroradiol* 1991;12:263–264.
221. Banna M, Aur R, Akkad S. Orbital granulocytic sarcoma. *Am J Neuroradiol* 1991;12:255–258.
222. Ginsberg LE. Neoplastic diseases affecting the central skull base: CT and MR imaging. *Am J Roentgenol* 1992;159:581–589.
223. Latack JT, Hutchinson RJ, Heyn RM. Imaging of rhabdomyosarcomas of the head and neck. *Am J Neuroradiol* 1987;8:353–359.
224. Scotti G, Harwood–Nash DC. CT of rhabdomyosarcomas of the skull base in children. *J Comput Asst Tomogr* 1982;6:33–39.
225. Raney RB Jr, Donaldson MH, Sutow WW, Lindberg RD, Maurer HM, Tefft M. Special considerations related to primary site in rhabdomyosarcoma: experience of the Intergroup Rhabdomyosarcoma Study, 1972–1976. *NCI Monogr* 1981;56:69–74.
226. Feldman BA. Rhabdomyosarcoma of the head and neck. *Laryngoscope* 1982;92:424–440.
227. Ruymann R. Rhabdomyosarcomas in children and adolescents. *Hematol Oncol Clin North Am* 1987;1:622–654.
228. Yousem DM, Lexa FJ, Bilaniuk LT, Zimmerman RA. Rhabdomyosarcomas in the head and neck. *Radiology* 1990;177:683–686.
229. Hasso AN, Vignaud J. Pathology of the paranasal sinuses, nasal cavity and facial bones. In: Newton TH, Hasso AN, Dillon WP, eds. *Computed tomography of the head and neck.* Clavadel, 1988:7.1–7.31.
230. Lloyd GAS, Phelps PD. Juvenile angiofibroma: imaging by MR, CT and conventional techniques. *Clin Otolaryngol* 1986;11:247–259.
231. Mirich DR, Blaser SI, Harwood-Nash DC, Armstrong DC, Becker LE, Posnick JC. Melanotic neuroectodermal tumor of infancy: clinical, radiologic, and pathologic findings in five cases. *Am J Neuroradiol* 1991;12:689–697.
232. Pierre-Kahn A, Cinalli G, Lellouch-Tubiana A, et al. Melanotic neuroectodermal tumor of the skull and meninges in infancy. *Pediatr Neurosurg* 1992;18:6–15.
233. Geyer JR. Infant brain tumors. In: Berger MS, eds. *Pediatric neuro-oncology. Neurosurgery clinics of North America.* Philadelphia: Saunders, 1992:781–791.
234. Jooma R, Kendall BE. Intracranial tumors in the first year of life. *Neuroradiology* 1982;23:267–274.
235. Duffner PK, Cohen ME. Treatment of brain tumors in babies and very young children. *Pediatr Neurosci* 1986;12:304–310.

whether the associated brain damage is the result of the presence of hydrocephalus in the developing brain or whether an injury *in utero* may have caused both the hydrocephalus and the associated malformation.

Prior to the age of 2 years, hydrocephalus is almost always accompanied by a progressive enlargement of the head. The Chiari malformations (with or without myelomeningocele), aqueductal stenosis, and aqueductal gliosis account for 80% of hydrocephalus in this age group. These anomalies are associated with 60% of all hydrocephalus regardless of age (20,27). Other relatively common causes of hydrocephalus in infancy include intrauterine infection, perinatal hemorrhage, and neonatal meningoencephalitis. Rare causes of hydrocephalus include congenital midline tumors, choroid plexus papillomas, and vein of Galen malformations (20).

In infants with hydrocephalus, the head tends to grow at an abnormal rate, producing macrocephaly within the first few months of life. The forehead is disproportionately large (frontal bossing), the skull is thin, the sutures are separated, the anterior fontanel is tense, and the scalp veins are dilated. Ocular disturbances are frequent and include paralysis of upward gaze, abducens nerve paresis, nystagmus, ptosis, and diminished pupillary light response. Spasticity of the lower extremities is common, resulting from disproportionate stretching and distortion of the myelinated paracentral corticospinal fibers that arise from the leg area of the motor cortex. These fibers have a longer distance to travel around the dilated ventricle than the corticospinal and corticobulbar fibers that supply the upper extremities and the face (20,28,29).

Children older than 2 years tend to present with neurologic symptoms resulting from increased intracranial pressure or with focal deficits referable to the primary lesion; these symptoms occur prior to significant changes in the head size. The most common causes of hydrocephalus in this age group are posterior fossa neoplasms and obstruction of the aqueduct. Although each of the specific lesions that result in hydrocephalus have some special features, certain clinical characteristics are common to all hydrocephalic patients. In most patients, the increased intracranial pressure results in an early-morning headache that improves with upright posture. Papilledema and strabismus are frequent. Pyramidal tract signs are more marked in the lower extremities, as described earlier. Hypothalamic–pituitary dysfunction is probably caused by compression of the hypothalamus, pituitary stalk, and pituitary gland by enlarged anterior recesses of the third ventricle. Affected patients may present with small stature, obesity, gigantism, amenorrhea or menstrual irregularities, hypothyroidism, or diabetes insipidus. Perceptual and motor deficits and visual spatial disorganization result from stretched fibers of the parietal and occipital cortex around the dilated posterior horns of lateral ventricles (20,28,29).

RADIOLOGIC DIAGNOSIS OF HYDROCEPHALUS

The radiologic diagnosis of hydrocephalus has evolved with the increasing sophistication of imaging modalities. Classically, the diagnosis was made on skull films by the presence of split sutures, increased craniofacial ratio, bulging of the anterior fontanel, and, occasionally, a "hammered silver" appearance of the calvarium when the hydrocephalus was chronic. Ultrasound, CT, and MR are much more sensitive than plain radiographs in the detection of hydrocephalus. The diagnosis of hydrocephalus is made when the ventricles are enlarged in the absence of atrophy. However, the differentiation of ventricular enlargement secondary to hydrocephalus and that resulting from white matter atrophy is not always easy; the differentiation is particularly difficult in the pediatric population. Several parameters have therefore been devised to aid in this determination. The parameters that favor hydrocephalus include (1) commensurate dilatation of the temporal horn with the lateral ventricles, (2) enlargement of the anterior or posterior recesses of the third ventricle, (3) narrowing of the mammillopontine distance, (4) narrowing of the ventricular angle, (5) widening of the frontal horn radius, and (6) effacement of cortical sulci (Fig. 8.1). It has also been suggested that an accentuated cerebrospinal fluid (CSF) "flow-void" (i.e., loss of signal of CSF) is seen in the third ventricle, aqueduct of Sylvius, and fourth ventricle of hydrocephalic patients as a result of hyperdynamic flow (30,31). Other authors, however, dispute the specificity of this finding (32).

The most reliable signs in the differentiation of hydrocephalus from the ex vacuo ventricular enlargement of white matter atrophy are *commensurate dilatation of the temporal horns* with the bodies of the lateral ventricles (Fig. 8.2) (33,34) and *enlargement of the anterior and posterior recesses of the third ventricle* (35,36) (Figs. 8.2, 8.3), both of which strongly suggest hydrocephalus. Several studies have shown that the temporal horns dilate considerably less than the bodies of the lateral ventricles in cerebral atrophy (33,37). The reason for the discrepancy in ventricular enlargement between the temporal lobe and the frontal, parietal, and occipital lobes is not fully understood. However, the small size of the temporal lobes and, in particular, the relatively small volume of white matter in the temporal lobes may play a role (34). This sign is not reliable in patients with significant temporal lobe atrophy, such as those with Down's syndrome. The Sylvian fissures should always be assessed for the degree of temporal lobe atrophy before enlargement of the temporal horns is used to make a diagnosis of hydrocephalus.

The disproportionate enlargement of the recesses of the third ventricle presumably results from the presence

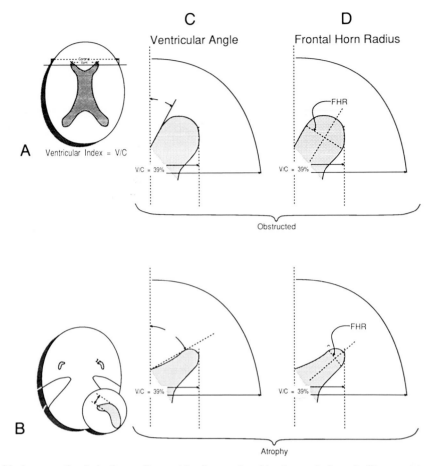

FIG. 8.1. Various methods in the radiographic diagnosis of hydrocephalus. **A:** The ventricular index is the ratio of the ventricular diameter at the level of the frontal horns to the diameter of the brain measured at the same level. This is not a very sensitive or specific measurement in the detection of hydrocephalus because the ventricular index enlarged in cerebral atrophy as well as in hydrocephalus. **B:** Enlargement of the temporal horns commensurately with the bodies of the lateral ventricles is probably the most sensitive and reliable sign in the differentiation of hydrocephalus from atrophy. There is significantly less dilatation of the temporal horns than of the bodies of the lateral ventricles in cerebral atrophy. **C:** The ventricular angle measures the divergence of the frontal horn. In theory, the angle made by the anterior or superior margins of the frontal horn at the level of the foramina of Monro is diminished when concentric enlargement of the frontal horns occurs. Compare the illustration of hydrocephalus (*top*) with that of atrophy (*bottom*). The ventricular index in both instances is 39%; however, the ventricular angle is markedly reduced in hydrocephalus. **D:** The frontal horn radius measures the widest diameter of the frontal horns taken at a 90° angle to the long axis of the frontal horn. The usefulness of this measurement is demonstrated by the markedly increased frontal horn radius in the patient with hydrocephalus (*top*) as opposed to the patient with atrophy (*bottom*). Overall, no one measurement is completely accurate in the diagnosis of hydrocephalus; the size of the temporal horns, ventricular angle, the frontal horn radius, and the size of the ventricles as compared to the cortical sulci should all be assessed.

of CSF, rather than brain tissue, bordering the ventricular wall. CSF presumably offers less resistance to ventricular expansion under conditions of increased intraventricular pressure. Enlargement of the anterior (chiasmal and infundibular) recesses seems to occur earlier and more severely than enlargement of the posterior (suprapineal) recess (36). The *mammilo-pontine distance* is decreased by downward displacement of the floor of the third ventricle (Fig. 8.3).

The *ventricular angle* (Fig. 8.1) measures the divergence of the frontal horns. The angle between the ante-

rior or superior margins of the frontal horns at the level of the foramina of Monro is diminished by concentric enlargement of the frontal horns (33). The diminution of the angle may be appreciated on either axial or coronal images. The concentric enlargement of the frontal horns eventually produces an appearance of "Mickey Mouse ears" on axial scans. This concentric enlargement of the frontal horns also causes enlargement of the so-called *frontal horn radius* (Fig. 8.1), which is determined by measuring the widest diameter of the frontal horns taken at a 90° angle to the long axis of the frontal horn (33).

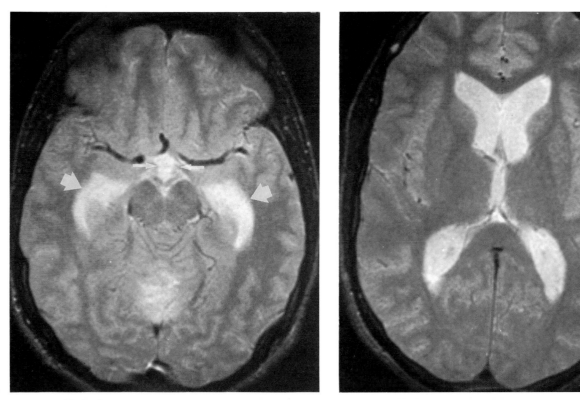

FIG. 8.2. Enlarged anterior recesses and commensurate dilatation of the temporal horns. Patient with medulloblastoma. **A:** Axial SE 2800/70 image shows enlarged temporal horns (*large arrows*) and dilated anterior recesses (*small arrows*) of the third ventricle. **B:** Axial SE 2800/70 at the level of the frontal horns shows that the temporal horns are dilated in proportion to the lateral ventricles.

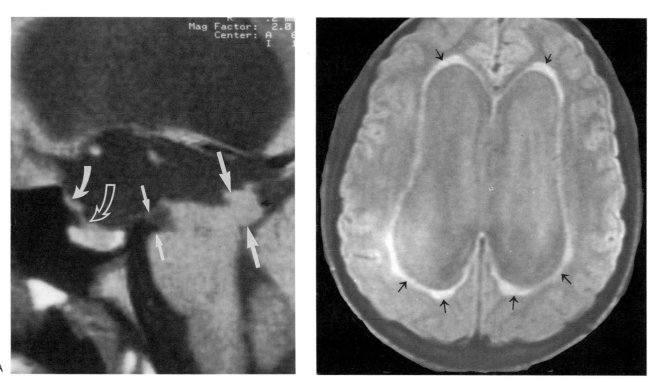

FIG. 8.3. Dilated anterior recesses of the third ventricle. **A:** Sagittal SE 600/20 image shows dilated chiasmatic (*closed curved arrow*) in infundibular (*open curved arrow*) recesses and decreased mamillo-pontine distance. The suprapineal recess is also dilated and is compressing the quadrigeminal plate (*large straight arrows*). **B:** Axial SE 2500/30 image shows irregular T2 prolongation (*arrows*) in the peri-ventricular white matter, diagnostic of transependymal CSF resorption.

The final indicator of hydrocephalus is *enlargement of the ventricular system to a degree that is disproportionate to the enlargement of the cortical sulci* (34). The theory behind this parameter is that increasing pressure within the ventricular system causes compression of the brain tissue against the inner table of the skull and consequent diminution of sulcal size. In pediatric patients, however, this parameter is often misleading because both atrophy and hydrocephalus can enlarge both the ventricles and sulci (38). Further complicating the radiologic assessment is the fact that the size of the ventricles and subarachnoid spaces is quite variable over the first 2 years of life (39).

The fact that both atrophy and hydrocephalus can cause enlargement of both ventricles and cortical sulci makes it difficult to differentiate hydrocephalus from atrophy by imaging studies alone (38). The failure of such measurements as the bicaudate index (40,41) and the Evans ratio (42,43) to differentiate hydrocephalus accurately from atrophy reflects this difficulty (44). This difficulty is complicated in infants by the wide variation in the normal ventricular size (39). Knowledge of the head size of the infant is essential; a large or enlarging head indicates hydrocephalus, whereas a small or diminishing head circumference is more compatible with atrophy. Monitoring of intracranial pressure is another important factor in the differentiation of hydrocephalus from atrophy. Radionuclide flow studies with technetium-99m DTPA may be useful (45,46). Patients with extraventricular obstructive hydrocephalus may demonstrate reflux of the radionuclide into the ventricles with a delay in flow over the convexities. Normally, flow should extend over the convexities within 24 hours (45,46).

The finding of *periventricular interstitial edema* resulting from transependymal flow of CSF is a further radiological finding that may be helpful in the diagnosis of hydrocephalus, particularly in children. When pressure within the ventricular system is increased, normal centripetal bulk flow of CSF into the ventricular system stagnates or reverses. Pressure gradients force intraventricular CSF into the extracellular spaces of the brain through the ependymal lining of the ventricles (18,20). CSF then flows through the brain parenchyma to the arachnoid villi or other sites of CSF absorption. The consequent increased water within the cerebral parenchyma can be detected both on CT and MR. On CT, it appears as hypodensity in the periventricular region. On MR, the increase in water appears as a rim of prolonged T1 and T2 relaxation times surrounding the lateral ventricles (Fig. 8.3B). This rim may not be appreciated on the long TR/TE sequences because the high signal intensity is indistinguishable from the ventricular CSF; a long TR, short TE image (Fig. 8.3B) is much more sensitive.

Although the parameters described in the preceding paragraphs are sometimes helpful in the diagnosis of hydrocephalus and in the differentiation of obstructive hydrocephalus from atrophy, in practice the diagnosis of hydrocephalus remains largely intuitive. In general, diffuse enlargement of the lateral ventricles with commensurate temporal horn enlargement (in the absence of significant enlargement of the Sylvian fissures or other evidence of temporal lobe atrophy), enlargement of the anterior recesses of the third ventricle, and a general rounding of the frontal horn shape in the proper clinical setting indicate hydrocephalus.

DISTORTIONS OF THE BRAIN AND VENTRICULAR SYSTEM RESULTING FROM HYDROCEPHALUS

Severe hydrocephalus may cause herniation of portions of the ventricular system or distortion of the adjacent brain. Such herniations and distortions can cause confusion in the interpretation of imaging studies and will therefore be discussed as a separate section.

The most common distortion resulting from severe hydrocephalus is herniation of the anterior recesses of the third ventricle. When they herniate, the chiasmatic and infundibular recesses can extend inferiorly into the suprasellar cistern in patients with moderate to severe hydrocephalus (Fig. 8.3A). The enlargement and inferior displacement of these recesses can compress the infundibulum and diminish flow within the hypothalamic–pituitary portal venous system, resulting in hypothalamic–pituitary dysfunction (47). Pulsations from the enlarged anterior recesses may erode the dorsum sellae, one of the classic plain film findings in hydrocephalus.

The suprapineal recess of the third ventricle is another common site of ventricular herniation. The dilated recess expands into the posterior incisural space, displacing the pineal gland inferiorly, and occasionally elevating the vein of Galen. When large, diverticulae sometimes extend inferiorly to compress the quadrigeminal plate, with consequent shortening of the tectum in the rostral-caudal direction (Fig. 8.3A) (48). The shortened, thickened tectum should not be mistaken for a neoplasm; isointensity with normal brain tissue on T2-weighted images and the absence of contrast enhancement exclude a tumor. The suprapineal recess may also enlarge further posteriorly and compress the tectum from the posterior direction, resulting in thinning of the tectum and narrowing of the aqueduct (48).

Severe hydrocephalus can cause the formation of *atrial diverticulae*, herniations of the ventricular wall through the choroidal fissure of the ventricular atrium into the supracerebellar and quadrigeminal cisterns. Atrial diverticulae can compress the mesencephalic tectum and can be mistaken for arachnoid cysts in the region of the quadrigeminal cistern (Fig. 8.4). Coronal images are very helpful in the evaluation of these patients,

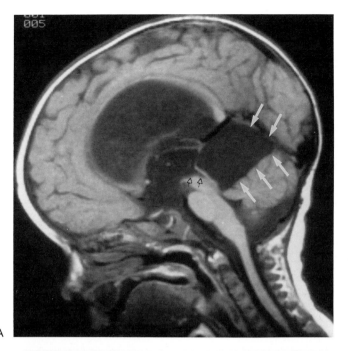

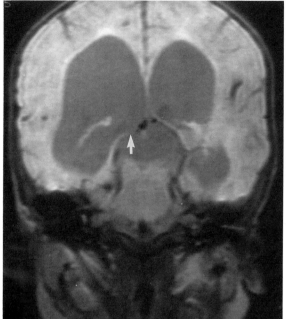

A

B

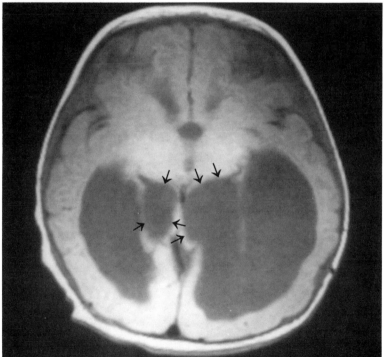

C

FIG. 8.4. Diverticulum of the atrium of the lateral ventricle. **A:** Sagittal SE 600/20 image shows severe hydrocephalus. The lateral ventricles are markedly enlarged, resulting in stretching of the corpus callosum and ballooning of the anterior recesses of the third ventricle. The proximal aqueduct is dilated (*open arrows*). A large cystic mass (*arrows*) is seen dorsal to the quadrigeminal plate. **B:** Coronal SE 2500/20 image shows continuity of the cystic mass in the quadrigeminal cistern with the atrium of the right lateral ventricle through the choroidal fissure (*arrow*), proving that it is an atrial diverticulum. The diverticulum disappeared after placement of a ventriculoperitoneal shunt. **C:** Axial SE 600/20 image in a different patient shows bilateral medial diverticulae (*arrows*) of the atria.

as they often demonstrate the continuity of the trigone of the lateral ventricle with the diverticulum.

When communicating hydrocephalus is severe, the cerebral hemispheres and temporal lobes, in particular, can enlarge markedly, compressing the quadrigeminal cistern. In some patients, the enlarged temporal lobes may compress the dorsal midbrain and quadrigeminal plate, giving the tectum a triangular shape on axial images and secondarily compressing the aqueduct (Fig. 8.5). In some

patients, the hydrocephalus may be primarily communicating in nature, with aqueductal narrowing being a secondary phenomenon (48–50).

SPECIFIC CATEGORIES OF HYDROCEPHALUS

Hydrocephalus can be divided into two major categories. The first is overproduction of CSF; all patients in

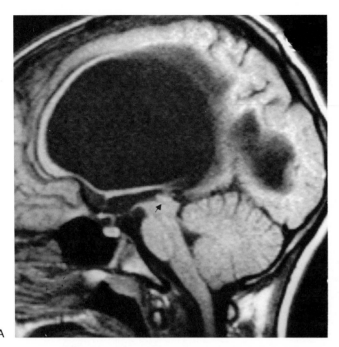
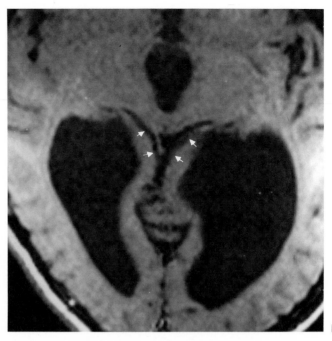

A   B

FIG. 8.5. Distortion of the tectum by the temporal lobes in severe hydrocephalus. **A:** Marked dilatation of the lateral ventricles is present. The third ventricle is only moderately enlarged. The aqueduct (*arrow*) is stenotic. **B:** Axial SE 700/33 image shows compression and distortion of the mesencephalic tectum (*arrows*) and aqueduct by dilated temporal lobes.

this category have choroid plexus papillomas, a rare tumor. The other major category is obstruction to normal CSF flow and absorption. The second category, *obstructive hydrocephalus*, is generally divided into *communicating hydrocephalus*, in which there is extraventricular obstruction to CSF flow or diminished absorption of CSF, and *noncommunicating hydrocephalus*, caused by intraventricular obstruction of CSF flow.

Both hydrocephalus secondary to overproduction of CSF and hydrocephalus secondary to disturbances of normal CSF flow and absorption are evaluated well by CT, MR, and ultrasonography in young infants with large fontanels. Noncommunicating (intraventricular obstructive) hydrocephalus, however, is probably best evaluated by MR. MR evaluates the posterior fossa better than either CT or sonography. CT is limited by beam-hardening artifact and the inability to image in more than one plane. Sonography is limited by decreased resolution that results from attenuation of the ultrasound signal over the long distance from the anterior fontanel to the cerebellum and fourth ventricle. Furthermore, the increased contrast resolution of MR allows better differentiation of subtle mass lesions from webs, membranes, and stenoses. As children grow, sonography becomes technically impossible and beam-hardening artifacts become progressively worse; thus, the superiority of MR is even clearer. Once hydrocephalus has been diagnosed and its cause established and treated, however, CT and sonography are adequate for following ventricular size in most cases.

Another advantage of MR over CT and sonography is

the ability to assess CSF flow qualitatively and quantitatively (32,51–55). On routine spin-echo MR scans, dynamic CSF flow can be detected by signal loss in areas of rapid or turbulent flow (30,51). By manipulating parameters, rapidly moving CSF can be made to appear bright while keeping the signal of stationary or slowly flowing CSF dark; the patency of the aqueduct can be assessed in this way (56). Finally, special techniques that take advantage of the change in phase angle of moving spins can be used to quantitate the flow of CSF through the foramina of Monro, aqueduct, foramen of Magendie, or brain stem cisterns (52,54,55).

In this section, the various causes of hydrocephalus are discussed. I have separated the various types of hydrocephalus. For each type of hydrocephalus, I discuss the most common causes, the mechanisms by which they cause hydrocephalus, the specifics of the radiologic appearance of each cause, and the appearance of the associated hydrocephalus.

Hydrocephalus Resulting from Excessive Formation of CSF (Choroid Plexus Papillomas)

Choroid plexus papillomas are large aggregations of choroidal fronds that are microscopically similar to normal choroid plexus; these neoplasms can produce great quantities of CSF (57,58). Choroid plexus papillomas account for 2% to 4% of childhood intracranial tumors. They usually present during infancy with signs of increased intracranial pressure; occasionally, however, they are found incidentally at postmortem examination.

In the past, the presence of hydrocephalus was thought to be related to the mass effect of the tumor, the presence of proteinaceous CSF, or hemorrhage into the CSF with subsequent obstruction of CSF flow (and an obstructive hydrocephalus). More recent preoperative and postoperative studies have substantiated earlier suggestions that, at least in some cases, oversecretion of CSF by the papilloma produces hydrocephalus (57,58).

The appearance of choroid plexus papillomas on CT and MR was discussed in Chapter 7. These tumors are most commonly located in the trigones of the lateral ventricles, with the bodies of the lateral ventricles, the third ventricle, and the fourth ventricle being the next most common sites. In contrast to adults, in whom the fourth ventricle is the most common site for these tumors, fourth ventricular choroid plexus papillomas are very rare in the pediatric age group. Resection of the tumor cures the hydrocephalus in these patients.

Hydrocephalus Secondary to Intraventricular Obstruction of CSF Flow (Noncommunicating Hydrocephalus)

Tumors

Noncommunicating hydrocephalus may result from obstruction of any portion of the ventricular system from the foramina of Monro to the foramina of Magendie and Luschka. The most common locations for obstruction are the locations where the CSF pathway is narrowest: the foramina of Monro, the posterior third ventricle, the aqueduct of Sylvius, the fourth ventricle, and the fourth ventricular outflow foramina. Tumors are the most common cause of noncommunicating hydrocephalus in the pediatric age group.

Tumors can grow into and obstruct the foramina of Monro from a number of locations. Tumors originating in the lateral ventricles (e.g., ependymomas, astrocytomas, or meningiomas) and tumors originating in the third ventricle (e.g., astrocytomas, choroid plexus papillomas, craniopharyngiomas, or teratomas) can grow into and obstruct the foramina of Monro (Fig. 8.6). Suprasellar tumors may occasionally grow upward to the foramina, pushing the floor of the third ventricle superiorly (Figs. 7.61). In patients with tuberous sclerosis, giant cell tumors, which originate adjacent to the foramina of Monro, often grow medially into the foramina to produce an obstruction (see Chapters 6 and 7).

Obstruction of the Sylvian aqueduct is a common cause of hydrocephalus. The most common cause of obstruction at this level in children is a tumor of the pineal region (see Chapter 7). Germ cell tumors (germinoma, endodermal sinus tumor, embryonal cell carcinoma, choriocarcinoma, teratoma), tumors of pineal origin (pineocytoma, pineoblastoma), astrocytomas (from the quadrigeminal plate or the tegmentum of the midbrain), meningiomas (from the tentorium), or varices of the vein of Galen may all present as a pineal region mass compressing the aqueduct. Most of these lesions are easily identified by CT; however, astrocytomas of the quadrigeminal plate are often subtle and difficult to identify on

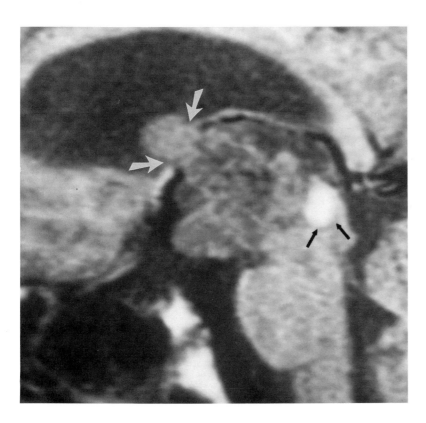

FIG. 8.6. Obstruction of the foramen of Monro and Sylvian aqueduct by tumor. A recurrent craniopharyngioma extends through the foramen of Monro (*white arrows*) and into the aqueduct (*black arrows*).

CT. On MR, they are easily identified as bulbous tectal masses with prolonged T2 relaxation (Fig. 8.7). Therefore, MRI is essential to differentiate benign aqueductal stenosis from stenosis secondary to a tectal astrocytoma in children with aqueductal stenosis.

Tumors of the fourth ventricle and cerebellum frequently have caused hydrocephalus by the time of presentation. The most common posterior fossa neoplasms in the pediatric age group are medulloblastomas, followed by cerebellar astrocytomas and ependymomas (see Chapter 7). Imaging studies will show the tumor in the fourth ventricle or cerebellum compressing the aqueduct and/or ventricle (Fig. 8.8). In contrast to cerebellar tumors, hydrocephalus is uncommon in brain stem neoplasms.

Arachnoid Cysts

Pathologic Characteristics

Arachnoid cysts are congenital lesions of the arachnoid membrane that expand by CSF secretion. Light and

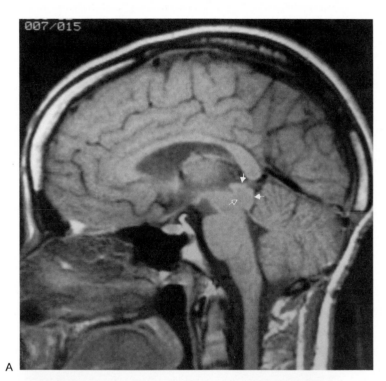

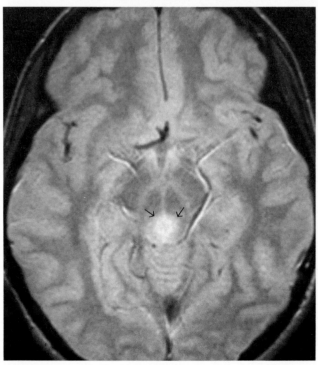

FIG. 8.7. Tectal astrocytoma. **A:** Sagittal SE 600/20 image shows a bulbous tectal mass (*closed arrows*) causing obstruction of the Sylvian aqueduct (*open arrow*). The ventricles are normal in size because of prior placement of a ventriculoperitoneal shunt. **B:** Axial SE 2500/30 image shows prolongation of T2 relaxation time (*arrows*) in the quadrigeminal plate, confirming the diagnosis of neoplasm.

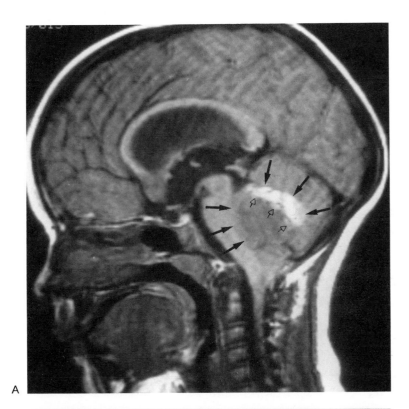

A

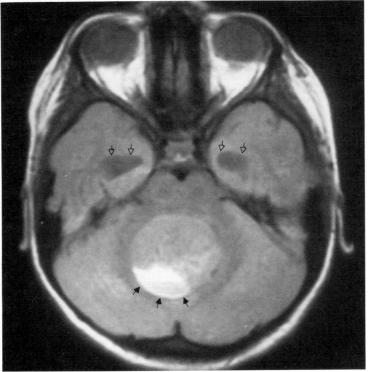

B

FIG. 8.8. Hydrocephalus secondary to medulloblastoma in the fourth ventricle. **A:** Sagittal SE 600/20 image shows a mass within the fourth ventricle (*arrows*) displacing the dorsal pons and the cerebellar vermis. The lateral ventricles, third ventricle and aqueduct are all dilated. The high signal area in the dorsal aspect of the tumor (*open arrows*) was hemorrhage, an unusual finding in medulloblastomas. **B:** Axial SE 2500/30 image shows the tumor with the dorsal hemorrhagic component (*arrows*). Note the dilated temporal horns (*open arrows*).

electron microscopic studies have conclusively demonstrated that congenital arachnoid cysts are intra-arachnoid in location; their inner and outer walls consist of sheets of arachnoid cells that join with normal arachnoid at the margins of the cyst (59,60). True arachnoid cysts differ from leptomeningeal cysts caused by trauma or inflammation (sometimes called arachnoid loculations, acquired arachnoid cysts, or secondary arach-

noid cysts) in that the latter are merely loculations of cerebrospinal fluid surrounded by arachnoidal scarring (59). Ultrastructural studies have shown that the cells lining true arachnoid cysts contain specialized membranes and enzymes for secretory activity (61). When true arachnoid cysts expand, therefore, the mechanism appears to be an accumulation of CSF secreted by cells in the cyst wall rather than by osmotically induced filtra-

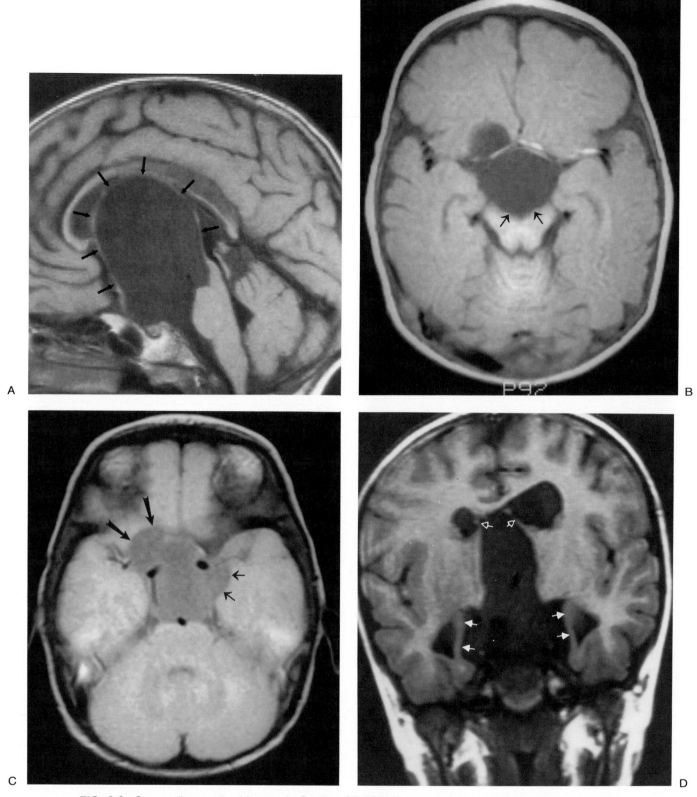

FIG. 8.9. Suprasellar arachnoid cyst. **A:** Sagittal SE 500/40 image shows the large suprasellar cyst extending upward from the suprasellar cistern (*arrows*) displacing the third ventricle superiorly and posteriorly. **B:** Axial SE 2000/40 image shows the cyst extending into the interpeduncular cistern (*arrows*), displacing the cerebral peduncles. **C:** Axial SE 2000/40 image shows the cyst extending laterally into the middle cranial fossa and displacing the uncus and parahippocampal gyrus (*small arrows*), and anteriorly (*large arrows*) into the anterior cranial fossa. Notice how the cyst extends beyond the vessels of the circle of Willis. This is a common imaging characteristic in suprasellar arachnoid cysts. **D:** Same patient after cyst-peritoneal shunt. Coronal SE 600/20 image shows the cyst extending upward and bulging between the leaves of the septum pellucidum (*open arrows*). Note once again the displacement of the medial temporal lobes (*closed arrows*) by the cyst.

tion or a ball-valve mechanism. The precise differences between arachnoid cysts that expand over time and those that remain stable in size have yet to be worked out (62).

Arachnoid cysts usually arise within and expand the margins of CSF cisterns that are rich in arachnoid. The Sylvian fissures are the most common location for arachnoid cysts, composing approximately 50% of these lesions. The suprasellar, quadrigeminal, cerebellopontine angle, and posterior infratentorial midline cisterns each account for approximately 10% of arachnoid cysts. The rest are situated in the interhemispheric fissure, cerebral convexity, and anterior infratentorial midline (60).

Clinical Characteristics

The physical and neurologic signs and symptoms caused by arachnoid cysts reflect their anatomic distribution and their effect on CSF flow. When small, arachnoid cysts are usually asymptomatic, and their discovery is almost always incidental. Large supratentorial cysts, suprasellar cysts, posterior fossa cysts, and quadrigeminal cysts may cause hydrocephalus. Large middle cranial fossa cysts present with seizures, headaches, or, rarely, hemiparesis (59). Suprasellar cysts may cause intracranial hypertension, craniomegaly, developmental delay, visual loss, precocious puberty, and the bobble head doll syndrome. Most of these signs and symptoms are the result of hydrocephalus (59,60,63).

Hydrocephalus is present in 30% to 60% of patients with arachnoid cysts and may be communicating or noncommunicating (63). It is found in up to 100% of children with posterior fossa arachnoid cysts; in a large number of these patients, the hydrocephalus results from defective CSF resorption and not mechanical obstruction to egress of CSF from the ventricles (64).

Imaging Characteristics

Arachnoid cysts appear on both CT and MR as sharply circumscribed, homogeneous, unilocular masses that are isointense to CSF on all imaging modalities and imaging sequences. On transfontanel sonography, they are sharply circumscribed, sonolucent masses with a well-defined posterior border and are enhanced through transmission.

Suprasellar arachnoid cysts can expand in all directions from the suprasellar cistern. They extend inferiorly into the sella turcica, laterally into the middle cranial fossae, and posteriorly into the interpeduncular and prepontine cisterns. As the cyst expands posteriorly, it fills the space previously occupied by the third ventricle and pushes the third ventricle superiorly (Fig. 8.9). In this process, it can disrupt the pituitary stalk and compress the hypothalamus. In very large cysts, the superior pole of the cyst can obstruct both foramina of Monro, causing hydrocephalus; it may even bulge further superiorly be-

tween the leaves of the septum pellucidum (Fig. 8.9). The posterior pole of the cyst may displace the pineal gland inferiorly and cover the entrance of the aqueduct. The optic nerves and chiasm can be stretched by the cyst, as well. Extension into the middle cranial fossae may be seen. Diagnosis is usually easily made by MR, with the midline sagittal image showing the cyst displacing the floor of the third ventricle superiorly (Fig. 8.9).

The major differential diagnoses of suprasellar arachnoid cysts are epidermoid tumors and cystic astrocytomas. A suprasellar epidermoid tumor may have signal characteristics identical to an arachnoid cyst. Epidermoids are generally less sharply defined than arachnoid cysts, however, and are somewhat heterogeneous; however, there are cases in which differentiation by spin echo MR imaging is impossible. If diffusion imaging and magnetization transfer imaging (see section on epidermoids in Chapter 7) are not available, cisternography, using intrathecal water-soluble contrast (Iohexol 180 mg of iodine per ml, 3 ml injected intrathecally via lumbar puncture) may be necessary to differentiate epidermoids from arachnoid cysts. After intrathecal injection of contrast, the patient is scanned after being placed in the head-down position (30°) for 2 min. A sharp border between the lesion and surrounding CSF is seen with arachnoid cysts (Fig. 8.10), whereas irregular interdigitation into the interstices of the mass is noted with epidermoids (Fig 7.26). Cystic astrocytomas are more easily differentiated. Intravenous administration of paramagnetic contrast will show an enhancing solid tumor component in cystic

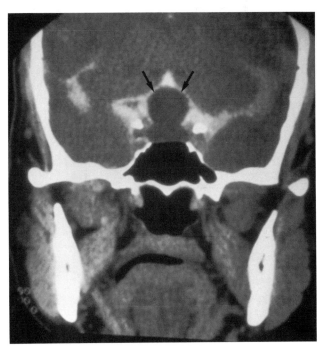

FIG. 8.10. Suprasellar arachnoid cyst. Iohexol cisternogram shows the sharply defined walls (*arrows*) of the arachnoid cyst (compare with Fig. 7.26).

astrocytomas; arachnoid cysts do not enhance and do not have mural nodules.

Cysts of the middle cranial fossa differ somewhat in appearance, depending upon size. Approximately 20% are small, biconvex, or semicircular lesions with little mass effect and no expansion of bone (60,63). These small cysts can be missed on CT because of bone artifact and volume averaging.

Approximately 50% of middle cranial fossa cysts are of moderate size (Fig. 8.11). They occupy the anterior and middle portions of the temporal fossa and frequently displace the tip of the temporal lobe posteriorly, superiorly, and medially. They cause a characteristic flat medial border of the Sylvian fissure and open the lips of the fissure laterally. The temporal fossa is usually mildly expanded by these lesions.

Approximately 30% of middle cranial fossa cysts are large, occupying nearly the whole temporal fossa, sometimes extending to the frontal fossa and convexity. These large cysts cause a marked mass effect with compression of adjacent brain and midline shift. When located anteriorly, they can extend into the orbit via the optic canal. Subdural and intracystic hemorrhages, which may follow trauma or occur spontaneously, frequently complicate middle cranial fossa arachnoid cysts. The bleeding is probably caused by the disruption of cortical veins, which frequently traverse the cyst near its periphery. These veins bleed readily with slight manipulation at the time of surgery (65,66). Concurrent subdural or intracystic hemorrhage should be carefully ruled out in any patient with signs of arachnoid cyst and acute progression of symptoms. Specific attention should be paid to the temporal fossa in any patient with clinical signs consistent with an arachnoid cyst and radiographic evidence of a temporal fossa hemorrhage. Similarly, the possibility of concurrent subdural hematoma should be considered whenever a Sylvian cyst appears to be separated from the inner table of the calvarium (60,63). Finally, middle cranial fossa arachnoid cysts may rupture into the subdural space after trauma as a result of preexisting or traumatic communication (67).

Approximately 25% of arachnoid cysts occur in the posterior fossa (Fig. 8.12). These lesions are usually large (greater than 5 cm) at the time of presentation (60,64,68). Although the cysts can occur anywhere in the posterior fossa, the cerebellopontine angle and inferior

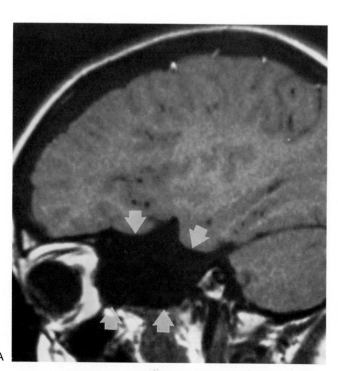

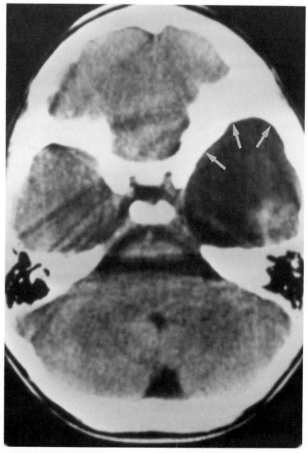

FIG. 8.11. Middle cranial fossa arachnoid cyst. **A:** Parasagittal SE 600/25 image shows displacement of the temporal lobe by the hypointense cyst (*arrows*). **B:** Axial CT image shows expansion of the middle cranial fossa (*arrows*) by the hypodense cyst.

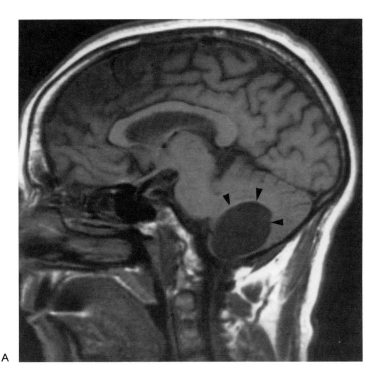

A

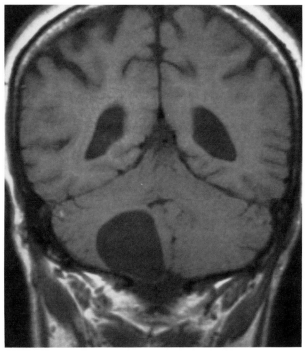

B

FIG. 8.12. Posterior fossa arachnoid cyst. **A:** Sagittal SE 600/20 image in this inferior paramedian arachnoid cyst shows a well-demarcated, sharply defined margin (*arrowheads*). Note the mass is isointense with CSF. **B:** Coronal SE 600/20 image localizes the mass slightly better than axial images.

midline are the most common locations. The major importance of these lesions is in their differentiation from the cysts of the Dandy-Walker complex. This distinction is usually made clinically. Patients with arachnoid cysts present with signs of cerebellar dysfunction (ataxia, dysdiadochokinesis) secondary to compression of the cerebellum by the cyst, whereas patients with the Dandy-Walker complex present either with hydrocephalus or developmental delay (69). Radiologically, the sharply defined walls of the posterior fossa arachnoid cysts are readily distinguishable. Most important, posterior fossa arachnoid cysts are clearly separate from the vallecula and fourth ventricle in all imaging planes, whereas the Dandy-Walker cyst is the enlarged fourth ventricle.

Therapy

Arachnoid cysts can be treated either by fenestration or by cyst-peritoneal shunting. The radiologic appearance after shunting is usually that of complete or nearly complete decompression of the cyst. After adequate treatment of the cyst, the associated hydrocephalus usually resolves as well.

Aqueductal Stenosis

After the initial closure of the neural tube, its lumen has a relatively uniform dimension throughout the neu-

ral axis. As the brain and spinal cord mature, the lumen of the neural tube expands in some areas, such as the cerebral ventricles, and narrows in others, such as the spinal canal and Sylvian aqueduct. The lumen of the aqueduct decreases in size, beginning in the second month of fetal life and continuing until birth (70). This narrowing appears to be caused by growth pressures upon the aqueduct from adjacent mesencephalic structures.

Aqueductal stenosis can be developmental or acquired (71) and is present in approximately 20% of patients with hydrocephalus. Its incidence ranges from 0.5 to 1 per 1,000 births with a recurrence rate in siblings of 1% to 4.5% (19). The normal mean cross-sectional area of the aqueduct at birth is 0.5 mm^2 with a range of 0.2 mm^2 to 1.8 mm^2 (72). In aqueductal stenosis, the aqueduct is focally reduced in size; narrowing generally occurs either at the level of the superior colliculi or at the intercollicular sulcus (72).

The onset of symptoms is usually insidious; it may occur at any time from birth to adulthood. As in all types of hydrocephalus, the symptoms depend upon the cause of the hydrocephalus and the age of the patient at the time of onset.

In many instances, aqueductal stenosis is accompanied by branching of the aqueduct into dorsal and ventral channels; the dorsal channel is often divided into a group of several ductules. This condition has been termed aqueductal forking (73). Forking of the aqueduct is often accompanied by fusion of the quadrigeminal bodies, fusion of the third nerve nuclei, and molding or beaking of the tectum. In some patients, the shape of the molded tectum is congruent with the shape of the medial aspect of the adjacent temporal lobes, which are markedly expanded by hydrocephalus (Fig. 8.5). This congruency has motivated some authors to postulate that aqueductal stenosis may be a secondary phenomenon in some patients, resulting from communicating hydrocephalus and secondary compression of the quadrigeminal plate by the dilated cerebral hemispheres (49,50,74).

The CT appearance of benign aqueductal stenosis is dilatation of the lateral and third ventricles with a normal-sized fourth ventricle. This appearance may be misleading, however, since the fourth ventricle is normal in a large percentage of patients with communicating hydrocephalus. Moreover, as stated earlier, tectal astrocytomas that are large enough to obstruct the aqueduct can be missed on routine CT scans. In all patients with suspected aqueductal stenosis the posterior third ventricle should be carefully scrutinized for the presence of a mass. The MR findings in aqueductal stenosis are more specific but are nonetheless quite variable. Patients with severe hydrocephalus generally have a stenosis in the proximal aqueduct, either at the level of the superior colliculi or at the entrance to the aqueduct immediately inferior to the

posterior commissure (Fig. 8.5) (48). In patients with mild hydrocephalus, the level of obstruction is more often in the distal portion of the aqueduct. In patients with distal aqueductal stenosis, the proximal aqueduct tends to be dilated and the quadrigeminal plate is displaced posteriorly and stretched by the dilated proximal aqueduct (Figs. 8.13 and 8.14). Benign aqueductal stenosis and neoplastic aqueductal stenosis can be easily differentiated by MR. Tectal and tegmental gliomas that compress and obstruct the aqueduct appear as bulbous masses that have high signal intensity on T2-weighted images (Fig. 8.7).

A special case of distal aqueductal stenosis is the *aqueductal web*, which is a thin membrane of brain tissue situated in the distal aqueduct, restricting the flow of CSF into the fourth ventricle. It has been suggested that the membrane may be the result of a small glial occlusion of the caudal aqueduct that becomes an attenuated sheet of tissue secondary to prolonged pressure from and dilatation of the canal above it (75). The imaging appearance is characteristic, consisting of a thin membrane of tissue separating a dilated aqueduct from a normal-sized fourth ventricle (Fig. 8.14). The importance of recognizing aqueductal webs lies in the possibility of perforating the membrane via ventriculoscopy or via stereotactic surgery, obviating the need of an indwelling shunt.

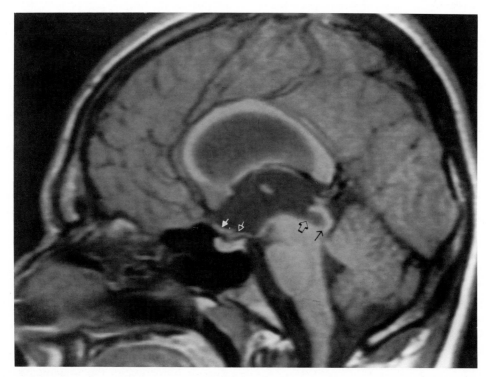

FIG. 8.13. Distal aqueductal stenosis with mild hydrocephalus. Sagittal SE 600/20 image shows mild dilatation of the lateral ventricles in the midline and moderate dilatation of the third ventricle with ballooning of the chiasmatic (*closed white arrow*) and infundibular (*open white arrow*) recesses. The proximal aqueduct is dilated (*open black arrow*) and the quadrigeminal plate is thin and posteriorly displaced. The stenosis is in the distal aqueduct (*thin black arrow*).

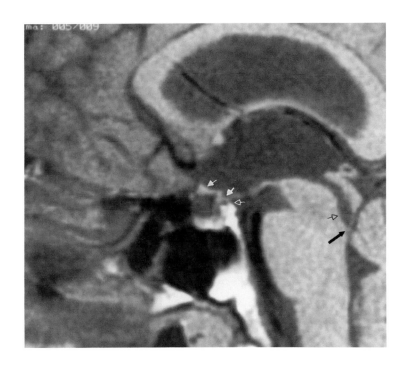

FIG. 8.14. Aqueductal web. This is a special form of aqueductal stenosis in which a small slip of tissue is stretched across the distal aqueduct (*arrow*). Characteristically, the portion of the aqueduct immediately rostral to the web is slightly dilated (*open black arrow*). Note the dilated anterior recesses of the third ventricle (*white arrows*). The infundibular recess can be seen adjacent to, and possibly eroding, the dorsum sellae (*open white arrow*).

Aqueductal Gliosis

Aqueductal gliosis is a postinflammatory process that is usually secondary to a perinatal infection or hemorrhage (71,73). It is becoming more prevalent as newborns with bacterial meningitis or intracranial hemorrhage survive at increasing rates. As in benign aqueductal stenosis, the onset of symptoms, which are those of hydrocephalus, is insidious. The ependymal lining of the aqueduct is destroyed and marked fibrillary gliosis of adjacent tissue is evident.

On imaging studies, differentiation of aqueductal stenosis from aqueductal gliosis is not possible. The appearance is identical on both MR and CT.

Congenital Anomalies

Among congenital malformations of the brain, two anomalies are by far the most common causes of hydrocephalus. The more common of these, the Chiari malformations, have been extensively discussed in Chapter 5 and will therefore be covered only briefly in this section. The *Chiari II malformation* accounts for approximately 40% of all hydrocephalic children (27). Although there is still some dispute as to the cause of hydrocephalus in these patients, the most generally accepted theory is that of Russell (73). Russell demonstrated that adequate flow of CSF exists between the ventricles and the spinal canal in patients with Chiari II malformations but that the connection between the lumbar subarachnoid space and the subarachnoid space over the cerebral convexities is poor. The implication is that disturbance in

CSF flow is most likely the result of the abnormal location of the exit foramina of the fourth ventricle below the foramen magnum, within the cervical spinal canal. Since the spinal canal absorbs much less CSF, hydrocephalus develops. The associated myelomeningocele seems to act as a release valve for the increased intracranial pressure; therefore, hydrocephalus becomes prominent only after repair of the myelomeningocele. It is an important clinical concept that patients with the myelomeningocele/Chiari II malformation who develop occipital headaches at night probably have a shunt malfunction. Fatal shunt malfunctions may result from apneic spells caused by brain stem compression. Symptoms of brain stem compression in patients with the Chiari II malformation are often interpreted as resulting from compression of the medulla by the neural arches of C1 and C2 or by the foramen magnum. These patients may be subjected to unnecessary decompressions of the foramen magnum and C1-2 instead of adjustment or replacement of the ventriculoperitoneal shunt. It is important to recognize that the fourth ventricle is normally a thin vertical slit in the Chiari II malformation (see Figs. 5.79, 5.80). The presence of a normal-appearing or enlarged fourth ventricle in these patients suggests a shunt malfunction or an isolated fourth ventricle that needs CSF diversion (see Fig. 5.83).

Hydrocephalus is present in 70% to 80% of patients with the *Dandy-Walker malformation* (see Chapter 5) (76,77). However, hydrocephalus is uncommonly present at birth and frequently does not become evident until after infancy. The reason for the delayed appearance of hydrocephalus in Dandy-Walker patients has not been established. It has been suggested that the large posterior fossa cyst makes these patients more susceptible to subarachnoid hemorrhage resulting from minor trauma; the subarachnoid blood may then impede the absorption of CSF, resulting in hydrocephalus (76). Two points about the Dandy-Walker malformation are worth emphasizing. First, contrary to common belief, some of the fourth ventricular outflow foramina are generally patent in patients with the Dandy-Walker malformation (76,78); the accompanying hydrocephalus, therefore, is most commonly communicating. Furthermore, in the absence of associated anomalies, these patients can have normal intelligence and lead normal lives if their hydrocephalus is controlled (79–81). Examination by MR (Fig. 8.15) is of great prognostic significance because MR is more sensitive than other imaging modalities in the detection of areas of damaged or dysgenetic brain (79,80).

Treatment, which consists of diversion of CSF from the posterior fossa cyst to the peritoneum, usually decompresses the ventricular system. Most surgeons now shunt both the ventricular system and the posterior fossa cyst to the peritoneum, since long-term results appear to be better (79,81).

The Isolated Fourth Ventricle

When both the aqueduct of Sylvius and the fourth ventricular outflow foramina are occluded, the fourth ventricle becomes "isolated" from the remaining ventricular system and from the CSF circulation of the subarachnoid space. Continued CSF production by the choroid plexus of the fourth ventricle leads to a progressive cystic dilatation of the ventricle; the dilated ventricle can then act as an expanding mass in the posterior fossa. The isolated or "trapped" fourth ventricle appears to result from mechanical or inflammatory changes that obstruct the aqueduct or the fourth ventricular outlet foramina after shunting of the lateral ventricles for communicating hydrocephalus, aqueductal stenosis, or obstruction of the outlets of the fourth ventricle (82). Thus, CSF from the fourth ventricle cannot drain through the shunt catheter or through normal CSF pathways; the ventricle becomes "isolated."

The clinical presentation depends upon the baseline neurologic status of the patient. In those patients who have moderate to severe preexisting neurologic deficits, the preexisting deficits are accentuated by the isolated fourth ventricle without the appearance of posterior fossa signs or symptoms. Patients with normal or near normal baseline neurologic examinations tend to present with signs and symptoms of a posterior fossa mass. A history of a recent ataxia, diplopia, or increasing drowsiness is common (83). Occasionally, patients are mildly symptomatic or asymptomatic, and the isolated fourth ventricle can be an incidental finding (82). In these asymptomatic patients, a steady state is presumably reached between production and absorption of the CSF within the posterior fossa, resulting in the absence of signs of increased intracranial pressure.

On imaging studies, the isolated fourth ventricle ap-

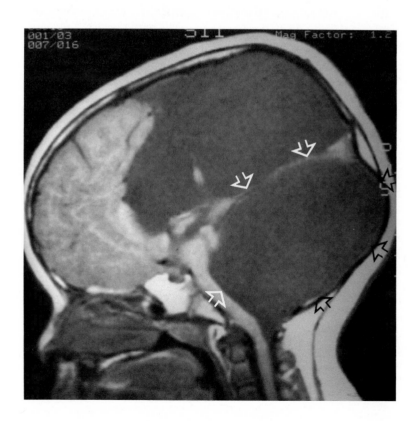

FIG. 8.15. Congenital hydrocephalus secondary to the Dandy-Walker malformation. This patient shows the classic findings of a large posterior fossa with a massive fourth ventricle (*arrows*) filling the posterior fossa and elevating the tentorium. This patient also has callosal hypogenesis with a large interhemispheric cyst.

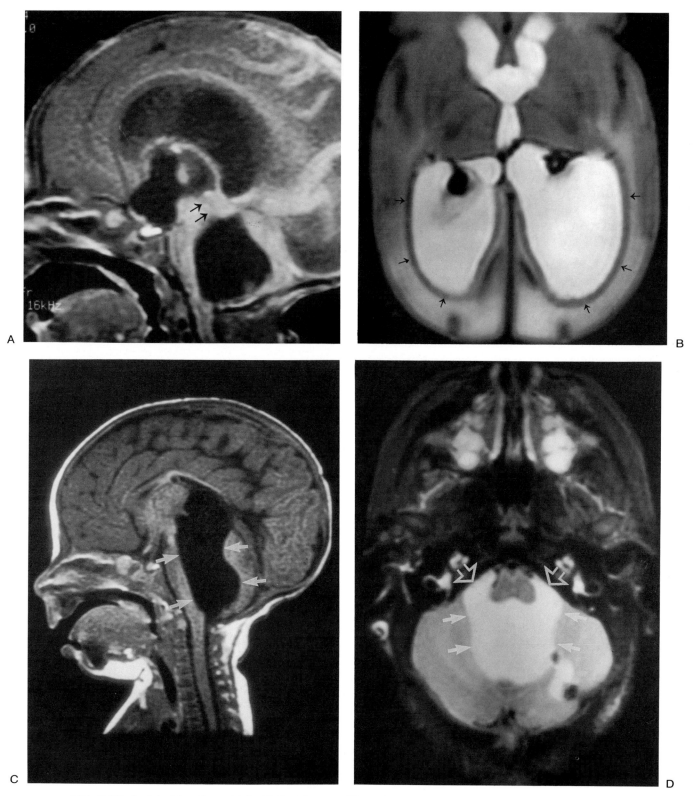

FIG. 8.16. Isolated fourth ventricle. Patient born at 28 weeks who had a grade III intraventricular hemorrhage. **A:** Sagittal SE 500/11 image shows a markedly dilated lateral, third, and fourth ventricles. Note that the aqueduct (*arrows*) is narrow despite the marked hydrocephalus. **B:** Axial SE 3000/120 image shows marked hydrocephalus and hemosiderin staining of the ependyma (low signal, *arrows*). Note the simplified gyral pattern of a 31-week premature infant. **C:** At age 7 months, the lateral and third ventricles are decompressed. However, the fourth ventricle (*arrows*) is enlarged and extends through the tentorial incisura into the supratentorial space. Note that the cisternal magna and basilar cisterns are small, indicating that the obstruction is in those locations. **D:** Axial SE 3000/120 image shows markedly dilated fourth ventricle (*closed arrows*) and foramina of Luschka (*open arrows*).

pears as a large rounded or pear-shaped midline cystic structure (Fig. 8.16) in the posterior fossa (82–84). The lateral and third ventricles are small or only moderately enlarged if the ventriculoperitoneal shunt is functioning. The aqueduct may be completely stenotic (Fig. 8.17), or the distal aqueduct may be dilated. Treatment is the installation of a fourth-ventricle to peritoneal shunt. After shunting, there is usually rapid reversal of posterior fossa signs, if they had been present or progressive. In patients with preexisting neurologic deficits, a return to baseline is generally observed. Occasionally, further treatment, such as a posterior fossa decompression, may be necessary (82,83).

Hydrocephalus Secondary to Extraventricular Obstruction of CSF (Communicating Hydrocephalus)

Communicating hydrocephalus represents approximately 30% of all childhood hydrocephalus (19). After leaving the foramina of the fourth ventricle, CSF normally enters the cisterna magna and basilar cisterns and then progresses into the cerebral and cerebellar subarachnoid spaces. Normal CSF drainage is jeopardized if the cisterns or the arachnoid villi over the cerebral cortex are obstructed by thickened arachnoid or meninges. In general, it is not possible to determine the level of the

extraventricular obstruction to CSF flow from imaging studies.

Impaired flow of CSF through the subarachnoid spaces may result from intracranial hemorrhage, bacterial infections, or granulomatous meningitis. Certain features seen on imaging studies can help to differentiate the different causes of the hydrocephalus. For example, hemorrhage often leaves a transient hemosiderin staining of the parenchyma, ependyma, or pia-arachnoid (superficial siderosis). The hemosiderin will appear black on long TR spin echo images (Fig. 8.16B) (85,86) and especially so on gradient echo images (87). Although hemosiderin will remain at the site of hemorrhage for months or years after parenchymal hemorrhages, it is absorbed much more quickly from the ependyma and arachnoid (Fig. 8.16). Both infectious and carcinomatous meningitis may result in meningeal enhancement (Figs. 8.18, 8.19) after administration of intravenous contrast (88–90). Differentiation of subarachnoid tumor from infection, however, is not currently possible by radiologic methods.

Hemorrhage

In premature infants, intraventricular hemorrhage is common, particularly in babies with a gestational age of

A
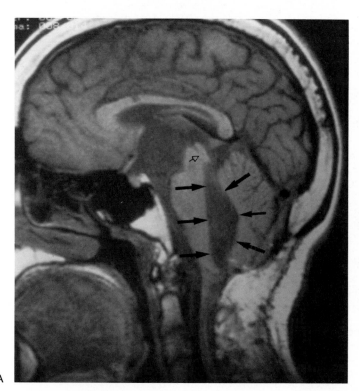

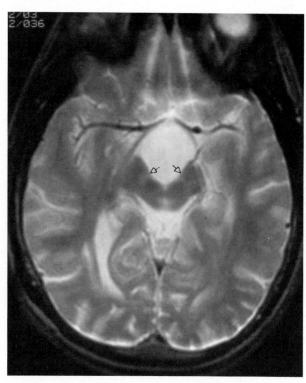
B

FIG. 8.17. Isolated fourth ventricle. Patient with history of staphylococcal meningitis. A: The fourth ventricle is markedly enlarged (arrows) and is posteriorly displacing the vermis. The aqueduct is stenotic (open arrow). The lateral ventricles are normal in size. There is an arachnoid loculation in the interpeduncular cistern. B: Axial SE 2500/70 image shows the arachnoid loculation in the interpeduncular cistern, splaying the cerebral peduncles (arrows).

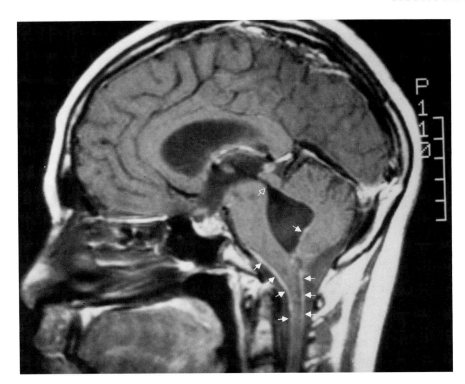

FIG. 8.18. Hydrocephalus secondary to cryptococcal meningitis. Sagittal SE/20 image after enhancement with paramagnetic contrast reveals mild dilatation of the lateral ventricles, moderate dilatation of the third ventricle, and marked enlargement of the fourth ventricle. The aqueduct is patent, as demonstrated by the flow void (*open white arrow*). Note the enhancement of the roof of the fourth ventricle, the dorsal and ventral surfaces of the medulla, and the cervical spinal cord (*closed white arrows*).

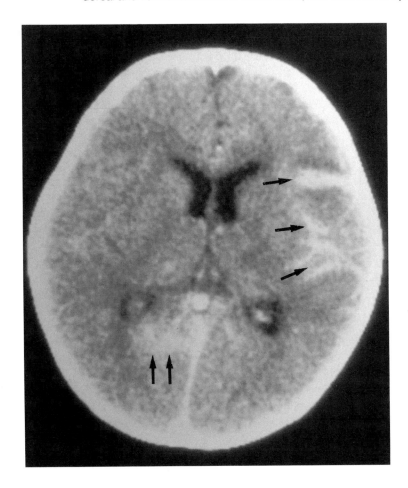

FIG. 8.19. Hydrocephalus secondary to tuberculous meningitis. Enhancement of the meninges (*arrows*) is common in granulomatous or carcinomatous meningitides.

32 weeks or less. Hydrocephalus is a frequent sequel of intraventricular hemorrhages. In the acute phase, the hydrocephalus is most commonly the result of red blood cells obstructing the ventricular system or the arachnoid villi; this acute hydrocephalus has no prognostic implications. Scarring and fibrosis begin to appear in the subarachnoid spaces approximately 10 days after the hemorrhagic event (91). The fibrosis tends to be most prominent in the region of the cisterna magna. This adhesive arachnoiditis is the cause of the subacute hydrocephalus that occurs after germinal matrix hemorrhage in premature infants (Fig. 8.16). The presence of subacute hydrocephalus imparts a poor functional prognosis to the infant. For further discussion of hemorrhage in premature infants and the radiologic manifestations, see Chapter 4.

Subarachnoid hemorrhage in full-term infants is most often caused by trauma (see Chapter 4). The causes of hydrocephalus acutely and subacutely in these patients are similar to the causes of hydrocephalus in premature infants with intraventricular hemorrhage; however, the prognostic value of the hydrocephalus is not as great in this group as in the premature infants.

Meningitis

Inflammation of the leptomeninges may lead to obstruction of the CSF pathways (see Chapter 12). In the acute phase, hydrocephalus is caused by clumping of purulent fluid in the CSF flow pathways. Another component of acute hydrocephalus may result from inflammation of the arachnoid granulations (19,21,92). In the chronic phase, organization of exudate and blood results in fibrosis of the subarachnoid spaces with subsequent obstruction to normal CSF flow and resultant hydrocephalus (21,92).

Clinically significant hydrocephalus is uncommon in bacterial or viral meningitis, but significantly more common in granulomatous and fungal meningitides. Hydrocephalus appears to be related to the duration and severity of the meningeal infections; in general, the longer the delay in treatment, the worse the prognosis for the patient. As a general rule, bacterial meningitis tends to produce cerebral cortical arachnoiditis, whereas granulomatous or parasitic meningitides produce cisternal obstruction (Fig. 8.18, 8.19) (19,21). Rarely, viral meningitides may result in obstruction at either point. Ventricular dilatation, which presumably results from transiently diminished CSF absorption, is the most common finding on CT scans or unenhanced MR scans in patients with bacterial meningitis. Gadolinium-enhanced MR scans often show localized or diffuse meningeal enhancement in bacterial and fungal meningitides (see Fig. 8.18 and examples in Chapter 11) (89).

Hydrocephalus Resulting from CSF Seeding of Tumor

A number of neoplastic processes can involve the subarachnoid space diffusely (see Chapter 7). The most common of these in children are medulloblastoma, germinoma, leukemia, and lymphoma. This is in contrast to adults where adenocarcinoma is the most common tumor to show diffuse meningeal involvement (93).

Older patients typically present with headache, stiff neck, and cranial nerve palsies. Hydrocephalus occurs only later in the course of the disease. As with infectious meningitis, ventricular enlargement is the most common manifestation of this process on CT and unenhanced MR scans. Occasionally, diffuse meningeal enhancement may be seen on CT scans enhanced with iodinated contrast. Significant enhancement of the subarachnoid spaces is typically seen on contrast-enhanced MR scans (88,90,94).

Venous Hypertension

Obstruction of the cerebral veins and sinuses has been alleged to be responsible for communicating hydrocephalus in infants (95–97). It appears that the increased intracranial venous pressure may produce either hydrocephalus or pseudotumor cerebri, depending upon the patient's age (95). Hydrocephalus is more likely if the patient is less than 18 months of age, whereas pseudotumor cerebri is noted if the patient is more than 3 years of age. This difference is thought to result from an expansile calvarium and softer, less myelinated parenchyma in the infant, which allows greater ventricular dilatation under high pressure (98–101). Once the cerebrum is myelinated and the sutures are fused or the calvarium is artificially prevented from expanding, intracranial hypertension occurs without ventricular enlargement and results in pseudotumor cerebri (95,98).

A number of disorders involving the skull base have ventricular enlargement as a part of the syndrome, including achondroplasia (102,103), craniofacial syndromes that result in multisutural craniosynostosis (Apert's syndrome, Carpenter's syndrome, Pfeiffer's syndrome, Crouzon's syndrome; see Chapter 5), and the Marshall-Smith syndrome (a syndrome of accelerated osseous maturation and CNS malformations) (97,104–106). It has been postulated that the ventricular enlargement in all these syndromes (Fig. 8.20) results from diminished venous outflow through the small jugular foramina, which, in turn, results from hypoplasia of the skull base; these theories are supported by experimental evidence in the case of achondroplasia (107,108). The mechanism of this ventricular enlargement is believed to be an increase in superior sagittal sinus pressures, leading to a decreased pressure gradient across the arachnoid

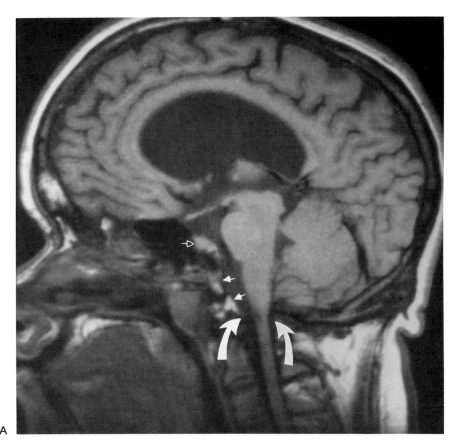

A

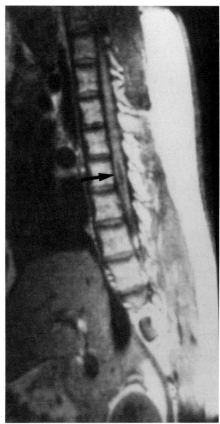

B

FIG. 8.20. Ventricular enlargement in achondroplasia. **A:** Axial SE 600/20 image shows marked enlargement of the lateral ventricles and stretching of the corpus callosum. The skull base (formed from enchondral bone) is quite small in achondroplasts. This is manifest in a small foramen magnum (*curved arrows*) and small clivus (*small white arrows*). The sella turcica and pituitary gland (*open white arrow*) lie substantially below the planum sphenoidale, another characteristic of achondroplasia. **B:** Another manifestation of achondroplasia is a narrow spinal canal. The small syrinx within the thoracic cord (*arrow*) may be a result of trauma or of altered CSF dynamics at the narrowed foramen magnum (see Chapter 10).

villi, from the subarachnoid spaces to the superior sagittal sinus. The resultant increased intracranial pressure results in expansion of the calvarium and ventricles in infants until the pressure normalizes (105,106). Progressive head enlargement in infants can also result from thrombosis of the dural venous sinuses (Fig. 8.21), presumably via the same mechanism. MR venography can be helpful to detect obstruction of the dural venous sinuses in patients with increased CSF pressures with no other obvious cause (Fig. 8.21). However, MR venography cannot determine pressure differential across narrowings in the dural venous sinuses, and, in fact, the 2D time-of-flight technique that is typically used can show apparent narrowings in the distal transverse and sigmoid sinuses that result only from complex flow in those areas. In general, a normal MR venogram can definitively exclude the diagnosis of venous sinus obstruction. However, an abnormal MR venogram should always be confirmed by a catheter venogram; preferentially, the pressure differential across the stenosis should be measured.

Normal Pressure Hydrocephalus (NPH)

Normal pressure hydrocephalus is a form of hydrocephalus in which a pressure gradient exists between ventricle and brain parenchyma, despite the fact that CSF pressure is within the normal range. Intermittent high pressure probably results in a compromise of normal compensatory pressure mechanisms (109,110). The fluctuating high pressures may combine with impaired regional cerebral blood flow to cause ventricular enlargement and parenchymal destruction (19). The most common cause of NPH is communicating hydrocephalus with incomplete arachnoidal obstruction to CSF drainage. Primary events leading to normal pressure hydrocephalus include neonatal intraventricular hemorrhage, spontaneous subarachnoid hemorrhage, intracranial trauma, infections, and surgery (111); it is most commonly seen in children who have underlying neurologic pathology such as sequelae of meningitis or perinatal asphyxia (112). Normal pressure hydrocephalus, therefore, is not merely a disease of adults but occurs in children as

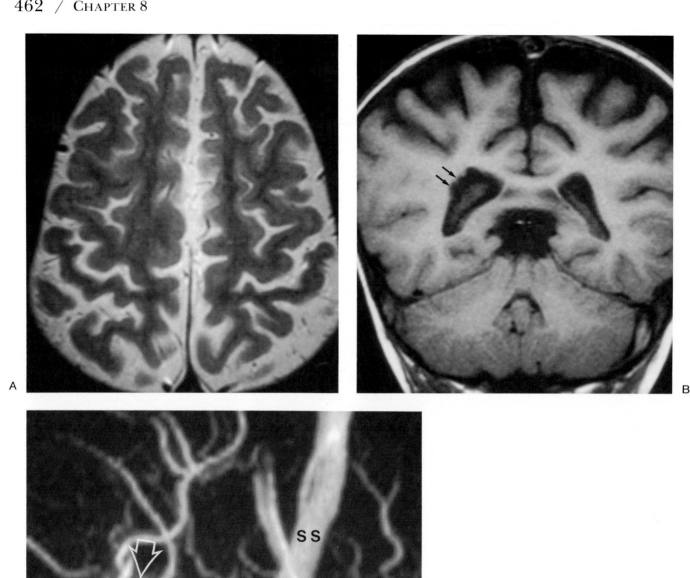

FIG. 8.21. Enlargement of the ventricles and subarachnoid spaces secondary to venous obstruction. **A, B:** Axial SE 2800/70 image shows very prominent subarachnoid spaces and lateral ventricles. In addition, subependymal veins (*arrows*) are dilated. **C:** Maximum intensity projection from MRA (oblique view) shows occlusion of the right transverse sinus (*open arrows*) and left sigmoid sinus (*closed arrows*). SS, superior sagittal sinus. TS, transverse sinus. J, jugular bulb.

well. The appearance of normal pressure hydrocephalus in children on MR and CT is indistinguishable from that of other forms of communicating hydrocephalus.

BENIGN ENLARGEMENT OF THE SUBARACHNOID SPACES IN INFANTS

The CT and MR pattern of enlarged CSF spaces and normal to slightly increased ventricular size (Fig. 8.22) in infants with macrocephaly or rapid head growth is fairly common (113–116). This phenomenon has been variously called benign extra-axial collections of infancy, external hydrocephalus, extraventricular obstructive hydrocephalus, benign subdural effusions of infancy, benign macrocephaly of infancy, and benign enlargement of the subarachnoid spaces. The significance of this finding and, indeed, the actual location of these fluid collections (subarachnoid versus subdural) has been a subject of much debate (113,115,116).

In the absence of underlying brain anomalies, children with benign enlargement of the subdural and subarachnoid spaces usually develop normally (116). Their head circumference tends to be in the high normal range at birth but increases rapidly during the first few months of life; it is generally well above the 95th percentile at the time of presentation (usually between the ages of 2 and 7 months). It is important to recognize that, in the absence of developmental delay or signs or symptoms of increased intracranial pressure, this rapid head growth may not represent hydrocephalus or the presence of subdural hematomas. In fact, when followed without interven-

tion, the head growth curve of affected infants tends to stabilize along a curve parallel to the 95th percentile by the age of 18 months; both the size of the extra-axial spaces and the head circumference often return to normal after the second birthday (115). Cisternography has demonstrated slow flow over the cerebral convexities in these patients (114); the enlarged subarachnoid spaces are therefore proposed to result from delayed maturation of the arachnoid villi. Histologic examination in affected patients has shown thickening of the arachnoid, which is postulated to be a reactive change that helps to increase resorption of CSF (117).

Enlarged subarachnoid spaces can be caused by a number of factors, including ACTH and corticosteroid therapy (118,119), dehydration, malnutrition (35), total parenteral nutrition, and cancer chemotherapy, in addition to the mechanisms discussed previously in this chapter. The presence of these factors should be ruled out before the diagnosis of benign enlargement of the subarachnoid spaces is made.

Imaging studies are often not helpful in the distinction of benign macrocephaly of infancy from hydrocephalus or, for that matter, from atrophy. As discussed earlier, scrutiny of the anterior and posterior recesses of the third ventricle and the temporal horns may be helpful in the differentiation from hydrocephalus (Fig. 8.23). Symmetry of the extra-axial collections is an important finding, especially on CT; asymmetry is unusual in benign macrocephaly and may indicate the presence of traumatic subdural hematomas (120). In the absence of clinical signs or symptoms, cisternography is probably not indicated.

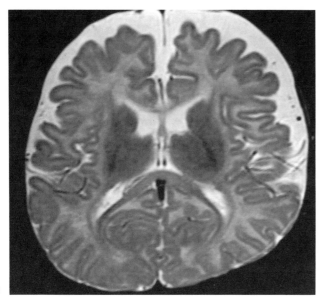
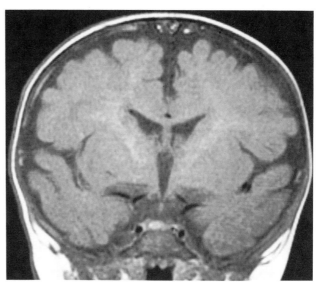

A   B

FIG. 8.22. Benign enlargement of the subarachnoid spaces. Axial SE 3000/120 (**A**) and coronal SE 600/16 images (**B**) in a 5-month-old infant with macrocephaly. The ventricles are prominent and the subarachnoid spaces are large.

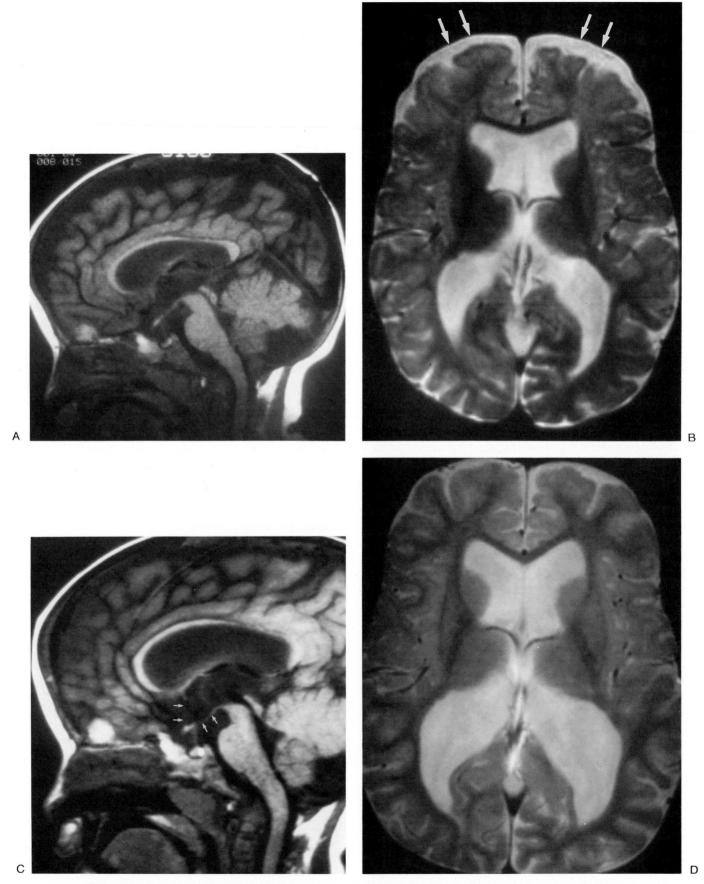

FIG. 8.23. Macrocephaly secondary to hydrocephalus. **A, B:** Sagittal SE 550/15 and axial SE 2800/70 images in a 12-month-old infant show prominent ventricles and large subarachnoid spaces (*arrows*). Differentiation between hydrocephalus and benign enlargement of the subarachnoid spaces is difficult by imaging. **C, D:** Follow-up images at age 20 months show new outward convexity of the anterior and inferior walls (*arrows*) of the third ventricle, despite normalizing of the size of the subarachnoid spaces.

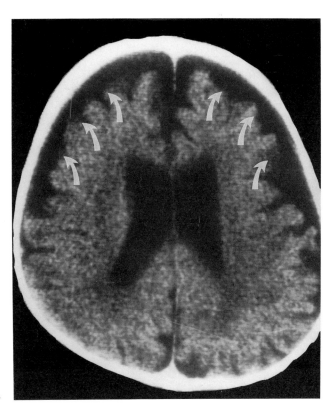
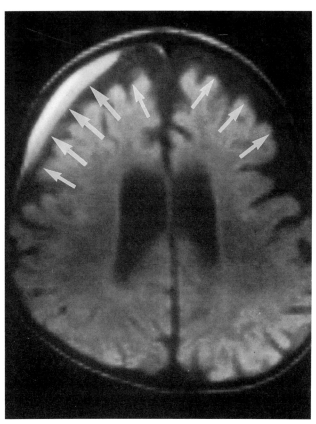

A

B

FIG. 8.24. Benign enlargement of the subarachnoid spaces with associated subdural hematoma. The subdural blood cannot be distinguished from the large subarachnoid spaces (*arrows*) on the axial CT image (**A**). On the SE 2000/40 MR image (**B**), a crescent of hyperintensity (*large arrows*), representing blood, is present peripheral to the large subarachnoid spaces.

Occasionally, patients with clinical courses and CT scans strongly suggestive of benign macrocephaly of infancy have had bloody subdural collections, superimposed upon large subarachnoid spaces, detected on MR scans (Fig. 8.24) (35,121). Wilms and colleagues have reported that infants with bloody subdural collections have a higher incidence of difficult births or postnatal traumatic incidents and are more likely to have symptoms of increased intracranial pressure, such as vomiting and somnolence (121). However, the author has seen several cases in which extensive investigations have revealed no evidence of significant trauma. It is possible that the large CSF spaces in these patients may make them more susceptible to subdural hematoma formation secondary to rather mild trauma, similar to the condition encountered in patients with middle cranial fossa arachnoid cysts (60,66).

TREATMENT OF HYDROCEPHALUS AND THE RESULTING COMPLICATIONS

Severe, long-lasting hydrocephalus will cause damage to the brain. In dogs, the brain is not permanently dam-

aged until the cerebral mantle is compressed to a thickness of less than 4 mm (122). Persistent compression of the brain results in gliosis, cortical distortion, damages to neurons, tearing of axons in the internal capsule, and myelin destruction (21,122,123). Therefore, treatment of uncompensated hydrocephalus is mandatory.

Hydrocephalus is usually treated by CSF diversion in the form of a ventriculoperitoneal or a ventriculoatrial shunt. These shunt systems are composed of a ventriculostomy tube, a reservoir, and a peritoneal tube. The ventriculostomy tube is inserted either into the frontal or occipital horn of the lateral ventricle through a small hole in the calvarium. This is attached to the reservoir, which lies subcutaneously over the calvarial defect. The peritoneal tube is run subcutaneously from the reservoir into the peritoneal cavity. The radiologist is usually asked to assess the function of the shunt by determining the position of its tip and the reduction in ventricular size resulting from its placement. In general, the tip of the ventriculostomy tube should lie within the lateral ventricle in the region of the foramen of Monro (Fig. 8.25). The tube is hypointense on both T1- and T2-weighted MR images (Fig. 8.25) and is dense on CT (Fig. 8.26). Some diminution in ventricular size should be ap-

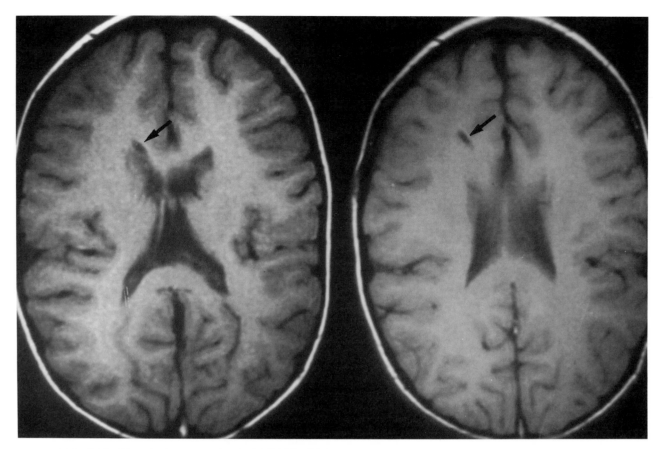

FIG. 8.25. Ventriculostomy tube. Axial SE 600/20 images show the hypointense shunt catheter (*arrows*) coursing through the right frontal lobe into the right frontal horn.

parent soon after the placement of a shunt; if the ventricular size is unchanged after 2–3 days, the patency of the shunt system should be questioned. If the cerebral mantle measures 2 cm or more after shunting, patients usually attain average intellectual development (21).

Shunt Malfunctions

Shunt malfunctions are manifested clinically by symptoms of increased intracranial pressure, persistent bulging of the anterior fontanel, and excessive rate of head growth in the infant. On imaging studies, shunt malfunction is usually manifested by increasing ventricular size (Fig. 8.26). However, some patients have considerable scarring in and around the ventricular walls, causing a decreased compliance of the brain; such patients may show no enlargement or minimal enlargement of the ventricular system in the presence of shunt malfunction [see the subsequent section on the slit ventricle syndrome (124,125)]. The most common cause of malfunction is occlusion of the ventricular catheter by choroid plexus or glial tissue that grows into the lumen of the catheter. This diagnosis can only be inferred from imaging studies, which will show enlarging lateral ventri-

cles in spite of a well-placed ventriculostomy tube and intact connections of the shunt system. Disconnection of the shunt components can occur at any point within the system; it most commonly occurs where the various components are joined. Although the site of shunt malfunction (ventricular portion versus peritoneal portion) can often be determined clinically, plain film studies of shunt components, positive contrast plain film radiography, or radionuclide studies are sometimes necessary (45,46,126,127). The "scout" film from a CT scan will sometimes show a disconnection at the valve that is not appreciated on the axial images; therefore, the scout film should always be analyzed. In addition to showing the location of obstruction or disconnection, shunt function studies are of value when symptoms of shunt malfunction are vague and clinical testing of shunt function is equivocal.

Using special techniques described in Chapter 1, CSF flow can be analyzed by MR techniques (52,54). When used properly, the CSF flow techniques can be used to analyze flow in ventricular catheters and in connecting tubing (128,129). Parameters are set to detect flow that is more rapid than a certain minimum velocity. If flow is seen within the shunt tubing, therefore, one may confidently conclude that a rate of flow above that minimum

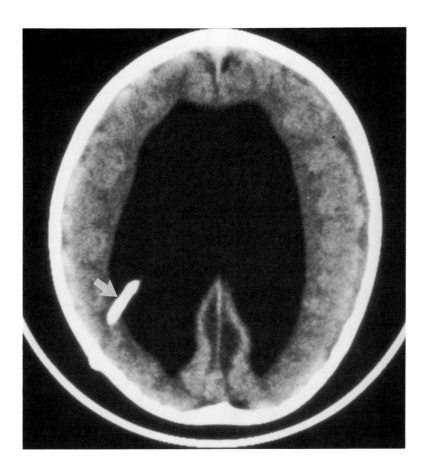

FIG. 8.26. CT of a shunt malfunction. Ventricles are markedly enlarged despite the presence of the ventriculostomy tube (*arrow*) in the right lateral ventricle. The catheter has a high attenuation compared to brain tissue.

is present within the shunt system. However, CSF production and, therefore, CSF flow vary from minute to minute (130). Consequently, a negative study (a study showing no flow) is indeterminate. CSF may be flowing through the shunt at a velocity below the minimum detectable rate (129). A more conventional radionuclide or positive contrast study becomes necessary.

Infection

The risk of infection resulting from ventricular shunting has decreased steadily over the years and is now generally between 1% and 5% (19). The major clinical manifestation of shunt infection is fever, which is usually intermittent and low grade. Anemia, dehydration, hepatosplenomegaly, and stiff neck can also be presenting signs. Shunt infection may also manifest itself by swelling and redness over a portion or all of the shunting tract or by such generalized symptoms as peritonitis. The only aspect of shunt infection that is visualized on imaging studies is that of *ventriculitis*, which is seen on contrast-enhanced imaging studies as enlarged lateral ventricles with an irregular, enhancing ventricular wall; the ventricles are often spanned by septations (Fig. 8.27). Patients with ventricular septae are more difficult to treat because each loculation must be drained separately. The capabil-

ity of imaging in three planes, by either sonography or MR, is extremely helpful in identifying and localizing each loculation within the ventricular system. Occasionally, after severe ventriculitis, the multiple loculations can cause distortion of the brain, resulting in a confusing image (Fig. 8.27).

Subdural Hematomas

Significant *subdural hematomas* (Fig. 8.28) are unusual after shunting. When present, their appearance is similar to that of traumatic subdural hematomas (see Chapter 4); however, surgical decompression of postshunt subdural hematomas is very uncommon, as the ventricular decompression results in a considerable buffer to increases in intracranial pressure. Because it is very sensitive to the presence of very small fluid collections, MR will often show small subdural hematomas in patients who have recently been shunted (Fig. 8.29). These small hematomas are almost never of clinical significance. Large subdural fluid collections, which can result in increased intracranial pressure, are usually seen in children over 3 years of age after overly vigorous drainage of markedly enlarged ventricles. The use of high-pressure valves in the shunting of these patients has reduced the incidence of significant subdural hematomas.

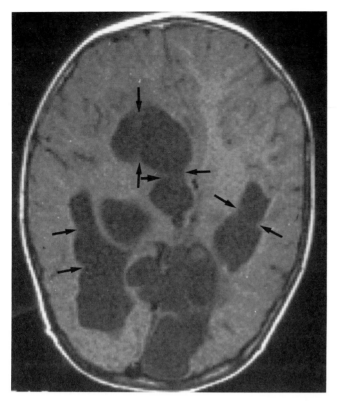

FIG. 8.27. Severe ventriculitis. Axial SE 500/40 image shows multiple septae within the ventricular system (*arrows*) causing multiple loculations of cerebrospinal fluid. These images can result in confusion unless the multiple loculations and septae are recognized.

Using contrast-enhanced MR or CT, chronic subdural hematomas can be distinguished from *postshunt meningeal fibrosis* [meningeal callus (131)], in which a thick collagenous scar develops in the subdural space, presumably as a reaction to chronic subdural hematoma (131–133). Whereas chronic subdural hematomas will not enhance after administration of contrast, meningeal fibrosis enhances dramatically (Fig. 8.30), presumably as a result of vascular granulation tissue intermixed with the collagen bundles in the subdural space (133).

Slit Ventricle Syndrome

Shunted hydrocephalic patients may become symptomatic from shunt failure without evidence of ventricular enlargement on ultrasound, CT, or MR. Patients who exhibit this phenomenon have been labeled as having the "slit ventricle syndrome" (125,134–137). Some debate exists as to what constellation of clinical and/or pathologic findings define this syndrome (125,138). It has become clear that there are multiple different entities lumped together under this name; therefore, affected patients require one of several different treatments (139).

Rekate (134) has attempted to classify the various disorders that have been given the name *slit ventricle syndrome.* He divides them into (1) extreme low-pressure headaches, probably from siphoning of CSF from the brain by the shunt; (2) intermittent obstruction of the

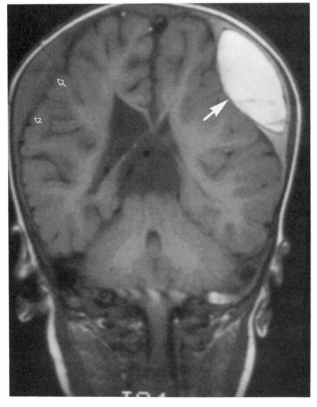

A

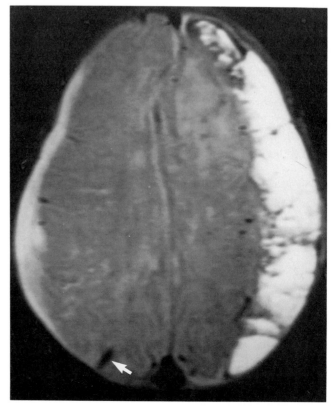

B

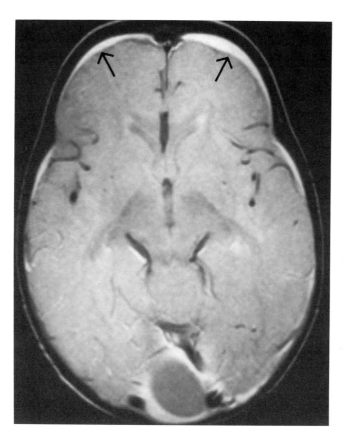

FIG. 8.29. Small bilateral subdural hematomas after placement of a ventriculoperitoneal shunt (*arrows*). It is not uncommon to see these small collections in patients who have been recently shunted because MR is extremely sensitive to extra-axial fluid collections. These small hematomas are of no clinical significance.

The syndrome most commonly referred to by the name *slit ventricle syndrome* is the result of decreased intracranial volume, resultant diminished CSF buffering capacity (diminished ability to compensate for the normal variations in intracranial pressure), diminished brain compliance, and, possibly, intermittent or partial shunt obstruction (124,125). Most affected patients have diminished intracranial volume secondary to premature sutural synostosis from prior shunting. Patients typically present with recurrent, transient symptoms of shunt failure. Treatment is bitemporal craniectomies that expand the volume of intracranial CSF. Theoretically, the expanded intracranial space is better able to compensate for the transient changes in intracranial pressure that accompany the variations in CSF production.

One finding on imaging studies that may help in the determination of which patients have diminished buffering capacity is that of calvarial thickening (Fig. 8.31). Such thickening may or may not be associated with premature synostosis of the cranial sutures; either way, the result is a diminished reservoir of CSF to buffer the normal variations in intracranial pressure (125).

It is less important for the radiologist to know all the possible causes of small ventricles in a symptomatic patient than to realize that the presence of very small ventricles after placement of a ventriculoperitoneal shunt is not diagnostic of, or even suggestive of, the slit ventricle syndrome. Small ventricles are not, in the majority of cases, a problem; they are the desired result of many surgeons after ventriculoperitoneal or ventriculoatrial shunting and, even when they are extremely small, their only implication in the vast majority of patients is that the shunt is functioning.

proximal shunt catheter; (3) normal volume hydrocephalus (in which the buffering capacity of the CSF is diminished, see following paragraph); (4) intracranial hypertension associated with working shunts (probably linked to venous hypertension); and (5) headaches in shunted children unrelated to intracranial pressure or shunt function. Thus, shunted patients may experience a number of disorders, with very different treatments, that can cause headaches without detectable ventricular enlargement. Other than category (3), which may show calvarial thickening, these categories cannot be differentiated by imaging methods.

Other Complications

Other complications resulting from ventriculoperitoneal shunting are much less common. Complications within the abdomen include ascites, pseudocyst formation, perforation of a viscus or of the abdominal wall, and intestinal obstruction (45,140). Very rarely, patients may develop a granulomatous reaction adjacent to the shunt tube either within or near the ventricle (141). These granulomatous lesions appear as irregular, contrast-enhancing masses along the course of the shunt tube. Calcification may be noted within the mass.

FIG. 8.28. Subdural hematomas complicating ventriculoperitoneal shunt placement. **A:** Coronal SE 700/20 image shows bilateral convexity hematomas. The hematoma over the right convexity (*open arrows*) is chronic, having been present since the shunt placement several weeks earlier. A subacute hematoma is present over the left convexity (*closed white arrow*). The subacute hematoma presumably still has methemoglobin present and is therefore of high signal intensity on the short TR/TE sequence. **B:** Axial SE 2500/70 image. Both the older right convexity subdural and the newer left convexity subdural are of high signal intensity on this T2-weighted image. The shunt catheter is seen entering the brain in the right occipital region (*arrow*).

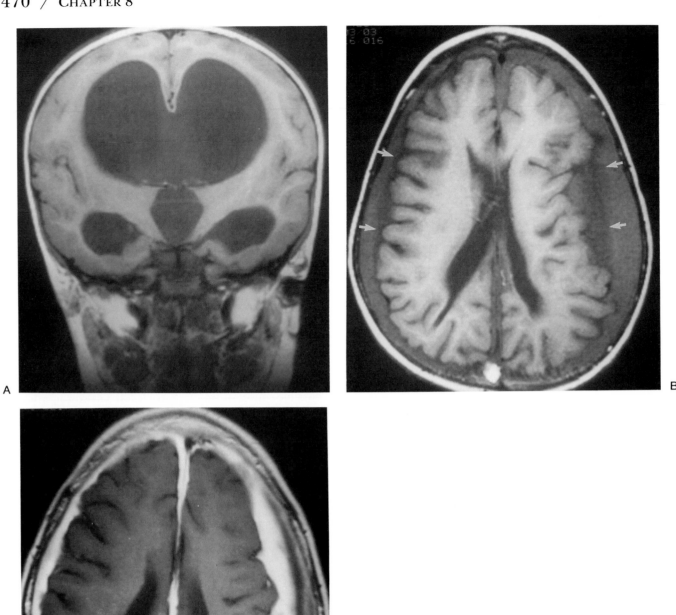

FIG. 8.30. Postshunt meningeal fibrosis. Patients with a pineal germinoma. **A:** Severe hydrocephalus prior to shunting or surgery. **B:** Noncontrast axial SE 600/20 image 1 year after surgery and shunting shows decompressed ventricles and intermediate intensity material in the subdural space. Note the more hypointense subarachnoid space (*arrows*) medially. **C:** Postcontrast image shows marked enhancement of the subdural material, suggesting the diagnosis of postshunt meningeal fibrosis.

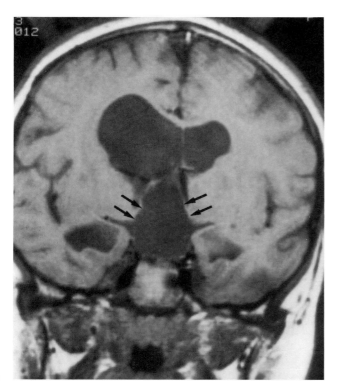

A

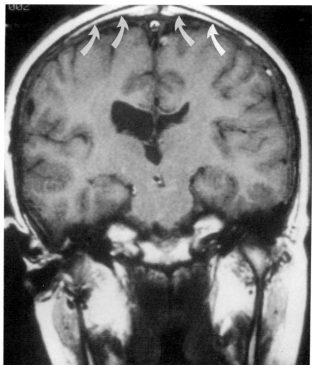

B

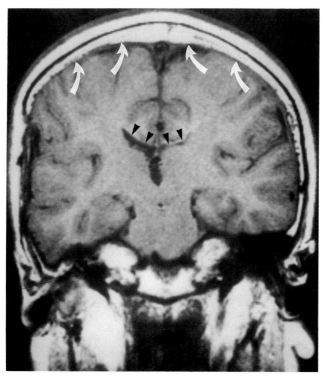

C

FIG. 8.31. Calvarial thickening associated with the slit ventricle syndrome. **A:** A suprasellar arachnoid cyst (*arrows*) is associated with hydrocephalus. Note the thin diploic space of the calvarium. **B:** Five months after shunting of the cyst, the ventricles are smaller and the calvarium (*arrows*) is thicker. **C:** After 2 years, the ventricles (*black arrowheads*) are small, the subarachnoid spaces small, and the calvarium (*white arrows*) very thick.

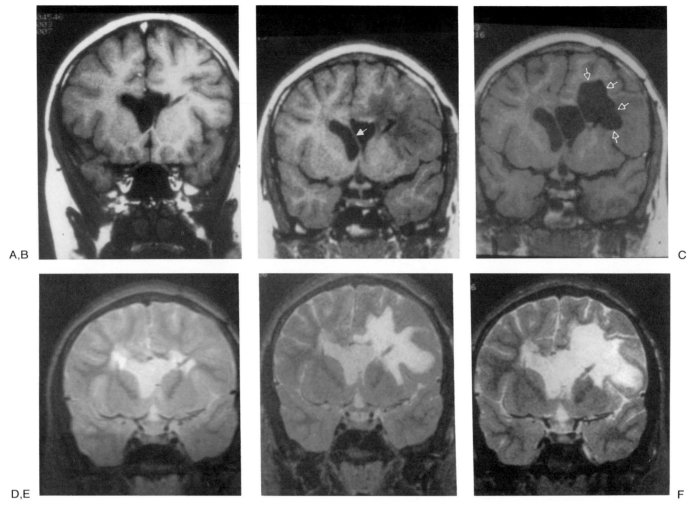

FIG. 8.32. Interstitial edema and cyst formation secondary to shunt malfunction. **A, D:** Coronal SE 600/20 (A) and 2500/70 (D) images through the frontal horns at a time when the patient was asymptomatic reveal a well-decompressed left lateral ventricle and minimal periventricular high signal intensity. **B, E:** Six months later, there is interstitial edema around the shunt tube, as manifested by prolonged T1 and T2 relaxation in the white matter. The left lateral ventricle is now larger than on the previous study and the septum pellucidum has shifted back toward the midline (*arrow*). **C, F:** One month later, there is frank cyst formation in the hemispheric white matter surrounding the shunt tube (*open arrows*). There has been further enlargement of the left lateral ventricle. All changes disappeared after shunt revision.

One final appearance of shunt malfunction should be mentioned. Rarely, when the ventricular end of the shunt becomes partially occluded, CSF may track along this shunt and enter the interstices of the centrum semiovale. On these occasions, the CT and MR appearance is that of edema (low density in the white matter on CT, prolonged T1 and T2 relaxation time in the white matter on MR) in the area around the shunt. Eventually, an actual cyst may form in the white matter surrounding the ventricular catheter (Fig. 8.32). It should be recognized that the presence of edema in these patients is not the result of infection or tumor but is a sign of shunt malfunction. The edema and cyst will resolve after shunt revision.

REFERENCES

1. Osaka K, Handa R, Matsumoto S, Yasuda M. Development of the cerebrospinal fluid pathway in the normal and abnormal human embryos. *Childs Brain* 1980;6:26–38.
2. Truwit CL, Barkovich AJ. Pathogenesis of intracranial lipoma: an MR study in 42 patients. *AJNR* 1990;11:665–674.
3. Dooling EC, Chi Je G, Gilles FH. Ependymal changes in the human fetal brain. *Ann Neurol* 1977;1:535.
4. Cutler RWP, et al. Formation and absorption of cerebrospinal fluid in man. *Brain* 1968;91:707–720.
5. McComb JG. Recent research into the nature of cerebrospinal fluid formation and absorption. *J Neurosurg* 1983;59:369–383.
6. McComb JG. Cerebrospinal fluid physiology of the developing fetus. *AJNR* 1992;13:595–599.
7. Greitz D, Franck A, Nordell B. On the pulsatile nature of intracranial and spinal CSF-circulation demonstrated by MR imaging. *Acta Radiol* 1993;34:1–8.

8. Greitz D. *Cerebrospinal fluid circulation and associated intracranial dynamics. A radiologic investigation using MR imaging and radionuclide cisternography.* (Ph.D. Thesis) Karolinska Institute, 1993.

9. Greitz D, Wirestam R, Franck A, Nordell B, Thomsen C, Ståhlberg F. Pulsatile brain movement and associated hydrodynamics studied by magnetic resonance imaging. The Monroe-Kellie doctrine revisited. *Neuroradiology* 1992;34:370–380.

10. Olivero WC, Rekate HL, Chizek JH, et al. Relationship between intracranial and sagittal sinus pressure in normal and hydrocephalic dogs. *Pediatr Neurosci* 1988;14:196–201.

11. McCormick JM, Yamada K, Rekate HL, Miyake H. Time course of intraventricular pressure change in a canine model of hydrocephalus: its relationship to sagittal sinus elastance. *Pediatr Neurosurg* 1992;18:127–133.

12. Welch K, Friedman V. The cerebrospinal fluid valves. *Brain* 1960;83:454–469.

13. Bradbury MWB, Cole DF. The role of the lymphatic system in drainage of cerebrospinal fluid and aqueous humor. *J Physiol* 1980;299:353–365.

14. McComb JG, Hyman S. Lymphatic drainage of cerebrospinal fluid in the primate. In: Johansson BB, Owman C, Widner H, eds. *Pathophysiology of the blood-brain barrier.* Amsterdam: Elsevier, 1990:421–438.

15. McComb JG, Hyman S, Weiss MH. Lymphatic drainage of cerebrospinal fluid in the cat. In: Shapiro K, Marmarou A, Portnoy H, eds. *Hydrocephalus.* New York: Raven, 1984:83–98.

16. James AE, Strecker EP, Sperber E, et al. An alternative pathway of cerebrospinal fluid absorption in communicating hydrocephalus. *Radiology* 1974;111:143–146.

17. Zervas NT, Lisczak TM, Mayberg MR, et al. Cerebrospinal fluid may nourish cerebral vessels through pathways in the adventitia that may be analogous to systemic vasa vasorum. *J Neurosurg* 1982;56:475–481.

18. Milhorat TH. Classifications of the cerebral edemas with reference to hydrocephalus and pseudotumor cerebri. *Childs Nerv Syst* 1992;8:301–306.

19. Gabriel RS, McComb JG. Malformations of the central nervous system. In: Menkes JH, ed. *Textbook of child neurology.* Philadelphia: Lea and Febiger, 1985:234–253.

20. Milhorat TH. Hydrocephaly. In: Myrianthopoulos NC, ed. *Malformations.* New York: Elsevier, 1987:285–300.

21. Friede RL. *Developmental neuropathology,* 2nd ed. Berlin: Springer-Verlag, 1989.

22. Weller RO, Schulman K. Infantile hydrocephalus, clinical, histological, and ultrastructural study of brain damage. *J Neurosurg* 1972;36:255–260.

23. Shirane R, Sato S, Sato K, et al. Cerebral blood flow and oxygen metabolism in infants with hydrocephalus. *Childs Nerv Syst* 1992;8:118–123.

24. Hill A, Volpe JJ. Decrease in pulsatile flow in the anterior cerebral arteries in infantile hydrocephalus. *Pediatrics* 1982;69:4–10.

25. Bannister CM, Chapman SA. Ventricular ependyma of normal and hydrocephalic subjects: a scanning electron microscopic study. *Dev Med Child Neurol* 1980;22:725–731.

26. Rosseau GL, McCullough DC, Joseph AL. Current prognosis in fetal ventriculomegaly. *J Neurosurg* 1992;77:551–555.

27. Laurence KM. The pathology of hydrocephalus. *Ann R Coll Surg Engl* 1959;24:388.

28. Warkany J, Lemire RJ, Cohen MM Jr. *Mental retardation and congenital malformations of the central nervous system.* Chicago: Yearbook, 1981.

29. Yakovlev PI. Paraplegias of hydrocephalics. *Am J Ment Defic* 1947;51:561–577.

30. Bradley WG Jr, Kortman KE, Burgoyne B, Eng D. Flowing cerebrospinal fluid in normal and hydrocephalic states: appearance on MR images. *Radiology* 1986;159:611–616.

31. Bradley WG Jr, Whittemore AR, Kortman KE, et al. Marked cerebrospinal fluid void: indicator of successful shunt in patients with suspected normal-pressure hydrocephalus. *Radiology* 1991;178:459–466.

32. Sherman JL, Citrin CM, Gangarosa RE, Bowen BJ. The MR appearance of CSF flow in patients with ventriculomegaly. *AJNR* 1986;7:1025–1031.

33. Heinz ER, Ward A, Drayer BP, DuBois PJ. Distinction between obstructive and atrophic dilatation of ventricles in children. *J Comput Assist Tomogr* 1980;4:320–325.

34. LeMay M, Hochberg FH. Ventricular differences between hydrostatic hydrocephalus and hydrocephalus ex vacuo by computed tomography. *Neuroradiology* 1979;17:191–195.

35. Barkovich AJ, Edwards MSB. Applications of neuroimaging in hydrocephalus. *Pediatr Neurosurg* 1992;18:65–83.

36. El Gammal T, Allen MB Jr, Brooks BS, Mark EK. MR evaluation of hydrocephalus. *AJNR* 1987;8:591–597.

37. Sjaastad O, Skalpe IO, Engeset A. The width of the temporal horn and the differential diagnosis between pressure hydrocephalus and hydrocephalus ex vacuo. *Neurology* 1969;19:1087–1093.

38. Fitz CR, Harwood-Nash DC. Computed tomography of hydrocephalus. *Comput Tomogr* 1978;2:91–108.

39. Kleinman PK, Zito JL, Davidson RI, Raptopoulos V. The subarachnoid spaces in children: normal variations in size. *Radiology* 1983;147:455–457.

40. Gomori JM, Steiner I, Melamed E, Cooper G. The assessment of changes in brain volume using combined linear measurements. A CT scan study. *Neuroradiology* 1984;26:21–24.

41. Hahn FJY, Rim K. Frontal ventricular dimensions on normal computed tomography. *AJR* 1976;126:593–596.

42. Haug G. Age and sex dependence of the size of normal ventricles on computed tomography. *Neuroradiology* 1977;14:201–204.

43. Evans WA. An encephalographic ratio for estimating ventricular enlargement and cerebral atrophy. *Arch Neurol Psychiatr* 1942;47:931–937.

44. Gooskens RHJM, Gielen CCAM, Hanlo PW, Faber JAJ, Willemse J. Intracranial spaces in childhood macrocephaly: comparison of length measurements and volume calculations. *Dev Med Child Neurol* 1988;30:509–519.

45. Guertin SR. Cerebrospinal fluid shunts. Evaluation, complications, and crisis management. *Pediatr Clin North Am* 1987;34:203–217.

46. Howman-Giles R, McLaughlin A, Johnston I, Whittle I. A radionuclide method of evaluating shunt function and CSF circulation in hydrocephalus. Technical note. *J Neurosurg* 1984;61:604–605.

47. Kim CS, Bennett DR, Roberts TS. Primary amenorrhea secondary to noncommunicating hydrocephalus. *Neurology* 1969;19:533–537.

48. Barkovich AJ, Newton TH. Aqueductal stenosis: evidence of a broad spectrum of tectal distortion. *AJNR* 1989;10:471–475.

49. Borit A, Sidman RL. New mutant mouse with communicating hydrocephalus and secondary aqueductal stenosis. *Acta Neuropathol* 1972;21:316–331.

50. Williams B. Is aqueductal stenosis the result of hydrocephalus? *Brain* 1973;96:399–412.

51. Sherman JL, Citrin CM. Magnetic resonance of normal CSF flow. *AJNR* 1986;7:3–6.

52. Nitz WR, Bradley WG Jr, Watanabe AS, et al. Flow dynamics of cerebrospinal fluid: assessment with phase-contrast velocity MR imaging performed with retrospective cardiac gating. *Radiology* 1992;183:395–405.

53. Quencer RM, Post MJD, Hinks RS. Cine MR in the evaluation of normal and abnormal CSF flow: intracranial and intraspinal studies. *Neuroradiology* 1990;32:371–391.

54. Levy LM, Di Chiro G. MR phase imaging and cerebrospinal fluid flow in the head and spine. *Neuroradiology* 1990;32:399–406.

55. Enzmann DR, Pelc NJ. Normal flow patterns of intracranial and spinal cerebrospinal fluid defined with phase-contrast cine MR imaging. *Radiology* 1991;178:467–474.

56. Atlas SW, Mark AS, Fram EK. Aqueductal stenosis: evaluation with gradient echo rapid MR imaging. *Radiology* 1988;169:449–453.

57. Milhorat TH, Hammock MK, Davis DA, Fenstermacher JD. Choroid plexus papilloma: I. Proof of cerebrospinal fluid overproduction. *Childs Brain* 1977;5:273–277.

58. Eisenberg HM, McComb JG, Lorenzo AV. Cerebrospinal fluid overproduction and hydrocephalus associated with choroid plexus papilloma. *J Neurosurg* 1974;40:381–385.

59. Harsch GR, Edwards MSB, Willson CB. Intracranial arachnoid cysts in children. *J Neurosurg* 1986;64:835–842.

60. Naidich TP, McLone DG, Radkowski MA. Intracranial arachnoid cysts. *Pediatr Neurosci* 1986;12:112–122.
61. Go KG, Houthoff HJ, Blaauw EH, et al. Arachnoid cysts of the Sylvian fissure. Evidence of fluid secretion. *J Neurosurg* 1984;60:803–810.
62. Becker T, Wagner M, Hoffman E, Warmuth-Metz M, Nadjmi M. Do arachnoid cysts grow? A retrospective CT volumetric study. *Neuroradiology* 1991;33:341–345.
63. Naidich TP, Gado M. Hydrocephalus. In: Newton TH, Potts DG, eds. *Ventricles and cisterns.* St Louis: CV Mosby, 1978:Chap 107.
64. DiRocco C, Caldarelli M, DiTrapani G. Infratentorial arachnoid cysts in children. *Childs Brain* 1981;8:119–133.
65. Dyck P, Gruskin P. Supratentorial arachnoid cysts in adults: a discussion of two cases from a pathophysiologic and surgical perspective. *Arch Neurol* 1977;34:276–279.
66. Galassi E, Tognetti F, Gaist G, et al. CT scan and metrizamide cisternography in arachnoid cysts of the middle cranial fossa: classification and pathophysiological aspects. *Surg Neurol* 1982;17:363–369.
67. Cullis PA, Gilroy J. Arachnoid cyst with rupture into the subdural space. *J Neurol Neurosurg Psychiatr* 1983;46:454–456.
68. Little JR, Gomez MR, MacCarty CS. Infratentorial arachnoid cysts. *J Neurosurg* 1973;39:380–386.
69. Barkovich AJ, Kjos BO, Norman D, Edwards MSB. Revised classification of posterior fossa cysts and cyst-like malformations based on results of multiplanar MR imaging. *AJNR* 1989;10:977–988.
70. Turkewitsch N. Die Entwicklung des Aquaeductus Cerebri des Menschen. *Morphologisches Jahrbuch* 1935;76:421–477.
71. Lapras C, Tommasi M, Bret P. Stenosis of the aqueduct of Sylvius. In: Myrianthopoulos NC, ed. *Malformations.* New York: Elsevier, 1987:301–322.
72. Woollam DHM, Millen JW. Anatomical considerations in the pathology of stenosis of the cerebral aqueduct. *Brain* 1953;76:104–112.
73. Russell DS. *Observations on the pathology of hydrocephalus.* London: His Majesty's Stationery Office, 1949.
74. Raimondi AJ, Clark SJ, McLone DG. Pathogenesis of aqueductal occlusion in congenital murine hydrocephalus. *J Neurosurg* 1976;45:66–77.
75. Turnbull I, Drake C. Membranous occlusion of the aqueduct of Sylvius. *J Neurosurg* 1966;24:24–33.
76. Hirsch JF, Pierre-Kahn A, Renier D, Sainte-Rose C, Hoppe-Hirsch E. The Dandy-Walker malformation: a review of 40 cases. *J Neurosurg* 1984;61:515–522.
77. Raimondi AJ, Sato K, Shimoji T. *The Dandy-Walker syndrome.* Basel: Karger, 1984.
78. Hart MN, Malamud N, Ellis WG. The Dandy-Walker syndrome. A clinico-pathological study based on 28 cases. *Neurology* 1972;22:771–780.
79. Osenbach K, Menezes AH. Diagnosis and management of the Dandy-Walker malformation: 30 years of experience. *Pediatr Neurosurg* 1992;18:179–189.
80. Maria BL, Zinreich SJ, Carson BC, Rosenbaum AE, Freeman JM. Dandy-Walker syndrome revisited. *Pediatr Neurosurg* 1987;13:45–51.
81. Bindal AK, Storrs BB, McLone DG. Management of the Dandy-Walker syndrome. *Pediatr Neurosci* 1990–91;16:163–169.
82. Scotti G, Musgrave MA, Fitz CR, Harwood-Nash DC. The isolated fourth ventricle in children: CT and clinical review of 16 cases. *Am J Roentgenol* 1980;135:1233–1238.
83. James HE. Spectrum of the isolated fourth ventricle in posthemorrhagic hydrocephalus of the premature infant. *Pediatr Neurosurg* 1990–1991;16:305–308.
84. Hall TR, Choi A, Schellinger D, Grant EG. Isolation of the fourth ventricle causing transtentorial herniation: neurosonographic findings in premature infants. *Am J Roentgenol* 1992;159:811–815.
85. Gomori JM, Grossman RI, Goldberg HI, Zimmerman RA, Bilaniuk LT. Intracranial hematomas: imaging by high field MR. *Radiology* 1985;157:87.
86. Gomori JM, Grossman RI, Goldberg HI, et al. High field spin echo MR imaging of superficial and subependymal siderosis secondary to neonatal intraventricular hemorrhage. *Neuroradiology* 1987;29:339.
87. Unger EC, Cohen MS, Brown TR. Gradient echo imaging of hemorrhage at 1.5T. *Mag Res Imag* 1989;7:163–167.
88. Rippe DJ, Boyko OB, Friedman HS, et al. Gd-DTPA-enhanced MR imaging of leptomeningeal spread of primary intracranial CNS tumors in children. *AJNR* 1990;11:329–332.
89. Mathews VP, Kuharit MA, Edwards MK, D'Amour PG, Azzarelli B, Dreesen RG. Gadolinium enhanced MR imaging of experimental bacterial meningitis: evaluation and comparison with CT. *AJNR* 1988;9:1045–1050.
90. Matthews VP, Broome DR, Smith RR, Bognanno JR, Einhorn LH, Edwards MK. Neuroimaging of disseminated germ cell tumors. *AJNR* 1990;11:319–324.
91. Bagley C. Blood in the cerebrospinal fluid. Resultant functional and organic alterations in the central nervous system. A. Experimental data. *Arch Surg* 1928;17:18–38.
92. Hughes CP, Gado M. Pathology of hydrocephalus and brain atrophy. In: Newton TH, Potts DG, eds. *Radiology of the skull and brain.* St Louis: CV Mosby, 1977:Chapter 97.
93. Little JR, Dale AJD, Okazaki H. Meningeal carcinomatosis: clinical manifestations. *Arch Neurol* 1974;30:138–143.
94. Kochi M, Mihara Y, Takada A, et al. MRI of subarachnoid dissemination of medulloblastoma. *Neuroradiology* 1991;33:264–267.
95. Rosman NP, Shands KN. Hydrocephalus caused by increased intracranial venous pressure: a clinicopathological study. *Ann Neurol* 1978;3:445–450.
96. Kalbag RM, Woolf AL. *Cerebral venous thrombosis.* London: Oxford, 1967.
97. Sainte-Rose C, LaCombe J, Peirre-Kahn A, et al. Intracranial venous sinus hypertension: cause or consequence of hydrocephalus in infants? *J Neurosurg* 1984;60:727–736.
98. Epstein F, Hochwald GM, Ransohoff J. Neonatal hydrocephalus treated by compressive head wrapping. *Lancet* 1973;1:634.
99. Hochwald GM, Epstein F, Malhan C, et al. The role of skull and dural in experimental feline hydrocephalus. *Dev Med Child Neurol* 1972;14(Suppl 27):65–69.
100. Shapiro K, Fried A, Takei F, Kohn I. Effect of the skull and dura on neural axis pressure–volume relationships and CSF hydrodynamics. *J Neurosurg* 1985;63:76–81.
101. Shapiro K, Fried A, Maramou A. Biomechanical and hydrodynamic characterization of the hydrocephalic infant. *J Neurosurg* 1985;63:69–75.
102. Hecht JT, Butler IJ. Neurologic morbidity associated with achondroplasia. *J Child Neurol* 1990;5:84–97.
103. Kao SCS, Waziri MH, Smith WL, Sato Y, Yuh WTC, Franken EA Jr. MR imaging of the craniovertebral junction, cranium, and brain in children with achondroplasia. *Am J Roentgenol* 1989;153:565–569.
104. Pappas CTE, Rekate HL. Cervicomedullary junction decompression in a case of Marshall-Smith syndrome. *J Neurosurg* 1991;75:317–319.
105. Moss ML. The pathogenesis of artificial cranial deformation. *Am J Phys Anthropol* 1958;16:269–286.
106. Moss ML. Functional anatomy of cranial synostosis. *Childs Brain* 1975;1:22–33.
107. Steinbok P, Hall J, Flodmark O. Hydrocephalus in achondroplasia: the possible role of intracranial venous hypertension. *J Neurosurg* 1989;71:42–48.
108. Lundar T, Bakke SJ, Nornes H. Hydrocephalus in an achondroplastic child treated by venous decompression at the jugular foramen. Case report. *J Neurosurg* 1990;73:138–140.
109. DiRocco C, et al. Continuous interventricular cerebrospinal fluid pressure recording in hydrocephalic children during wakefulness and sleep. *J Neurosurg* 1975;42:683.
110. DiRocco C, et al. Cerebrospinal fluid pressure studies in normal pressure hydrocephalus and cerebral atrophy. *Eur Neurol* 1976;14:119.
111. Stein BM, Fraser RA, Tenner MS. Normal pressure hydrocephalus: complication of posterior fossa surgery in children. *Pediatrics* 1972;49:50–52.

112. Barnett GH, Hahn JF, Palmer J. Normal pressure hydrocephalus in children and young adults. *Neurosurgery* 1987;20:904–907.

113. Barlow CF. CSF dynamics in hydrocephalus—with special attention to external hydrocephalus. *Brain Dev* 1984;6:119–127.

114. Briner S, Bodensteiner J. Benign subdural collections of infancy. *Pediatrics* 1980; 67:802–804.

115. Carolan PL, McLaurin RL, Tobin RB, Tobin JA, Egelhoff JC. Benign extra-axial collections of infancy. *Pediatr Neurosci* 1986;12:140–144.

116. Nickel RE, Gallenstein JS. Developmental prognosis for infants with benign enlargement of the subarachnoid spaces. *Dev Med Child Neurol* 1987;29:181–186.

117. Kim D, Choi J, Yoon S, Suh J, Kim T. Hypertrophic arachnoid membrane in infantile external hydrocephalus: neuroradiologic and histopathologic correlation. *Radiology* 1993;189(P):195.

118. Gordon N. Apparent cerebral atrophy in patients on treatment with steroids. *Dev Med Child Neurol* 1980;22:502–506.

119. Ito M, Takao P, Okumo T, Mikawa H. Sequential CT studies of 24 children with infantile spasms on ACTH therapy. *Dev Med Child Neurol* 1983;25:475–480.

120. Maytal J, Alvarez LA, Elkin CM, Shinnar S. External hydrocephalus: radiologic spectrum and differentiation from cerebral atrophy. *AJNR* 1987;8:271–278.

121. Wilms G, Vanderschueren G, Demaerel PH, et al. CT and MR in infants with pericerebral collections and macrocephaly: benign enlargement of the subarachnoid spaces versus subdural collections. *Am J Neuroradiol* 1993;14:855–860.

122. Yamada H, Yokota A, Furuta A, Horie A. Reconstitution of shunted mantle in experimental hydrocephalus. *J Neurosurg* 1992;76:856–862.

123. Wright LC, McAllister JP II, Katz SD, et al. Cytological and cytoarchitectural changes in the feline cerebral cortex during experimental infantile hydrocephalus. *Pediatr Neurosurg* 1990–91;16:139–155.

124. Oi S, Matsumoto S. Infantile hydrocephalus and the slit ventricle syndrome in early infancy. *Childs Nerv Syst* 1987;3:145–150.

125. Epstein F, Lapras C, Wisoff JH. "Slit ventricle syndrome": Etiology and treatment. *Pediatr Neurosci* 1988;14:5–10.

126. Evans RC, Thomas MD, Williams LA. Shunt blockage in hydrocephalic children. The use of the valvogram. *Clin Radiol* 1976;27:489.

127. Sweeney LE, Thomas PS. Contrast examination of cerebrospinal fluid malfunction in infancy and childhood. *Pediatr Radiol* 1987;17:177–183.

128. Martin AJ, Drake JM, Lemaire C, Henkelman RM. Cerebrospinal fluid shunts: flow measurements with MR imaging. *Radiology* 1989;173:243–247.

129. Castillo M, Hudgins PA, Malko JA, Burrow BK, Hoffman JC Jr. Flow-sensitive MR imaging of ventriculoperitoneal shunts: in vitro findings, clinical applications, and pitfalls. *AJNR* 1991;12:667–672.

130. Minns RA, Brown JK, Engleman HM. CSF production rate: "real time" estimation. *Z Kinderchir* 1987;47:36–40.

131. Falhauer K, Schmitz P. Overdrainage phenomena in shunt treated hydrocephalus. *Acta Neurochir (Wien)* 1978;45:89–101.

132. Emery JL. Intracranial effects of long-standing decompression of the brain in children with hydrocephalus and meningomyelocele. *Dev Med Child Neurol* 1965;7:302–309.

133. Destian S, Heier LA, Zimmerman RD, et al. Differentiation between meningeal fibrosis and chronic subdural hematoma after ventricular shunting: value of enhanced CT and MR scans. *AJNR* 1989;10:1021–1026.

134. Rekate HL. Classification of slit-ventricle syndrome using intracranial pressure monitoring. *Pediatr Neurosurg* 1993;19:15–20.

135. Hyde-Rowan MD, Rekate HL, Nulsen FE. Reexpansion of previously collapsed ventricles: the slit ventricle syndrome. *J Neurosurg* 1982;56:536–539.

136. Epstein FJ, Fleisher AS, Hochwald GM, Ransohoff J. Subtemporal craniectomy for recurrent shunt obstruction secondary to small ventricles. *J Neurosurg* 1974;41:29–31.

137. Epstein FJ, Hochwald GM, Wald A, Ransohoff J. Avoidance of shunt dependency in hydrocephalus. *Dev Med Child Neurol* 1975;Suppl 17:71–77.

138. Serlo W, Heikkinen E, Saukkonen A-L, Wendt L. Classification and management of the slit ventricle syndrome. *Childs Nerv Syst* 1985;1:194–199.

139. Benzel EC, Reeves JD, Kesterson L, Hadden TA. Slit ventricle syndrome in children: clinical presentation and treatment. *Acta Neurochir (Wien)* 1992;117:7–14.

140. Davidson RI. Peritoneal bypass in the treatment of hydrocephalus: historical review of abdominal complications. *J Neurol Neurosurg Psychiatry* 1976;39:640–648.

141. Citrin CM, Hammock MK. Computed tomographic representation of granulomatous reaction from intraventricular shunt. *Comput Tomogr* 1979;3:177–180.

CHAPTER 9

Congenital Anomalies of the Spine

NORMAL AND ABNORMAL EMBRYOGENESIS OF THE SPINE: AN OVERVIEW

Understanding the normal embryonic developmental sequence of the spine is invaluable to understanding spinal anomalies. Furthermore, combining a knowledge of embryology with an understanding of the anatomic relationships in the mature congenital lesion allows insight into the time and stage of development at which the normal sequence was altered; this insight leads to a better understanding of developmental lesions. Normal development of the spine will therefore be discussed in some detail.

Neurulation

On about the 15th day of embryonic life, ectodermal cells proliferate to form a plate, the primitive streak, along the surface of the embryo. A rapidly proliferating group of cells forms at one end of the primitive streak; this nodular proliferation, surrounding a small primitive pit (known as Hensen's node) defines the cephalic end of the primitive streak. At days 15 and 16, cells enter the primitive pit and migrate cephalad in the midline; these cells form the notochordal process, which will eventually become the notochord. The notochord induces the formation of a plate of ectodermal cells in the dorsal midline, beginning immediately cephalad to Hensen's node (Fig. 9.1). The edges of this structure, the neural plate, are contiguous with the superficial ectoderm from which the plate differentiated.

At approximately 17 days of gestation, the lateral portions of the neural plate begin to thicken bilaterally, forming the neural folds. The thinner midline portion of the plate is called the neural groove. Contractile filaments resembling myosin are concentrated in the neuroepithelial cells at the base of the neural groove and in the cells along the lateral edges of the neural folds. As these

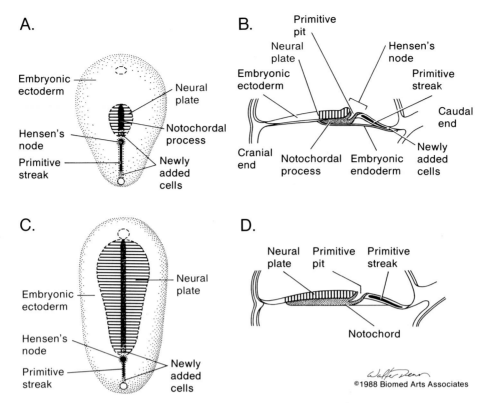

FIG. 9.1. Schematic showing the development of the neural plate. The primitive streak forms along the surface of the embryo by about 15 days of embryonic life. A small primitive pit lies at what will become the cephalic end of the primitive streak; a nodular proliferation of cells surrounding the primitive pit becomes known as Hensen's node. On about days 15 and 16, cells enter the primitive pit and migrate cephalically in the midline to form the notochordal process, which will eventually become the notochord. The notochordal process and notochord induce formation of a plate of ectodermal cells dorsally in the midline; this is the neural plate.

filaments contract, the neural folds bend dorsally along the entire length of the neural groove, bringing the edges of the neural folds toward one another in the midline. The more lateral contractile filaments, which are now located dorsally, contract and bend the neural folds even more medially (Fig. 9.2). Closure of the neural tube

(known as neurulation) probably begins in the rhombencephalon (brain stem area), where microvilli project medially from the most dorsal cells of the neural folds on either side. Cell recognition and adhesion occur, closing the tube at that point. Immediately following closure, the overlying ectoderm separates from the neural tissue and

FIG. 9.2. Normal and abnormal neurulation. **A–E:** Normal neurulation. **A:** The neural plate is composed of neural ectoderm that is continuous with cutaneous ectoderm on either side. The cells at the junction of the neural ectoderm and cutaneous ectoderm will eventually differentiate into neural crest cells. **B:** At approximately 17 days of gestation, the lateral portions of the neural plate begin to thicken, forming the neural folds (**C**). Contractile filaments located in the neuroepithelial cells in the neural folds contract, causing the neural folds to bend dorsally along the entire length of the neuraxis, bringing the edges of the neural folds toward one another in the midline (**D**). Neurulation (closure of the neural tube) begins when the neural folds meet in the midline. At the time of closure, the overlying ectoderm separates from the neural tissue and fuses in the midline, forming a continuous ectodermal covering of the neural structures. At the same time, the neural crest cells are extruded from the neural tube to form a transient structure immediately dorsal to the tube. **E:** Eventually these neural crest cells will migrate to form dorsal root ganglia and multiple other structures. **F–G:** Abnormal neurulation. **F:** When there is premature disjunction of neural ectoderm from cutaneous ectoderm, the surrounding mesenchyme gains access to the inner surface of the neural tube. When mesenchyme comes in contact with this primitive ependymal lining, it evolves into fat. This is believed to be the process underlying the formation of spinal lipomas (*F*). Complete nondisjunction of cutaneous ectoderm from neural ectoderm results in the formation of myelomeningoceles (Fig. 9.4). **G:** Focal nondisjunction results in a persistent epithelium-lined connection between the central nervous system and the skin. This persistent connection has been labeled a dorsal dermal sinus.

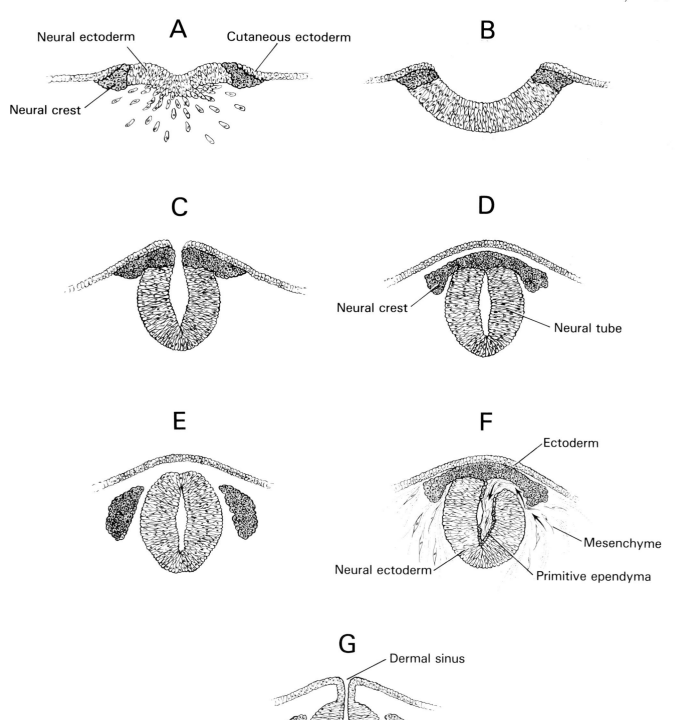

A

Neural ectoderm

Cutaneous ectoderm

Neural crest

B

C

D

Neural crest

Neural tube

E

F

Ectoderm

Mesenchyme

Neural ectoderm

Primitive ependyma

G

Dermal sinus

the edges of the ectoderm meet in the midline and close, forming a continuous ectodermal covering of the neural structures. The accepted theory suggests that progressive folding and closure of the neural structures and separation from ectoderm then proceed both cranially and caudally from the point of initial closure, closing the neural tube in both directions. However, new evidence indicates that the neural tube may close at multiple independent sites (1–3); if confirmed, the multisite closure may have significant impact upon our understanding of many anomalies of the CNS (3). The most cephalic end of the neural tube, the *anterior neuropore*, closes at the lamina terminalis at approximately 24 days of gestation. The most caudal end of the neural tube, the *posterior neuropore*, closes by approximately 27 days of gestation. The exact site of the posterior neuropore is debatable but most likely lies in the lower lumbar region (4–9).

Canalization and Retrogressive Differentiation

The neural tube develops caudal to the posterior neuropore and elongates further by another process known as canalization. In this process, a *caudal cell mass,* composed of undifferentiated, pleuripotential cells, forms in the tail fold as a result of fusion of neural epithelium (at the caudal end of the embryo) with the notochord. Ventral to the caudal cell mass, with the notochord interposed, lies the cloaca. The cloaca will form the cells of the anorectal and lower genitourinary tract structures.

By the time the embryo is 30 days old, multiple microcysts and clumps of cells begin to appear in the caudal cell mass. These microcysts coalesce to form an ependyma-lined tubular structure that unites with the neural tube above (Fig. 9.3). This process is not as organized as the process of neurulation; the multiple acces-

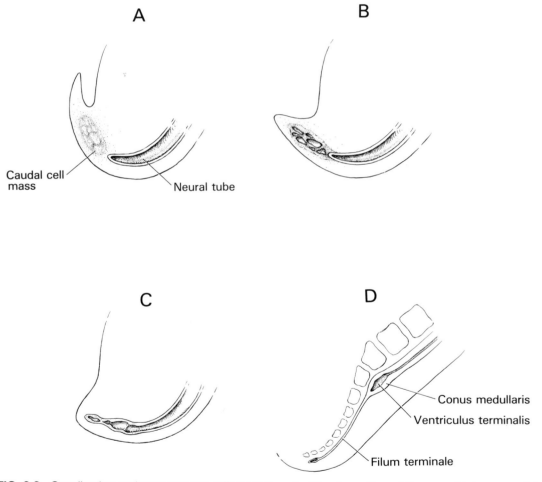

FIG. 9.3. Canalization and retrogressive differentiation. **A:** After formation of the neural tube, a caudal cell mass forms in the tail fold as a result of fusion of neural epithelium at the caudal end of the embryo with the notochord. **B:** By the age of 30 days, multiple cysts and clumps of cells appear in the caudal cell mass. **C:** These cysts coalesce to form a tubular structure that unites with the neural tube above. **D:** At about 38 days, the cell mass and central lumen of the caudal neural tube decrease in size through cell necrosis in a process known as retrogressive differentiation. The segment formed by this process eventually forms the distal-most conus medullaris, the filum terminale, and the ventriculus terminalus **(D)**.

sory lumina and ependymal rests in the normal filum terminale and distal conus medullaris of the adult are believed to result from the disorder of this process.

The final stage in the formation of the distal spinal cord begins at about 38 days of gestation, at which time the cell mass and central lumen of the caudal neural tube decrease in size as a result of cell necrosis. This process has been named *retrogressive differentiation* (Fig. 9.3). The caudal segment (formed by canalization and retrogressive differentiation) eventually becomes the most caudal portion of the conus medullaris, the filum terminale, and a focal dilatation of the central canal (within the conus medullaris) known as the *ventriculus terminalis* (4–10).

Formation of the Vertebral Column

Formation of the vertebral column was discussed in Chapter 2 and illustrated in Figure 2.23. A review of the subject is given here, as well, for the convenience of the reader. Development of the vertebral column can be divided into three periods. The first of these is *membrane development*. At about the 25th gestational day, the notochord separates from the primitive gut and neural tube to create two zones, the ventral subchordal, and dorsal epichordal zones. These zones are filled with mesenchyme that migrates to them from its initial position lateral to the neural tube.

The mesenchyme situated lateral to the closing neural tube organizes into somites that are separated by small intersegmental fissures. Each somite is divided into a medial (medial sclerotome) and a lateral (lateral myotome) portion. The medial sclerotome contributes to the formation of the vertebrae, while the lateral myotome gives rise to the paraspinous musculature. After the neural tube has closed and becomes separated from the superficial ectoderm, mesenchyme also migrates dorsal to the neural tube to form the precursors of the neural arches (in addition to the meninges and paraspinous muscles).

During the second stage of vertebral development (known as *chondrification*), the sclerotomes separate transversely along the previously mentioned intersegmental fissures. The inferior half of one sclerotome then fuses with the superior half of the subjacent sclerotome across the fissure to form a vertebral body. This process proceeds bilaterally and symmetrically so that the fusion of the sclerotomes on each side forms half of the vertebral body on that side. As a consequence of this resegmentation, the intersegmental arteries and veins become located in the center of the new vertebral bodies. Notochordal remnants persist between the newly formed vertebral bodies and become incorporated into the intervertebral discs as the nuclei pulposi. Portions of the thoracic sclerotomes later migrate ventrolaterally to form ribs.

In the final stage of vertebral development (*ossification*), the chondral skeleton ossifies to complete the formation of the vertebrae. Ossification starts in three centers, one in the middle of the vertebral body and one in each vertebral arch. The formation of the vertebrae at the caudal end of the embryo proceeds by a different, less organized process. A mass of cells composed of notochord, mesenchyme, and neural tissue merely divides into somites to form the sacral and coccygeal levels. Regression results in reduction and fusion of most of these segments. As in development of the caudal neural tube, this apparent disorganization of the caudal cell mass leads to frequent anomalous development. Caudal regression syndromes, lipomas, and teratomas can result (11,12).

Anomalies of Spinal Formation: Concepts

Embryologic Theories

Embryologic explanations of anomalies of the developing spine are continually evolving. As new facts are discovered, old theories sometimes have to be discarded and new ones developed. In contrast to mathematical theories, embryologic theories cannot be proved correct; they can only be verified or disproved. In clinical medicine a theory is useful if it explains observations and helps to organize a classification; the ability to predict future observations is an added bonus. The classification scheme used in this chapter is based primarily upon a theory of spinal dysraphism developed by David McLone and Thomas Naidich when they worked together at the Children's Memorial Hospital in Chicago. At present, it is the best theory I have found for classifying and explaining anomalies of the spine.

Neurulation Anomalies

The process of separation of the neural tube from the overlying ectoderm during closure of the neural tube is known as *disjunction*. After disjunction, the overlying ectoderm fuses in the midline, dorsal to the closed neural tube. At the same time, perineural mesenchyme migrates into the newly created space between the neural tube and cutaneous ectoderm, surrounds the neural tube, and is induced to form the meninges, the bony spinal column, and the paraspinous musculature (13). The mesenchyme always remains isolated from the newly formed central canal of the spinal cord because the neural tube closes immediately prior to, or simultaneously with, disjunction.

Defective disjunction can explain a number of diverse pathologic lesions. For example, focal unilateral premature disjunction of the neural ectoderm from the cutaneous ectoderm (prior to closure of the neural tube) would allow the perineural mesenchyme to gain access to the neural groove and come in contact with the primitive ependymal lining of the groove. Mesenchyme that is exposed to the interior of the neural tube appears to be induced to form fat (14). Therefore, focal premature disjunction of neural ectoderm from the superficial ectoderm could explain spinal lipomas and lipomyelomeningoceles (Fig. 9.2F). Spinal lipomas situated rostral to the filum terminale seem to be formed in this manner. Lipomas caudal to the conus medullaris more likely form from other processes, such as abnormal development of the caudal cell mass.

Other anomalies of the spine can be explained by defects in disjunction. Dermal sinus tracts may be the consequence of a focal failure of disjunction, resulting in a focal ectodermal–neuroectodermal tract (Fig. 9.2G). The tract should prohibit mesenchyme from migrating between the neural ectoderm and cutaneous ectoderm at that site, forming a focal spina bifida, as is commonly seen in patients with dermal sinus tracts. Moreover, the adhesion between the ectoderm and neural ectoderm could explain the correlation of the dermatomal level of the cutaneous lesion with the neuroectodermal level of the central nervous system connection of the tract. Myelomeningoceles can be explained as a large area of nondisjunction (Figs. 9.2 and 9.4). These concepts will be discussed in more detail in later sections of this chapter.

Relationships of Spinal Anomalies to Other Systemic Anomalies

As discussed earlier, the caudal cell mass forms in close anatomic proximity to the cloaca, the region of origin of the lower genitourinary tract and the anorectal structures. As a result of this close embryologic relationship, patients with anorectal and urogenital anomalies have a high incidence of lumbosacral hypogenesis, myelocystoceles, and tethered spinal cords with thick fila terminale or terminal lipomas (15). Moreover, the notochord is associated with the induction of normal formation of visceral structures, as well as the neural tube. Therefore, patients with spinal anomalies secondary to abnormal formation of the notochord will often have anomalies of the upper gastrointestinal tract or the respiratory tract. Finally, it is important to remember that the development of the vertebral column is influenced by many of the same factors that influence development of the spinal cord. Therefore, any condition that results in vertebral anomalies—such as the VATER syndrome (16), the Klippel-Feil syndrome (17), and the lumbosacral hypogenesis (18)—should be investigated for associated anomalies of the spinal cord.

TERMINOLOGY

The term *spinal dysraphism* refers to a heterogeneous group of spinal anomalies. In spite of their heterogeneity, all lesions within this group have incomplete midline closure of mesenchymal, osseous, and nervous tissue (9).

Spina bifida refers to incomplete closure of the bony elements of the spine (lamina and spinous processes) posteriorly (19,20).

Spina bifida aperta (spina bifida cystica) refers to a posterior protrusion of all or part of the contents of the spinal canal through a bony spina bifida. Included under this heading are (1) the simple meningocele, an extension of dura and arachnoid (but no neural tissue) through the posterior spina bifida; (2) the myelocele, a midline plaque of neural tissue that lies exposed at and is flush with the skin surface; and (3) the myelomeningocele, a

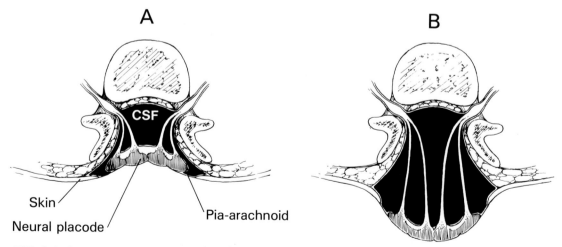

FIG. 9.4. Myelocele and myelomeningocele. **A:** Myelocele. The neural placode is a flat plaque of neural tissue that is exposed to the air. The dura is deficient posteriorly; the pia and arachnoid line the ventral surface of the placode and dura, forming an arachnoid sac that is continuous with the subarachnoid space superiorly and inferiorly. Both the dorsal and ventral roots arise from the ventral surface of the placode. **B:** Myelomeningocele. This is identical to the myelocele with the exception that there is an expansion of the ventral subarachnoid space which posteriorly displaces the placode.

myelocele that has been elevated above the skin surface by expansion of the subarachnoid space ventral to the neural plaque.

Occult spinal dysraphisms are a group of lesions that develop beneath an intact dermis and epidermis [i.e., there is no exposed neural tissue (21)]. A subcutaneous mass is frequently present in these patients, usually the result of a subcutaneous lipoma or a simple meningocele. Included in the category of occult spinal dysraphism are meningoceles, most cases of diastematomyelia and the split notochord syndrome, dorsal dermal sinuses, the tight filum terminale syndrome, spinal lipomas, and myelocystoceles.

IMAGING TECHNIQUES

The spine can be imaged using a variety of techniques. Sonography, CT, and MR can all give exquisite images of the diverse anatomic anomalies that characterize these entities (14,17,18,21–53). An understanding of the characteristic anatomic features that distinguish these various entities is therefore more important than the imaging modality in the diagnosis and presurgical planning of these entities.

An important concept to remember, however, is that multiple spinal anomalies are often present in individual patients. For example, a patient with a myelomeningocele may have syringohydromyelia, diastematomyelia, a tight filum terminale, and a dorsal dermal sinus as well. Therefore, it is important to image the entire spine if a cutaneous anomaly or vertebral anomaly suggests the presence of a malformation. The ability to image the entire spinal cord in the sagittal and coronal planes in a very few sequences is an advantage of MR that other modalities cannot match. Typical MR sequences for spine imaging are discussed in Chapter 1.

ABNORMALITIES OF NEURULATION

Disorders Resulting from Nondisjunction

Myelocele and Myelomeningocele

Myeloceles and myelomeningoceles most likely result from a localized lack of closure of the neural tube, result-

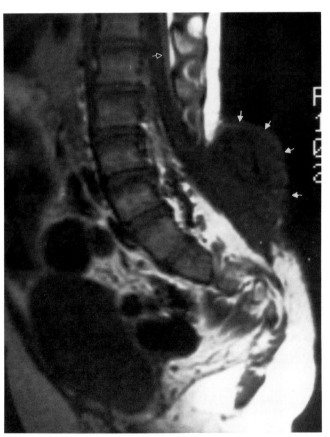 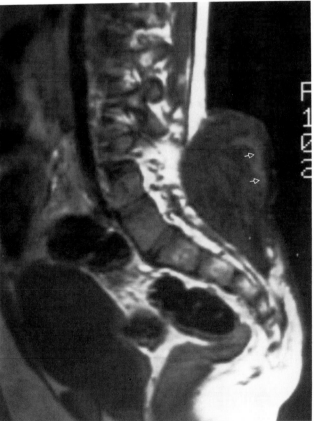

A   B

FIG. 9.5. Myelomeningocele. **A:** Sagittal SE 600/20 image shows a stretched, thin spinal cord coursing caudally in the dorsal aspect of the spinal canal (*open arrows*). A large meningocele is seen dorsal to the L4 and L5 vertebral bodies and the sacrum (*closed arrows*). **B:** Parasagittal image shows the neural placode (*open arrows*) pushed dorsally by the expansive subarachnoid space. This child was exceptional in that most patients with myelomeningoceles are surgically repaired within the first 48 hours of life and are not imaged prior to their surgery.

ing from a lack of expression of complex carbohydrate molecules on the surface of the neuroectoderm cells (54). In the affected zone, the neural folds do not fuse in the midline to form the neural tube; instead the neural tube remains open and the neural folds remain in continuity with cutaneous ectoderm at the skin surface (nondisjunction). The open spinal cord, located at the skin surface in the posterior midline, is referred to as the *neural placode*. The posterior (dorsal) surface of the placode is made up of the tissue that would normally form the internal, ependymal lining of the neural tube. The anterior (ventral) surface of the placode corresponds to what would normally be the external surface of the spinal cord (pia mater) (Fig. 9.4).

As a result of the lack of closure of the neural tube, the neural tissue cannot separate from the cutaneous ectoderm; it therefore remains attached to the skin along the lateral surface of the placode. The newborn presents with a placode of reddish neural tissue in the middle of the back that is exposed to the air because of the absence of overlying skin.

Because the placode never separates from the cutaneous ectoderm, mesenchyme cannot migrate into the area posterior to the neural ectoderm; it is forced to remain anterolateral to the nervous tissue. Thus, the pedicles and lamina (which are formed from this mesenchyme) are everted, facing posterolaterally instead of posteromedially (Fig. 9.4). As a result of the external rotation of the lamina and pedicles, the spinal canal undergoes a fusiform enlargement throughout the extent of the spinal bifida. The maximum enlargement of the canal occurs when the laminae are in the sagittal plane; further rotation of the lamina diminish the size of the canal (9).

The vertebral bodies can be nearly normal or can have anomalies of segmentation ranging from single hemivertebrae to a jumbled mass of malsegmented ossifications. Segmentation anomalies result in a short radius kyphoscoliosis in approximately one-third of patients with myelomeningoceles (9). Another 65% of affected patients develop a (less severe) kyphoscoliosis as a result of a neuromuscular imbalance (55,56).

In patients with lumbar or lumbosacral myelomeningoceles, the spinal cord is always tethered. The nerve roots in affected patients radiate in a spoke–wheel pattern as they leave the placode and travel rostrally, laterally, and caudally to their respective neural foramina.

Imaging studies are rarely performed in the newborn with a myelocele or myelomeningocele (Fig. 9.5). The exposed placode is obvious upon visual examination and is usually repaired within 48 hours. After repair, the infants typically have a neurologic deficit that is stable. They should not further deteriorate if the accompanying hydrocephalus, which is almost always present, is controlled. Neuroradiologic examination of these patients is indicated if they deteriorate neurologically, in spite of adequate treatment of hydrocephalus, or if they present

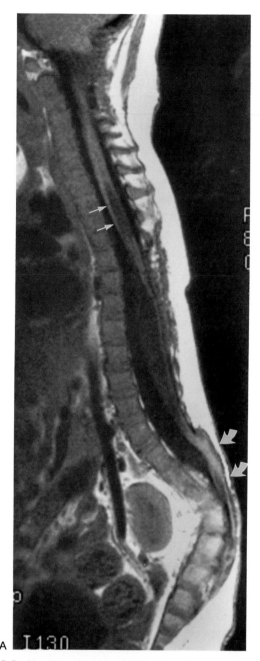

FIG. 9.6. Hemimyelocele. **A:** Sagittal SE 600/20 image shows a repaired myelomeningocele (*curved arrows*) at the thoracolumbar level and focal syringohydromyelia (*straight arrows*) in the cervicothoracic spinal cord.

with an unusual neurologic examination, such as an asymmetric deficit (which should make one suspect a hemimyelocele).

Hemimyelocele

Cameron (57), Emery and Lendon (58), and Pang (59) have shown that between 31% and 46% of patients with myelomeningoceles have an associated diastematomye-

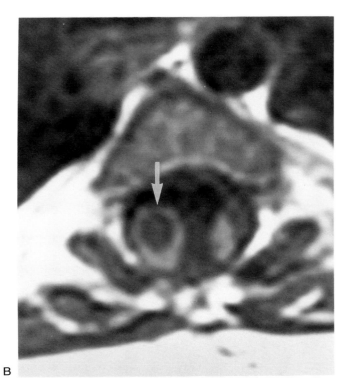 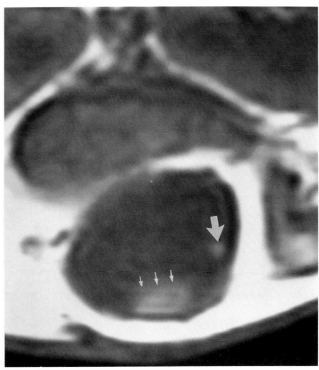

FIG. 9.6. (*Continued*.) **B:** Axial SE 800/20 image reveals a diastematomyelia in the thoracic region. The right hemicord (*arrow*) is dilated by hydromyelia. **C:** At the level of the myelomeningocele repair, the right hemicord is a flattened placode (*small arrows*) that is tethered to the dura and epidural fat. The smaller left ventral hemicord (*large arrow*) was not appreciated at the time of repair.

lia. The spinal cord may be split above (31%), below (25%), or at the same level (22%) as the myelomeningocele (58). In addition to the patients with frank diastematomyelia, 5% of patients with myelomeningocele have a duplication of the central canals of the spinal cord cephalic to and at the level of the placode, indicating a mild form of splitting that is insufficient to affect the gross contour of the cord (58).

The hemimyelocele, a special form of myelomeningocele with diastematomyelia, is observed in ~10% of patients with myelomeningoceles (58,60). In the hemimyelocele, one of the two hemicords exhibits a small myelomeningocele that tends to lie on one side of the midline, whereas the other hemicord either is normal, is tethered by a thickened filum terminale (Fig 9.6), or has a smaller myelomeningocele at a much lower level. The two hemicords usually lie in separate dural tubes that are separated by a fibrous or bony spur. Occasionally, the two hemicords lie within a single dural tube that becomes deficient at the level of the hemimyelocele. In general, affected patients have impaired neurologic function on the side of the hemimyelocele but normal or nearly normal function on the normal side (60). Imaging studies (Fig. 9.6) will show the splitting of the spinal cord, the extent and symmetry (or lack thereof) of the myelomeningocele, the presence or absence of the bony spur, and any other anomalies that may alter the surgical ap-

proach. Diastematomyelia is more fully discussed later in this chapter.

Postoperative Complications

After repair of a myelomeningocele (or any form of spinal dysraphism), patients usually have a stable neurologic deficit. Deterioration in neurologic function, therefore, suggests the presence of a complication. There are five major causes of postoperative neurologic deterioration in this group of patients: (1) The spinal cord and placode may be tethered by scar or by a second, previously unrecognized malformation; (2) the dura may be pulled too tightly when approximated over the placode, forming a constricting dural ring; (3) the cord may be compressed by a dermoid or epidermoid tumor or an arachnoid cyst; (4) ischemia may occur because of vascular compromise; (5) there may be syringohydromyelia (61,62).

Retethering of the cord by scar is a diagnosis that can only be made by exclusion of other causes. The purpose of imaging patients after the repair of myelomeningoceles is to identify one of these causes. If no other cause for neurologic deterioration is identified, the clinical diagnosis of retethering is made. The diagnosis of retethering may be suggested or verified by demonstrating di-

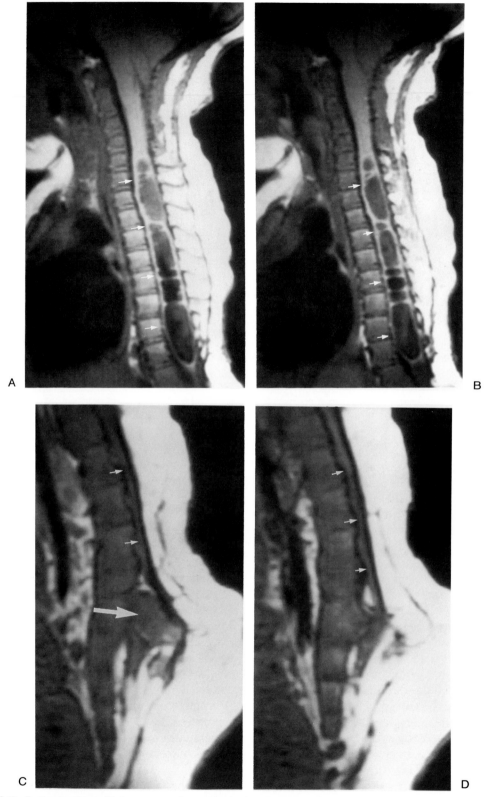

FIG. 9.7. Patient with multiple causes of neurologic deterioration after myelomeningocele repair at birth. **A, B:** Sagittal SE 600/20 images show multiloculated hydromyelia (*arrows*) in the lower cervical and upper thoracic spinal cord. **C, D:** Sagittal SE 600/20 image in the lower thoracic region shows thinning of the cord (*small arrows*), another possible cause of neurologic deterioration, and a large bony spur (*large arrow*).

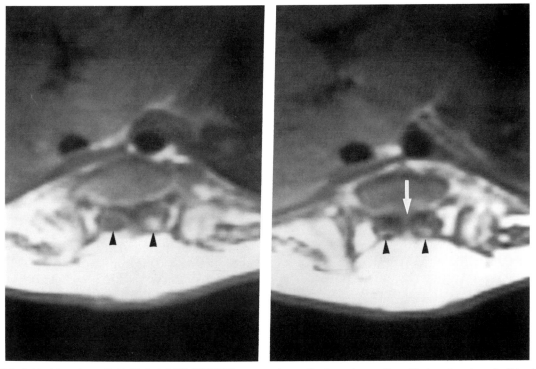

E   F

FIG. 9.7. *(Continued.)* **E, F:** Axial SE 800/20 images show diastematomyelia, with two hemicords (*black arrowheads*) and a bony spur (*white arrow*). The right hemicord is dilated by hydromyelia.

minished motion of the cervical spinal cord by phase contrast MR imaging (63). However, more experience with the technique is necessary to establish the sensitivity and specificity of the phase contrast examination in making this diagnosis.

Associated malformations are common. Diastematomyelia (Figs. 9.6, 9.7) and dermal sinuses are seen in up to 35% of patients with myelomeningoceles. Hydrocephalus and the Chiari II hindbrain malformation are almost invariably associated. Therefore, patients with neurologic deterioration after myelomeningocele repair must have their entire craniospinal axis evaluated. We typically perform a sagittal and axial T1-weighted study of the brain, followed by a coronal study of the entire spine (to rule out a split spinal cord malformation). Finally, sagittal images are obtained from the foramen magnum to the conus medullaris to rule out intrinsic or extrinsic anomalies.

Dermoids and epidermoids can appear as developmental tumors or as tumors that result from lumbar puncture or myelomeningocele repair (61,64–67). They appear on imaging studies as intraspinal masses that may be intramedullary or adherent to the spinal cord, the roots of the cauda equina, or the wall of the thecal sac (27,28,30,68). It is not possible to distinguish among these lesions by CT or myelography; on MR, some der-

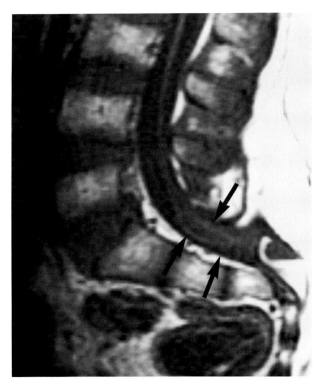

FIG. 9.8. Epidermoid tumor and hydromyelia in a patient who underwent myelomeningocele repair at birth. The epidermoid (*arrows*) is difficult to detect by MR.

moids will show a markedly shortened T1 relaxation time. More commonly, both epidermoids and dermoids are difficult to identify by MR because they are nearly isointense with cerebrospinal fluid (Fig. 9.8); however, compression of the adjacent cord or displacement of nerve roots by the tumor will indicate presence of the mass (28).

Arachnoid cysts can be congenital (true cysts) or acquired (arachnoid loculations), as described in Chapter 8. They can occur at any level and may be dorsal or ventral to the cord. Because they are filled with CSF, they are isointense to the subarachnoid space and must be identified on MR by their mass effect upon the adjacent spinal cord (Fig. 9.9). Although cysts too small to exhibit mass effect will not be detected, myelography is rarely necessary, as cysts that do not have mass effect will not produce symptoms.

Ischemic segments of spinal cord are identified by a severe, abrupt diminution in the caliber of the cord at the level of the ischemic insult. This abrupt narrowing can be identified by sonography, CT myelography, or MR. A narrowing of the dural sac, suggesting that the meninges have been approximated too tightly at the time of the closure of the lesion, is difficult to demonstrate by MR and is more easily seen by myelography and sonography.

Hydromyelia is present in between 29% and 77% of patients with myelomeningoceles (Figs. 9.7, 9.8) (57,58,69). The exact frequency depends upon the efficacy of treatment of the patient's hydrocephalus (69–72). The hydromyelia is probably a result of the passage of cerebrospinal fluid through the obex from the fourth ventricle into the central canal of the spinal cord: Hydromyelia is not usually seen caudal to the placode. Hydromyelia is most easily diagnosed by MR, where it appears as a dilated (CSF-intensity) central canal, causing a fusiform enlargement of the cord, most frequently in the lower cervical or upper thoracic region. The hydromyelia can also involve a short segment beginning a small distance above the site of the placode or may involve the entire central canal from the cervicomedullary junction down to the placode.

Untreated hydromyelia can cause the rapid development of *scoliosis* (47,69–73). In patients with myelomeningocele and hydrocephalus, a rapidly developing scoliosis may be the sign of a nonfunctioning shunt or an encysted fourth ventricle. Because scoliosis in these patients may result from shunt malfunction, encystment of the fourth ventricle, or hydromyelia unrelated to the above, all patients with scoliosis that is rapidly progressive, has an atypical curve, or is associated with neurologic deficits should have imaging studies of the entire craniospinal axis to eliminate these curable causes of scoliosis. Magnetic resonance is the imaging study of choice in these circumstances (47,73,74).

The Chiari II Malformation

The Chiari II malformation is an anomaly of the cervical spinal cord, brain stem, and hindbrain that is observed in varying degrees in all patients with myelomeningoceles. Because of the close association of Chiari II malformations with myelomeningoceles, a brief discussion is appropriate in this section, in spite of the fact that this malformation is discussed extensively in Chapter 5.

The Chiari II malformation can be best considered as an entity in which the posterior fossa is too small (75). As a result of the small bony posterior fossa, normal contents of the posterior fossa are distorted as they are squeezed out through the tentorial incisura and the foramen magnum. The brain stem is stretched inferiorly and narrowed in the anteroposterior diameter, often lying at the foramen magnum or in the cervical spinal canal. The cervical spinal cord is displaced inferiorly, and the upper cervical nerve roots have to ascend toward their respective neural foramina. The medulla is also displaced inferiorly. In 70% of patients, it folds caudally at the cervicomedullary junction, dorsal to the cervical spinal cord (which is tethered by the dentate ligaments and therefore limited in its vertical descent), forming a characteristic cervicomedullary kink (Figs. 5.79, 5.80). The cerebellar vermis often herniates inferiorly, forming a tongue of tissue posterior to the medulla that usually extends down to the C2 or C4 level. Rarely, it extends down into the upper thoracic segments of the canal. The cerebellum wraps around the brain stem (Fig. 5.81). The fourth ventricle is vertical in orientation (Figs. 5.79, 5.80), extending inferiorly between the medulla and cerebellar vermis; occasionally it extends down below the medulla, posterior to the cervical spinal cord, in a cystlike fashion (Fig. 5.83). The quadrigeminal plate is stretched posteriorly and inferiorly (Figs. 5.79–5.81) (76–81).

Dorsal Dermal Sinuses

Dorsal dermal sinuses are epithelium-lined dural tubes that extend inward from the skin surface for varying distances and frequently connect the body surface with the central nervous system or its coverings. This anomaly seems to result from a focal area of incomplete disjunction of cutaneous ectoderm from neural ectoderm during the process of neurulation (Fig. 9.2). When the spinal cord later becomes surrounded by mesenchyme and undergoes its relative ascent with respect to the spinal column, this adherence remains and forms a long, epithelium-lined tract. The incidence of dermal sinuses is low in the cervical region, where the neural folds first fuse into the primitive neural tube, and relatively great in the lumbosacral and occipital regions, which are

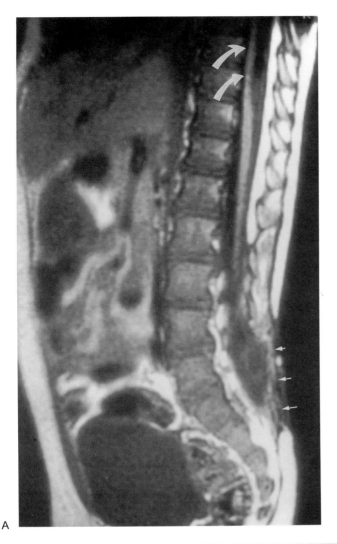

A

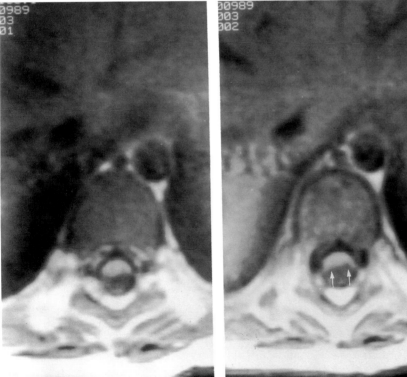

B,C

FIG. 9.9. Patient who had myelomeningocele repair at birth, now with worsening neurologic exam secondary to arachnoid cyst. **A:** The site of repair (*small arrows*) is identified at the lumbosacral level on this SE 600/20 image. A narrowing (*large curved arrows*) of the mid-thoracic spinal cord is suggested. This patient emphasizes the need to image the entire spinal cord. **B, C:** The spinal cord is distorted by the dorsally located arachnoid cyst.

the last portions of the neural tube to close. In a series of 120 cases of dorsal dermal sinuses, 1 was sacrococcygeal, 72 were lumbosacral, 12 thoracic, 2 cervical, and 30 occipital; the remaining 10 were mostly ventral to the skull and spinal column (82).

Dorsal dermal sinuses occur equally frequently in males and females and are usually encountered in early childhood through the third decade of life. Physical examination reveals a midline (rarely paramedian) dimple or pinpoint ostium that is frequently associated with a hyperpigmented patch, hairy nevus, or capillary angioma (83). The patients become symptomatic either by infection or because of compression of neural structures by an associated dermoid or epidermoid tumor. Meningitis or abscesses in the subcutaneous, epidural, subdural, subarachnoid, and/or subpial spaces may intervene as a result of bacterial ascent through the sinus tract (84–86). Occasionally, the meningitis is chemical in nature, resulting from the release of cholesterol crystals or other contents of dermoid or epidermoid cysts into the cerebrospinal fluid (87).

Pathologically, dermal sinuses are thin, epithelium-lined channels that course inward from the skin surface through the subcutaneous tissues, extending intraspinally in one-half to two-thirds of cases. The sinus may reach the dura without passing through it; in such cases, the dura and arachnoid are tented dorsally at the attachment of the sinus tract to the dura. This tenting may be the only manifestation of the sinus tract on myelography. If they pass through the dura, the sinuses may empty into the subarachnoid space or may traverse the subarachnoid space to terminate within the conus medullaris, filum terminale, a nerve root, a fibrous nodule on the dorsal aspect of the cord, or a dermoid or epidermoid cyst (Fig. 9.10) (88–90). About half of dorsal dermal sinuses end in dermoid or epidermoid tumors. Conversely, 20% to 30% of dermoids and epidermoids are associated with dermal sinus tracts (89–93). Dermal sinuses can be midline or paramedian in location. Those with midline orifices are usually associated with midline dermoid tumors. Paramedian orifices are more commonly associated with epidermoids, which can be located laterally in the epidural, subdural, or subarachnoid spaces. In some patients the dermal sinus courses horizontally beneath the skin to the dura mater. In others it courses subcutaneously for some distance before reaching the dura and then ascends within the spinal canal to the level of the conus medullaris. The exact course of the sinus seems to vary from patient to patient. Therefore, the complete course of each dermal sinus must be defined by narrow, contiguous sections above the level of the external orifice.

The bony abnormalities associated with dermal sinuses are variable. Bone abnormalities may be absent if the dermal sinus extends intraspinally through a ligamentous defect at the interspace between two spinous

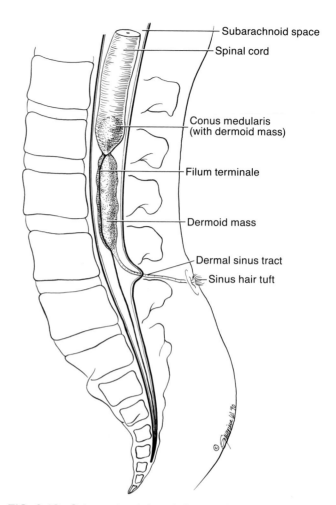

FIG. 9.10. Schematic of dorsal dermal sinus. A tuft of hair, nevus, or hemangioma frequently marks the ostium of the sinus. The dura is often tented when the sinus penetrates the dura. The sinus may terminate in a CNS structure, the dura, or external to the dura. Dermoid or epidermoid tumors develop along the course of the sinus in 50% of affected patients. (Reprinted with permission from ref. 28.)

processes. In other cases, the sinus may be associated with a groove in the upper surface of the spinous process and lamina of the vertebra, a hypoplastic spinous process, a single bifid spinous process, focal multilevel spina bifida, or a laminar defect (85,89,91).

When a dermoid or epidermoid tumor is present, the nerve roots are frequently bound down to the capsule of the cyst. The cord may be displaced and compressed by extramedullary dermoids or epidermoids, or expanded by intramedullary lesions (Figs. 9.11, 9.12) (9,28). Nerve roots may be clumped because of adhesive arachnoiditis from previous infections or ruptures of a dermoid (Fig. 9.13). If abscesses form, they may remain confined near the tract and entry site of the sinus or may extend cephalad and caudad for considerable distances (28,86).

Sonography, CT, and MR can all demonstrate the subcutaneous and extracanalicular extent of the dermal

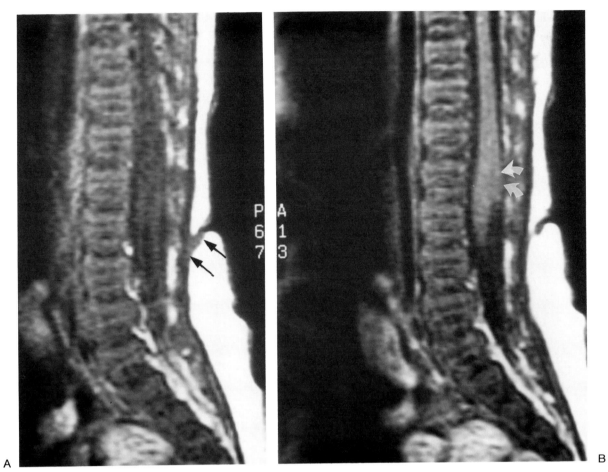

FIG. 9.11. Dorsal dermal sinus with dermoid in conus medullaris. **A:** Sagittal SE 500/15 image shows the dermal sinus (*arrows*) coursing through subcutaneous fat. **B:** Curved arrows show a focal expansion of the conus medullaris posteriorly. This was in intramedullary dermoid.

sinus tract (Figs. 9.11, 9.12). CT and MR will both demonstrate intramedullary dermoid and epidermoid tumors (Figs. 9.11, 9.12). However, only CT with intrathecal contrast will demonstrate the intraspinal portions of the dermal sinus and small extramedullary (epi)dermoids. The intrathecal portions of the sinus tracts are small and hypointense; therefore, they are essentially invisible on MR (Figs. 9.11, 9.12). Spinal (epi)dermoids (Figs. 9.11–9.13) are nearly isointense to cerebrospinal fluid on all imaging sequences and are therefore difficult to visualize with MR. Ruptured dermoid and epidermoid tumors are also difficult to identify by MR, as no distinct mass is seen. Instead, the subarachnoid space has a "smudgy," slightly heterogeneous appearance (Fig. 9.13) that cannot be differentiated from arachnoiditis by MR techniques. The use of strongly T1-weighted images (28) and the administration of paramagnetic contrast [which results in enhancement of sinus tracts that have previously been infected (23)] may help to identify tumors, if present. In addition, fast spin echo sequences, which allow excellent resolution of the spinal nerve roots, can show the deviation of the roots around the

mass, giving a strong indication of its presence. However, if the intraspinal anatomy is not clearly defined after high-quality MR, a CT myelogram should be performed. If only one examination is performed in patients with a dermal sinus, it should be CT myelography.

Disorders Resulting from Premature Disjunction: Spinal Lipomas

Spinal lipomas are masses of fat and connective tissue that appear at least partially encapsulated and have a connection with the leptomeninges or the spinal cord (94). Grossly, the lipomas are homogeneous masses of mature fat cells that are separated into globules by strands of fibrous tissue. The proportion of fibrous tissue is much greater near the interface of the cord and lipoma and considerably less near the skin surface (90,95). Calcification and ossification are infrequently seen (90,96).

Spinal lipomas can be divided into three principal groups: (1) intradural lipomas (4%); (2) lipomyeloceles/lipomyelomeningoceles (84%); and (3) fibrolipomas of

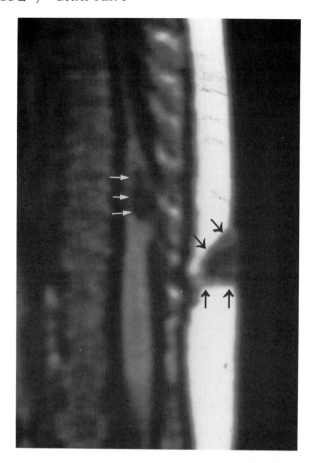

FIG. 9.12. Dorsal dermal sinus with intramedullary dermoid in thoracic spinal cord. Sagittal SE 500/25 image shows the sinus as a defect (*black arrows*) in the subcutaneous fat. The intramedullary dermoid (*white arrows*) is hypointense compared to the spinal cord. Note that the sinus tract is not seen in its intraspinal course. (Reprinted with permission from ref. 28.)

the filum terminale (12%). Group 2 can be further divided into terminal lipomas, which are always associated with a thickened filum terminale and are better classified as anomalies of the caudal cell mass, and dorsa lipomyeloceles/lipomyelomeningoceles (97). Fibrolipomas of the filum terminale are also best classified as anomalies of the caudal cell mass and are discussed in that section of this chapter. In contrast, intradural lipomas and dorsal lipomyelomeningoceles are postulated to result from a premature separation of cutaneous ectoderm from neuroectoderm during the process of neurulation (Fig. 9.2). This premature separation permits the surrounding mesenchyme to enter the ependyma-lined central canal of the neural tube, which has not yet closed. The presence of the mesenchyme impedes the closure of the neural folds and results in an open neural placode at the site of premature disjunction. Moreover, the mesenchyme that enters the central canal differentiates into fat. This same mesenchyme, if exposed to the exterior of the cord,

differentiates into meningeal tissue, bone, and paraspinous muscles. The junction between the internal and external surfaces of the cord therefore determines the junction between the meninges and the fat. The faulty disjunction between neural ectoderm and cutaneous ectoderm that results in the formation of spinal lipomas may also explain the frequent association of lipomas with dorsal dermal sinuses that, as described earlier, result from a focal area of faulty disjunction.

MR is the imaging modality of choice for the evaluation of patients with spinal lipomas. The short T1 relaxation time of fat results in a characteristic high signal intensity of the lipoma on short TR sequences. MR allows the full extent of the lipoma and its relationship to the neural placode, spinal cord, and roots of the cauda equina to be fully evaluated.

Intradural Lipomas

Intradural lipomas, which constitute slightly less than 1% of primary intraspinal tumors, are juxtamedullary masses that are totally enclosed in an intact dural sac. They are slightly more frequent in females and exhibit three age peaks: the first 5 years of life (24%), the second and third decades (55%), and the fifth decade (16%) (98). Cervical and thoracic intradural lipomas most frequently present with a slow, ascending monoparesis or paraparesis, spasticity, cutaneous sensory loss, and defective deep sensation. Radicular pain is uncommon. Lumbosacral intradural lipomas typically present with flaccid paralysis of the legs and sphincter dysfunction (98). The skin and the adjacent subcutaneous tissues overlying the lipoma are most often normal.

Intradural lipomas occur most commonly in the cervical and thoracic spine (cervical, 12%; cervicothoracic, 24%; thoracic, 30%) but may occur anywhere in the spinal cord or cauda equina (97,99,100). Most of these lesions occur in the dorsal aspect of the cord, but 25% are lateral or anterolateral in location (90,92,96,98,101, 102). Hydromyelia and syringomyelia are present in approximately 2%.

Intradural lipomas are actually subpial–juxtamedullary lesions (Fig. 9.14) (98). The spinal cord is open in the midline dorsally with the lipoma situated in the opening between the unopposed lips of the placode. The lipoma fills the space between the central canal and the pia, which is frequently lifted from the cord surface as the lipoma projects into the subarachnoid space. In the 45% of patients in whom the lipoma is exophytic, the exophytic component tends to be at the upper or lower pole of the lipoma. No lipoma has been described that is fully encompassed by cord (9,98).

Although the bony spinal canal can be normal in patients with intradural lipomas, a focal enlargement of the spinal canal and, occasionally, the adjacent neural fo-

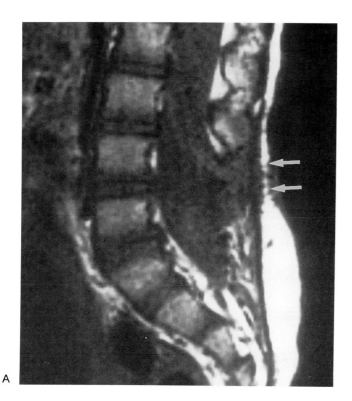

A

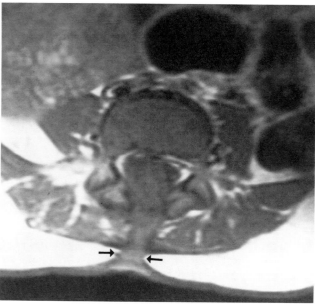

B

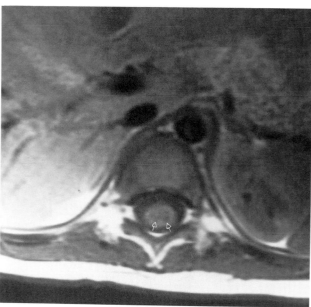

C

FIG. 9.13. Dorsal dermal sinus. **A:** Sagittal SE 800/20 image shows the large dermal sinus (*arrows*). There is marked heterogeneity of the subarachnoid space rostral to the sinus. However, it cannot be determined from this study whether the heterogeneous signal is the result of clumping of nerve roots from prior infection or from dermoid or epidermoid tumor. At surgery, this patient was found to have a large epidermoid extending all the way up into the spinal cord. **B:** Axial SE 1000/20 images clearly show the sinus tract extending from the skin (*arrows*) through a spina bifida into the subarachnoid space. The intermediate intensity within the spinal canal was found to be epidermoid tumor at surgery. **C:** Axial SE 1000/20 image of the caudal spinal cord, immediately above the conus. The marbled areas of low signal intensity (*white arrows*) were found to be epidermoid tumor at surgery.

A

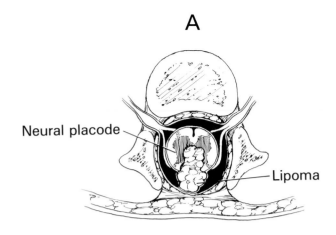

Neural placode

Lipoma

B

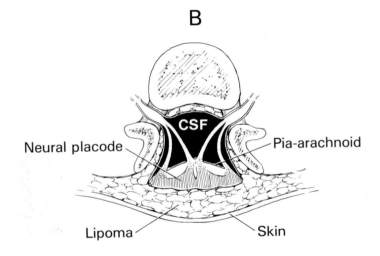

CSF

Neural placode

Pia-arachnoid

Lipoma

Skin

C

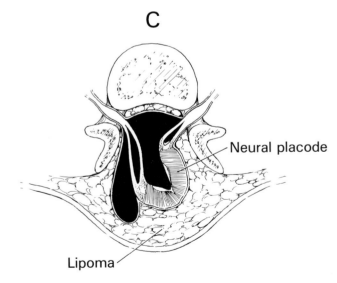

Neural placode

Lipoma

Fig 9.14. Schematic illustrating spinal lipomas and lipo-myelomeningoceles. **A:** Subpial-juxtamedullary (intra-dural) lipoma. The spinal cord is open in the midline dorsally with the lipoma situated between the unapposed lips of the placode. **B:** Lipomyelocele. This lesion is very similar to a myelocele with two additional characteristics. The lipoma lies dorsal to and is attached to the surface of the placode. This lipoma is continuous with subcutaneous fat. Equally important is the fact that an intact skin layer overlies the lesion, making this an occult spinal dysraphism. **C:** Lipomyelomeningocele with rotation of the neural placode. When the lipoma is asymmetric, it extends into the spinal canal and causes the ventral meningocele to herniate posteriorly and the dorsal surface of the placode to rotate to the side of the lipoma. This rotation brings the contralateral dorsal roots (in this case the right dorsal root) into the midline posteriorly, putting it at increased risk for surgical trauma. Moreover, the left roots are markedly shortened by this rotation, limiting the mobility of the cord and impeding the neurosurgeon from completely untethering it.

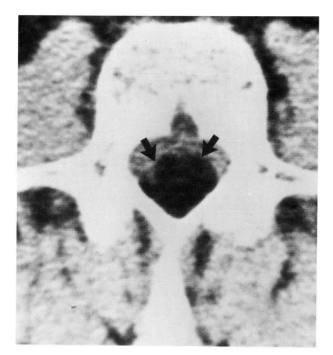

FIG. 9.15. Intradural lipoma. Axial CT image shows a low attenuation mass (*arrows*) in the dorsal aspect of the spinal canal.

ramina is more common (14). Often a narrow and very localized spina bifida is observed at the level of the lipoma. There are generally no segmentation anomalies of the vertebral bodies.

Intradural lipomas appear on imaging studies as focal, round to oval masses that most often lie dorsal to the spinal cord (Figs. 9.15, 9.16) and may expand the spinal canal (Fig. 9.16). Lipomas have a very low attenuation on CT and therefore can be detected on studies without intrathecal contrast (Fig. 9.15). They are easily identified on T1-weighted MR images by their lobulated shape and high signal intensity (Fig. 9.16). Compression of adjacent neural structures is best identified by MR.

Lipomyeloceles and Lipomyelomeningoceles

Lipomyelomeningoceles are lipomas that are tightly attached to the dorsal surface of a neural placode and extend dorsally through a bony spina bifida to be continuous with subcutaneous fat (14,103). These lesions constitute approximately 20% of skin-covered lumbosacral masses and between 20% and 50% of cases of occult spinal dysraphism (104,105). Patients are typically female and present before the age of 6 months, but occasionally

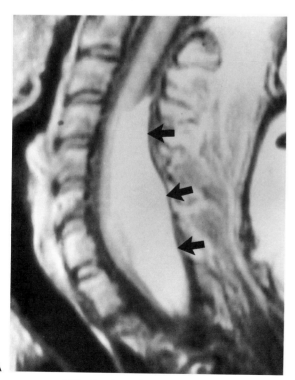
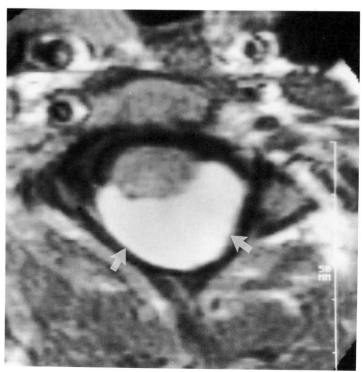

A   B

FIG. 9.16. Intradural lipoma. Sagittal **(A)** and axial **(B)** T1-weighted images show the hyperintense lipoma (*arrows*) dorsal to the compressed spinal cord. The spinal canal is expanded by the mass.

the condition goes undetected into adulthood (97,106). Affected patients present with a rather soft lumbosacral mass, sensory loss in the sacral dermatomes, bladder dysfunction, motor loss, orthopedic deformities of the foot, and leg pain. Because patients with lumbosacral masses often come to attention early, 45% are neurologically normal on initial examination. However, 88% of children not operated upon eventually develop progressive neurologic symptoms (97,106).

Lipomyelomeningoceles and *lipomyeloceles* usually occur in the lumbosacral region of the cord and tether the cord at that level. Anatomically, lipomyelomeningoceles and lipomyeloceles are very similar to myelomeningoceles and myeloceles, respectively, with two important additional characteristics: (1) A lipoma is attached to the dorsal surface of the placode, and (2) an intact skin layer overlies the lesion.

Patients with lipomyeloceles have a normal-sized subarachnoid space ventral to the placode; the cord and the junction between the placode and the lipoma, therefore, are within the spinal canal (Figs. 9.17, 9.18). The lipoma is continuous with extraspinal fat and extends into the canal through the spina bifida; the focus of continuity with extraspinal fat is sometimes quite small (Fig. 9.17) but is always present. The spinal cord can have a number of different shapes, depending upon the morphology of the lipoma. If the intracanalicular portion of the lipoma is ovoid, the cord is crescent shaped, with the concave aspect facing posteriorly, arching around the ventral surface of the lipoma. On the other hand, if the intracanalicular portion of the lipoma extends laterally on both sides of the cord, the placode may have the shape of an arrowhead, pointed posteriorly between the lateral extensions of fat.

In patients with lipomyelomeningoceles an expansion of the spinal subarachnoid space ventral to the placode causes the placode, cord, subarachnoid space, and dura to herniate posteriorly (Fig. 9.19). Similar to lipomyeloceles, a lipoma is attached to the dorsal aspect of the placode; this lipoma extends posteriorly to blend with the subcutaneous fat. Depending upon the degree of posterior herniation of the spinal cord, the junction between the placode and lipoma may be entirely posterior to the spinal canal, or partly within and partly posterior to the canal. The dura is deficient in the zone of the spina bifida and does not pass posterior to the neural elements to form a closed dural tube as it does elsewhere. Instead, the dura is attached to the lateral border of the neural placode, posterior to the dorsal nerve roots as they emerge from the cord (Fig. 9.14). A continuous layer of pia arachnoid continues superiorly and inferiorly with the subarachnoid space, lining the deep surface of the dura and the ventral surface of the placode (Fig. 9.14). The dorsal surface of nervous tissue is therefore exposed to the lipoma, external to the dural sac and subarachnoid space (14,96,103). The dorsal and ventral nerve roots

exit from the ventral surface of the placode (Fig. 9.14B). The nerve roots traverse the subarachnoid space, not the lipoma, as they pass toward their nerve root sleeves.

The dorsal surface of the placode, adjacent to the lipoma, has no ependymal lining; instead it is covered by a relatively thick layer of connective tissue mixed with islands of glial and smooth muscle fibers (96). The lipoma lies immediately external to the connective tissue in the extradural space. The lipoma may be localized to the levels of the spina bifida or may extend upward along the dorsal placode and underlie an outwardly normal-appearing spinal canal. Moreover, the lipoma can enter the central canal of the spinal cord and pass upward within it to form an apparently isolated intradural lipoma at higher levels. The lipoma can also extend upward within the extradural portion of the spinal canal, forming an apparent epidural lipoma. In both of these situations, the use of MR, especially in the sagittal plane, helps to trace the lipoma to its caudal origin near the myeloschisis (Fig. 9.20).

At the level of the placode, the spinal canal is generally large and is almost invariably associated with a focal spinal bifida (107). Butterfly vertebrae and segmental anomalies of the vertebral bodies may be found in as many as 43% of affected patients, and abnormalities of the sacrum, including confluent sacral foramina and partial sacral agenesis, occur in up to 50% (100,107).

The lipoma is asymmetric in approximately 40% of patients. If the asymmetric lipoma extends into the spinal canal, it causes the meningocele to herniate posteriorly and the dorsal surface of the placode to rotate to the side of the lipoma (Fig. 9.18). Such rotation and herniation bring the contralateral dorsal roots and dorsal root entry zones into the midline posteriorly, putting them at increased risk for surgical trauma (Figs. 9.18, 9.19). Moreover, the nerve roots in affected patients are unequal in length. Those that originate posterior to the spinal canal are very long, whereas those that originate from the intracanalicular portion of the placode are very short. These short nerve roots limit the mobility of the cord and impede complete untethering of the cord.

ANOMALIES OF THE CAUDAL CELL MASS

As discussed in the embryology section at the beginning of this chapter, the lowest portion of the spinal cord (the conus medullaris), the filum terminale, and the lower lumbar and sacral nerve roots form the caudal cell mass by a process referred to as canalization and retrogressive differentiation. The nearby anorectal and lower genitourinary tract structures form from the cloaca, which develops in close proximity to the caudal cell mass at the same time. As a result, the anomalies listed in this section are commonly associated with anorectal and genitourinary anomalies (15). Anomalies of the caudal spine

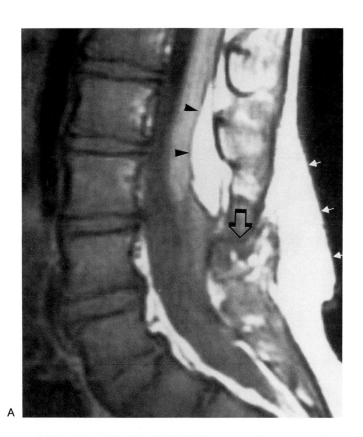

A

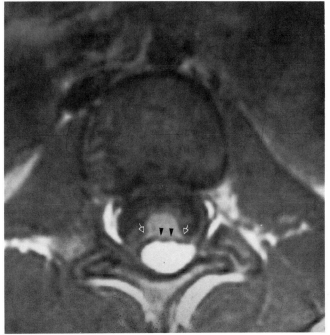

B

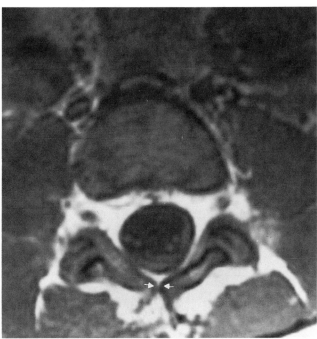

C

FIG. 9.17. Lipomyelocele. **A:** Sagittal SE 600/20 image shows an elongated lipoma dorsal to the spinal cord at the L2 and L3 levels (*arrowheads*). There is a spina bifida immediately caudal to the lipoma (*open arrow*). **B:** Axial SE 800/20 through the central portion of the lipoma. The junction of the lipoma with the placode (*black arrowheads*) is clearly seen. The dorsal nerve roots (*open arrows*) are seen exiting the cord immediately ventral to the lipoma. **C:** Axial SE 800/20 image caudal to the lipoma. The nerve roots are seen to course caudally through the subarachnoid space. A small spinal bifida (*white arrows*) is present. The subcutaneous lipoma (*white arrows* in *A*) was continuous with the dorsal lipoma within the spinal canal through this small spina bifida.

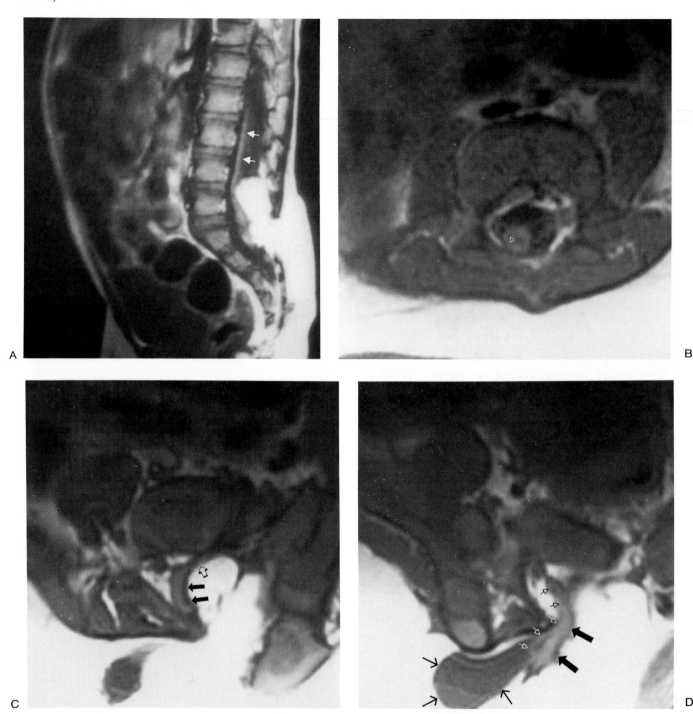

FIG. 9.18. Lipomyelocele. **A:** The spinal cord (*white arrows*) is tethered by a large lipoma that extends from the subcutaneous fat through a spina bifida into the dorsal subarachnoid space. **B:** Rostral to the lipomyelocele, an area of prolonged T1 relaxation (*arrow*) is seen in the center of the spinal canal. This focus of prolonged T1, which is believed to be a small hydromyelia, is seen in about 25% of patients with tethered spinal cords. **C:** Subcutaneous fat herniates into the spinal canal through the spinal bifida. The placode (*closed black arrows*) is rotated to the right, contralateral to the fat that is invaginating on the left. The left dorsal nerve root (*open black arrow*) courses immediately anterior to the lipoma and is at risk for surgical trauma. **D:** At a slightly more caudal level, the placode (*thick black arrows*) herniates even further posteriorly adjacent to the lipoma. The right dorsal nerve root (*open arrows*) is seen coursing lateral to the placode toward its neural foramen. The meningocele (*thin black arrows*) herniates posteriorly into the subcutaneous tissues of the back. Multiple nerve roots are seen floating within the meningocele.

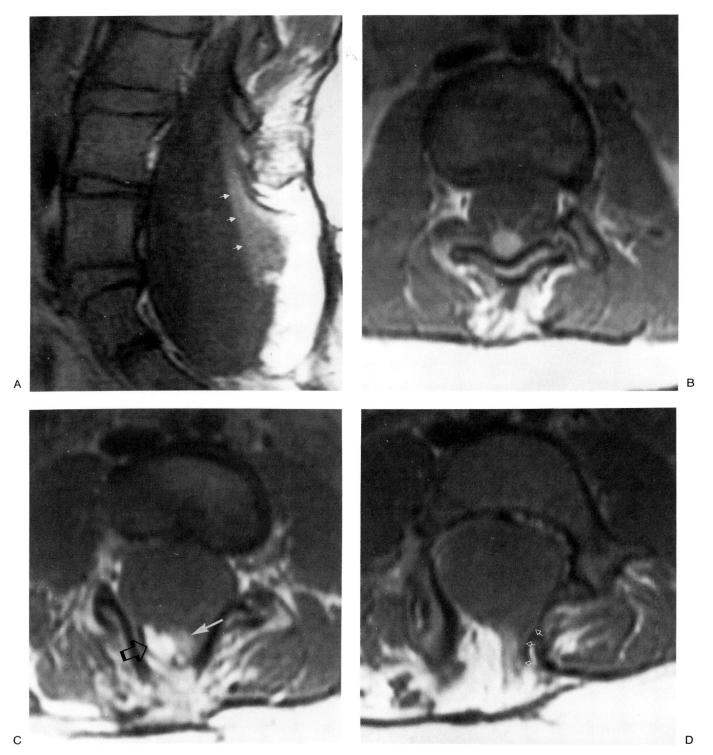

FIG. 9.19. Lipomyelomeningocele. **A:** Sagittal SE 600/20 image acquired with a temporomandibular joint coil shows a large expansion of cerebrospinal fluid ventral to the neural placode (*arrows*) that is attached to a dorsal lipoma. **B:** Axial SE 1000/20 image rostral to the lipoma shows a normal-appearing cord that is displaced posteriorly within the spinal canal. **C:** At the most rostral level of the lipoma, the spinal cord is seen to unfold into a neural placode (*white arrow*). Because the lipoma (*open black arrow*) is invaginating into the spinal canal on the right side, the placode is rotated. **D:** The lipoma is larger at this level. The left dorsal nerve root is seen originating from the placode adjacent to the lipoma and courses ventrally toward its neural foramen (*open arrows*). The posterior elements are widely bifid at this level and the spinal canal is expanded by the large meningocele.

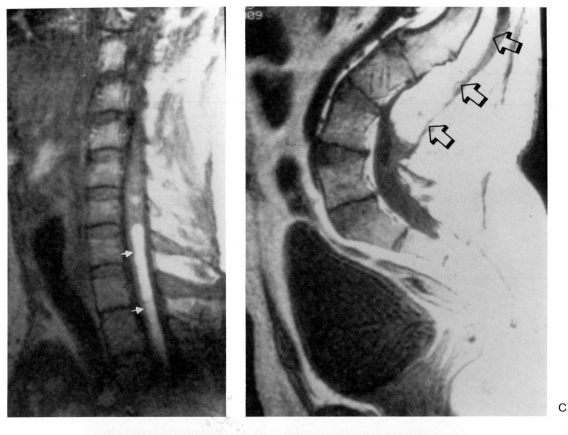

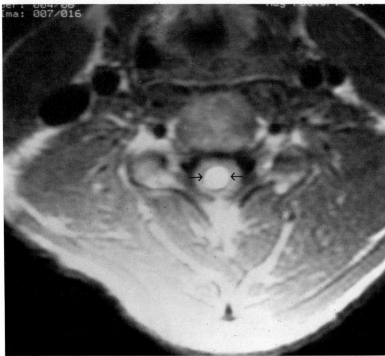

FIG. 9.20. Rostral extension of lipoma through the central canal of the spinal cord. **A:** Sagittal SE 600/20 image of the cervical spine shows a lipoma (*arrows*) within the spinal cord. **B:** Axial SE 1000/20 image confirms the location of the lipoma (*arrows*) within the central canal of the spinal cord. **C:** SE 600/20 image of the lumbar spine shows a marked spinal deformity at the site of repair of a lipomyelomeningocele (*arrows*). The lipoma entered the cord at the level of the placode and extended upward through the central canal of the spinal cord, thereby mimicking the appearance of a purely intramedullary lipoma.

should always be suspected in patients with anorectal and genitourinary anomalies and vice versa.

Normal Position of the Conus Medullaris

Early in embryogenesis, the spinal cord extends to the caudal end of the spinal canal. At that time, each neural segment is at precisely the same level as the corresponding segment of spinal canal. Each nerve root courses directly laterally toward its neural foramen. As the embryo matures, the most distal portion of the cord undergoes retrogressive differentiation; moreover, the vertebral bodies grow more quickly than the remaining cord. This combination of factors produces a relative ascent of the spinal cord within the spinal canal.

The exact level of the conus medullaris at the time of birth is debated; however, by the age of 3 months, it is usually positioned above the middle of the L2 vertebral level (32,53,108). In several series involving a total of more than 1,000 patients, the inferior-most aspect of the conus was observed above the L2–L3 level in more than 98% of cases and at the L3 level in less than 2% (32,53,109). Therefore, if the conus is at or below the level of the L2–L3 disc space, it should be considered abnormal and a search should be made for a tethering mass, bony spur, or thick filum.

Fibrolipomas of the Filum Terminale

The normal filum terminale is a long, thin fibrous filament that is both intra- and extradural. It starts at the tip of the conus medullaris and extends caudally, through the bottom of the subarachnoid space, through the dura mater, to insert on the dorsal aspect of the first coccygeal vertebra (94). Fibrolipomas of the filum probably result from a minor anomaly in the sequence of canalization and retrogressive differentiation; the exact nature of the insult is not known. Filum fibrolipomas are often asymptomatic. Emery and Lendon found incidental lipomas in 6% of autopsied patients with presumably normal spines. Moreover, they found fibrolipomas at autopsy in 67 out of 100 patients with myelomeningoceles (94). The fibrolipomas may be limited to the intradural filum, may be limited to the extradural filum, or may involve both portions.

Fibrolipomas can be seen incidentally on imaging studies of both children and adults referred for other reasons (52,110). They appear on CT as small foci of hypoattenuation and on MR as areas of high signal intensity within the enlarged filum on short TR/TE images (Fig. 9.21). The natural history of such patients with respect to the potential for the development of symptoms of a tethered spinal cord is not clear. It is the author's experience that patients with a short section of filum containing minimal fat are rarely symptomatic, but those patients with larger accumulations of filar fat are found to have some degree of neurologic impairment if a detailed history and physical examination are performed.

The Tight Filum Terminale Syndrome

The syndrome of the tight filum terminale denotes a complex of neurologic and orthopedic deformities associated with a short, thick filum terminale and a low position of the conus medullaris. It is probably the result of incomplete retrogressive differentiation, with failure of involution of the terminal cord and/or failure of lengthening of the nerve fibers that form the filum. Patients can present with new onset of symptoms at any age; the author has seen several sexagenarians become suddenly symptomatic from their tethered spinal cord. All patients suffer from difficulty with locomotion, ranging from muscle stiffness to actual weakness; all exhibit abnormal lower-extremity reflexes. The patients can also exhibit bladder dysfunction, sensory changes, orthopedic deformities of the lower extremities (most commonly clubfoot), and back pain (particularly with exertion). Bowel dysfunction is uncommon. Although scoliosis frequently accompanies this syndrome, it is rarely the sole complaint (9,111–113). Symptoms are frequently worse in the mornings and after exercise. The clinical symptomatology is believed to be due to stretching of nerve fibers, resulting in abnormal oxidative metabolism in the conus medullaris and nerve roots. An increased incidence of tethered spinal cords is seen in lumbosacral hypogenesis and in the VATER syndrome (16,114).

The normal filum terminale measures 2 mm or less in diameter at the L5–S1 level (9,46). Although at one time thought to vary with the age of the patient, recent studies performed by MR and sonography indicate that the conus should be at its normal level (between the middle of T11 and the middle of L2) by age 2 months (32,53), and probably at birth (32). Although patients with a normal conus level can have a tethered cord, the presence of the conus below the L2–L3 disk space is always abnormal (32,53,108).

Plain radiographs typically show a small spina bifida occulta; scoliosis is present in approximately 20% of affected patients (102,111,115,116). Imaging studies will typically show a thickened filum; it nearly always has a diameter greater than 2 mm at the L5–S1 level (46). The conus medullaris is almost always low-lying, being tethered by the tight filum (35,46). However, occasionally the conus is at a normal level in these patients (46). An area of prolonged T1 relaxation, probably representing a dilated central canal, is seen in the center of the spinal cord on T1-weighted MR images in approximately 25% of affected patients. It is not known whether this area represents a mild hydromyelia or myelomalacia resulting from the metabolic abnormalities within the conus as a result of the tethering (46,117).

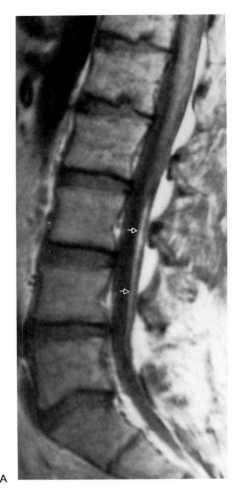

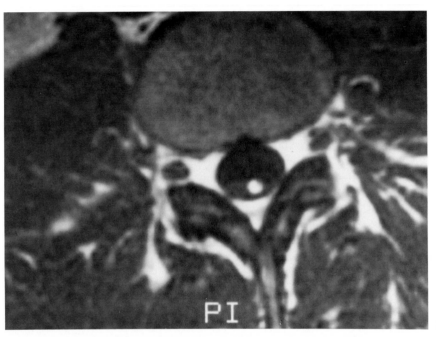

A   B

FIG. 9.21. Fibrolipoma of the filum terminale. **A:** Sagittal SE 600/20 image shows a thickened filum terminale demonstrating a short T1 relaxation time indicative of fat (*arrows*). Note that the conus medullaris is at the normal level. **B:** Axial SE 600/20 through the filum shows a thickened, fatty filum diagnostic of a fibrolipoma.

The dural sac is frequently widened and the dorsal dura is tense and tented posteriorly by the filum. The filum may be so closely applied to the dura posteriorly that it cannot be detected by myelography (9). Therefore, CT myelography or MR with thin sagittal and axial sections are the studies of choice. The thickness of the filum must be measured from axial images and should always be measured at the L5–S1 level, as the filum may be stretched, and therefore of normal thickness, at more rostral levels (46). In a series of 31 patients operated for the tethered cord syndrome, 55% had an obviously thick, fibrotic filum; 23% had a small fibrolipoma within the thickened filum; and 3% had a small filar cyst. In 13% of patients, no distinct filum was seen; rather, the spinal cord was markedly elongated, extending downward to the lower end of the dural sac and ending in a small lipoma at the caudal end of the thecal sac (Fig. 9.22) (118). Phase contrast MR may be useful to detect diminished

motion of the cervical spinal cord in patients with cord tethering (63).

Syndrome of Caudal Regression

The syndrome of caudal regression is composed of a spectrum of anomalies, including sirenomelia (fusion of the lower extremities), absence of the caudal-most vertebrae and spinal cord (lumbosacral agenesis), anal atresia, malformed external genitalia, exstrophy of the urinary bladder, bilateral renal aplasia, and pulmonary hypoplasia with Potter's facies. The syndrome seems to result from disturbances of the caudal mesoderm, including the caudal cell mass and cloaca, before the fourth week of gestation (119). The lack of formation of the caudal spinal cord and spinal column in patients with lumbosacral agenesis may be caused by maldevelopment of the

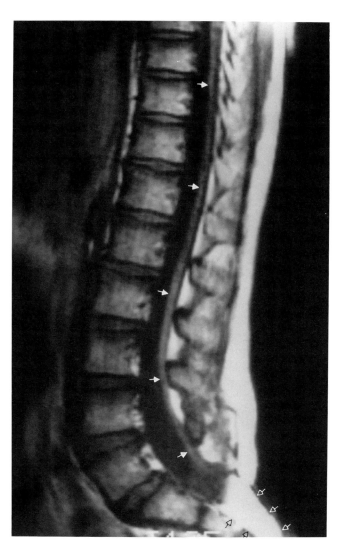

FIG. 9.22. Tethered spinal cord (tight filum terminale syndrome). Sagittal SE 600/20 image shows a very thin, elongated spinal cord (*closed white arrows*) extending all the way down into a terminal lipoma (*open arrows*). The thickness of the filum at the L5–S1 level is always greater than 2 mm in these patients.

lower portions of the spinal cord and notochord as a result of a toxic, infectious, or ischemic insult. As discussed earlier in the chapter, the notochord influences neurulation and the development of the vertebral bodies. The neural tube, dependent upon the notochord for proper formation, then strongly influences the development of the vertebral arches (114).

The incidence of caudal regression syndrome is approximately one in 7,500 births (119). The milder forms, including isolated sacral hypogenesis or anal atresia, are more common than the more severe forms. Approximately one-sixth of infants with caudal regression syndrome have diabetic mothers (120). Clinical signs at presentation range from isolated deformities of the feet or

minor distal muscle weakness to complete sensorimotor paralysis of both lower extremities (114). The more severely affected patients almost always have anal atresia or severe genitourinary anomalies. Motor deficits, which are almost always more severe than the sensory loss, correspond to the level of vertebral loss (within one level) unless an associated myelomeningocele is present. In most patients, sensation is intact caudally for several segments below the vertebral loss; therefore, perineal sensation can be preserved despite severe leg weakness, sphincter disorder, and sacral agenesis. Almost all patients have a neurogenic bladder (9). The clinical scenario of sphincter dysfunction and lower-extremity motor deficits results in a tentative clinical diagnosis of tethered spinal cord in many of the less severely affected patients.

The degree of spinal agenesis is variable, ranging from a partial or total unilateral sacral agenesis (with an oblique lumbosacral joint) to total agenesis of the lumbar and sacral spine (18). The caudal-most two or three vertebral bodies are often fused (Fig. 9.23). The bony canal immediately rostral to the last intact vertebra may be severely narrowed as a result of bony excrescences originating from the vertebral bodies, from fibrous bands connecting the bifid spinous processes, or from stenosis of the dural tube. Surgical release of such dural stenosis and duraplasty may achieve an improvement of neurologic function (114). The major neural anomaly is hypoplasia of the distal spinal cord, which is more severe ventrally than dorsally, resulting in a characteristic "wedge" shape of the cord terminus (Figs. 9.23, 9.24) (18). Diminished numbers of anterior horn cells are present in the distal cord, and sacral nerve roots are abnormally small. Below the level of the last intact vertebra, scattered nerve fibers pass through dense fibrous tissue (90,121). The spinal cord may be tethered in sacral agenesis. The embryologic basis for this association is not certain, but it is interesting to speculate that an abnormality of the notochord may result in faulty retrogressive differentiation (producing the tethered spinal cord) while at the same time causing lack of induction of the more caudal vertebral bodies.

On imaging studies, the diagnosis of caudal regression is easily made. Plain films allow diagnosis of the bony hypogenesis but do not show associated cord tethering or dural stenosis, if present. Sagittal MR images are helpful in detecting hypogenesis or dysgenesis of the caudal vertebral bodies (Figs. 9.23–9.25). Moreover, assessment of the level and shape of the conus medullaris will determine whether tethering is present. MR reveals a characteristic blunted or, often, "wedge-shaped" appearance of the terminus of the spinal cord in those patients in whom the cord is not tethered (Figs. 9.23, 9.24) (18). When this appearance is seen on sagittal images, the sacrum should always be scrutinized to assess for the presence and de-

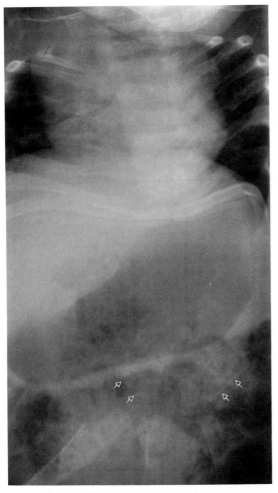

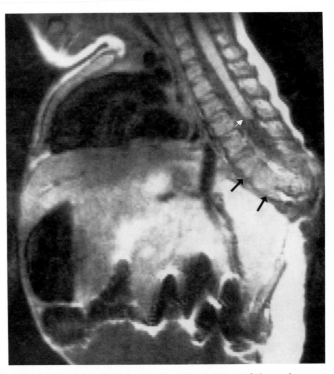

A

B

FIG. 9.23. Severe caudal regression. **A:** Anteroposterior plain film demonstrates termination of the spinal column at the T8 level. The bones of the pelvis (*arrows*) can be vaguely seen through the bowel gas. **B:** Sagittal SE 500/40 image shows fusion of the most caudal three vertebral bodies (*black arrows*). The lowest vertebral body is dysplastic. The terminus of the spinal cord has a blunted "wedge" shape (*white arrow*), which is characteristic of this anomaly.

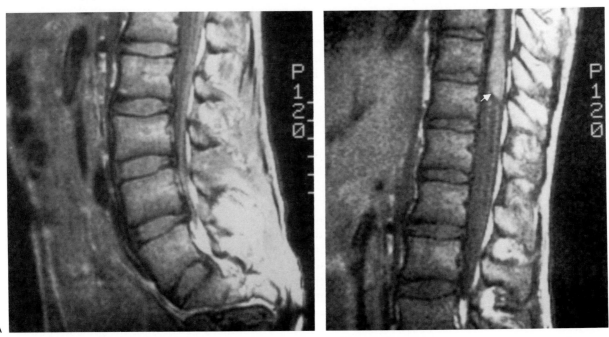

A

B

FIG 9.24. Mild caudal regression. **A:** The spinal column is normal except for the sacrum. S2 is dysplastic and the S3, S4, and S5 segments and the coccyx are absent. **B:** The cord terminus (*arrow*), situated at the mid-T11 level, has the characteristic (wedge) shape of caudal regression.

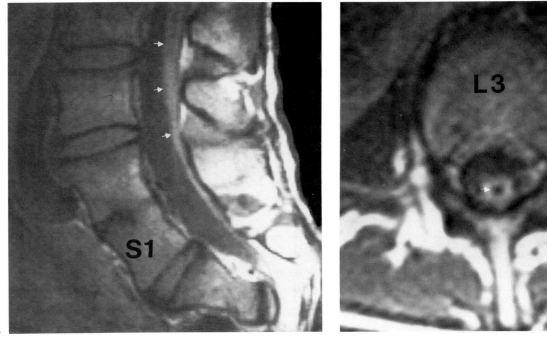
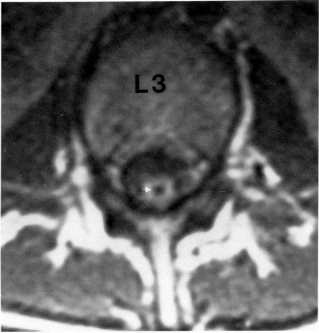
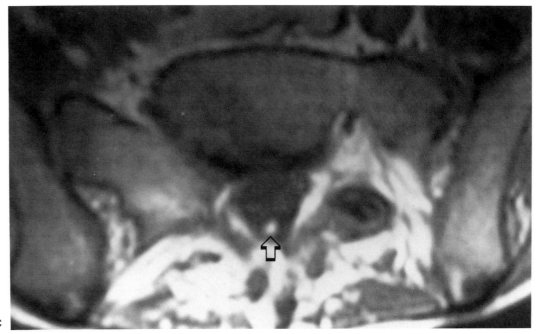

FIG. 9.25. Caudal regression with a tethered cord. **A:** Sagittal SE 540/30 image shows fusion of L5 and S1, dysplastic S3 and absence of S4, S5, and the coccyx. The caudal spinal cord (*arrows*) is thin and stretched inferiorly. It is difficult to determine where the conus medullaris ends and the filum terminale begins. A vague area of decreased intensity is seen within the spinal cord at the L3 level, suggestive of mild hydromyelia. **B:** Axial SE 700/30 image at the L3 level reveals focal hydromyelia (*arrow*). This is seen in approximately 25% of patients with tethered spinal cords and does not necessarily require treatment when it is minimal, as in this patient. **C:** Axial SE 700/30 image at the S1 level shows a thickened filum terminale (*open arrow*) containing fatty elements (note the short T1 relaxation time).

gree of hypogenesis. The distal cord has a tapered appearance when tethered (Fig. 9.25). Axial images should be obtained through the levels immediately adjacent to the level of regression to demonstrate the presence of bony spinal stenosis.

Myelocystocele and Terminal Myelocystocele

The myelocystocele (also known as syringocele) is the least common form of spinal dysraphism with posterior spina bifida (122). This anomaly is an occult spinal dysraphism in which the hydromyelic spinal cord and the arachnoid are herniated through a posterior spina bifida, creating an unusual type of myelomeningocele (Figs. 9.26, 9.27). The most common form, the terminal myelocystocele, is truly an anomaly of the caudal cell mass and is associated with anomalies of the anorectal system, lower genitourinary system, and vertebrae, such as anal

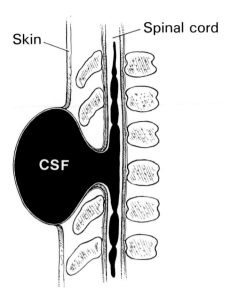

FIG. 9.27. Schematic of myelocystocele. This is an occult, skin-covered, spinal dysraphism in which the spinal cord (which has a syringohydromyelia) and the arachnoid are herniated through a posterior spina bifida. The cyst is in continuity with the central canal of the spinal cord. Myelocystoceles can occur at any level. Localized expansion of the subarachnoid space is not a necessary component and is uncommon in myelocystoceles that occur at locations other than the cord terminus.

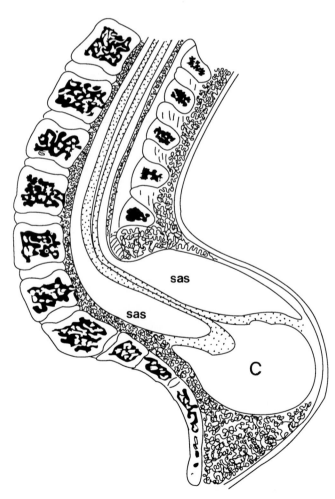

FIG. 9.26. Schematic of terminal myelocystocele. Hydromyelia is always present in the spinal cord. At the cord terminus, the central canal opens into a large cyst (c). This cyst is below a region of bony spina bifida and expanded subarachnoid space (sas) that surrounds the distal spinal cord.

atresia, cloacal exstrophy, lordosis, scoliosis, and partial sacral agenesis (15). Myelocystoceles in other areas of the spinal cord are of unknown cause, but clearly not the result of disturbances of the caudal cell mass. They are discussed in this section for convenience. Patients present with cystic, skin-covered masses that most commonly involve the lumbosacral spine (terminal myelocystocele), although they can occur at the cervical or thoracic levels.

In the terminal myelocystocele, the spinal cord traverses a meningocele and inserts within its posterior wall (Fig. 9.26). At the junction line between the placode and the meninges, the pia covering the spinal cord is reflected along the wall of the meningocele, creating a closed cavity filled with cerebrospinal fluid. In all forms of myelocystocele, a hydromyelic cavity lies within the cord. At the level of the myelocystocele this hydromyelic cavity dilates into a large ependyma-lined cyst that protrudes beyond the reflection of the pia in such a manner that it can be extra-arachnoidal in location (Figs. 9.26, 9.27).

Imaging studies demonstrate direct continuity of the meningocele with the subarachnoid space and the presence of a cyst with the central canal of the spinal cord (Fig. 9.28) (41,43,122). Because the cyst doesn't communicate with the meningocele, myelography will demonstrate only the meningocele (if present), which is much smaller in volume and at a different level from the clinically apparent mass. Imaging studies show that the clini-

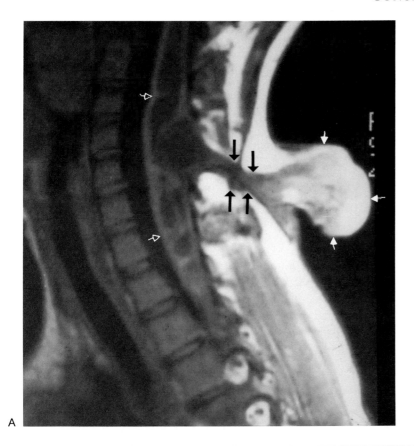

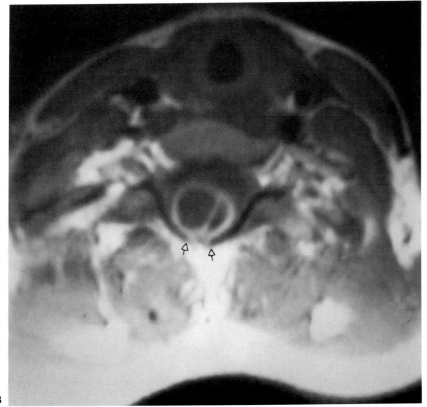

FIG. 9.28. Cervical myelocystocele. **A:** Sagittal SE 600/20 image through the cervical spine shows syringohydromyelia of the cord with multiple septations within the syrinx (*open white arrows*). The ependyma-lined cyst is seen to extend posteriorly through a spina bifida into the subcutaneous tissues (*black arrows*) forming a skin-covered dorsal mass (*closed white arrows*). **B:** Axial SE 800/ 20 immediately caudal to the dorsal cyst shows the multiple loculations within the spinal cord and a bony spina bifida (*open black arrows*). The subarachnoid space ventral to the spinal cord is expanded.

cally apparent mass is a second cyst that is thin-walled and has no internal structure (Figs. 9.28, 9.29) (41,43,44,122,123). The cyst may show delayed opacification with water-soluble intrathecal contrast, similar to a hydromyelia. The ependyma-lined (hydromyelia) cyst is frequently the larger of the two cysts; it is typically situated posteriorly and inferiorly to the meningocele but occasionally extends rostrally outside the meningocele.

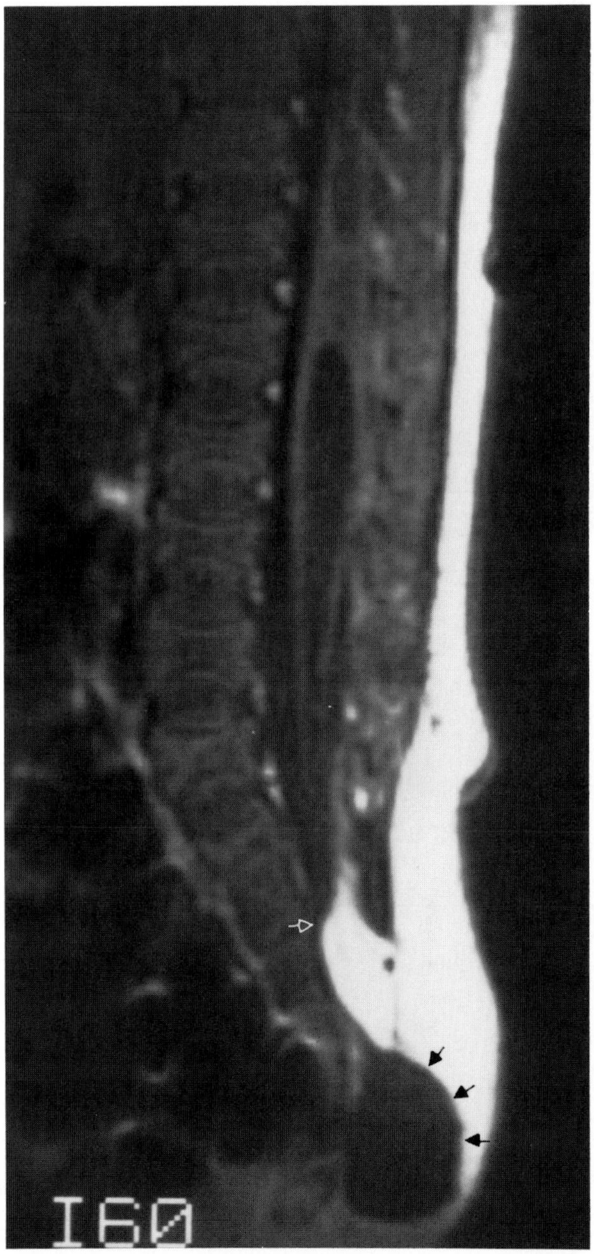

Anterior Sacral Meningoceles

Anterior sacral meningoceles are anomalies characterized by a focal erosion or hypogenesis of segments of the sacrum and coccyx with herniation of a CSF-filled meningeal sac through the defect into the pelvis. They account for ~5% of retrorectal tumors and are usually diagnosed in the second and third decades of life. In children, males and females are equally affected (9,40). Symptoms are produced as a result of pressure on the pelvic viscera, causing constipation, urinary frequency and incontinence, dysmenorrhea, dyspareunia, or pain in the lower back or pelvis. Furthermore, pressure may be exerted on nerve roots, resulting in sciatica, diminished rectal and detrusor tone, or numbness and paresthesia in the lower sacral dermatomes. Finally, fluid shifts between the sac and the spinal subarachnoid space can cause intermittent high-pressure headache (when supine), nausea, vomiting (especially during defecation), or low-pressure headache (while in the erect position).

The embryogenesis of anterior sacral meningoceles is not determined. A relatively simple form arises in patients with neurofibromatosis type I and in patients with Marfan syndrome. A more complex familial form—which is associated with a partial sacral agenesis, imperforate anus or anal stenosis, and a tethered spinal cord—has been described (124). The sacral dural sac is usually widened; it communicates with the pelvic cyst through a (usually) narrow neck that is situated within the sacral defect. The meningoceles may be large or small, simple or multiloculated, devoid of neural tissue or traversed by nerve roots within the wall or lumen of the sac (40,124–126). The identification of traversing nerve roots is crucial, since the neck of the meningocele cannot be simply ligated in their presence.

Bony anomalies consist of a widened sacral canal, scalloping of the anterior wall of the sacrum, and sacral scoliosis (126). The curved appearance of the residual sacrum, which is scalloped beneath the defect, gives the appearance of scimitar sacrum or a sickle-shaped sacrum on sagittal images; this appearance is highly suggestive of an anterior sacral meningocele (125).

Imaging studies show a deficient sacrum and a variably sized cyst extending into the pelvis through an enlarged sacral foramen. Continuity of the cyst with the thecal sac must be demonstrated to make the diagnosis. On MR studies, the continuity is best demonstrated in the sagittal plane (Fig. 9.30) (40). If CT is used, contrast should be injected intrathecally to show optimally the continuity of the meningocele with the subarachnoid space. Whatever imaging technique is used, the most important features to demonstrate are (1) tethering of the

FIG. 9.29. Terminal myelocystocele in a newborn. This newborn infant had a sacral mass. Sagittal SE 600/20 image shows an expanded, syringohydromyelic spinal cord that appears to terminate at the mid-sacral level (*white arrow*). A large cystic mass is seen caudal to the apparent cord termination (*black arrows*). At surgery, this terminal cyst was found to communicate with the dilated central canal of the spinal cord, resulting in the classification of this anomaly as a myelocystocele.

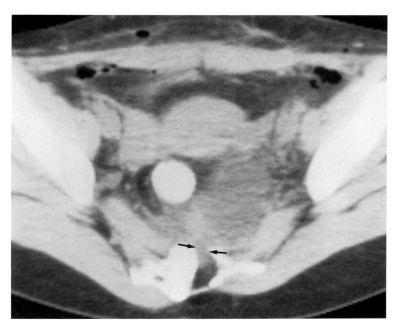
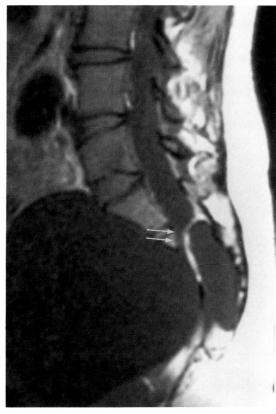

A B

FIG. 9.30. Anterior sacral meningocele. **A:** CT scan through the sacrum shows a cystic mass extending through an enlarged sacral foramen (*arrows*) into the pelvis. **B:** Sagittal SE 600/20 image shows the anterior sacral meningocele extending into the pelvis from the sacrum. A thin connection (*arrows*) with the thecal sac is shown. It is important in these anomalies to determine whether nerve roots of the cauda equina are floating within the meningocele before the meningocele is ligated.

cord and the associated tethering lipoma or dermoid, if present, and (2) whether nerve roots traverse the sacral defect.

Sacrococcygeal Teratomas

Sacrococcygeal teratomas are rare congenital tumors, thought to arise from rests of totipotential cells in the caudal cell mass, that involve the lower sacrum. Females are affected more commonly than males, by a four-to-one preponderance. The tumors may present as an external mass protruding from the gluteal cleft or from the perineum, or they may intrude into the pelvis, causing radicular pain, constipation, or urinary frequency and incontinence. Histologically, approximately two-thirds of these tumors are mature teratomas; the other one-third is split relatively evenly between immature teratomas and anaplastic carcinomas (9). In general, sacral teratomas are large, well-encapsulated, lobulated masses, having both solid and cystic portions. Approximately 5% are predominantly cystic.

Sacrococcygeal teratomas have been classified by their location (127–129). Type I tumors (47%) are situated al-

most entirely posteriorly and have only a minimal presacral portion. Type II tumors (35%) are also largely posterior in location but have a significant pelvic extension. Type III tumors (8%) are visible from the exterior as a mass but are mainly in the pelvis and abdomen. Type IV (10%) tumors are entirely presacral without any external mass. The sacral canal is involved in 2% of affected patients.

If a sacral malformation is associated with a sacrococcygeal teratoma, it suggests the rare familial form of tumor, which has an autosomal dominant inheritance, a slight female preponderance, and prominent sacrococcygeal defects. Anorectal stenosis, vesicoureteral reflux, and cutaneous stigmata are frequently present in patients with the familiar form.

The sporadic and familial forms are indistinguishable on imaging studies. Bony erosions in the sacrum, when present, outline the entire soft tissue component, whether dorsal to the sacrum or intrapelvic. Depending upon the percentage of solid components, cystic components, and calcification, the tumors are variably heterogeneous. Adequate CT evaluation necessitates opacification of the bowel, the ureters, and bladder by the use of contrast agents to evaluate the relationship of the tumor to the pelvic viscera. Contrast agents are not necessary if MR is used. The MR appearance of the tumor is variable, depending upon its composition. Most often these lesions are extremely heterogeneous as a result of high signal from fat, intermediate signal from soft tissue, and low signal from calcium on T1-weighted images (Fig. 9.31). The tumors are usually lobulated and sharply demarcated. When mostly cystic (Fig. 9.31C), contrast administration may be necessary to identify a solid component in the wall of the cyst.

ANOMALIES OF DEVELOPMENT OF THE NOTOCHORD

The Split Notochord Syndrome

Classification

The term *split notochord syndrome* refers to a spectrum of anomalies that are believed to be sequelae of splitting or deviation of the notochord with a persistent connection between the ventrally located endoderm and the dorsally located ectoderm (130). The most severe form of this syndrome is a fistula (the *dorsal enteric fistula*) through which the intestinal cavity communicates with the dorsal skin surface in the midline, traversing the prevertebral soft tissues, the vertebral bodies, the spinal canal and its contents, and the posterior elements of the spine (130–132). The extreme case of the dorsal enteric fistula is a dorsal bowel hernia in which a portion of bowel is herniated into a skin- or membrane-covered dorsal sac after passing through a combined anterior and posterior spina bifida. Often the bowel lumen is open to the skin surface. Because any portion of the dorsal enteric fistula may become obliterated or persist, apparently isolated diverticula, duplications, cysts, fibrous cords, and/or sinuses may be present at any point along the tract. The *dorsal enteric sinus* is the remnant of the posterior part of the tract and forms a blind tract with a midline opening to the dorsal external skin surface (130,131). *Dorsal enteric enterogenous cysts* (which are derived from the intermediate part of the tract) are enteric-lined cysts that may be prevertebral, postvertebral, or intraspinal (130,131). *Dorsal enteric diverticula* are tubular or spherical diverticula that arise from the dorsal mesenteric border of the bowel. These diverticula represent a persistence of a portion of the tract between the gut and the vertebral column. Because the bowel segments migrate inferiorly and rotate, it is not uncommon to trace dorsal enteric diverticula far upward from the small bowel through the mesentery and diaphragm into the mediastinum. Occasionally, these diverticula will extend to the anterior surface of the vertebra or into the spinal canal (130). If there is involution of the portion of

the diverticulum near the gut, a prevertebral *dorsal enteric cyst* is formed (131). Finally, in some patients, the dorsal enteric fistula may close at multiple sites. In these patients, one may find combined, noncommunicating elements of the split notochord syndrome; for example, intestinal diverticula, mediastinal enteric cysts, and intraspinal enterogenous cysts may be present.

Embryology

A review of some embryology aids in the understanding of split notochord malformations. During the second week of gestation, the embryo consists of a flat, two-layered disc. The developing ectoderm lies dorsally, in contact with the amniotic cavity. The primitive endoderm lies ventrally, in contact with the yolk sac. During the third week of life, a thickening occurs in the dorsal midline as a result of a focal rapid proliferation of cells; this area has been called Hensen's node. Cells proliferate and migrate from Hensen's node, separating the ectoderm from the endoderm and eventually forming the notochord. If the ectoderm fails to separate completely from the endoderm (leaving a strand or adhesion), the notochord must either split around the adhesion or deviate to the left or right of it (133,134). The mesoderm, which normally surrounds the notochord to form the vertebral bodies, is split or deviated by the anomaly, resulting in a persistent connection between the dorsal surface of the gut and the dorsal, midline surface of the body. As the embryo grows and the gut migrates, the adhesion can become quite long, and the structures connected by it may become quite distant topographically. Because the notochord may split or deviate around the adhesion, the connection of the cyst to the vertebrae may be in the midline or paramedian. Moreover, because all or part of the connection may involute, only portions of the connection may be present (133,134).

Clinical and Imaging Characteristics

Patients with *dorsal enteric fistula* usually present as newborns with a bowel ostium or an exposed pad of mucous membrane in the dorsal midline. These openings pass meconium and then feces. *Dorsal bowel herniations* present as large, midline, dorsal sacs that are partly covered by skin and partly covered by mucous membrane; the vertebral column around the sac is duplicated (Fig. 9.32) (132). *Dorsal enteric cysts* present as masses either in the mediastinum or in the abdomen. None of the previously mentioned lesions present primarily as a neurologic problem and will therefore not be discussed further in this book. The reader is referred to standard pediatric and pediatric radiology texts for further information.

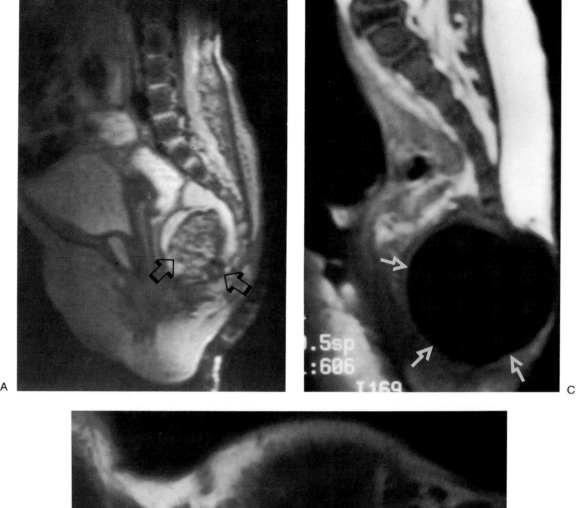

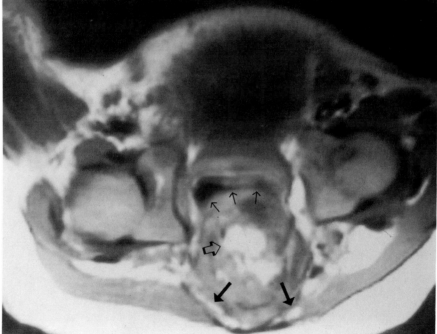

FIG. 9.31. Sacrococcygeal teratomas. **A:** A heterogeneous presacral mass (type IV teratoma) is seen on this SE 2000/40 image (*arrows*). **B:** Axial SE 800/20 image shows that the heterogeneous mass contains fat (*open arrow*), and displaces the rectum anteriorly (*small arrows*) and the sacrum posteriorly (*large arrows*). The low signal intensity within the mass may represent calcium. **C:** Sagittal SE 500/12 image of a different patient shows a largely cystic mass (type III teratoma, *arrows*) centered at the coccyx.

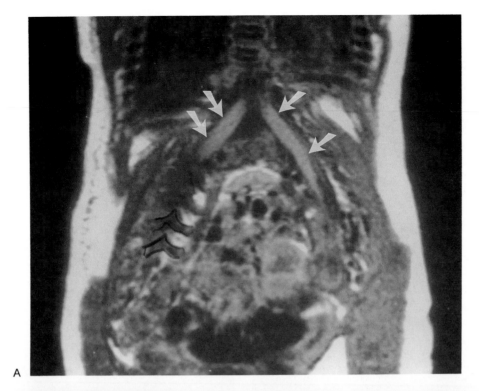

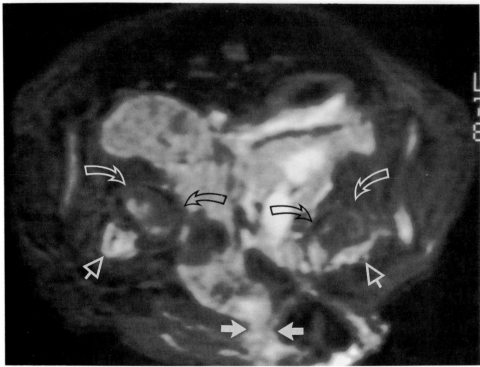

FIG. 9.32. Dorsal enteric fistula. **A:** Coronal SE 600/20 image shows a split spinal column and spinal cord (*arrows*) framing the bowel. **B:** Axial GE 600/15 image shows two spinal columns (*open curved arrows*), two spinal canals (*open straight arrows*), and the high-intensity bowel extending dorsally between them to open (*solid arrows*) at the skin surface. (This case courtesy Dr. Rosiland Dietrich, Irvine, CA.)

Intraspinal Enteric Cysts

Intraspinal enteric cysts infrequently present in newborn infants; they most commonly present in adolescents or young adults with intermittent or progressive local and radicular pain that is worsened by elevating intraspinal pressure. Eventually, myelopathy ensues, with spinal cord compression with both local and distal long-tract symptomatology. By the time these patients are imaged, marked compression of the spinal cord is usually evident (29,135).

Enteric cysts are usually single, smooth, and unilocular, occurring primarily in the lower cervical and thoracic regions. Rarely, they occur in the lumbar spine or in the cerebellopontine angle (136,137). The fluid within them may be nearly identical to cerebrospinal fluid or may be milky, cream-colored, yellowish, or xanthochromic. These lesions are usually intradural, extramedullary, and situated ventral or ventrolateral to the cord. The cord is usually markedly narrowed and displaced posteriorly or to one side by the mass. Less frequently, the cyst may be dorsal or dorsolateral to the cord, within the cord, or within the cleft of a diastematomyelia (135,137).

Plain spine radiographs usually show an enlarged spinal canal at the site of the enteric cyst. Newborns and infants who are symptomatic from intraspinal enteric cysts sometimes exhibit vertebral anomalies, including hemivertebrae, lack of segmentation, partial fusions, and scoliosis in the region of the cyst (such changes are more common with mediastinal or abdominal dorsal enteric cysts). Older patients usually exhibit no vertebral changes other than focal enlargement of the canal resulting from local pressure effects (135).

Imaging studies typically show a cyst of CSF intensity lying ventral to and compressing the adjacent spinal cord (Fig. 9.33) (29,135,137). However, the cyst may lie dorsal to the cord or partially or completely within the cord; it is most important to define the cyst and its relationship to the spinal cord. The cyst contents may be similar to cerebrospinal fluid or may be proteinaceous, shortening the T1 relaxation time and resulting in relatively (compared to cerebrospinal fluid) high intensity on T1-weighted images (Fig. 9.34). The identification of anomalies of the adjacent vertebral bodies aids in identification of the abnormal level. The abnormal vertebrae and the cysts are easily identified by myelography or by CT with intrathecal contrast (Fig. 9.33). On MR, identification of the abnormal vertebrae is facilitated by obtaining coronal images through the vertebral bodies (Fig. 9.34). The cyst may be difficult to detect if its contents are very similar to cerebrospinal fluid. However, the displacement and distortion of the spinal cord by the cyst facilitates detection. In addition to evaluating the spine, it is important to look for associated fistulae and mediastinal or abdominal cysts.

Diastematomyelia

Definition

The term diastematomyelia refers to a sagittal division of the spinal cord into two symmetric or asymmetric hemicords, each containing a central canal, one dorsal horn (giving rise to a dorsal nerve root), and one ventral horn (giving rise to a ventral nerve root). Both hemicords are surrounded by a layer of pia (9,26,90,138–141). The division may involve the entire thickness of the cord or may only affect the anterior or posterior half of the cord (partial diastematomyelia) (17,134,142). Partial division is frequently observed in the transitional zones superior and inferior to an area of complete diastematomyelia (9,38,134,141).

Clinical Presentation

The signs and symptoms of diastematomyelia may appear at any time of life. Females are affected much more commonly than males (38,59,143). Cutaneous stigmata (e.g., hypertrichosis, nevi, lipomas, dimples, and hemangiomas) overlie the spine in more than half of cases. Orthopedic problems of the feet, particularly clubfoot, are also present in about half of affected patients. Neurologic symptoms are nonspecific, indistinguishable from other causes of cord tethering (9,38,59,134,143–145).

Embryology

Diastematomyelia most likely develops as a result of a split notochord (134,142). If the cells forming the notochord, in the course of their migration from Hensen's node, encounter an obstacle, such as an adhesion between the primitive ectoderm and endoderm, the notochordal cells must course laterally around the obstacle on one side or split and go around on both sides at the same time. As a consequence of this detour, the notochord develops either a lateral notch or a central cleft. Because the notochord influences the development of the vertebral bodies, any alteration of the notochord could result in an abnormality of the vertebral bodies, such as a hemivertebra (if the notochord were notched) or a butterfly vertebra (if the notochord had a cleft). Similarly, a split notochord could induce the formation of two neural plates, which may go on to form two hemicords. Surrounding mesenchyme can migrate into the space between the hemicords, forming a fibrous, cartilaginous, or bony spur. Moreover, one can imagine in this setting that the distal notochord could be split, resulting in two separate foci of canalization and retrogressive differentiation. This sequence of events could explain the rare cases of diastematomyelia affecting only the conus medullaris and filum terminale.

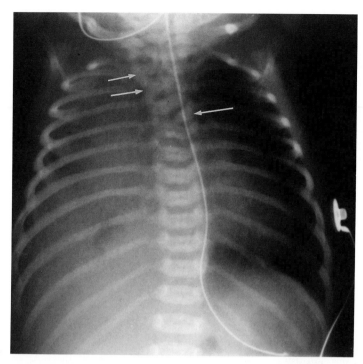

A

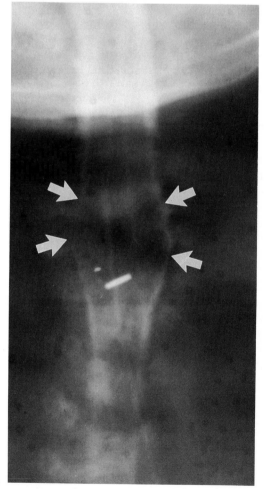

B

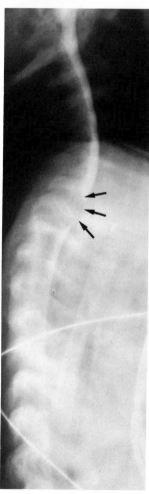

C

FIG. 9.33. Intraspinal enteric cyst. **A:** AP plain film shows multiple vertebral body anomalies (*arrows*) in the upper thoracic and lower cervical spine. **B, C:** AP and lateral films from a myelogram show the cord to be displaced posteriorly by a ventral intradural, extramedullary mass (*arrows*).

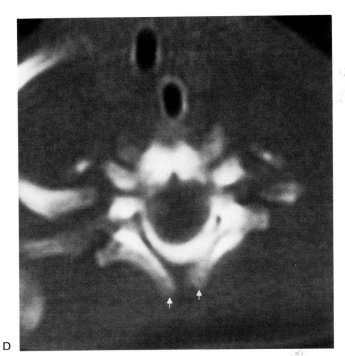
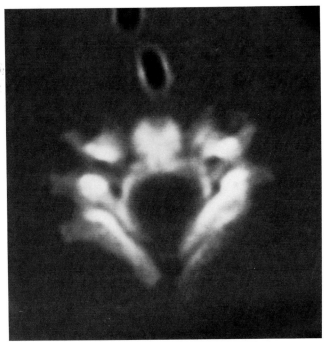

D

E

FIG. 9.33. (*Continued.*) **D, E:** Axial postmyelogram CT reveals a posterior spina bifida (*white arrows*) and the ventral mass adjacent to a butterfly vertebra. The spinal canal is enlarged at this level. The ventral mass has completely effaced the ventral subarachnoid space at this level, making it difficult to determine whether the mass is intramedullary or extramedullary. (This case courtesy of Dr. S. Chuang, Toronto, Ont).

Pathology and Imaging

The level of the cleft is variable, but it is most commonly in the lumbar region. Upper thoracic clefts are unusual, and cervical clefts are rare (59,146,147). It is possible that the cervical and upper thoracic clefts are more common than is generally accepted but remain asymptomatic because they are less likely to cause tethering of the cord than clefts that are located more caudally. (The segmental level of the spinal cord much more closely coincides with the segmental level of the adjacent vertebrae in the cervical and upper thoracic levels.) The two hemicords reunite caudal to the cleft in most patients (38). Occasionally, however, the cleft will extend unusually low and the hemicords remain distinct with two separate conus medullaris and two fila terminale. Imaging of the cleft is optimally performed by MR in the coronal plane, using either T1- or T2-weighted images. Bony and cartilaginous spurs are most easily identified on T2-weighted images or on CT.

In 50% to 60% of patients with diastematomyelia, the two hemicords, each covered by an intact layer of pia, travel through a single subarachnoid space surrounded by a single dural sac (148). Each hemicord has its own anterior spinal artery. This form of diastematomyelia is not accompanied by a bony spur, but it always has a fibrous band coursing through the most inferior portion

of the cleft, inserting in the dura (134); patients are rarely symptomatic unless hydromyelia (Fig. 9.35) or tethering (Fig. 9.36) are present (59,109,134). Imaging studies (Fig. 9.36) in these patients show the split cord and the vertebral anomalies, if present, but rarely show the fibrous band (59).

In the other 40% to 50% of patients, the arachnoid and the dura split into two separate arachnoid and dural tubes, each surrounding the corresponding hemicord. Thus, each hemicord has its own pial, arachnoid, and dural sheath for several spinal sections (134,140,148). Patients with two separate dural sheaths nearly always have a bony or cartilaginous spur at the most inferior portion of the cleft; the spur may originate from a lamina or from the vertebral body (Fig. 9.37). If the myelogram or imaging study appears to show the spur at a more rostral level, a second spur, present in ~5% of patients with diastematomyelia, is likely to be present (Fig. 9.38) (48,134,140,148). The bony spur forms from cartilage and has multiple ossification centers. Therefore, depending upon the age of the patient and the number of ossification centers, the spur can be nonossified cartilage, cartilaginous with multiple small ossification centers arranged linearly between the two hemicords, a bony strut attached to the wall of the spinal canal by a synchondrosis, or a complete osseous bridge joining the vertebral body with the posterior elements (141). The spur

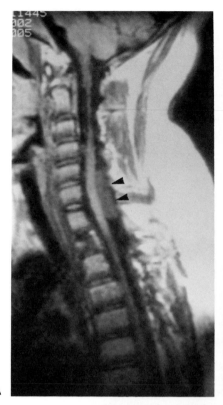

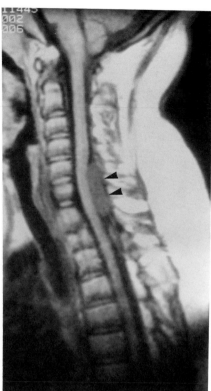

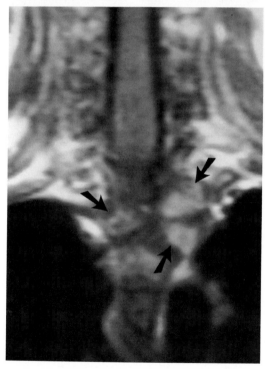

FIG. 9.34. Intraspinal enteric cyst. **A, B:** Sagittal SE 600/20 images show a mass (*arrowheads*) dorsally in the cervical subarachnoid space compressing the spinal cord. **C:** Coronal SE 600/20 image shows several hemivertebrae (*arrows*) at the level of the cyst.

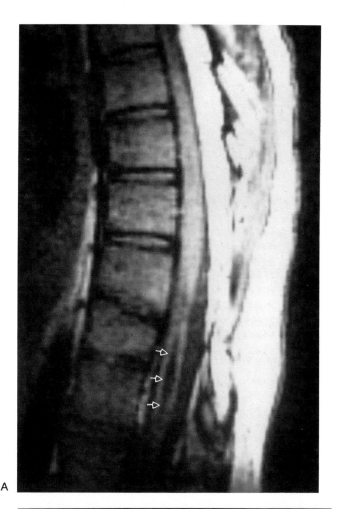

A

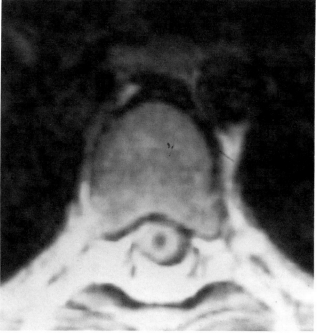

B

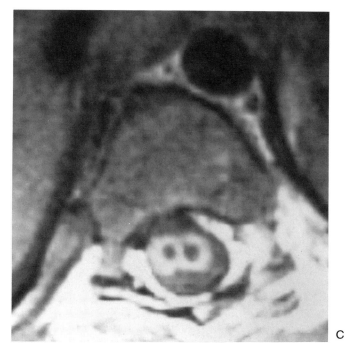

C

FIG. 9.35. Diastematomyelia with hydromyelia. **A:** Sagittal SE 600/20 image shows a dilated central canal (*arrows*). **B:** Axial SE 1000/20 image in the mid-thoracic region confirms the presence of hydromyelia. **C:** Axial SE 1000/20 at the upper lumbar level shows diastematomyelia with extension of the syrinx into both hemicords.

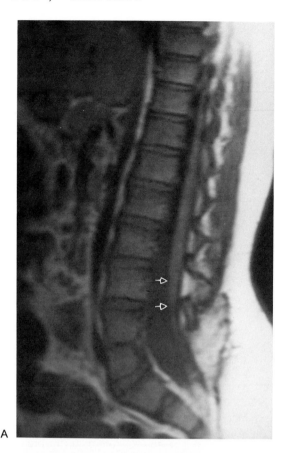

A

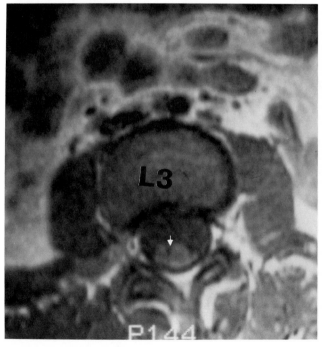

B

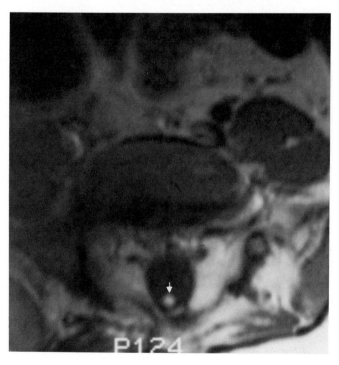

C

FIG. 9.36. Diastematomyelia without bony spur but with tethering of cord. **A:** Sagittal SE 600/20 image reveals tethering of the cord (*arrows*) that is situated posteriorly in the spinal canal; the conus medullaris lies at approximately the L3–L4 level. There is a lack of segmentation of L5 and S1. **B:** At the L3 level there is a cleft (*white arrow*) within the tethered cord, dividing it into two hemicords. **C:** At the level of the L5–S1 disc, a thickened, fat-infiltrated filum terminale is seen (*arrow*). When the filum is thicker than 2 mm at the L5–S1 level, tethering of the cord is strongly suggested. Tethering of the cord and thickening of the filum is seen in more than half of patients with diastematomyelia.

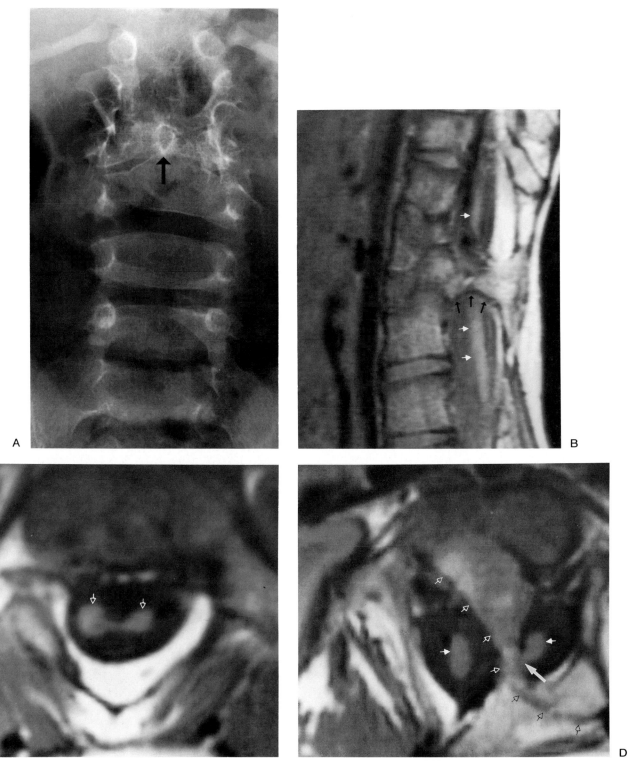

FIG. 9.37. Diastematomyelia with bony spur and meningocele manqué. **A:** AP plain film of the lumbar spine. There are segmentation anomalies of T12 to L3. The laminae of T12, L1, and L2 are fused. A large central bony spur is seen at the L2 level (*arrow*). **B:** Sagittal SE 600/20 through the thoracolumbar spine. Portions of the spinal cord (*white arrows*) are seen above and below the large bony spur that extends from the body of L2 posteriorly (*black arrows*). **C:** Axial SE 800/20 image slightly rostral to the bony spur. The single spinal cord is in the process of diving into two hemicords (*open arrows*). **D:** Axial SE 800/20 image at the level of the spur. The left hemicord is connected to the dura by a small extension of neural tissue (*large solid arrow*) known as a meningocele manqué. The spur (*open arrows*) extends from the body of L2 to the left lamina of L2. The left lamina is everted and thickened. At this level, the two hemicords (*small solid arrows*) are contained within separate dural sacs. Caudal to the spur, the two separate dural sacs will once again fuse into a single dural sac. In this patient, the two hemicords also reunited caudal to the cleft.

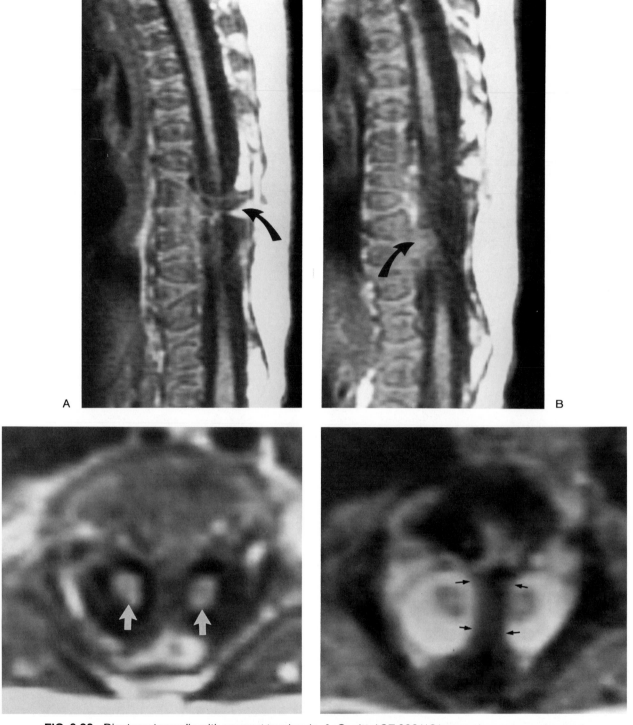

FIG. 9.38. Diastematomyelia with spurs at two levels. **A:** Sagittal SE 600/12 image shows a spur (*curved arrow*) at the mid-thoracic level. This spur is several levels rostral to the lowest level of the split spinal cord, suggesting that a second spur is present. **B:** Adjacent image shows a possible spur (*curved arrow*) at the lower thoracic level. **C:** Axial SE 600/12 image at the level of the upper spur shows the two hemicords (*arrows*) separated by a poorly defined spur. **D:** The spur (*arrows*) is much better demonstrated by this GRE 600/15 image.

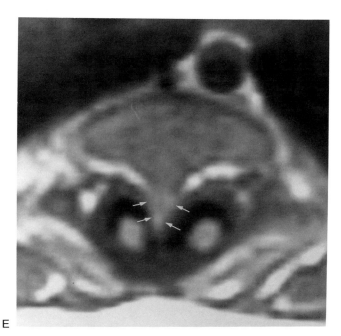

FIG. 9.38. (*Continued.*) **E:** Axial SE 600/12 image shows the lower spur (*arrows*). Note that the posterior part of the spur is fibrous and therefore poorly seen by MR.

may be isointense or slightly hyperintense compared to cerebrospinal fluid on T1-weighted images if nonossified; it is hyperintense on T1-weighted images if ossified (Fig. 9.37) because of the high signal from the marrow. Bony, cartilaginous, and fibrous spurs all appear hypointense on T2-weighted spin echo and gradient echo (Fig. 9.38) images. The CT attenuation will vary, depending upon the stage of ossification.

Usually the bony spur is in the midline sagittal plane and divides the canal into two fairly equal halves. However, scoliosis may rotate the spur such that the two hemicanals are oriented more anteriorly and posteriorly (Fig. 9.39) (140). Occasionally, the spur may cross the spinal canal obliquely and insert into an externally rotated lamina or a pedicle, creating a significant asymmetry in the two hemicanals; in these patients the larger canal is usually posterior. MR imaging is especially helpful in patients with rotoscoliosis (Fig. 9.39). An initial coronal image is obtained. Oblique sagittal and oblique axial planes of imaging are then defined parallel and perpendicular, respectively, to the straight segments of spine, as described in Chapter 1.

It must be emphasized that even osseous spurs can be missed on short TR spin echo MR images. Therefore, patients with two hemicords should be imaged using T2-weighted images (which facilitate identification of bone) in the axial plane or with CT. Resection of the spur is critical to relieve the tethering of the cord and improve the patient's deficits (59).

Associated spinal anomalies are very commonly present in affected patients. The conus medullaris is situated below the L2 level and the filum is thickened in more than 75% of patients with diastematomyelia (Fig. 9.36) (59,149). Myeloceles/myelomeningoceles (of the undivided spinal cord) are present in 15% to 25%, whereas hemimyeloceles (myeloceles/myelomeningoceles of one of the hemicords) are present in 15% to 20% of affected patients (59). Lipomas, dermal sinuses, (epi)dermoid tumors, and tethering adhesions (meningocele manqué) are reported commonly, but in less than 20% of patients (59). The meningocele manqué (Fig. 9.37) is a very subtle finding on imaging studies and will be seen only if the radiologist is actively looking for it (59,145,150,151). The appearance is that of a small band of tissue extending from the hemicord to the dura and mimicking a nerve root; only a portion of the band may be visible on the imaging study (59,150). Hydromyelia is found in about half of patients with diastematomyelia. When present, the hydromyelic cavity may extend from the spinal cord above the cleft into one or both hemicords (Fig. 9.35) (149). The importance of the high incidence of associated anomalies is that the radiologist cannot be satisfied with identification of the diastematomyelia but must scrutinize the imaging examination in an attempt to identify other lesions that may lead to neurologic deterioration in the patient.

The spinal column is nearly always abnormal in patients with diastematomyelia (Figs. 9.37, 9.39) (38,109). The lamina are often thick and fused with the ipsilateral or contralateral lamina of adjacent vertebrae; fusion with contralateral laminae of the adjacent level is known as *intersegmental laminar fusion*. Spina bifida is almost always present. The association of an intersegmental laminar fusion with spina bifida is seen in ~60% of patients with diastematomyelia and is essentially pathognomonic for this anomaly. The intersegmental laminar fusion is almost always at the level of the diastematomyelia (38,139). Anomalies of the vertebral bodies (Fig. 9.39)—including hemivertebrae, butterfly vertebrae, block vertebrae, and decreased disc height—are observed in a high proportion of cases. Kyphoscoliosis (Fig. 9.39) resulting from the osseous anomalies is seen in more than half of patients. Diastematomyelia is responsible for ~5% of congenital scolioses (143).

MALFORMATIONS OF UNKNOWN ORIGIN

All the anomalies described in this chapter are actually of unknown origin. Those anomalies discussed up to this point can be explained by reasonable theories, permitting a classification based upon their embryogenesis. At this time, however, no reasonable theory has been proposed that explains simple meningoceles and lateral meningoceles, which can develop anywhere along the spinal canal.

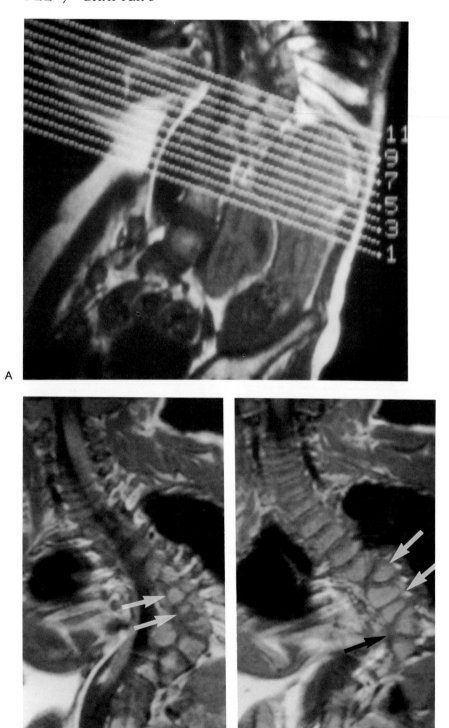

FIG. 9.39. Diastematomyelia with roto-scoliosis. **A:** Coronal image showing the oblique plane proscribed for axial images. **B, C:** Coronal SE 600/20 images show vertebral anomalies (*arrows*) at the level of the most severe spinal curve.

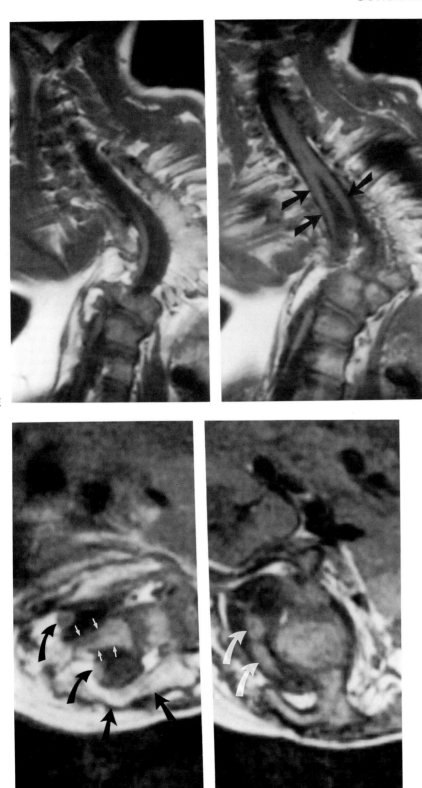

FIG. 9.39. (*Continued.*) **D, E:** Images posterior to those in (B) and (C) show the spinal cord splitting into two hemicords (*arrows*). **F, G:** Oblique axial SE 600/20 images show the hemicords (*curved arrows*) aligned anterior and posterior to each other, split around a spur (*small white arrows*) that is nearly horizontal. Note the markedly thick laminae (*straight black arrows*).

Simple Meningoceles

Simple meningoceles are composed of a herniation of dura, arachnoid, and cerebrospinal fluid that extends into the subcutaneous tissues of the back. The overlying skin is intact unless secondary skin ulcerations arise. By definition, the simple meningocele does not contain nervous tissue, although occasionally a nerve root may enter the sac before leaving it to reenter the spinal canal en route to its respective neural foramen (90). Rarely, a nerve root may become adherent to the wall of the sac. The conus medullaris tends to be in its normal position within the spinal canal. The filum terminale occasionally extends into the neck of the sac.

Simple meningoceles are lined with arachnoid. Arachnoidal adhesions occasionally occur within the sac and, when unusually thick, may partially obliterate the neck of the sac (152). Because the sac communicates with the subarachnoid space, it may change in size with patient position or with Valsalva maneuver.

The bony abnormalities accompanying simple meningoceles are usually limited. They may range from absence of a single spinous process to a localized spina bifida or to a multisegmental spina bifida with enlargement of the spinal canal.

The purpose of imaging studies in these patients is (1) to detect the meningocele, (2) to determine its shape, (3) to define associated anomalies of the bony spinal canal, (4) to determine the presence or absence of nervous tissue within the sac, and (5) to assess the relationship of the sac to the conus medullaris and the filum terminale. Although sonography demonstrates most of these details, MR and CT myelography give the most information. Because it is noninvasive, MR is the imaging procedure of choice in the evaluation of these patients.

Lateral Meningoceles

Lateral thoracic meningoceles are CSF-filled protrusions of dura and arachnoid that extend laterally through an enlarged neural foramen and then anteriorly through the adjacent intercostal space into the extrapleural aspect of the thoracic gutter. Males and females are equally affected and most commonly present during the fourth and fifth decades of life. Although usually asymptomatic, these patients may have pain, vague sensory deficits, hyperreflexia, or slight weakness. Neurofibromatosis is present in approximately 85% of patients with lateral thoracic meningoceles (152,153).

Patients with lateral thoracic meningoceles frequently have a sharply angled scoliosis in the upper thoracic spine, usually convex toward the meningocele, which is located near the apex of the curvature (153). Scalloping of the pedicles, laminae, and vertebral bodies adjacent to the meningocele often result in an enlarged spinal canal (Fig. 9.40).

The size of the meningocele varies markedly from small, nearly undetectable meningeal protrusions to enormous cystic masses filling an entire hemithorax. When large, they may compromise the ventilation of the neonate. Most remain static in size, but occasionally they show slow growth. The meningocele may disappear after shunting of hydrocephalic lateral ventricles (154).

The position of the cord with respect to the meningocele sac is variable. When scoliosis is present, the cord tends to be situated on the side opposite the sac. More rarely, the cord may be pulled toward the sac or into the sac by nerve roots at that level (9).

Lumbar lateral meningoceles are protrusions of dura and arachnoid through one or several enlarged lumbar neural foramina into the lumbar subcutaneous tissue and retroperitoneum. They often occur in a setting of Marfan syndrome or neurofibromatosis but may be seen as isolated anomalies. The meningoceles may be unilateral or bilateral, may involve a single neural foramen or multiple adjacent neural foramina, and may displace adjacent structures. Lumbar meningoceles are similar to those in the thorax in that they are commonly associated with an expanded spinal canal, erosion of the posterior surface of the vertebral bodies, thinning of the neural arches, and enlargement of the neural foramina.

CONGENITAL TUMORS OF THE SPINE

Teratomas

Teratomas are neoplasms containing tissues belonging to all three germinal layers at sites where these tissues do not normally occur. Excluding sacrococcygeal teratomas (discussed earlier in the chapter), these neoplasms constitute 0.15% of all intraspinal tumors (9). Males and females are affected equally, usually presenting with pain and myelopathy. All ages are affected.

Two basic theories have been proposed for the pathogenesis of teratomas. They may arise by multiplication of displaced germ cells or of cells left behind during the migration of Hensen's node that can give rise to any of the three germinal layers of tissue (105,155,156). Alternatively, teratomas might arise from rests of tissues that have escaped the control of those factors in early embryonic development that determine cell line. Tissue growth therefore produces diverse tissues that can be more or less well differentiated (157).

The appearance of spinal teratomas is extremely variable. The tumor may be solid, partially or wholly cystic, unilocular, or multilocular. When cysts are present, they may be thin or thick walled and the fluid within them may be clear, milky, or dark. Bone and cartilage may be present, sometimes in the form of a well-defined bone or tooth. Teratomas may be intra- or extramedullary. Whatever their location, they usually fill the spinal canal at the time of presentation and will produce a complete

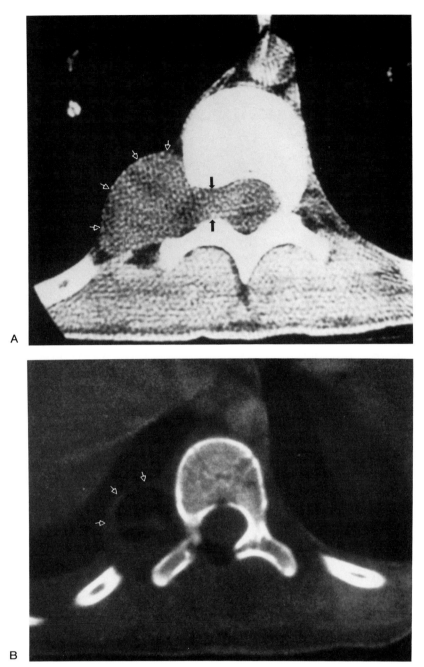

FIG. 9.40. Lateral meningocele. **A:** The right neural foramen (*black arrows*) is widened by this CSF-filled dural diverticulum. The lateral meningocele is seen extending laterally to the posterior mediastinum and laterally displacing the pleura (*white arrows*). **B:** Intrathecal air, injected by lumbar puncture, is seen to fill the meningocele (*arrows*), proving that it is filled with CSF and differentiating it from a solid tumor.

block at myelography. When they are extramedullary, the tumors are often closely adherent to the cord, with a poorly defined cleavage plane formed by tumor, connective tissue, and reactive gliosis. In such cases, it is difficult to differentiate the extramedullary tumor from an intramedullary one. When teratomas occur in the lumbar region, the roots of the cauda equina are frequently adherent to the walls of the tumor as they are draped over it. Syringomyelia may appear above the level of the tumor secondary to restricted CSF flow. Malignant teratomas

are rare and cannot be differentiated from the more common benign variant by imaging.

The spinal canal may be normal or may be focally widened by erosion of the pedicles and laminae. Other bony anomalies are uncommon.

Dermoids and Epidermoids

Dermoids are uni- or multilobular tumors, sometimes cystic, that are lined by a squamous epithelium containing skin appendages, such as hair follicles, sweat glands, and sebaceous glands. Epidermoids are tumors lined by a membrane composed of only the superficial (epidermal) elements of the skin (90). Dermoids usually cause symptoms before the age of 20; they occur equally in males and females. Epidermoids develop slightly more slowly, begin to manifest symptoms in early adulthood (third to fifth decades), and are more common in males (92). Together, dermoid and epidermoid tumors constitute approximately 1% to 2% of spinal cord tumors at all ages and 10% of spinal cord tumors below the age of 15. Approximately 20% develop in association with dermal sinuses; of those not associated with dermal sinuses, epidermoids are slightly more common than dermoids (92). When not associated with dorsal dermal sinuses, dermoids and epidermoids may present as a slowly progressive myelopathy or as an acute onset of a chemical meningitis secondary to rupture of the inflammatory cholesterol crystals from the cyst into the cerebrospinal fluid (87,92).

Dermoid and epidermoid tumors most commonly arise from congenital dermal or epidermal rests or from focal expansion of a dermal sinus. They may also be acquired as iatrogenic lesions resulting from implantation of viable dermal and epidermal elements by spinal needles not provided with trocars (65,158) or as a result of surgery (61,67).

Epidermoids are distributed fairly uniformly along the spine (upper thoracic, 17%; lower thoracic, 26%; lumbosacral, 22%; and cauda equina, 35%) (92). Dermoids, on the other hand, are much more common in the lumbosacral area (60%) and cauda equina (20%), but they are quite infrequent in the cervical and thoracic regions (92). Sixty percent of (epi)dermoids are extramedullary and 40% are intramedullary (93).

Although they range in size from tiny subpial growths to huge mass lesions, at the time of clinical presentation, dermoid and epidermoid cysts almost always cause a complete spinal block to intrathecal contrast when myelography is performed (93). On imaging studies, dermoids almost always have the appearance of fat on CT, showing low attenuation. However, the appearance is variable on MR, sometimes showing high intensity on T1-weighted images but more commonly having low to intermediate intensity on T1-weighted images and high intensity on T2-weighted images (see Figs. 9.11 and 9.12 in the section on dermal sinuses in this chapter). The lack of a fatty signal may be a result of secretions from sweat glands within the tumor causing an increased water content. Epidermoids also have a variable signal intensity on MR, most commonly isointense to cerebrospinal fluid but sometimes hyperintense; this variability is similar to that seen in intracranial epidermoids, as described in Chapter 7. Small epidermoids are difficult to diagnose on both MR and CT because they are difficult to differentiate from surrounding cerebrospinal fluid on both im-

aging modalities. Using MR, larger epidermoids can be identified by slightly altered signal intensity and the displacement of the spinal cord or nerve roots by the mass (Fig. 9.41). The administration of intrathecal contrast greatly facilitates detection of the tumor and its relationship to the spinal cord and nerve roots by CT. Neither dermoids nor epidermoids enhance after administration of intravenous contrast unless they are or have been infected. Infection is much more common if the tumors have developed in association with dermal sinuses.

Hamartomas

Hamartomas are malformations composed of an abnormal mixture of those tissue elements that normally occur at the tumor site. Because they grow and develop at the same rate as normal tissues, hamartomas are unlikely to result in compression of adjacent parenchyma; therefore, neurologic deficits and hydrocephalus are usually not present (9,159).

Hamartomas are composed of mesodermal elements, such as bone, cartilage, fat, and muscle. They appear as midline, dorsal, skin-covered masses that are located in the mid-thoracic, thoracolumbar, or lumbar regions and may be associated with cutaneous angiomas. Spina bifida is present in ~60% of patients, and the spinal canal is widened in 80%. Rarely, hamartomas may contain functioning choroid plexus and present with syringohydromyelia (Fig 9.42).

SYRINGOHYDROMYELIA

Definition

Although syringohydromyelia is usually a disease of adults, it can occur in children and, furthermore, is often associated with (and likely the result of) a congenital anomaly of the spine or the cervicomedullary junction. Therefore, I have included the topic in this chapter. Syringohydromyelia is characterized by the presence of longitudinally oriented CSF-filled cavities and gliosis within the spinal cord. When the cavity is a dilated central canal of the spinal cord, the term *hydromyelia* has been applied. The term *syringomyelia* has been reserved for spinal cord cavities extending lateral to, or independent of, the central canal. On detailed pathologic or radiologic examination, most cavities are found to involve both parenchyma and central canal. The term *syringohydromyelia* reflects this difficulty in classification. Some have used the terms *syringomyelia* and *syrinx* in a general manner to represent any spinal cord cyst. I shall use these terms in the same general sense in this chapter, recognizing that in some patients *syringomyelia* is not precisely correct (49,160–162).

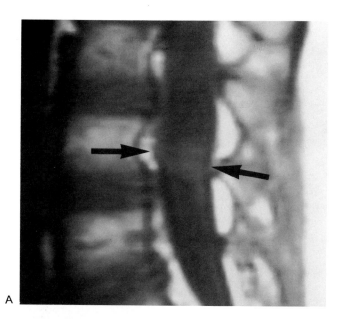

FIG. 9.41. Intraspinal epidermoid. A: Sagittal SE 600/12 image shows no definite abnormality, although some heterogeneity (*arrows*) is present within the canal at the L4 level. B: SE 2500/30 image shows slightly increased intensity (*arrows*) at the L3–L4 level. C: SE 2500/80 image shows hyperintensity (*arrows*), probably secondary to displacement of the cauda equina, at the L3–L5 levels. D, E: Axial SE 600/15 images show the roots of the cauda equina (*arrows*) displaced laterally into a ring around the central epidermoid tumor.

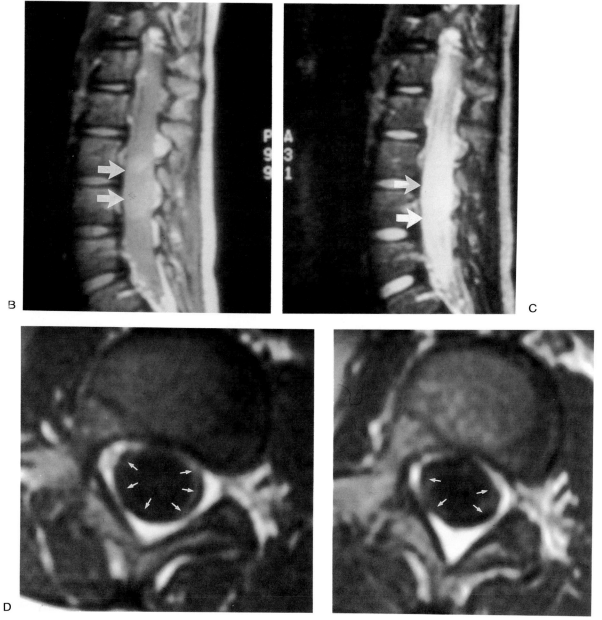

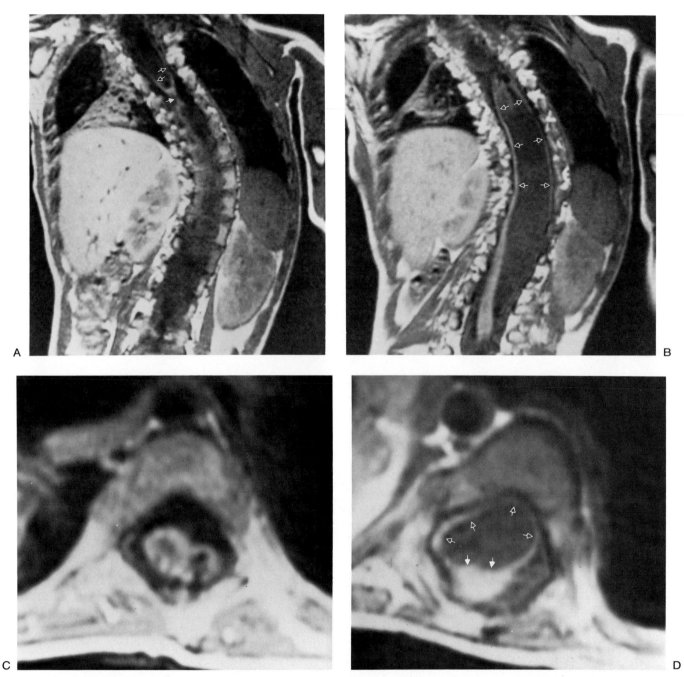

FIG. 9.42. Spinal cord hamartoma with associated syringomyelia. **A, B:** Coronal SE 600/20 images show a dilated spinal cord with CSF intensity within it (*open arrows*), both rostral and caudal to a focal heterogeneous narrowing of the cord at the mid-thoracic level (*closed white arrow*). The hamartoma was located at the site of the narrowing. **C:** Axial SE 1000/20 at the level of the hamartoma shows heterogeneity of signal and a bilobed appearance to the cord resulting from the tumor and the associated syringomyelia. This hamartoma, which contained functioning choroid plexus, is believed to be the cause of the severe syringomyelia. **D:** Axial SE 1000/20 image in the lower thoracic region. The ventral aspect of the spinal cord is markedly thinned and expanded by the syrinx cavity (*open arrows*). The dorsal cord (*closed arrows*) is compressed and displaced posteriorly by the syrinx.

Clinical Presentation and Course

Syringomyelia uncommonly presents in childhood. In children, syringes are most commonly enlarged central canals of the spinal cord (true hydromyelia) and associated with Chiari II (more commonly) or Chiari I (less commonly) malformations (69). Presenting symptoms are similar to those in adults, with anesthesia and weakness of the upper limbs, scoliosis, and unsteadiness of gait (69). Children may also develop dilated central canals in association with the tight filum terminale syndrome. However, the central canal does not seem to be under increased pressure in this group of patients. Therefore, the term *syringomyelia* does not seem appropriate. Children with spinal cord tumors can develop associated syringomyelia or hydromyelia; typically, the syrinx will resolve after resection of the tumor. Spinal cord tumors of childhood are discussed in Chapter 10.

Most commonly, symptoms of syringomyelia begin in late adolescence or early adulthood and progress irregularly with long periods of stability. In traumatic syringo-

myelia, a latent period of 20–30 years is not uncommon before the onset of symptoms is noted (163). The clinical presentation is variable, depending upon the cross-sectional and vertical extent of cord destruction. The classical presentation is of segmental weakness with atrophy of the hands and arms, loss of tendon reflexes, and segmental anesthesia of the dissociative type (loss of pain and temperature sense with preservation of the sense of touch) over the neck, shoulders, and arms (164). Pain is often severe and may be most intense in an analgesic limb (anesthesia dolorosa). In practice, symptoms are often unilateral, confined to the lower extremities, or absent (165,166). The clinical course is equally unpredictable. Long periods of stability of symptoms can be followed by acute deterioration. Lesions at the level of the foramen magnum, such as the Chiari I malformation, arachnoiditis, or a foramen magnum tumor, frequently are present in patients with syringomyelia (166,167). It may be difficult to differentiate symptoms of syringomyelia from those of brain stem compression by the accompanying lesion.

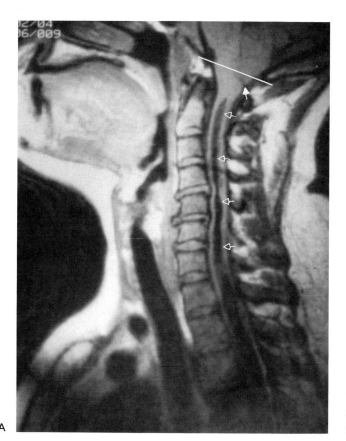 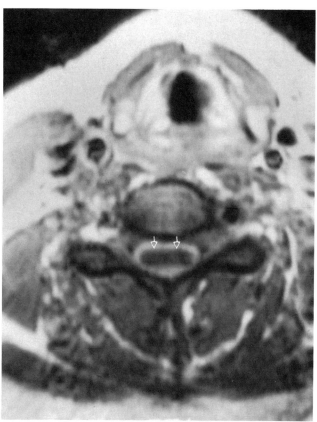

A B

FIG. 9.43. Syringohydromyelia secondary to Chiari I malformation. **A:** A long segment of low attenuation is seen in the center of the dilated spinal cord (*open white arrows*). The patient has a Chiari I malformation with the cerebellar tonsils (*closed white arrow*) extending below the foramen magnum (marked by the white line). **B:** Axial SE 1000/20 image through the cervical spine shows the large syringohydromyelic cavity (*arrows*) causing expansion of the cervical spinal cord.

Causes and Classification

Syringomyelia has many causes, just as cystic spaces in the brain may be of diverse origin. The shape and structure of the spinal cord and spinal canal have a strong influence on the appearance of the syrinx, making the pathologic (and imaging) appearance of the cavities and the clinical signs similar, regardless of the underlying cause (49).

A classification system based upon the way the syrinx communicates with the central canal has been adopted (168). *Communicating* syringomyelia is postulated to communicate with the fourth ventricle via the obex at some time during the development of the spinal cord cyst, allowing fluid transmission to the syrinx cavity via this communication. Thus, communicating syringes should be centrally located; however, in reality, these hydromyelic cavities often dissect into, and are thus eccentric within, the surrounding spinal cord tissue (49,161). Communicating syringomyelia is the form that is associated with the Chiari malformations (Fig. 9.43) and with syndromes with decreased size of the foramen magnum, such as achondroplasia (Fig. 9.44) (169,170). Gardner (171,172) has postulated that continued communication

between the fourth ventricle and central canal is the result of a failure of the foramina of the fourth ventricle to open at the eighth or ninth week of fetal life. He describes a "water hammer effect" (caused by CSF pulsations) that is transmitted to the central canal through the obex, causing the canal to dilate. Rupture of the ependymal lining results in cyst extension into the substance of the spinal cord (Fig. 9.45B). Gardner's theory was modified by Williams (173,174), who favored a pressure differential between the intracranial and spinal cerebrospinal fluid as the cause for formation of the syrinx (Fig. 9.45C). Williams speculated that coughing and other maneuvers that produce increased intrathoracic and intra-abdominal pressure result in spinal epidural venous distention. Distention of the veins within the confined space of the spinal canal causes a rapid rostral displacement of spinal fluid. In patients with the Chiari I malformation or other causes of obstruction within the CSF spaces, the initial surge forces cerebrospinal fluid into the intracranial space; however, the cerebrospinal fluid does not drain out immediately, because of a ball-valve effect that results from the obstructing lesion. The result of the fluid shift is a craniospinal pressure dissociation. The higher intracranial pressure, according to Wil-

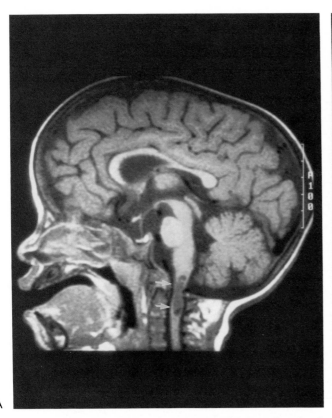

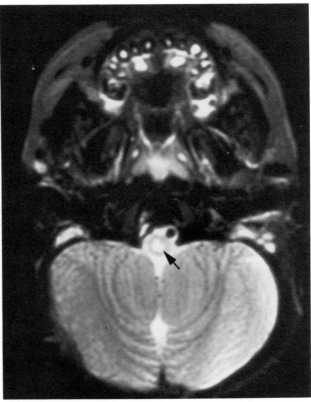

A

B

FIG. 9.44. Syringomyelia secondary to achondroplasia. **A:** Sagittal SE 600/12 image shows small clivus, long infundibulum, and big ventricles, as described in Chapter 8. A focal, well-defined region of hypointensity (*arrows*) is seen extending from the foramen magnum to the bottom of C2. The craniocervical junction is compressed by the narrow foramen magnum. **B:** Axial SE 3000/120 image confirms the intramedullary cyst (*arrow*) at the craniocervical junction.

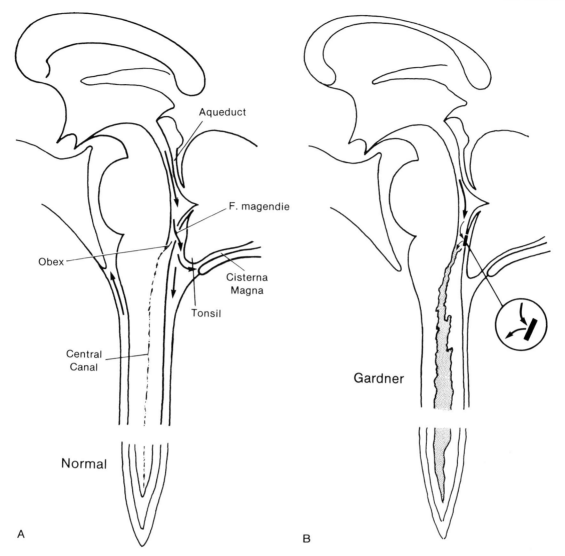

FIG. 9.45. Diagrammatic representations of pathophysiologic theories concerning syringohydromyelia. **A:** In the normal situation, cerebrospinal fluid flows from the aqueduct into the fourth ventricle, out the fourth ventricular foramina and into the cisterna magna, basilar cisterns and spinal subarachnoid space. The central canal of the spinal cord is usually incompletely patent in older children and adults. **B:** Gardner's theory suggests that there is a lack of perforation of the foramen of Magendie (*blocked arrow* in inset) that forces cerebrospinal fluid through the obex into the central canal of the spinal cord.

liams, forces fluid through the obex into the central canal of the spinal cord (173). Furthermore, Williams speculated that the engorgement of the epidural veins by increased thoracoabdominal pressure compresses the subarachnoid space and spinal cord, forcing fluid upward within the syrinx cavity (Fig. 9.45C). If enough fluid is forced upward with sufficient force, the syrinx cavity will be extended. A rapid upward acceleration of contrast within syrinx cavities and in the subarachnoid space has been demonstrated with coughing, Valsalva, and respiration (173,175).

Ball and Dayan (176) have speculated that cerebrospinal fluid enters the central canal via the perivascular spaces of Virchow and Robin. They postulated that in-

creased pressure in the spinal subarachnoid space is generated by an obstructing lesion (such as the ectopic cerebellar tonsils in the Chiari I malformation) that acts as a one-way valve and allows cerebrospinal fluid to escape from the basal cisterns into the spinal canal but blocks its return. They proposed that the increased intraspinal pressure then drives cerebrospinal fluid into the central canal (Fig. 9.45D), resulting in an increased intraspinal CSF pressure compared to the brain.

Aboulker (177) proposed a theory somewhat analogous to that of Ball and Dayan. Referring to animal experiments that demonstrate that 30% of cerebrospinal fluid is produced in the central canal of the cord, he postulated that stenosis at the foramen magnum or else-

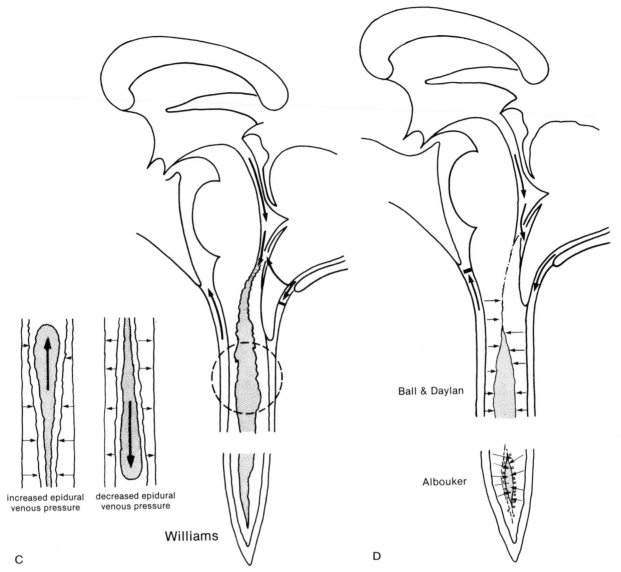

C

increased epidural
venous pressure   decreased epidural
                      venous pressure

Williams

Ball & Daylan

Albouker

D

FIG. 9.45. *(Continued.)* **C:** Williams suggests that there is CSF flow cephalad from the spinal subarachnoid space into the intracranial cisterns but that flow is partially blocked in the cephalo-caudal direction. He suggests that this cranial-spinal pressure association leads to cerebrospinal fluid being "sucked" into the central canal of the cord from the fourth ventricle, initiating the syrinx. He further proposes that the fluid within the syrinx moves both rostrally and caudally as a result of changes in epidural venous pressure; when engorged, these veins compress the subarachnoid space and spinal cord, forcing fluid upward within the syrinx cavity. Rapid accelerations result in extension of the syrinx cavity. **D:** Both Ball and Dayan and Aboulker believe that the craniospinal pressure dissociation is present but reversed in direction from that proposed by Williams. These authors believe that increased CSF pressure in the spinal CSF space results in cerebrospinal fluid filtering from the subarachnoid space into the central canal through the spinal cord.

where in the canal inhibits CSF flow toward intracranial areas of resorption and causes increased CSF pressure in the spinal canal. The cerebrospinal fluid, driven by high intraspinal pressure, then filters into the spinal cord, either through the parenchyma or along the posterior nerve roots. Long-standing spinal cord edema may eventually cause cavitation within the cord parenchyma (Fig. 9.45D).

The other forms of syringomyelia that have been described are *traumatic syringomyelia, tumor-associated syringomyelia, syringomyelia secondary to arachnoiditis,* and *"idiopathic" syringomyelia* (168). Clearly, communication with the fourth ventricle via the obex is not the underlying mechanism of the formation of the syrinx in all cases. However, extension of the cavity within the cord [or even into the brain stem or thalami,

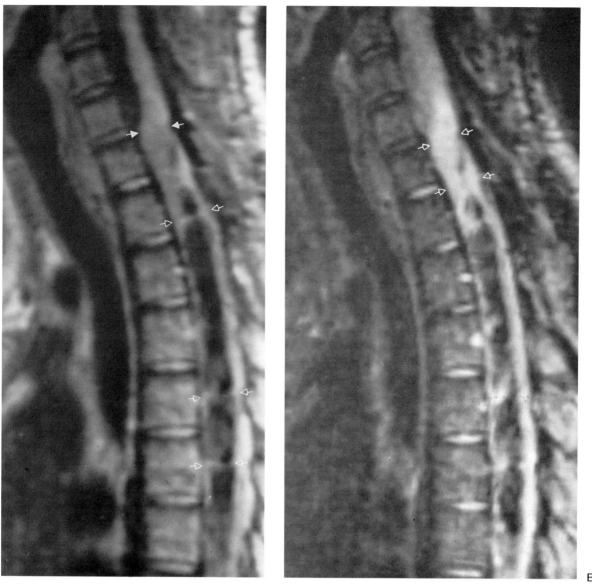

FIG. 9.46. Syringohydromyelia with septations and T2 prolongation in adjacent cord. **A:** Sagittal SE 1500/40 image shows a dilated spinal cord up to approximately the C6 level (*white arrows*) and a large syrinx with multiple septations (*open white arrows*) extending caudally into the thoracic spine. **B:** SE 1500/80 image shows a marked increased signal intensity in the portion of the spinal cord that lies immediately rostral to the syrinx cavity (*arrows*). This was found surgically to be an area of microcystic myelomalacia. The fluid within the syrinx cavity remains low in signal intensity as a result of the pulsatile motion within the cavity.

a condition known as *syringobulbia* (178,179)] may well occur via the same mechanism once the cavity is established. Williams's proposed mechanism of (1) an obstructing lesion causing a pressure dissociation above and below it and (2) extension of the cavities as a result of CSF accelerations from increased thoracoabdominal pressure and distention of the epidural venous plexus (Fig. 9.45C) explains the clinical observation that these cavities frequently extend after severe coughing, straining, or sneezing. Moreover, the observation that foramen magnum decompression often cures the syringomyelia

without any other therapy supports the theory that syringes are primarily caused by disturbed CSF dynamics.

Imaging

MR is the diagnostic modality of choice in the diagnosis and evaluation of treatment of syringohydromyelia and syringobulbia (49,179). To assess syringes properly by standard MR imaging, it is necessary to obtain 3-mm-thick sagittal short TR/TE images, followed by axial, 5-

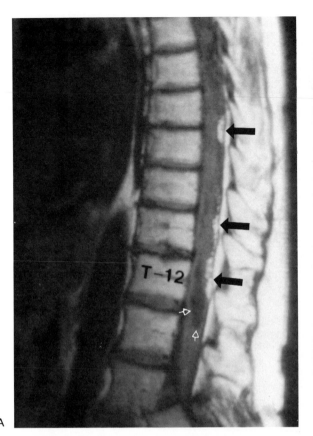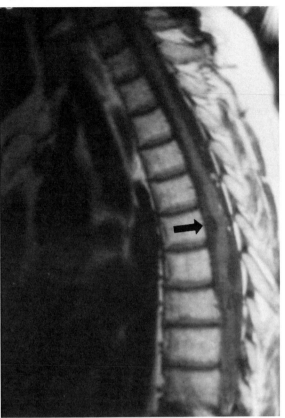

A   B

FIG. 9.47. Syringomyelia resulting from arachnoiditis. **A:** This patient has had a previous pantopaque myelogram. Note the multiple droplets of pantopaque (*black arrows*) layering posteriorly within the subarachnoid space. A syrinx (*open white arrows*) is present within the conus medullaris. **B:** Sagittal SE 600/20 in the upper thoracic spine shows a focal indentation (*arrow*) upon the spinal cord by a CSF loculation. These arachnoidal loculations, which disrupt normal CSF dynamics, are frequently seen in syringomyelia associated with trauma or infection.

mm, short TR/TE images. The syrinx cavity can be missed if only sagittal images are obtained. The syrinx appears on MR images as a CSF-intensity collection within the cord (Figs. 9.43, 9.44, 9.46, 9.47). If the cavity extends into the medulla (Fig. 9.48), syringobulbia is diagnosed. The involved region of spinal cord or medulla is usually enlarged by the process. Often there are multiple incomplete septations within the syrinx cavity, giving a "beaded" appearance (Fig. 9.46). If long TR sequences are used, increased signal intensity may be seen within the parenchyma at the rostral or caudal end of the cavity (Fig. 9.46). This high signal intensity should not be misinterpreted as tumor; the prolonged T2 relaxation time results from microcystic or gliotic changes at the end of the syrinx cavity, presumably caused by the pulsations of the cyst upon the adjacent cord. If flow compensation techniques are not used, the syrinx cavity may have a low signal intensity on long TR/TE sequences (Fig. 9.46) as a result of CSF pulsations within the cavity (49,180). If CT myelography is used to evaluate the spinal cord in these patients (only if MR is unavailable or contraindicated), it is necessary to obtain delayed images to visual-

ize the cavity. The patient should be scanned 4 hours after infusion of the water-soluble contrast. After 4 hours, contrast will usually have diffused into the cavity. If a syrinx is suspected clinically and it is not detected on the initial scan or the 4-hour delayed scan, a 12-hour delayed or even a 24-hour delayed scan should be obtained. Even with delayed imaging, however, CT myelography is much less sensitive to syringomyelia and does not show the rostral and caudal extent as well as MR.

Syringes can be eccentric within the spinal cord, even exophytic, in all forms of syringomyelia (Fig. 9.42) (37). In less severe cases, differentiation is made by examining consecutive axial images and seeing progressive eccentricity of the cyst and thinning of the cord peripheral to the cyst. When it is very eccentric or very large, the remnant of compressed spinal cord peripheral to the syrinx cavity may be impossible to see on an MR scan; therefore, the syrinx may be impossible to differentiate from an arachnoid cyst. In practice, the differentiation is not important for the treating physician, however.

Techniques have been developed that allow assessment of CSF flow in the cerebral ventricles and at the

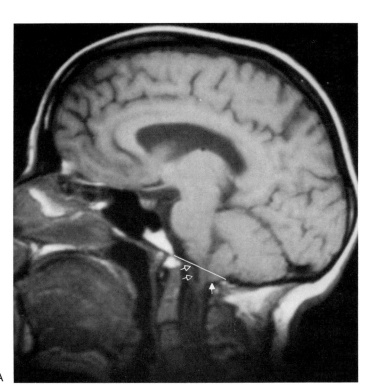

A

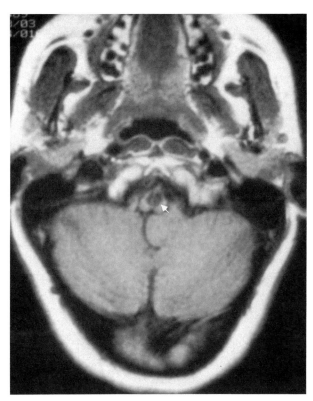

B

FIG. 9.48. Syringobulbia. **A:** Sagittal SE 600/20 image of the brain shows the cerebellar tonsils (*arrow*) extending below the foramen magnum (Chiari I malformation). Syringohydromyelia is present in the spinal cord. Additionally, there is a curvilinear area of low attenuation (*open arrows*) within the medulla. **B:** Axial SE 600/20 image through the medulla shows the area of low attenuation (*arrow*) to be within the medulla. This is a classic appearance for syringobulbia.

foramen magnum by phase contrast MR (181–183). The technique currently used at UCSF, and illustrated in Fig. 9.49, is described in Chapter 1. Using this technique, flow dynamics of cerebrospinal fluid through the foramen magnum or past an obstructive lesion within the spinal canal can be evaluated and quantified. It has been demonstrated that the foramen magnum obstruction in Chiari I malformations is reduced when the head is in extension (184). Therefore, all CSF flow studies should be performed with the patient's head flexed.

Static MR imaging and MR CSF flow studies can also be used to assess the foramen magnum after decompression. The MR appearance of the decompressed foramen magnum is that of a widened foramen; the posterior margin of the foramen is located high above its normal position secondary to removal of bone. Some "kinking" of the cervicomedullary junction and "slumping" of the cerebellum into the enlarged foramen magnum is commonly seen (185,186). Some CSF should be seen anterior to the cervicomedullary junction and posterior to the cerebellum at all levels. The CSF flow study should show unimpeded flow through the foramen with the head in the flexed position.

In all patients in whom a syrinx is discovered radiologically, a search should be made for the underlying cause

of the syrinx. First, the foramen magnum should be evaluated; the position of the cerebellar tonsils should be noted. The tonsils should lie no more than 5 mm below the level of the foramen magnum as measured on sagittal images (187,188) (see Chapter 5 for a more detailed discussion of tonsillar ectopia). MR of the craniocervical junction may also show stenosis of the foramen magnum (as in achondroplasia), masses at the level of the foramen magnum (such as schwannomas and meningiomas), or arachnoidal adhesions. Any mass or narrowing can cause craniospinal pressure dissociation. If arachnoiditis, either from previous trauma or from infection, is the cause of syringohydromyelia, arachnoid loculations can usually be identified at some point within the spinal canal. Although the loculations are isointense with free-flowing cerebrospinal fluid, they can be identified by their mass effect upon the spinal cord (Fig. 9.47). The cord will be slightly displaced and deformed by adjacent loculations.

As mentioned earlier in this section, mild dilatation of the central canal is seen by MR in up to 25% of patients with a tethered spinal cord (Figs. 9.18, 9.25) (46). The exact cause of this dilatation is not known. However, in these patients, the mild dilatation of the central canal is not felt to be significant and the cause of the tethering

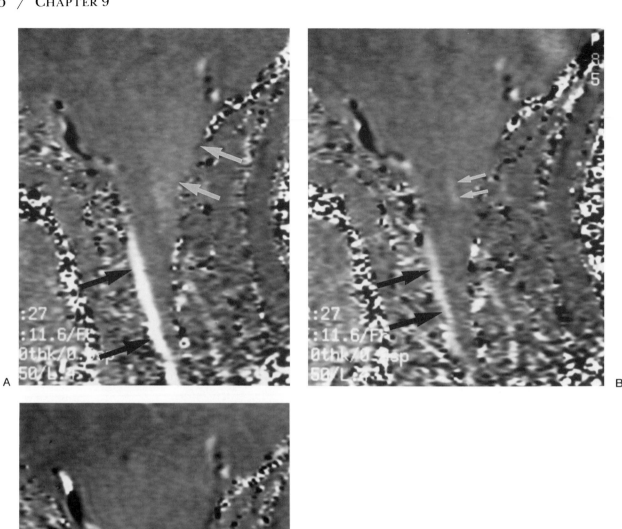

A

B

C

FIG. 9.49. Phase contrast CSF flow study in a patient with Chiari I and syringohydromyelia. Flow sensitivity is in the superior–inferior plane. **A:** In early systole, the cerebrospinal fluid in the ventral cervical subarachnoid space (*black arrows*) is moving caudally and therefore gives high signal intensity. No flow is seen at the foramen magnum or dorsal cervical subarachnoid space. The cerebellar tonsils (*white arrows*) are also slightly high in intensity, indicating that they are moving caudally also. **B:** Later in systole, flow is slower in the subarachnoid space (*black arrows*). Flow through the foramen of Magendie is shown by the white arrows. **C:** In diastole, flow in the cervical subarachnoid space (*black arrows*) and the foramen of Magendie (*white arrows*) moves rostrally.

should be dealt with primarily. Only if symptoms persist after the release of the tethered cord should the dilated central canal be evaluated further.

If patients do not have a known history of prior severe trauma and an obstructing lesion cannot be demonstrated, they should be studied by MR with intravenous contrast. A significant number of patients who have previously been labeled as having "idiopathic" syringomyelia have been shown to harbor small spinal cord neoplasms by contrast-enhanced MR. Moreover, a small but significant number of patients with syringomyelia and cerebellar tonsillar ectopia (the Chiari I malformation) have spinal cord neoplasms as well (49). Such patients will not improve unless the neoplasm, which is the primary cause of their syrinx, is treated. If the patient has not improved after foramen magnum decompression, paramagnetic contrast should always be given on the follow-up MR scan.

REFERENCES

1. Golden J, Chernoff G. Intermittent pattern of neural tube closure in two strains of mice. *Teratology* 1993;47:73–80.
2. O'Rahilly R, Müller F. *Neurulation in the normal human embryo.* Presented at: CIBA Foundation Symposium No. 181, May 1993.
3. Van Allen M, Kalousek D, Chernoff G, et al. Evidence for multisite closure of the neural tube in humans. *Am J Med Genet* 1993;47:723–743.
4. Muller F, O'Rahilly R. The first appearance of the human nervous system at stage 8. *Anat Embryol* 1981;163:1–13.
5. Muller F, O'Rahilly R. The first appearance of the major divisions of the human brain at stage 9. *Anat Embryol* 1983;168:419–432.
6. Muller F, O'Rahilly R. The first appearance of the neural tube and optic primordium in the human embryo at stage 10. *Anat Embryol* 1985;172:157–169.
7. Muller F, O'Rahilly R. The development of the human brain and the closure of the rostral neuropore at stage 11. *Anat Embryol* 1986;175:205–222.
8. Muller F, O'Rahilly R. The development of the human brain, the closure of the caudal neuropore, and the beginning of secondary neurulation at stage 12. *Anat Embryol* 1987;176:413–430.
9. Naidich TP, McLone DG, Harwood-Nash DC. Spinal dysraphism. In: Newton TH, Potts DG, eds. *Modern neuroradiology,* vol. 1: *Computed tomography of the spine and spinal cord.* San Anselmo, CA: Clavedel, 1983:299–353.
10. Muller F, O'Rahilly R. The first appearance of the future cerebral hemispheres in the human embryo at stage 14. *Anat Embryol* 1988;177:495–511.
11. Moe JH, Winter RB, Bradford DS, et al. *Scoliosis and other spinal deformities.* Philadelphia: WB Saunders, 1978.
12. Sensenig EC. The early development of the meninges of the spinal cord in human embryos. *Contrib Embryol* 1951;34:147–157.
13. McLone DG. The subarachnoid space: a review. *Childs Brain* 1980;6:113–130.
14. Naidich TP, McLone DG, Mutleur S. A new understanding of dorsal dysraphism with lipoma (lipomyeloschisis): radiological evaluation and surgical correction. *Am J Neuroradiol* 1983;4:103–116.
15. Warf BC, Scott RM, Barnes PD, Hendren WH III. Tethered spinal cord in patients with anorectal and urogenital malformations. *Pediatr Neurosurg* 1993;19:25–30.
16. Chestnut R, James HE, Jones KL. The VATER association and spinal dysraphia. *Pediatr Neurosurg* 1992;18:144–148.
17. Ulmer JL, Elster AD, Ginsberg LE, Williams DW III. Klippel-Feil syndrome: CT and MR of acquired and congenital abnormalities of cervical spine and cord. *J Comput Assist Tomogr* 1993;17:215–224.
18. Barkovich AJ, Raghavan N, Chuang SH. MR of lumbosacral agenesis. *Am J Neuroradiol* 1989;10:1223–1231.
19. Schut L, Pizzi FJ, Bruce DA. Occult spinal dysraphism. In: McLaurin RL, eds. *Myelomeningocele.* New York: Grune & Stratton, 1977:349–368.
20. French BN. The embryology of spinal dysraphism. *Clin Neurosurg* 1983;30:295–340.
21. Anderson FM. Occult spinal dysraphism: diagnosis and management. *J Pediatr* 1968;73:163–178.
22. Korsvik HE, Keller MS. Sonography of occult dysraphism in neonates and infants with MR imaging correlation. *Radiographics* 1992;12:297–306.
23. Algra PR, Hageman LM. Gadopentate dimeglumine-enhanced MR imaging of spinal dermal sinus tract. *Am J Neuroradiol* 1991;12:1025–1026.
24. Altman NR, Altman DH. MR imaging of spinal dysraphism. *Am J Neuroradiol* 1987;8:533–538.
25. Aoki S, Machida T, Sasaki Y, et al. Enterogenous cyst of cervical spine: clinical and radiological aspects (including CT and MR). *Neuroradiology* 1987;29:291–293.
26. Arredondo F, Haughton VM, Hemmy DC, Zeleya B, Williams AL. The computed tomography appearance of diastematomyelia. *Radiology* 1980;136:685–688.
27. Awwad EE, Backer R, Archer CR. The imaging of an intraspinal cervical dermoid tumor by MR, CT, and sonography. *Comput Radiol* 1987;11:169–173.
28. Barkovich AJ, Edwards MSB, Cogen PH. MR evaluation of spinal dermal sinus tracts in children. *Am J Neuroradiol* 1991;12:123–129.
29. Brooks BS, Duvall ER, El Gammal T, Garcia JH, Gupta KL, Kapila A. Neuroimaging features of neurenteric cysts: analysis of nine cases and review of the literature. *Am J Neuroradiol* 1993;14:735–746.
30. Brunberg JA, Di Pietro MA, Venes JL, et al. Intramedullary lesions of the pediatric spinal cord: correlation of findings from MR imaging, intraoperative sonography, surgery, and histologic study. *Radiology* 1991;181:573–579.
31. Davis PC, Hoffman JC Jr, Ball TI, et al. Spinal abnormalities in pediatric patients: MR imaging findings compared with clinical, myelographic, and surgical findings. *Radiology* 1988;166:679–685.
32. DiPietro MA. The conus medullaris: normal US findings throughout childhood. *Radiology* 1993;188:149–153.
33. Gryspeerdt GL. Myelographic assessment of occult forms of spinal dysraphism. *Acta Radiol* 1963;1:702–717.
34. Gusnard DA, Naidich TP, Yousefzadeh DK, Haughton VM. Ultrasonic anatomy of the normal neonatal and infant spine: correlation with cryomicrotome sections and CT. *Neuroradiology* 1986;28:493–511.
35. Hall WA, Albright AL, Brunberg JA. Diagnosis of tethered cords by magnetic resonance imaging. *Surg Neurol* 1988;30:60–64.
36. Harwood-Nash DC, Fitz CR, Resjo M, Chuang S. Congenital spinal and cord lesions in children and computed tomographic metrizamide myelography. *Neuroradiology* 1978;16:69–70.
37. Heinz ER, Curnes J, Friedman A, Oakes J. Exophytic syrinx, an extreme form of syringomyelia: CT, myelographic, and MR imaging features. *Radiology* 1992;183:243–246.
38. Hilal SK, Marton D, Pollack E. Diastematomyelia in children: radiographic study of 34 cases. *Radiology* 1974;112:609–621.
39. Lantos F, Epstein F, Kory LA. MR imaging of intradural spinal lipoma. *Neurosurgery* 1987;20:469–472.
40. Lee K, Gower DJ, McWhorter JM, Albertson DA. The role of MR imaging in the diagnosis and treatment of anterior sacral meningocele. *J Neurosurg* 1988;69:628–631.
41. Naidich TP, Fernbeck SK, McLone DG, Shkolnik A. John Caffey Award. Sonography of the caudal spine and back: congenital anomalies in children. *Am J Neuroradiol* 1984;5:221–234.
42. Naidich TP, Doundoulakis SH, Poznanski AK. Intraspinal masses: efficacy of plain spine radiography. *Pediatr Neurosci* 1985–1986;12:10–17.
43. Naidich TP, Radkowsky MA, Britton J. Real time sonographic display of caudal spine anomalies. *Neuroradiology* 1986;28:512–527.
44. Peacock WJ, Murovic JA. Magnetic resonance imaging in myelocystoceles: report of two cases. *J Neurosurg* 1989;70:804–807.

45. Quencer RM, Montalvo BM, Naidich TP, Donovan Post MJ. Intraoperative sonography in spinal dysraphism and syringohydromyelia. *Am J Neuroradiol* 1987;8:329–337.
46. Raghavan N, Barkovich AJ, Edwards MS, Norman D. MR imaging in the tethered cord syndrome. *Am J Neuroradiol* 1989;10: 27–36.
47. Samuelsson L, Bergstrom K, Thomas KA, Hemmingson A, Wallensten R. MR imaging of syringohydromyelia and Chiari malformations in myelomeningocele patients with scoliosis. *Am J Neuroradiol* 1987;8:539–546.
48. Scotti G, Musgrave MA, Harwood-Nash DC, Fitz CR, Chuang SH. Diastematomyelia in children: metrizamide and CT metrizamide myelography. *Am J Neuroradiol* 1980;1:403–410.
49. Sherman JL, Barkovich AJ, Citrin CM. The MR appearance of syringohydromyelia: new observations. *Am J Neuroradiol* 1986;7:985–995.
50. Sigal R, Denys A, Halimi P, Shapiro L, Doyon D, Boudghene F. Ventriculus terminalis of the conus medullaris: MR imaging in four patients with congenital dilatation. *Am J Neuroradiol* 1991;12:733–737.
51. Tadmore R, Davis KR, Roberson G, Chapman PH. The diagnosis of diastematomyelia by computed tomography. *Surg Neurol* 1977;8:434–436.
52. Uchino A, Mori T, Ohno M. Thickened fatty filum terminale: MR imaging. *Neuroradiology* 1991;33:331–333.
53. Wilson DA, Prince JR. MR imaging determination of the location of the normal conus medullaris throughout childhood. *Am J Roentgenol* 1989;152:1029–1032.
54. McLone DG, Knepper PA. Role of complex carbohydrates and neurulation. *Pediatr Neurosci* 1985–1986;12:2–9.
55. Pigott H. The natural history of scoliosis in myelodysplasia. *J Bone Joint Surg [Br]* 1980;62B:54–58.
56. Hoppenfeld S. Congenital kyphosis in myelomeningocele. *J Bone Joint Surg [Br]* 1967;49:276–280.
57. Cameron AH. The Arnold-Chiari and other neuroanatomical malformations associated with spina bifida. *J Pathol Bacteriol* 1957;73:195–211.
58. Emery JL, Lendon RG. The local cord lesion in neurospinal dysraphism (meningomyelocele). *J Pathol* 1973;110:83–96.
59. Pang D. Split cord malformation: part II: clinical syndrome. *Neurosurgery* 1992;31:481–500.
60. Duckworth T, Sharrard WJ, Lister J, Seymour N. Hemimyelocele. *Dev Med Child Neurol* 1968;10(suppl 16):69–75.
61. McLone DG, Dias MS. Complications of myelomeningocele closure. *Pediatr Neurosurg* 1991–1992;17:267–273.
62. McLone DG, Herman JM, Gabrieli AP, Dias L. Tethered cord as a cause of scoliosis in children with a myelomeningocele. *Pediatr Neurosurg* 1990–1991;16:8–13.
63. Levy LM, DiChiro G, McCullough DC, Dwyer AJ, Johnson DL, Yang SSL. Fixed spinal cord: diagnosis with MR imaging. *Radiology* 1988;169:773–778.
64. Chadduck WM, Roloson GJ. Dermoid of the filum terminale of a newborn with myelomeningocele. *Pediatr Neurosurg* 1993;19: 81–83.
65. Halcrow SJ, Crawford PJ, Craft AW. Epidermoid spinal cord tumor after lumbar puncture. *Arch Dis Child* 1985;60:978–979.
66. Kirsch WM, Hodges FJ III. An intramedullary epidermal inclusion cyst of the thoracic cord associated with a previously repaired meningocele. *J Neurosurg* 1966;24:1018–1020.
67. Scott RM, Wolpert SM, Bartoshesky LE, Zimbler S, Klauber GT. Dermoid tumors occurring at the site of previous myelomeningocele repair. *J Neurosurg* 1986;65:779–783.
68. Vion-Drury J, Vincentelli F, Jiddane M, et al. MR imaging of epidermoid cysts. *Neuroradiology* 1987;29:333–338.
69. Hoffman HJ, Neil J, Crone KR, et al. Hydrosyringomyelia and its management in childhood. *Neurosurgery* 1987;21:347–351.
70. Hall PV, Lindseth R, Campbell R, Kalsbeck JE, Desousa A. Scoliosis and hydrocephalus in myelocele patients; the effects of ventricular shunting. *J Neurosurg* 1979;50:174–178.
71. Hall PV, Campbell RL, Kalsbeck JE. Meningomyelocele and progressive hydromyelia: progressive paresis in myelodysplasia. *J Neurosurg* 1975;43:457–463.
72. Batnitzky S, Hall PV, Lindseth RE, Wellman HN. Meningomyelocele and syringohydromyelia: some radiologic aspects. *Radiology* 1976;120:351–357.
73. Barnes PD, Brody JD, Jaramillo D, Akbar JU, Emans JB. Atypical idiopathic scoliosis: MR imaging evaluation. *Radiology* 1993;186:247–253.
74. Nokes SR, Murtaugh FR, Jones JD III, et al. Childhood scoliosis: MR imaging. *Radiology* 1987;164:791–797.
75. McLone DG, Knepper PA. The cause of Chiari II malformation: a unified theory. *Pediatr Neurosci* 1989;15:1–12.
76. MacKenzie NG, Emery JL. Deformities of the cervical cord in children with neurospinal dysraphism. *Dev Med Child Neurol* 1971;25[suppl]:58–67.
77. Naidich TP, McLone DG, Fulling KH. The Chiari II malformation, part IV: the hindbrain deformity. *Neuroradiology* 1983;25: 179–197.
78. Wolpert SM, Anderson M, Scott RM, Kwan ES, Runge VM. The Chiari II malformation: MR imaging evaluation. *Am J Neuroradiol* 1987;8:783–791.
79. Variend S, Emery JL. Cervical dislocation of the cerebellum in children with meningomyelocele. *Teratology* 1976;13:281–290.
80. Emery JL, MacKenzie N. Medullo-cervical dislocation deformity (Chiari II deformity) related to neurospinal dysraphism (meningomyelocele). *Brain* 1973;96:155–164.
81. Daniel PM, Strich SJ. Some observations on the congenital deformity of the central nervous system known as the Arnold-Chiari malformation. *J Neuropathol Exp Neurol* 1958;17:256–266.
82. Wright RL. Congenital dermal sinuses. *Prog Neurol Surg* 1971;4: 175–191.
83. Haworth JC, Zachary RB. Congenital dermal sinuses in children: their relation to pilonidal sinuses. *Lancet* 1955;2:10–14.
84. Walker AE, Bucy PC. Congenital dermal sinuses: source of spinal meningeal infection and subdural abscesses. *Brain* 1934;57:401–421.
85. Mount LA. Congenital dermal sinuses as a cause of meningitis, intraspinal abscess and intracranial abscess. *JAMA* 1949;139: 1263–1268.
86. Bean JR, Walsh JW, Blacker HM. Cervical dermal sinus and intramedullary spinal cord abscess: case report. *Neurosurgery* 1979;5:60–62.
87. Scotti G, Harwood-Nash DC, Hoffman HJ. Congenital thoracic dermal sinus: diagnosis by computer assisted metrizamide myelography. *J Comput Assist Tomogr* 1980;4:675–677.
88. Schwartz HG. Congenital tumors of the spinal cord in infants. *Ann Surg* 1952;136:183–192.
89. Matson DD. *Neurosurgery of infancy and childhood,* 2nd ed. Springfield, IL: Charles C Thomas, 1969.
90. Friede RL. *Developmental neuropathology,* 2nd ed. Berlin: Springer-Verlag, 1989.
91. Harwood-Nash DC, Fitz CR. Normal spine, abnormal spine, myelography, mass lesions of the spinal canal. In: Harwood-Nash DC, Fitz CR, eds. *Neuroradiology in infants and children.* St Louis: CV Mosby, 1976:1054–1227.
92. List CF. Intraspinal epidermoids, dermoids, and dermal sinuses. *Surg Gynecol Obstet* 1941;73:525–538.
93. Guidetti B, Gagliardo FM. Epidermoid and dermoid cysts: clinical evaluation and late surgical results. *J Neurosurg* 1977;47:12–18.
94. Emery JL, Lendon RG. Lipomas of the cauda equina and other fatty tumors related to neurospinal dysraphism. *Dev Med Child Neurol* 1969;11[suppl 20]:62–70.
95. Ehni G, Love JG. Intraspinal lipomas: report of cases, review of the literature, and clinical and pathologic study. *Arch Neurol Psychiatr* 1945;53:1–28.
96. Leveuf JB. Spina bifida avec tumeur. In: Leveuf J, ed. *Études sur le spina bifida.* Paris: Masson, 1937:93–106.
97. Chapman PH. Congenital intraspinal lipomas: anatomic considerations and surgical treatment. *Childs Brain* 1982;9:37–47.
98. Guiffre R. Intradural spinal lipomas: review of the literature (99 cases) and report of an additional one. *Acta Neurochir* 1966;14: 69–95.
99. Knierim DS, Wacker M, Peckham N, Bedros AA. Lumbosacral intramedullary myolipoma. *J Neurosurg* 1987;66:457–459.
100. Dubowitz V, Lorber J, Zachary RB. Lipoma of the cauda equina. *Arch Dis Child* 1965;40:207–213.
101. Schroeder S, Lackner K, Weiand G. Lumbosacral intradural lipoma. *J Comput Assist Tomogr* 1981;5:274.

102. Jones PH, Love JG. Tight filum terminale. *Arch Surg* 1956;73: 556–566.
103. McLone DG, Mutleur S, Naidich TP. Lipomeningoceles of the conus medullaris. In: American Society for Pediatric Neurosurgeons, eds. *Concepts in pediatric neurosurgery,* vol. 3. Basel: Karger, 1983:170–177.
104. Villarejo FJ, Blazquez MG, Gutierrez-Diaz JA. Intraspinal lipomas in children. *Childs Brain* 1976;2:361–370.
105. Lemire RJ, Graham CB, Beckwith JB. Skin-covered sacrococcygeal masses in infants and children. *J Pediatr* 1971;79:948–954.
106. Bruce DA, Schut L. Spinal lipomas in infancy and childhood. *Childs Brain* 1979;5:192–203.
107. Gold LH, Kieffer SA, Peterson HO. Lipomatous invasion of the spinal cord associated with spinal dysraphism: myelographic evaluation. *Am J Roentgenol* 1969;107:479–485.
108. Barson AJ. The vertebral level of termination of the spinal cord during normal and abnormal development. *J Anat* 1970;106: 489–497.
109. James CCM, Lassman LP. *Spinal dysraphism: spina bifida occulta.* New York: Appleton-Century-Crofts, 1972.
110. McLendon RE, Oakes WJ, Heinz ER, Yeates AE, Burger PC. Adipose tissue in the filum terminale: a CT finding that may indicate tethering of the spinal cord. *Neurosurgery* 1988;22:873–876.
111. Holtzman RN, Stein BM. *The tethered spinal cord.* New York: Thieme-Stratton, 1985.
112. Pang D, Wilberger JE Jr. Tethered cord syndrome in adults. *J Neurosurg* 1982;57:32–37.
113. Pang D. Tethered cord syndrome in adults. In: Holtzman RNN, Stein BM, eds. *The tethered spinal cord.* New York: Thieme-Stratton, 1985:99–115.
114. Pang D, Hoffman HJ. Sacral agenesis with progressive neurological deficit. *Neurosurgery* 1980;7:118–126.
115. Love JG, Daly DD, Harris LE. Tight filum terminale: report of condition in three siblings. *JAMA* 1961;176:31–33.
116. Hendrick EB, Hoffman HJ, Humphreys RP. The tethered spinal cord. *Clin Neurosurg* 1983;30:457–463.
117. Tani S, Yamada S, Knighton RS. Extensibility of the lumbar and sacral cord. Pathophysiology of the tethered spinal cord in cats. *J Neurosurg* 1987;66:116–123.
118. Hendrick EB, Hoffman HJ, Humphreys RP. Tethered cord syndrome. In: McLaurin RL, ed. *Myelomeningocele.* New York: Grune & Stratton, 1977:369–376.
119. Kallen B, Winberg J. Caudal mesoderm pattern of anomalies: from renal agenesis to sirenomelia. *Teratology* 1974;9:99–112.
120. Passarge E. Congenital malformations and maternal diabetes. *Lancet* 1965;1:324–325.
121. Rusnak SL, Driscoll SG. Congenital spinal anomalies in infants of diabetic mothers. *Pediatrics* 1965;35:989–995.
122. McLone DG, Naidich TP. Terminal myelocystocele. *Neurosurgery* 1985;16:36–43.
123. Vade A, Kennard D. Lipomyelomeningocystocele. *Am J Neuroradiol* 1987;8:375–377.
124. Naidich TP, McLone DG. Congenital pathology of the spine and spinal cord. In: Taveras JM, Ferrucci JT, eds. *Radiology,* vol. 3. Philadelphia: JB Lippincott, 1986:1–23.
125. Sherman RM, Caylor HD, Long L. Anterior sacral meningocele. *Am J Surg* 1950;79:743–747.
126. Dyck P, Wilson CB. Anterior sacral meningocele: case report. *J Neurosurg* 1980;53:548–552.
127. Schey WL, Shkolnik A, White H. Clinical and radiographic considerations of sacrococcygeal teratomas. An analysis of 26 new cases and review of the literature. *Radiology* 1977;125:189–195.
128. Noseworthy J, Luck EE, Kozakewich HPW. Sacrococcygeal germ cell tumor in childhood: an updated experience with 113 patients. *J Pediatr Surg* 1981;16:358–364.
129. Altman RP, Randolph JG, Lilly JR. Sacrococcygeal teratoma. *J Pediatr Surg* 1973;9:389–398.
130. Burrows FGO, Sutcliffe J. The split notochord syndrome. *Br J Radiol* 1968;41:844–847.
131. Bentley JFR, Smith JR. Developmental posterior enteric remnants and spinal malformations: the split notochord syndrome. *Arch Dis Child* 1960;35:76–86.
132. Hoffman CH, Dietrich RB, Pais MJ, Demos DS, Pribram HFW. The split notochord syndrome with dorsal enteric fistula. *Am J Neuroradiol* 1993;14:622–627.
133. Beardmore HE, Wigglesworth FW. Vertebral anomalies and alimentary duplications: clinical and embryological aspects. *Pediatr Clin North Am* 1958;5:457–473.
134. Pang D, Dias MS, Ahab-Barmada M. Split cord malformation, part I: a unified theory of embryogenesis for double spinal cord malformations. *Neurosurgery* 1992;31:451–480.
135. D'Almeida AC, Steward DJ Jr. Neurenteric cyst: case report and literature review. *Neurosurgery* 1981;8:596–599.
136. Harris CP, Dias MS, Brockmeyer DL, Townsend JJ, Willis BK, Apfelbaum RI. Neurenteric cysts of the posterior fossa: recognition, management, and embryogenesis. *Neurosurgery* 1991;29: 893–897.
137. LeDoux MS, Faye-Petersen OM, Aronin PA, Vaid YN, Pitts RM. Lumbosacral neurenteric cyst in an infant. *J Neurosurg* 1993;78: 821–825.
138. Han JS, Benson JE, Kaufman B, et al. Demonstration of diastematomyelia and associated abnormalities with MR imaging. *Am J Neuroradiol* 1985;6:215–219.
139. James CCM, Lassman LP. Diastematomyelia: a critical survey of 24 cases submitted to laminectomy. *Arch Dis Child* 1964;39:125–130.
140. Guthkelch AN. Diastematomyelia with median septum. *Brain* 1974;97:729–742.
141. Cohen J, Sledge CB. Diastematomyelia: an embryological interpretation with report of a case. *Am J Dis Child* 1960;100:257–263.
142. Rilleit B, Schowing J, Berney J. Pathogenesis of diastematomyelia: can a surgical model in the chick embryo give some clues about the human malformation? *Childs Nerv Syst* 1992;8:310–316.
143. Keim HA, Greene AF. Diastematomyelia and scoliosis. *J Bone Joint Surg [Am]* 1973;55A:1425–1435.
144. Gower DJ, Curling OD, Kelly DL Jr, Alexander E Jr. Diastematomyelia—a 40 year experience. *Pediatr Neurosci* 1988;14: 90–96.
145. Mathieu JP, Dube J. Diastematomyelia and diplomyelia. In: Myrianthopoulos NC, ed. *Malformations.* Amsterdam: Elsevier, 1987:435–442.
146. Wolf AL, Tubman DE, Seljeskog EL. Diastematomyelia of the cervical spinal cord with tethering in an adult. *Neurosurgery* 1987;21:94–97.
147. Beyerl BD, Ojemann RG, Davis KR, Hedley-Whyte ET, Mayberg MR. Cervical diastematomyelia presenting in adulthood. *J Neurosurg* 1985;62:449–453.
148. Naidich TP, Harwood-Nash DC. Diastematomyelia: hemicord and meningeal sheaths; single and double arachnoid and dural tubes. *Am J Neuroradiol* 1983;4:633–636.
149. Schlesinger AE, Naidich TP, Quencer RM. Concurrent hydromyelia and diastematomyelia. *Am J Neuroradiol* 1986;7:473–477.
150. Kaffenberger DA, Heinz ER, Oakes JW, Boyko O. Meningocele manqué: radiologic findings with clinical correlation. *Am J Neuroradiol* 1992;13:1083–1088.
151. Lassman LP, James CCM. Meningocele manqué. *Childs Brain* 1977;3:1–11.
152. Erkulvrawatr S, El Gammal T, Hawkins J, Green JB, Srinivasan G. Intrathoracic meningoceles and neurofibromatosis. *Arch Neurol* 1979;36:557–559.
153. Bunner R. Lateral intrathoracic meningocele. *Acta Radiol* 1959;51:1–9.
154. Mahboubi S, Schut L. Decrease in size of intrathoracic meningocele after insertion of a ventriculovenous shunt. *Pediatr Radiol* 1977;5:178–180.
155. Rosenbaum TJ, Loule EH, Onofrio BM. Teratomatous cyst of the spinal canal. *J Neurosurg* 1978;49:292–297.
156. Lemire RJ, Loeser JD, Leech RW, Alvord EC. *Normal and abnormal development of the human nervous system.* Hagarstown, MD: Harper & Row, 1975.
157. Pickens JM, Wilson J, Myers GG, Frunnet MD. Teratoma of the spinal cord: case report and review of the literature. *Arch Pathol* 1975;99:446–448.
158. Van Gilder JC, Schwartz HG. Growth of dermoids from skin implants to the nervous system and surrounding spaces of the newborn rat. *J Neurosurg* 1967;26:14–20.
159. Tibbs PA, James HE, Rorke LB, Schut L, Bruce DA. Midline

hamartomas masquerading as meningomyeloceles or teratomas in the newborn infant. *J Pediatr* 1976;89:928–933.

160. Peerless SJ, Durward QU. Management of syringomyelia: a pathophysiologic approach. *Clin Neurosurg* 1983;30:531–576.

161. Larroche J-C. Malformations of the nervous system. In: Adams JH, Corsellis J, Duchin EW, eds. *Greenfield's neuropathology.* New York: Wiley, 1984:396–402.

162. Harwood-Nash DC, Fitz CR. Myelography and syringohydromyelia in infancy and childhood. *Radiology* 1974;113:661–669.

163. Rossier AB, Foo D, Shillito J, Dyro FM. Posttraumatic cervical syringomyelia. *Brain* 1985;108:439–461.

164. Adams RD, Victor M. *Principles of neurology.* New York: McGraw-Hill, 1981.

165. Schlesinger EB, Antunes JL, Michelsen WJ, Louis KM. Hydromyelia: clinical presentation and comparison of modalities of treatment. *Neurosurgery* 1981;9:356–365.

166. Logue V, Edwards MR. Syringomyelia and its surgical treatment—an analysis of 75 patients. *J Neurol Neurosurg Psychiatry* 1981;44:273–284.

167. Saez RJ, Onofrio BM, Yanigihara T. Experience with the Arnold Chiari malformation 1960–1970. *J Neurosurg* 1976;45:416–422.

168. Barnett MJM. The epilogue. In: Barnett MJM, Foster JB, Hudgson P, eds. *Syringomyelia.* London: WB Saunders, 1973:302–313.

169. Hecht JT, Butler IJ. Neurologic morbidity associated with achondroplasia. *J Child Neurol* 1990;5:84–97.

170. Kao SCS, Waziri MH, Smith WL, Sato Y, Yuh WTC, Franken EA Jr. MR imaging of the craniovertebral junction, cranium, and brain in children with achondroplasia. *Am J Roentgenol* 1989;153:565–569.

171. Gardner WJ. Hydrodynamic mechanism of syringomyelia: its relationship to myelocele. *J Neurol Neurosurg Psychiatry* 1965;28:247–259.

172. Gardner W, Angel J. The mechanism of syringomyelia and its surgical correction. *Clin Neurosurg* 1975;6:131–140.

173. Williams B. On the pathogenesis of syringomyelia: a review. *J R Soc Med* 1980;73:798–806.

174. Williams B. The distending force in the production of "communication syringomyelia." *Lancet* 1969;2:189–193.

175. DuBoulay GH. Pulsatile movements of the CSF pathways. *Br J Radiol* 1966;19:255–262.

176. Ball MJ, Dayan AD. Pathogenesis of syringomyelia. *Lancet* 1972;2:799–801.

177. Aboulker J. La syringomyélie et les liquides intrarachidiens. *Neurochirurgie* 1979;24[suppl 2]:1–44.

178. Valentini MC, Forni C, Bracchi M. Syringobulbia extending to the basal ganglia. *Am J Neuroradiol* 1988;9:205–207.

179. Sherman JL, Citrin CM, Barkovich AJ. MR imaging of syringobulbia. *J Comput Assist Tomogr* 1987;11:407–411.

180. Sherman JL, Citrin CM. Magnetic resonance of normal CSF flow. *Am J Neuroradiol* 1986;7:3–6.

181. Quencer RM, Post MJD, Hinks RS. Cine MR in the evaluation of normal and abnormal CSF flow: intracranial and intraspinal studies. *Neuroradiology* 1990;32:371–391.

182. Enzmann DR, Pelc NJ. Normal flow patterns of intracranial and spinal cerebrospinal fluid defined with phase-contrast cine MR imaging. *Radiology* 1991;178:467–474.

183. Levy LM, Di Chiro G. MR phase imaging and cerebrospinal fluid flow in the head and spine. *Neuroradiology* 1990;32:399–406.

184. Tachibana S, Iida H, Yada K. Significance of positive Queckenstedt test in patients with syringomyelia associated with Arnold-Chiari malformations. *J Neurosurg* 1992;76:67–71.

185. Vaquero J, Martinez R, Arias A. Syringomyelia-Chiari complex: magnetic resonance imaging and clinical evaluation of surgical treatment. *J Neurosurg* 1990;73:64–68.

186. Barkovich AJ, Sherman JL, Citrin CM, Wippold FJ II. MR of postoperative syringomyelia. *Am J Neuroradiol* 1987;8:319–327.

187. Elster AD, Chen MYM. Chiari I malformations: clinical and radiologic reappraisal. *Radiology* 1992;183:347–353.

188. Barkovich AJ, Wippold FJ, Sherman JL, Citrin CM. Significance of cerebellar tonsillar ectopia on MR. *Am J Neuroradiol* 1986;7:795–799.

CHAPTER 10

Neoplasms of the Spine

Tumors of the spinal cord in children are slowly growing lesions with often subtle and slowly progressive clinical manifestations. The diagnosis of these neoplasms, therefore, has been somewhat difficult and has characteristically occurred late in the course of the disease. Magnetic resonance imaging has provided an extremely sensitive tool for assessing the symptoms referable to the spinal cord and earlier detection of pathologic change.

Although the neoplasms that involve the cord in the pediatric age group are similar to those affecting adults, the incidence and the presentation of the various tumors are often quite different. This chapter discusses the epidemiology, clinical manifestations, and pathologic/radiologic manifestations of intraspinal neoplasms in children.

GENERAL IMAGING CHARACTERISTICS OF SPINAL TUMORS

The introductory section of Chapter 7 discussed general characteristics of brain tumors. In that discussion the importance of determining whether a tumor is located within the brain (intraparenchymal) or outside the brain (extraparenchymal) was stressed. A similar distinction must be made in tumors of the spine: Does the tumor originate within the spinal cord (intramedullary tumor) or outside it (extramedullary tumor)?

Differentiating an intramedullary mass from an extramedullary mass is usually straightforward on MR and on CT with intrathecal contrast. *Intramedullary masses*

cause enlargement of the spinal cord as viewed in the sagittal, coronal, and axial planes. The spinal cord above and below the mass remains in its normal location within the spinal canal. The margins of the intramedullary mass may be sharply defined (particularly in congenital tumors, such as dermoids and epidermoids) or indistinct. *Extramedullary masses* are always sharply marginated. Small ones are usually clearly separated from the cord by cerebrospinal fluid. When large, the CSF space between the mass and the cord is obliterated; in addition, the mass may compress the cord. If it is compressed by a laterally located mass, the cord will appear enlarged if viewed in the sagittal plane; therefore, coronal and axial planes are optimal for imaging. If it is compressed by an anteriorly or posteriorly located mass, the cord will appear enlarged in the coronal plane. Imaging in the sagittal and axial planes is therefore optimal. Sometimes the site of tumor origin is clarified after tumor enhancement by intravenous administration of paramagnetic contrast.

A potential pitfall in the diagnosis of intramedullary tumors is in the differentiation of tumors from nonneoplastic processes in the spinal cord. In children, the major problem is in the differentiation of tumors from foci of demyelination. For example, acute disseminated encephalomyelitis and multiple sclerosis (see Chapter 3) can both present with signs and symptoms referable to a spinal cord lesion. In either disease, a region of focal cord enlargement with prolongation of T2 relaxation time may be identified (see Fig. 3.18). Demyelinating plaques may enhance after the administration of contrast.

Differentiation is most easily made by the shape and size of the lesion at the time of presentation. Neoplasms of the spine are round to ovoid in shape and often have associated cysts. They typically cause considerable enlargement in the cord diameter at the time of presentation because they rarely present when they are less than 2 cm in diameter. Plaques of demyelination are usually flame-shaped and rarely cause significant enlargement of the spinal cord. Associated cysts are almost never present. It is often helpful to image the brain to look for other characteristic foci of demyelination (Fig. 3.18); if present, they establish the diagnosis. If no other lesions are found and uncertainty persists as to whether an intramedullary lesion is tumor or plaque, a follow-up MR examination with and without paramagnetic contrast should be obtained 4–6 weeks after the initial examination. A tumor will be unchanged or larger, whereas a focus of demyelination should be smaller and the enhancement characteristics should be different from those on the first study. A delay of 6 weeks will not impact on the outcome of a patient with a tumor, but biopsy of an acute demyelinating plaque may leave the patient with a worse neurologic deficit.

INTRAMEDULLARY TUMORS

Intramedullary (intrinsic) neoplasms of the spinal cord make up approximately 6% to 10% of neoplasms of the central nervous system in children (1–4); they constitute approximately one-third of spinal neoplasms of childhood (4–6). All age groups are affected; however, the tumors are most frequently seen in patients toward the end of the first decade and beginning the second decade of life. Males and females are equally affected (2–4,6). Spinal neoplasms are relatively less common in children than adults; the ratio of intracranial to intraspinal neoplasms in children varies between 10:1 and 20:1 (as compared to 5:1 in adults) (4).

Patients with spinal cord neoplasms generally present for treatment months, or even years, after the onset of clinical symptoms (2,4,6–8). Often the patient's course

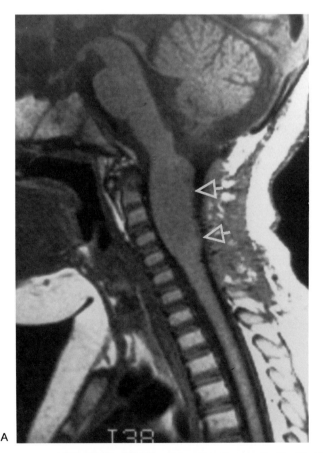

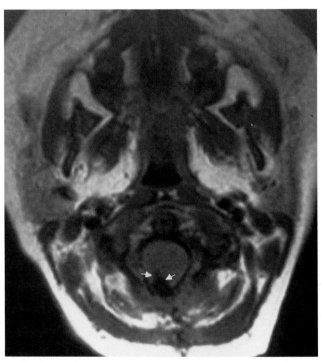

FIG. 10.1. Spinal cord astrocytoma. **A:** Sagittal SE 600/20 image shows expansion (*arrows*) of the cervical spinal cord from the cervicomedullary junction to the top of C5. The tumor is slightly hypointense compared to the normal spinal cord below it and the normal brain stem above it. There is a laminectomy defect posteriorly from a prior biopsy. **B:** Axial SE 800/20 image at the C1 level shows the enlarged spinal cord completely filling the spinal canal. The triangular shaped area (*arrows*) of low signal intensity in the dorsal spinal cord is from the prior biopsy.

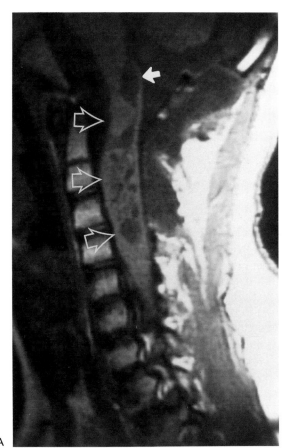

A

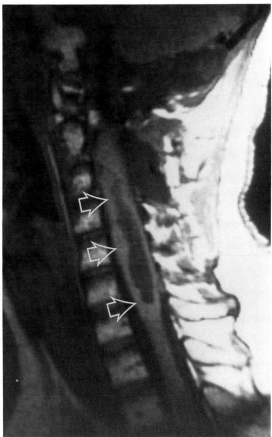

B

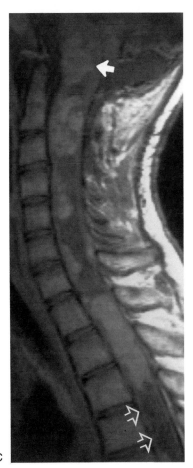

C

FIG. 10.2. Spinal cord astrocytoma. **A, B:** Sagittal SE 600/25 images show an expanded medulla (*solid arrow*) spinal cord (*open arrows*) from the cervicomedullary junction inferiorly to the C7 level. There is mixed low and intermediate signal intensity within the tumor. Presumably, the low signal intensity is a result of necrotic regions within the tumor. The patient has had a suboccipital craniectomy and C1–C7 laminectomy. **C:** Contrast-enhanced MR obtained 1 year later. The tumor has markedly expanded and spread through the spinal cord. The nodule of tumor at the C1 level (*arrow*) has markedly increased in size (compare with A). Moreover, a large tumor mass now extends from mid-T1 to mid-T3. Tumor-associated cyst (*open arrows*) is seen to extend from the T3 to the T4 level inferiorly.

has been punctuated by exacerbations and remissions of symptoms, which may result from alteration in the edema surrounding the neoplasm (2,4,7). Although weakness is the most common presenting complaint, 25% to 30% of these children have pain at their initial presentation (4). The most common type of pain, occurring in approximately 70% of patients, is *spinal pain*. This pain is dull and aching and is localized to bone segments adjacent to the tumor (4). The cause of this pain is unknown but may result from distention of the dural tube by the swollen spinal cord (4). The second most common type of pain seen in children is *root pain*, which is indistinguishable from pain caused by compression of a nerve root by an extramedullary process (4). Finally, some patients manifest *tract pain*, a vague, burning type of pain associated with paresthesias. The burning and paresthesias typically occur caudal to the tumor and are believed to result from infiltration of the lateral spinothalamic tracts by tumor (2,4,9).

Children of different age groups often present with very different symptomatology. Young children and infants often have severe pain, rigidity, and paraspinous muscle spasms (2,7,10), whereas older children more commonly present with progressive scoliosis or gait disturbance (3,4,7). Weakness of the extremities is a common finding in all patients. In cervical tumors, upper-extremity weakness may or may not be accompanied by weakness of the lower extremities. Although sensory levels may be present, they are less common in intramedullary tumors than in extramedullary ones. Sphincter dysfunction, when present, may not occur until late in the course of the illness (2,7,10).

Up to 15% of patients with spinal cord tumors patients may present with symptoms of increased intracranial pressure, most likely a result of either greatly elevated CSF protein content, which blocks the normal CSF pathways and impairs CSF resorption, or blockage of the foramen magnum by cervicomedullary tumors (11–14). The increased intracranial pressure usually does not misdirect the diagnostic work-up of these patients because all will manifest symptoms of an intraspinal process on physical examination.

Astrocytomas comprise approximately 60% and ependymomas 30% of intramedullary tumors in the pediatric age group (1,4). This relative incidence is reversed in adults, in whom more than half of intramedullary tumors are ependymomas. Malignant astrocytomas and glioblastomas of the cord are relatively more common in children than in adults (15). Intramedullary neoplasms tend to be located more rostrally in children than in adults (1,4). Nearly 50% of intramedullary tumors in children are cervical or cervicothoracic, as compared with 28% in adults. Intramedullary tumors in children usually occupy a small number of cord segments; however, the extent of cord involvement is often increased by the presence of cysts rostral or caudal to the tumor. Such peritumoral cysts have been reported in 40% of spinal cord astrocytomas (16).

Magnetic resonance is the modality of choice for imaging patients with suspected or known intramedullary neoplasms (17–21). MR will show an enlarged spinal cord (Figs. 10.1, 10.2) that exhibits prolongation of T2 and, to a lesser extent, T1 at the location of the tumor. The regions of prolonged T1 and T2 relaxation within the expanded cord may represent tumor, necrosis, or cyst; therefore, intravenous administration of paramagnetic contrast (Figs. 10.2–10.4) is essential. Contrast enhancement may be homogeneous (Fig. 10.3) or heterogeneous (Fig. 10.4). The region of contrast enhancement corresponds to the solid portion of the tumor and usually assists in distinguishing tumor (which enhances) from cyst and necrosis (which do not enhance; Figs. 10.2, 10.3). The reader should recognize, however, that the tumor margin usually extends beyond the enhancing tissue. It has been suggested that the margin of tumor enhancement corresponds to the margin of solid tumor in adult ependymomas (22). Verification of this observation in pediatric tumors has not been established.

In 20% to 40% of patients, cysts are present caudal or rostral to the solid portion of the tumor (4,16,18). These cysts may result from secretion of fluid by the tumor or by obstruction of normal CSF pathways within the cord and subarachnoid space. The solid portion of the tumor often cannot be differentiated from the cyst without the administration of IV paramagnetic contrast (Fig. 10.3). Axial and sagittal T1-weighted sequences may be of use in defining the full extent of the associated cyst. The full extent of the cyst is not critical information, however, because it usually resolves after resection of the tumor and elimination of the obstruction.

The differentiation of tumor-associated syringomyelia from congenital or posttraumatic syringomyelia is difficult, even impossible, without the use of contrast-enhanced MR. Reactive astrocytosis, which has the same

---

FIG. 10.3. Spinal cord ependymoma. **A:** Noncontrast sagittal SE 600/20 image shows enlargement of the spinal cord (*arrows*) with prolonged T1 relaxation within the cord extending from the upper thoracic spine inferiorly. **B:** Sagittal SE 1800/20 image shows the widened spinal cord (*arrows*) extending inferiorly through the widened spinal canal to the L2–L3 level. **C:** Sagittal SE 2000/70 image shows the tumor (*large arrows*) to be of high signal intensity uniformly to the L2–L3 level. The caudal end of the tumor is marked by a curvilinear rim of hypointensity (*small arrows*). **D:** After infusion of intravenous contrast, sagittal SE 600/20 image shows a focus of enhancement (*arrows*) from the T8–T9 interspace caudally to the body of T11. All the enlargement inferior to this, seen in B and C, was a proteinaceous cyst.

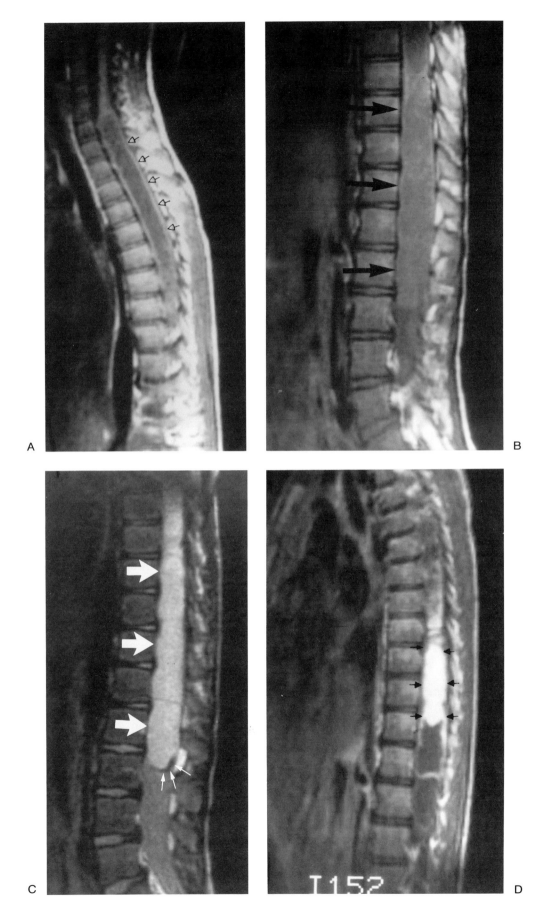

A

B

C

D

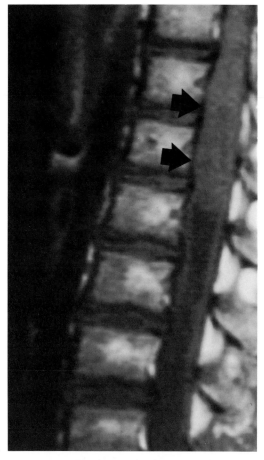
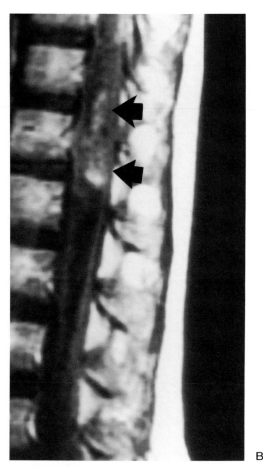

FIG. 10.4. Ependymoma of the conus medullaris. **A:** Sagittal SE 500/15 image shows slight expansion (*arrows*) of the caudal spinal cord. **B:** Postcontrast image shows heterogeneous enhancement (*arrows*) of the mass.

signal characteristics as tumor (prolonged T1 and T2), is frequently present at the caudal and rostral ends of benign syrinx cavities (23). Although the presence of such anomalies of the craniocervical junction as cerebellar tonsillar ectopia, occipitalization of the atlas, and the Klippel-Feil anomaly suggests that a syrinx is nonneoplastic, these anomalies can occur in conjunction with spinal cord tumors as well (23,24). Whether all patients with syringohydromyelia should have a contrast-enhanced scan, even if a Chiari malformation is present, is debatable. Certainly, if any question exists regarding the cause of the syrinx, paramagnetic contrast should be administered. If an area of contrast enhancement is present within or adjacent to the syrinx, the diagnosis of tumor-related cyst should be strongly considered. Rarely, an enhancing inflammatory mass can cause cavitary cord disease.

Spinal cord astrocytomas and ependymomas are difficult to differentiate by MR imaging (Figs. 10.2, 10.3). In general, ependymomas are more sharply circumscribed on postcontrast MR images. In addition, a finding of T2 shortening at the superior and inferior borders of the mass (Fig. 10.3), suggesting prior hemorrhage, is more common in ependymomas (25). In practice, preoperative differentiation of these tumors is of no clinical importance because the operative approach does not differ. It is much more important to determine whether the tumor is intramedullary or extramedullary and to identify accurately the level of the solid portion of the tumor.

Chapter 9 discusses congenital intramedullary tumors, such as lipomas, teratomas, hamartomas, dermoids, and epidermoids.

EXTRAMEDULLARY SPINAL TUMORS

Approximately two-thirds of all intraspinal tumors of childhood are extramedullary; of these, 50% are extradural and 10% to 15% are intradural (26,27). Extramedullary neoplasms can be classified in several different ways; they will be classified in this chapter by their site of origin. Clinically, extramedullary tumors present with signs of progressive myelopathy. Presentation is similar to intramedullary tumors in that weakness, predominantly of the lower extremities and trunk, is the most common presenting symptom. Diffuse back pain and radicular ("root") pain are frequently present. Torticollis, upper-extremity weakness, scoliosis, and urinary incontinence are other frequent signs and symptoms (3,9,10). The histologic type of tumor cannot be predicted by its clinical presentation.

CSF Seeding of Intracranial Neoplasms

The seeding of tumor from intracranial neoplasms via the cerebrospinal fluid occurs more frequently in the pediatric age group than in adults. This manner of tumor spread is most commonly observed in medulloblastomas (28). Up to one-third of patients with medulloblastoma will eventually seed tumor through the cerebrospinal fluid, most often to the spine (29). CSF-borne metastases appear to be more common in patients with differentiated medulloblastomas, that is, medulloblastomas with areas of glial, ependymal, and/or neuronal differentiation (30). The presence of metastases in the spinal canal indicates a much poorer prognosis for the patient.

Ependymomas, anaplastic gliomas, germinomas, choroid plexus tumors, and pineal gland tumors (pineoblastomas and pineocytomas) also frequently seed through the cerebrospinal fluid and deposit metastases in the spinal canal (28). Benign ependymomas typically do not have detectable spinal metastases at the time of the initial diagnosis. Spinal deposits from ependymomas occur more frequently after local recurrence of the tumor is detected and in anaplastic tumors (28); fourth ventricular ependymomas spread through the cerebrospinal fluid much more frequently than those located supratentorially. The fact that pineoblastomas and poorly differentiated pineocytomas metastasize to the cerebrospinal fluid is not surprising, since these neoplasms are intraventricular and, in the case of the pineoblastoma, closely resemble medulloblastomas.

As discussed in Chapter 7, contrast-enhanced MR is now the imaging study of choice in the search for CSF spread of tumor (31). If MR is contraindicated or unavailable, CT myelography should be performed. CSF-borne metastases have the same appearance on imaging studies independent of the histology of the tumor of origin. On CT and plain film myelography, the nerve roots and spinal cord are thickened and nodular and the thecal sac can be nodular and irregularly narrowed by adherent tumor (Figs. 10.5, 10.6). The lumbosacral region is most commonly affected. Sometimes metastases can completely coat the outer surface of the spinal cord, giving the appearance on myelography of a cord enlarged by an

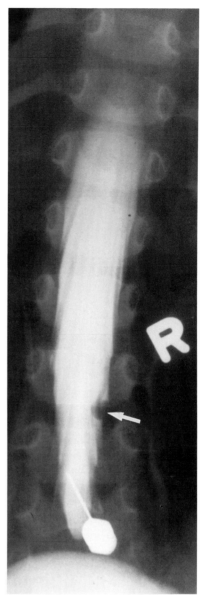

FIG. 10.5. Drop metastasis from a medulloblastoma. AP myelogram film shows a focal intradural extramedullary filling defect (*arrow*) adherent to the right side of the thecal sac at the L4–L5 level.

intramedullary process (30,32). The detection of subarachnoid seeding from intracranial tumors on MR is difficult without the use of intravenous contrast (33,34). Moreover, the use of higher doses of contrast (0.3 mmol/kg) of contrast may increase sensitivity of detection of CSF-borne metastases (35). After the infusion of paramagnetic contrast, subarachnoid metastases appear as nodular or diffuse extramedullary masses that enhance markedly (Figs. 10.7, 10.8) (31,33,34). Typical locations are the lower thoracic and lumbar regions. Enhancing nodules may be seen on the cord surface, roots of the cauda equina, and thecal sac. Even small metastases coating the nerve roots can be identified if thin sections (3 mm or less; see Chapter 1) are acquired. Veins on the surface of the conus medullaris may mimic metastases; they are differentiated by their characteristic location along the ventral and dorsal midline of the spinal cord and their long, curvilinear configuration.

As discussed in Chapter 7, artifacts are common on MR examinations of the spine in the first few weeks after posterior fossa craniectomy (36). These artifacts, presumably from postoperative spinal subdural collection and perhaps from "leakage" of contrast into the subarachnoid space, can be very difficult to differentiate from CSF spread of tumor. Therefore, *it is essential to stage the tumor preoperatively.*

Tumors of the Spinal Column

Although primary tumors of the vertebrae are rare in childhood and infancy, any tumor involving the spinal column may extend into the spinal canal and lead to myelopathy or radiculopathy.

Aneurysmal Bone Cysts

Aneurysmal bone cysts occur most commonly in children and young adults. They are not true neoplasms but are expansile vascular lesions of unknown cause (37). Approximately 20% of aneurysmal bone cysts involve the spine or sacrum; the cervical and thoracic regions are predominantly involved (38). Clinically, patients exhibit pain and stiffness in the affected portion of the spine; larger lesions present with evidence of cord compression (37,39).

The appearance of aneurysmal bone cysts on imaging studies reflects their gross pathology. These lesions are formed of large communicating cavities, filled with unclotted blood; their walls are formed by expanded, thin cortical bone. They are located primarily in the posterior elements and occasionally expand into the pedicles and vertebral body. On plain films and CT studies, aneurysmal bone cysts appear as expansile, cystic masses with eggshell-like peripheral calcification (39) (Fig. 10.9). Occasionally, faintly discernible trabeculae are seen within the mass. When large, the tumor mass extends laterally and anteriorly or posteriorly into the paraspinous soft tissues and into adjacent vertebrae. *Aneurysmal bone cysts are the only benign vertebral lesion that involve adjacent vertebrae* (40). Expansion can also occur into the spinal canal, causing compression of the spinal cord. On MR, aneurysmal bone cysts show variable signal intensities; they can be of high or medium signal intensity on T1-weighted images but are usually of high intensity on T2-weighted images. Fluid–fluid levels, if present, are

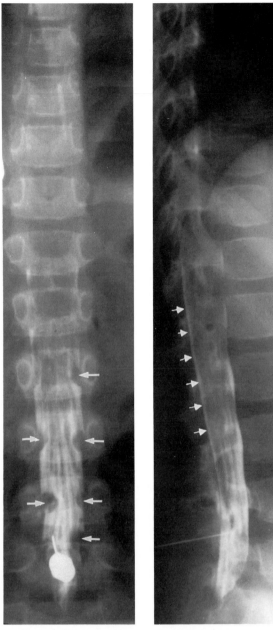

FIG. 10.6. Drop metastases from an anaplastic ependymoma. **A, B:** Anteroposterior and lateral films from a lumbar myelogram demonstrate multiple nodular filling defects (*arrows* in A) adherent to the wall of the thecal sac at several levels. The nerve roots are thickened and nodular. The distal spinal cord and conus medullaris are widened by tumor adherent to the cord, resulting in widening of the cord shadow and narrowing of the subarachnoid space (*arrows* in B).

very helpful in making the diagnosis (Fig. 10.9). The expansile nature of the tumor is apparent on MR, although the thin peripheral rim of calcification is difficult to see. An advantage of MR imaging is the ability to noninvasively assess the amount of spinal cord displacement or compression (41).

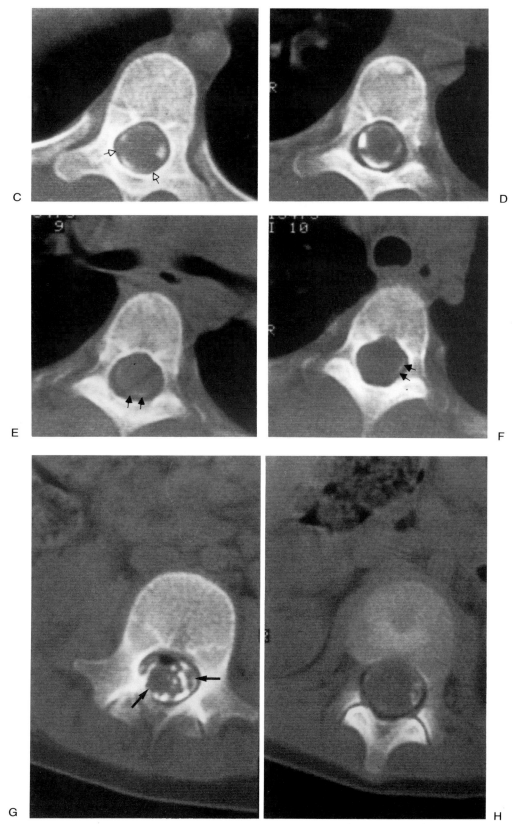

FIG. 10.6. (*Continued.*) **C–F:** Axial CT cuts through the lower spinal cord show nodular masses adherent to the cord (*open arrows*). These masses encroach upon the subarachnoid space and result in only a small amount of contrast (*closed arrows*) creeping by. **G–H:** At the mid-lumbar level, the nerve roots (*arrows*) are clumped and thickened as a result of the metastatic tumor that is coating them.

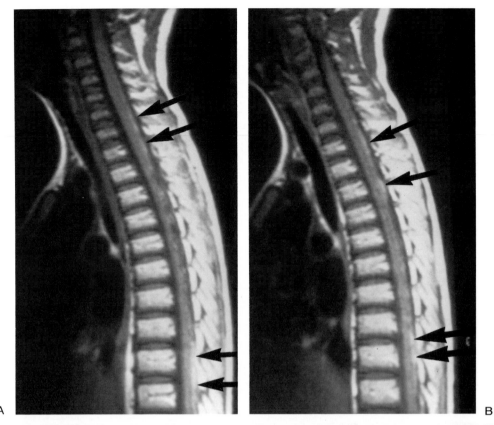

FIG. 10.7. Subarachnoid metastases from medulloblastoma. **A, B:** Postcontrast sagittal SE 600/20 images reveal multiple enhancing nodules on the dorsal surface of the spinal cord (*arrows*).

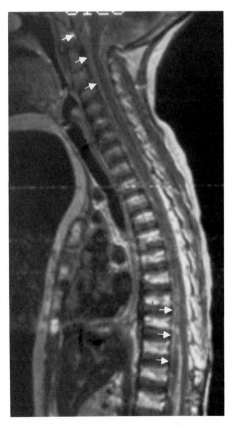
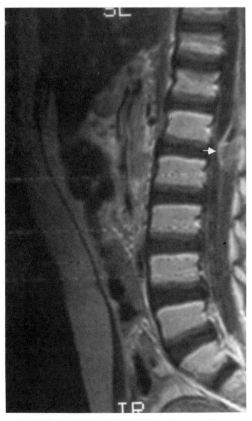

FIG. 10.8. Diffuse subarachnoid metastases. **A, B:** Postcontrast sagittal SE 600/20 images reveal enhancement in the basilar cisterns and the subarachnoid spaces surrounding the spinal cord for nearly the entire length of the cord (*arrows*). At times subarachnoid tumor can completely coat the spinal cord, giving the impression on myelography and CT of an intramedullary mass. Contrast-enhanced MR will, however, make the differentiation.

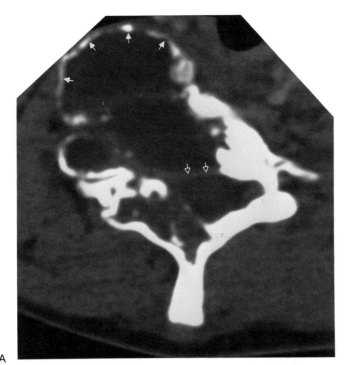

A

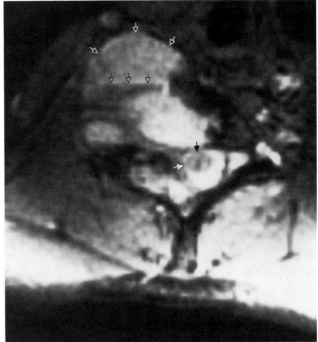

C

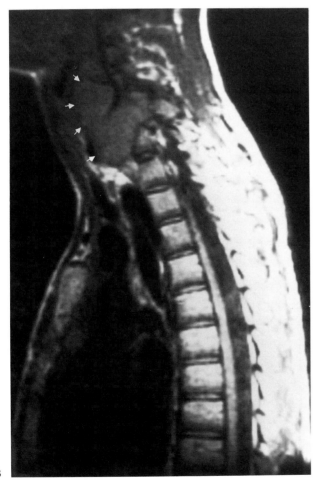

B

FIG. 10.9. Aneurysmal bone cyst. **A:** Axial CT scan shows an expansile lesion of the T7 vertebral body with a low-density center and eggshell-like peripheral calcification (*arrows*). The process involves the right lamina, right pedicle, and vertebral body, and extends into the paraspinous soft tissues. Open arrows point to an interface of the expansile lesion with the epidural space. **B:** Sagittal SE 600/20 image shows the mass (*arrows*) extending anteriorly and superiorly from the T6–T7 level. One of the characteristics of aneurysmal bone cysts is that they tend to involve multiple vertebral levels. **C:** Axial GE 100/50 (θ = 15°) through the lesion. The tumor (*open white arrows*) is of high signal intensity. An air–fluid level (*open black arrows*) is present. The relationship of the tumor to the spinal cord (*closed black arrow*) and the thecal sac (*closed white arrow*) is easily seen. (This case courtesy Dr. K. Maravilla, Seattle, WA.)

Langerhans' Cell Histiocytosis

Langerhans' cell histiocytosis consists of a spectrum of diseases, including eosinophilic granuloma, Letterer-Siwe disease, and Hand-Schüller-Christian disease. All three are characterized by the presence of abnormal histiocytes, known as Langerhans' cells (42). The cranial manifestations are discussed in Chapter 7. Lesions of the spinal column can occur in any of the forms of Langerhans' cell histiocytosis; however, patients with the severe forms of the disease have multiorgan involvement and chronic disability from their disease, so the diagnosis of the spine lesion is never in doubt. When involvement is limited to the spine, patients most commonly present with local pain developing over weeks to months; a history of trauma can often be elicited (43). Treatment is controversial on the rare occasions when patients manifest neurologic deficits (44). Imaging or radiographic studies often show vertebral collapse (Fig. 10.10) or a lytic vertebral lesion (Fig. 10.11) at the time of presentation. On MR, an appearance of two intervertebral discs in apposition without intervening vertebral body is the classic appearance (Fig. 10.10). Both CT and MR may show soft tissue extending into the spinal canal, although

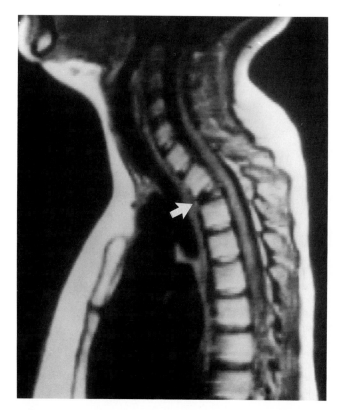

FIG. 10.10. Langerhans' cell histiocytosis. Sagittal SE 500/25 image shows near complete collapse of the T1 vertebral body (*large arrow*). The vertebral discs are in apposition without intervening vertebral body. Minimal soft tissue extends into the spinal canal.

the amount of tissue is typically small (37,39,45). Infusion of paramagnetic or iodinated contrast typically results in homogeneous enhancement of the abnormal tissue.

Osteogenic Sarcoma

Although osteogenic sarcomas account for approximately 20% of all sarcomas, they rarely affect the spine. Patients most commonly present in the second decade with localized pain or a mass (46). Osteosarcomas are distributed uniformly throughout the spinal column and have an extremely variable gross pathologic appearance, ranging from soft and friable to firm with marked calcification (38). The imaging findings vary as much as the gross pathology. On CT or plain films, the vertebral involvement may be purely lytic, predominantly sclerotic, or a combination of the two (39,47). Intrathecal contrast is often necessary to define the degree of involvement of the spinal canal. MR shows the tumor primarily as an area of prolonged T1 and T2 relaxation time when compared to normal bone marrow. Tumors that are heavily ossified may be dark on T2- and, especially, T2*-weighted images. As with other bony tumors of the spine, MR is the preferred way to assess extraosseous spread of tumor and the degree of cord displacement and cord compression (41).

Giant Cell Tumors

Giant cell tumors comprise approximately 4% of primary benign bone tumors (38). Although the peak incidence of these neoplasms is in the third decade, patients in their teens are sometimes affected. Involvement of the spine is most common at the sacrum. On imaging studies, giant cell tumors are destructive, lytic lesions with poorly defined, nonsclerotic margins. The involved bone is often expanded. Although they may extend to the cortical surface, giant cell tumors rarely break through the periosteum unless the affected vertebral body collapses (Fig. 10.12). Occasionally, the area of bony expansion or the associated soft tissue mass will extend into and narrow the spinal canal (Fig. 10.12). CT is the imaging study of choice to define the vertebral body involvement, but MR most accurately defines the status of the spinal cord. Enhancement is usually minimal after administration of intravenous iodinated or paramagnetic contrast.

Chordomas

Chordomas are extremely rare in the spinal canal of children; intracranial chordomas are discussed in Chapter 7. They arise from rests of notochord cells and primarily involve the clivus and the sacrum; only about

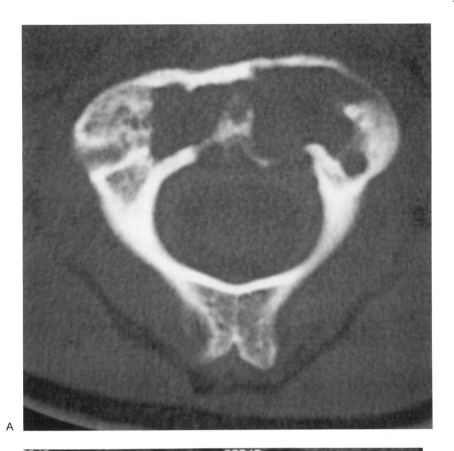

A

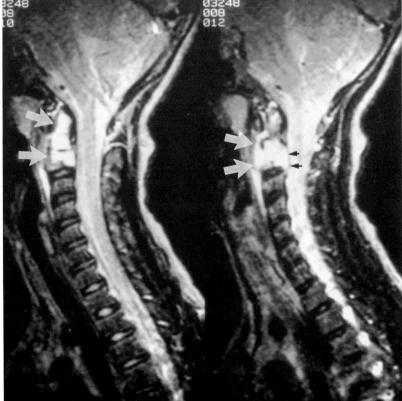

B,C

FIG. 10.11. Langerhans' cell histiocytosis. **A:** Axial CT image shows a lytic lesion of the C2 vertebral body. **B, C:** Sagittal GE 600/15 images show high intensity of the C2 vertebral body and odontoid (*large white arrows*). The vertebral body is expanded (*small black arrows*) and narrows the ventral subarachnoid space.

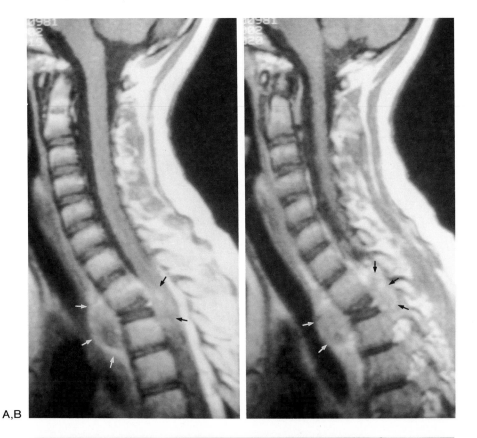

A,B

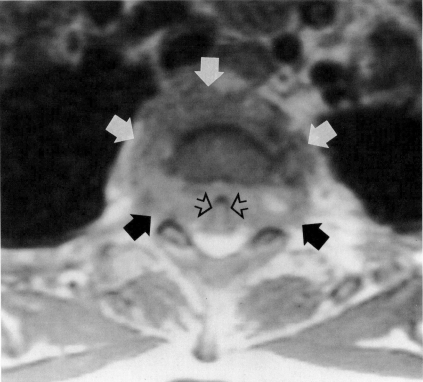

C

FIG. 10.12. Giant cell tumor. **A, B:** Sagittal SE 550/15 images show collapse of the T2 vertebral body with associated soft tissue mass anteriorly (*white arrows*) and posteriorly (*black arrows*). The size of the soft tissue mass makes Langerhans' cell histiocytosis less likely. **C:** Axial SE 660/16 image shows the large soft tissue mass (*large solid arrows*) compressing the spinal cord (*open black arrows*).

15% of chordomas involve the vertebrae (38). Chordomas grow slowly by erosion and compression of adjacent structures; they rarely metastasize. On imaging studies, chordomas appear as lytic lesions, causing destruction of one or more adjacent vertebrae. Sclerosis is commonly seen in the bone adjacent to the tumor. Extension to the paravertebral soft tissues is not uncommon; destruction of the intervertebral discs can occur when the vertebral bodies are involved. On CT, irregular spicules of calcification are almost always seen within the tumor mass (39). The MR appearance of chordomas is similar to other primary bone tumors; they are sharply defined, destructive lesions with prolonged T1 and T2 relaxation times when compared to nervous tissue. Contrast enhancement is variable; however, *the absence of contrast enhancement favors the diagnosis of chordoma*, as most other tumors of the pediatric spinal column show significant enhancement.

Ewing's Sarcoma

Ewing's sarcoma is the second most common primary bone tumor in childhood. Although it most commonly involves the spine as a metastasis from primary tumor elsewhere, it may occur as a primary osseous, or rarely extraosseous, spinal tumor. The most common age at presentation is the second decade; presentation with Ewing's sarcoma is rare before the age of 5 years and after the age of 30 years (47). CT or plain radiographs of Ewing's sarcoma reveal lytic lesions with poor margination and often a "moth-eaten" appearance. The "onionskin" appearance from periosteal reaction is more common in long bones than in the spine. MR studies show hypointensity compared to normal bone on T1-weighted images and a variable signal, ranging from hypo- to hyperintensity on T2-weighted images. Moderate, uniform enhancement is seen after administration of intravenous contrast (45). The appearance of intraosseous Ewing's sarcoma is identical to that of osseous leukemia and metastatic neuroblastoma. When it is extraosseous (Fig. 10.13), Ewing's sarcoma cannot be differentiated from other soft tissue tumors, including neuroblastoma (described in a later section in this chapter).

Osteoblastoma

Osteoblastomas account for less than 1% of primary bone tumors. The presenting symptoms, usually pain of many months duration, occur most commonly in males during the second and third decades of life. Because the tumors are usually 2 cm or greater in diameter when they present, pain secondary to compression of nerve roots or spinal cord is sometimes part of the presentation (38,48).

On imaging studies, osteoblastomas are well-defined, solitary masses that most commonly originate in the posterior elements (39,48). CT and plain films show lytic

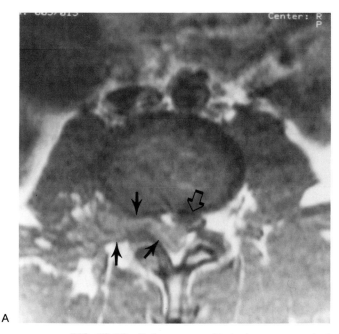
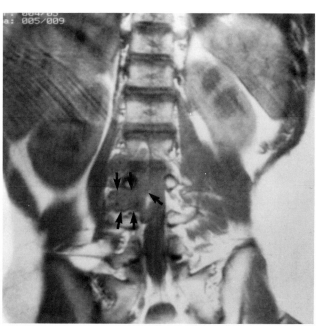

A

B

FIG. 10.13. Extraosseous Ewing's sarcoma. **A:** Axial SE 1000/20 image shows a soft tissue mass (*solid arrows*) extending from the paraspinous region through the right neural foramen into the epidural space. The thecal sac (*open arrow*) is pushed anteriorly and to the left by the mass. **B:** Coronal SE 600/20 image shows the tumor mass (*arrows*) extending through the neural foramen between the pedicles into the spinal canal and displacing the thecal sac to the left.

lesions with a variably thick sclerotic rim (Fig. 10.14); extension into surrounding soft tissues is common. Calcification or new bone formation may be seen within the lytic area (39). On MR, osteoblastomas are well-defined masses with prolonged T1 and T2 relaxation times as compared with normal bone. They most commonly occur in the articular facets, pedicles, and lamina (49,50). Contrast enhancement is variable. Occasionally, osteoblastomas may generate widespread edema in the surrounding bone, suggesting diffuse infiltration of tumor (51). CT studies are diagnostic.

Other Vertebral Tumors

Although hemangiomas of the spine and osteoid osteomas are not uncommon in children, they rarely present with neurologic manifestations. Chondrosarcomas, fibrosarcomas, paragangliomas, and bone metastases (other than neuroblastoma and Ewing's sarcoma, which are discussed in this chapter) are extremely uncommon in the spines of children. They will not be discussed in this text.

Meningeal Tumors

Meningiomas

Although meningiomas account for 25% to 45% of all spinal tumors, they are extremely uncommon in children with an incidence of 2% to 3% of pediatric intraspinal tumors (52). The histologic, clinical, and therapeutic features are similar to meningiomas occurring in later life. The tumors are primarily intradural and extramedullary, although they occasionally extend into the extradural compartment. Patients usually present with spinal cord or nerve root compression (39). Plain film and CT myelography reveal meningiomas to be smoothly marginated masses that are isodense to skeletal muscle. MR is the imaging modality of choice because it clearly demonstrates the homogeneous extramedullary lesions that are isointense with spinal cord and surrounded by cerebrospinal fluid. Short TR/TE sequences and long TR/TE sequences using cardiac gating and flow compensation gradients optimize lesion detection. Infusion of paramagnetic contrast results in homogeneous enhancement (17,34). Therefore, contrast-enhanced

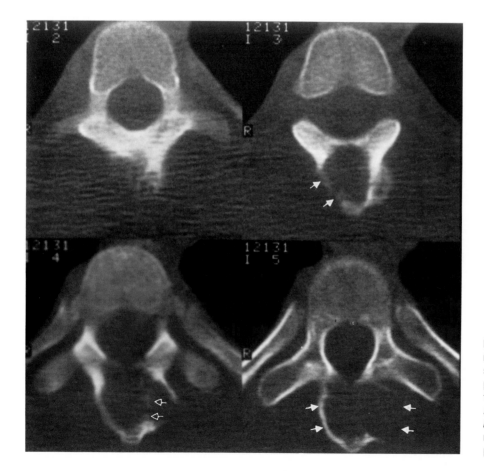

FIG. 10.14. Osteoblastoma of the spinous process. Multiple axial CT scans show an expansile lesion of the spinous process that markedly expands the cortex (*solid arrows*), especially on the left. A small amount of calcification (*open arrows*) is seen within the mass. There is no extension into the spinal canal in this particular case.

MR is the diagnostic modality of choice for both the initial diagnostic work-up and for postoperative studies.

Meningeal Cysts

Meningeal cysts, although not true neoplasms, may occur in childhood and act as expanding masses, causing cord compression. As discussed in Chapter 8, extraparenchymal meningeal cysts may be congenital (true arachnoid cysts) or acquired (arachnoid loculations). In children, most meningeal cysts are located dorsal to the thoracic spinal cord; they may be extradural or intradural. Extradural cysts may develop secondary to a congenital or an acquired dural defect with resultant herniation of arachnoid and cerebrospinal fluid through the defect (53,54). Intradural cysts may be the result of congenital deficiencies within the arachnoid or adhesions from prior infection or trauma. Presenting symptoms of both intra- and extradural cysts are usually intermittent pain and weakness, which may be accentuated in the upright position; the accentuation of symptoms may be related to gravitational filling of the cyst and subsequent cord compression (27). CT or plain film myelography of affected patients reveals an ovoid, sharply demarcated extramedullary mass that may show immediate or delayed filling by contrast, depending upon the size of the opening between the cyst and the subarachnoid space (Fig. 10.15) (53). Cord compression is assessed by its degree of deformity. On MR, the arachnoidal adhesions are difficult to identify. Instead the diagnosis can be made by identifying local displacement and compression of the spinal cord at the site of the arachnoid loculation. The cyst will almost always exhibit higher signal intensity than adjacent cerebrospinal fluid because the cyst fluid exhibits a relative lack of CSF pulsations.

Classification of Meningeal Cysts

Other types of meningeal cysts can occur in the spine. Nabors and colleagues (55) have proposed a classification for spinal meningeal cysts. *Type I cysts* are extradural meningeal cysts without nerve roots. This group is composed primarily of the thoracic extradural arachnoid cysts (herniating through dural rents) that commonly occur in adolescents and sacral meningoceles, which most commonly present with localized sacral pain in adults. *Type II cysts* are extradural meningeal cysts that contain nerve roots. Most type II cysts are Tarlov's cysts or spinal nerve root diverticula; they almost always present in adults. *Type III cysts* are intradural arachnoid cysts. In this group are the true arachnoid cysts and arachnoid loculations described in the prior paragraph. These cysts typically present in childhood or adolescence and are

most commonly located dorsal to the spinal cord at the thoracic level.

Tumors of the Nerve Roots and Nerve Root Sheaths

Although pathologists are not completely agreed on the terminology of tumors of the spinal nerve roots, we will adhere to the terminology of Russell and Rubenstein, who separate solitary, encapsulated lesions, which they call schwannomas, from tumors that are associated with neurofibromatosis (neurofibromas, in which the nerve itself cannot be easily separated from the nerve sheath) (56). *Schwannomas* are very uncommon in children (except when associated with neurofibromatosis type II [NF2], as discussed in Chapter 6) and will not be discussed here. Neurofibromas are composed of Schwann cells and fibroblasts. They are rare as isolated lesions and are most often seen in patients with neurofibromatosis type I (NF1). Patients with multiple spinal nerve or nerve sheath tumors are common in both NF1 and NF2. It has recently been shown that the nerve sheath tumors in NF1 are primarily neurofibromas and that those in NF2 are primarily schwannomas (57). Affected patients present with symptoms of nerve root or spinal cord compression. Plain film findings include vertebral anomalies and erosive changes with resulting neural foraminal enlargement. On plain film and CT myelography, neurofibromas appear as well-defined intradural, extramedullary masses that are hypodense or isodense to skeletal muscle. Those tumors that have extradural components often extend through the neural foramina. MR studies reveal tumors that are slightly hyperintense with respect to the skeletal muscle and show variable contrast enhancement on T1-weighted sequences; they are peripherally hyperintense with respect to skeletal muscle on the T2-weighted sequences (Figs. 6.15, 6.16, 10.16). Central areas of decreased signal intensity are often noted on T2-weighted images; these regions of short T2 may reflect dense central areas of collagenous stroma (58). Bone erosion will be appreciated when moderate or severe, causing canal enlargement, foraminal enlargement (Fig. 10.17), or both (Fig. 10.16). Enhancement after administration of intravenous contrast (CT or MR) is variable (Fig. 10.17, and see discussion in Chapter 6). When multiple neurofibromas are present, the spinal cord can be compressed between them, often to a virtual ribbon of tissue (Fig. 6.21). The compression is best demonstrated by MR in the axial or coronal plane.

Extraspinal Tumors Invading the Epidural Space

Tumors of the autonomic nervous system sometimes enter the spinal canal through an intervertebral fora-

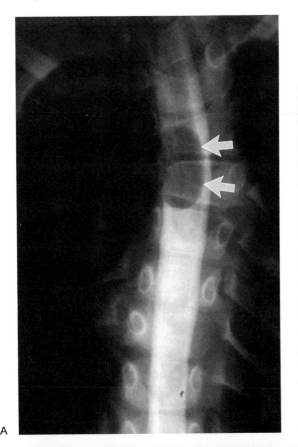

A

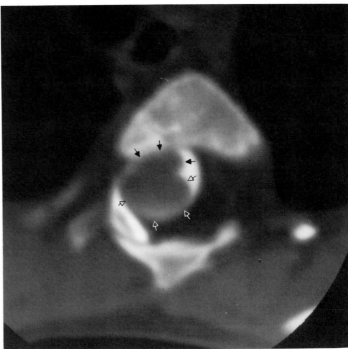

B

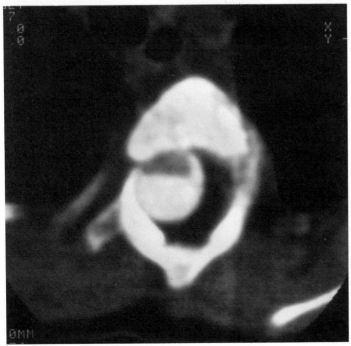

C

FIG. 10.15. Spinal arachnoid cyst. **A:** Anteroposterior film from a myelogram shows a large, lucent, smooth-walled filling defect (*arrows*) at the T3 and T4 levels. The patient has mild to moderate scoliosis as a result of a tethered spinal cord. **B:** Axial CT at the T3 level immediately after the myelogram shows a lucent mass (*open arrows*) dorsal to the spinal cord (*solid arrows*) that compresses the spinal cord and displaces it anteriorly. **C:** Axial CT scan obtained at the same level 4 hours after the myelogram shows the posterior mass to be completely filled with contrast, confirming the diagnosis of a cyst.

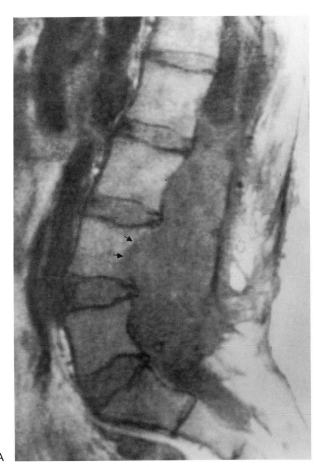

A

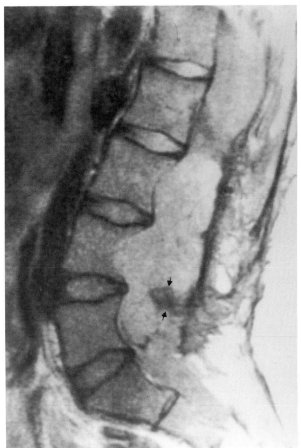

B

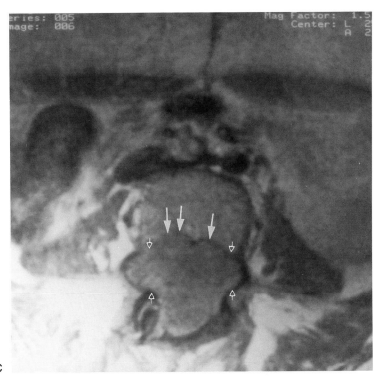

C

FIG. 10.16. Large spinal neurofibroma. **A:** Sagittal SE 1000/20 image shows a large mass extending from mid-L2 to the sacrum. There is marked erosion of the posterior body of L4 (*arrows*) by tumor. **B:** Sagittal SE 1000/70 image shows that most of the tumor becomes hyperintense on this T2-weighted image. However, there is a central area of low signal intensity (*arrows*) that is characteristic of neurofibromas. **C:** Axial SE 1000/20 image shows the marked expansion of the spinal canal by the tumor mass, which is widening both neural foramina (*open arrows*) and eroding the posterior vertebral body (*closed arrows*). This patient has undergone prior laminectomy.

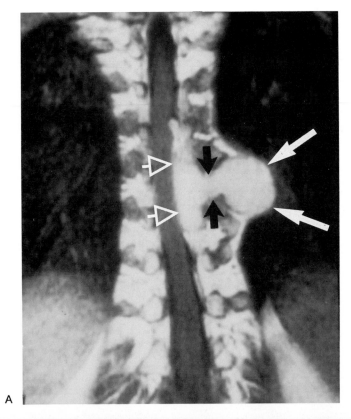

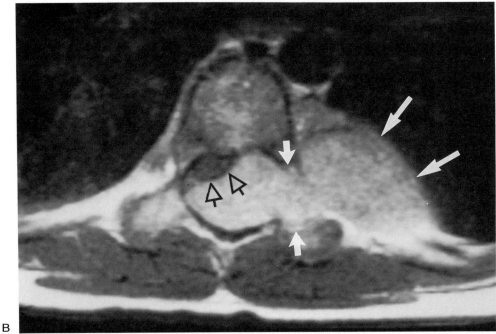

FIG. 10.17. Dumbbell neurofibroma. Postcontrast coronal **(A)** and axial **(B)** T1-weighted images show a large, uniformly enhancing mass compressing the spinal cord (*open arrows*), widening the neural foramen (*small solid arrows*) and extending into the paraspinous region (*large solid arrows*).

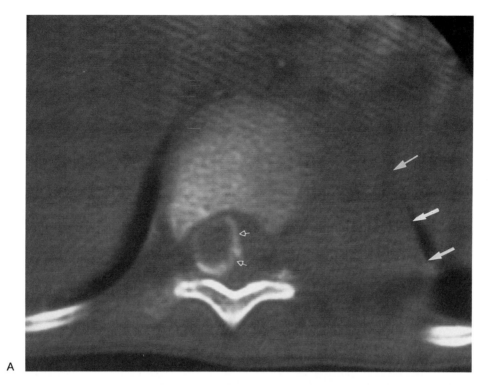

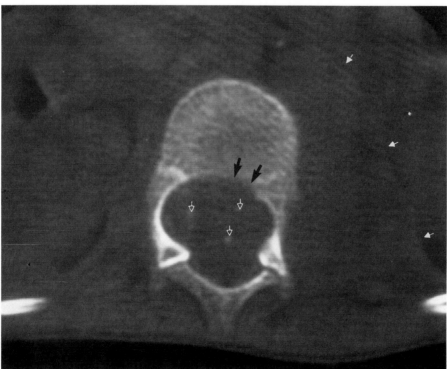

FIG. 10.18. Neuroblastoma. **A:** CT after myelography shows a large paraspinous mass (*solid white arrows*) extending through the neural foramen into the epidural space and compressing the thecal sac (*open white arrows*). The thecal sac and spinal cord are displaced to the right side of the spinal canal. **B:** Axial CT at slightly lower level again shows the paraspinous mass (*solid white arrows*). At this level, the spinal canal is expanded and the posterior vertebral body is eroded (*black arrows*). Small foci of calcification (*open white arrows*) are present within the tumor mass in the spinal canal.

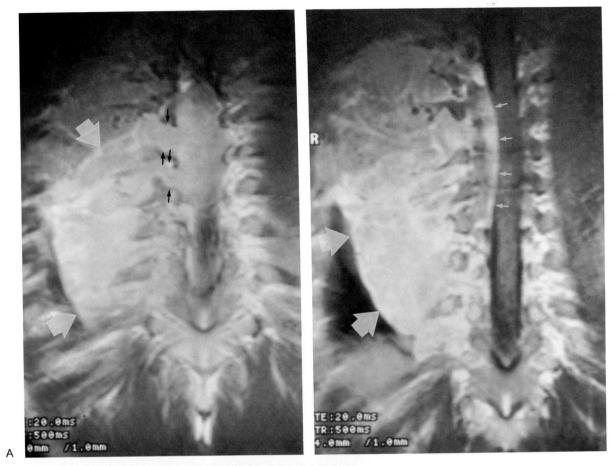

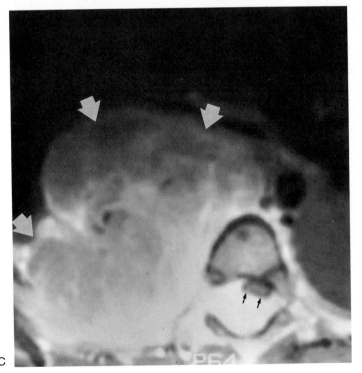

FIG. 10.19. Neuroblastoma. **A, B:** Postcontrast coronal SE 600/16 images show a large enhancing paraspinous mass (*large white arrows*) entering the spinal canal through neural foramina (*small black arrows*) and displacing (*small white arrows*) the spinal cord. **C:** Postcontrast axial SE 600/15 image shows enhancing tumor (*large white arrows*) filling the spinal canal and compressing the spinal cord (*small black arrows*) anterolaterally.

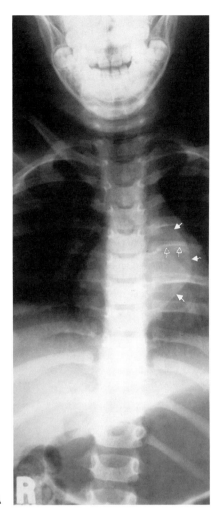

A

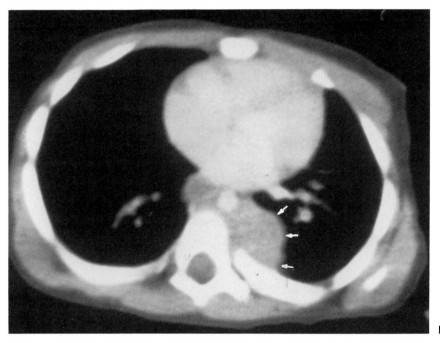

B

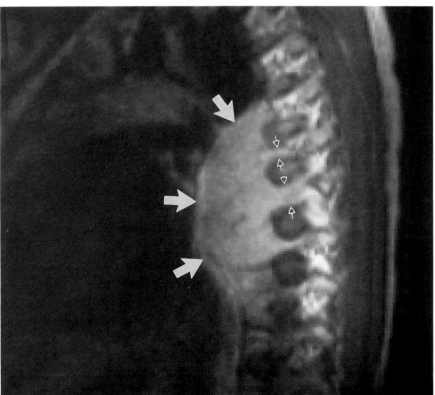

C

FIG. 10.20. Ganglioneuroma. **A:** AP chest x-ray shows a large paraspinous mass on the left (*solid arrows*). There is some widening of the interspace between the left seventh and eighth ribs and some erosion of the inferior left seventh rib (*open arrows*). **B:** Axial CT through the level of the mass shows the large paraspinous density (*open arrows*). It is difficult without the use of intrathecal contrast to assess the degree of invasion of the spinal canal. **C:** Sagittal SE 500/40 image through the mass (*large solid arrows*) shows the tumor extending into the neural foramina (*small open arrows*) and obliterating the fat that is usually present in the neural foramina.

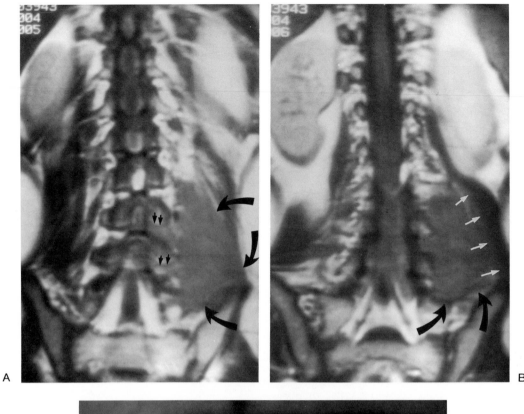

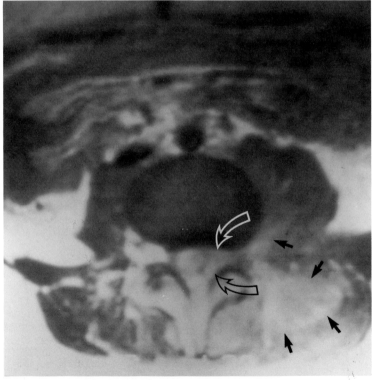

FIG. 10.21. Granulocytic sarcoma (leukemia). **A, B:** Coronal SE 550/15 images show a large para-spinous mass (*curved black arrows*) that displaces the iliopsoas muscle (*white arrows*) and extends into the neural foramina of L3–L4 and L4–L5 (*small black arrows*), replacing the normal high intensity of fat. **C:** Postcontrast axial SE 600/16 image shows enhancing tumor mass (*straight black arrows*) in the paraspinous muscles and extending through the left neural foramen into the epidural space (*open curved arrows*).

men. Such tumors tend to be of the neuroblastoma/ganglioneuroblastoma/ganglioneuroma spectrum.

Neuroblastoma

Neuroblastomas, the fourth most common tumors of childhood, are tumors of infancy and childhood that arise in the sympathetic nervous system. They most often originate in the adrenal medulla (40%) but can occur in the spinal sympathetic chain (25%, most commonly the upper lumbar area), the carotid ganglia, the aortic bodies, and the organ of Zukerkandl. Metastases to bone, including the spine, are frequent and sometimes result in spinal cord compression (59). Cord compression may also result from direct extension of tumor through neural foramina into the spinal canal; however, cord compression as an initial manifestation of the disease is rare (60).

When assessing affected patients for spinal cord or cauda equina compression, MR is the study of choice. If MR is not available or is contraindicated, CT myelography should be performed. CT will show a paraspinous mass extending through the neural foramen into the epidural space with displacement and compression of the thecal sac (Fig. 10.18). Destruction of the adjacent bone may be present. When cord compression results from extension of bony metastases, irregular destruction of the vertebral body is seen, with extension of the soft tissue mass into the spinal canal and displacement and compression of the thecal sac by the mass. MR optimally shows the paraspinous or bony mass and the extension of the tumor into the spinal canal, without the need for intrathecal contrast (Fig. 10.19). Prior to intravenous administration of paramagnetic contrast, the mass appears relatively homogeneous and is isointense to nervous tissue. After contrast administration, the mass enhances heterogeneously (Fig. 10.19). Coronal images are most helpful to visualize the full extent of tumor in the spinal canal and the resultant cord displacement and compression (Fig. 10.19).

The imaging appearance of metastases of neuroblastoma to the skull and skull base is discussed in Chapter 7.

Ganglioneuroma

Ganglioneuromas represent tumors of the sympathetic nervous system that are at the benign end of the neuroblastoma/ganglioneuroblastoma/ganglioneuroma spectrum. The predominant cell type is the mature ganglion cell. In contradistinction to neuroblastomas, which usually present in early childhood, ganglioneuromas often do not present until the second or third decade. Males and females are equally affected. The most frequent site of origin for ganglioneuromas is the posterior mediastinum; abdominal sites are also common, but the

neck and the pelvis are somewhat unusual locations (61,62). Ganglioneuromas do not metastasize; when the spinal canal is involved, it is the result of a "dumbbell" mass extending from the paraspinous region through the neural foramen into the epidural space (Fig. 10.20). Calcification is frequently present within the tumor. Although the calcification does not allow differentiation from neuroblastomas (Fig. 10.18), it does differentiate these masses from neurofibromas, schwannomas, and extraosseous Ewing's sarcomas, which rarely calcify.

Ganglioneuroblastoma

Ganglioneuroblastomas are tumors of the sympathetic nervous system that are intermediate between neuroblastoma and ganglioneuroma. In fact, some feel that ganglioneuroblastomas represent a stage in the maturation of neuroblastomas to ganglioneuromas (63). Ganglioneuroblastomas, which are considerably less common than neuroblastomas or ganglioneuromas, tend to present in young children; both sexes are affected equally. As with ganglioneuromas, the posterior mediastinum and abdomen are the most common sites of ori-

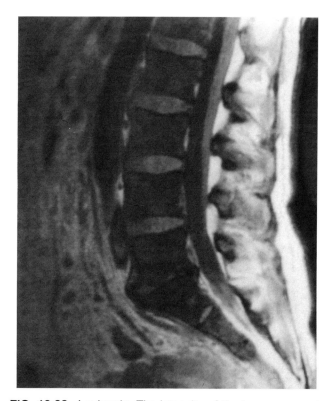

FIG. 10.22. Leukemia. The intensity of the bone marrow is much too low on this sagittal SE 600/20 image of a 15-year-old boy. The normal fat within the marrow has been replaced by either leukemic infiltrate or hematopoietically active red marrow, which has replaced the yellow marrow as a result of pancytopenia. The bone marrow should have a high signal intensity on short TR/TE images in adolescents.

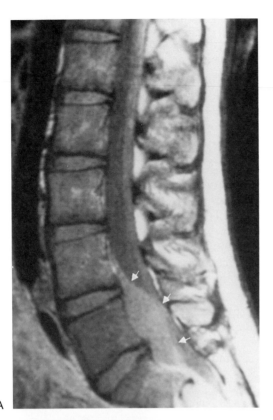

A

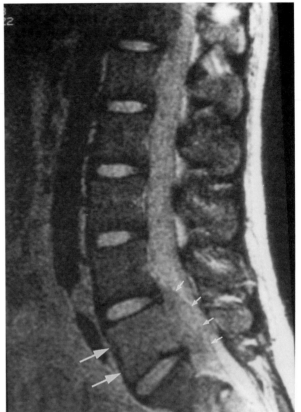

B

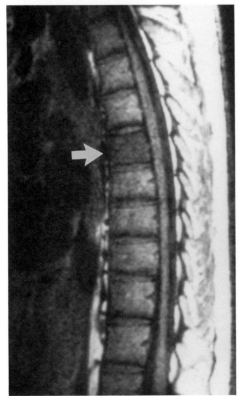

C

FIG. 10.23. Non-Hodgkin's lymphoma. **A:** Sagittal SE 600/20 image shows a mottled signal intensity of all the vertebral bodies. The L5 vertebral body is clearly abnormal in signal intensity, being uniformly hypointense. A soft tissue mass (*arrows*) is seen in the epidural space posterior to the bottom of L4, L5, and top of S1. At biopsy this was epidural lymphoma. **B:** Sagittal SE 2200/70 image shows the L5 vertebral body (*large arrows*) to have abnormally high signal intensity. The epidural lymphoma (*small arrows*) is more difficult to appreciate on this imaging sequence. **C:** Sagittal SE 600/20 image through the thoracic spine shows that the T7 vertebral body (*arrow*) is also involved by lymphoma.

gin. Although less histologically and biologically aggressive than neuroblastomas, their behavior is similar to neuroblastomas in that they can metastasize to bone or extend directly into the spinal epidural space through the neural foramina (39,59). Extension from either the vertebral bodies or the paraspinous sympathetic ganglia into the spinal canal can result in nerve root or spinal cord compression.

As the preceding paragraphs illustrate, all the tumors in the neuroblastoma/ganglioneuroblastoma/ganglioneuroma spectrum can have an identical appearance on imaging studies. When a paraspinous mass is seen in the suprarenal area extending into the spinal canal or if diffuse bony metastases are present, the most likely diagnosis is neuroblastoma. However, when a paraspinous mass is seen to extend through the neural foramen into the epidural space in the posterior mediastinum, lower abdomen, pelvis, or neck, the differentiation between the three tumors in this spectrum is not possible by imaging studies alone. If CT is performed, intrathecal contrast is necessary to define fully the extent of spinal epidural involvement. MR should be the imaging procedure of choice because the full extent of paraspinous and epidural tumor can be defined noninvasively and without the use of ionizing radiation. Moreover, the ability to obtain images in the coronal plane is invaluable in the assessment of spinal canal involvement.

Leukemia and Lymphoma

Leukemic involvement of the spinal epidural space is rarely symptomatic. However, most patients with symptomatic spinal epidural leukemic deposits are in the pediatric age group (27,37). Most leukemic deposits (known in acute myelogenous leukemia as granulocytic sarcomas or "chloromas," because of their characteristic green color) are direct metastases to the epidural space. Approximately half of the affected children are in complete hematologic remission when meningeal leukemia is detected. This phenomenon may be the result of an entrance of leukemic cells into the meninges from petechial hemorrhages superimposed upon the failure of antimetabolites to cross the blood-brain barrier; leukemic cells thus enter the central nervous system, survive, and proliferate. Patients with epidural leukemia usually present with signs of meningeal irritation. Occasionally, the leukemic masses attain sufficient size to cause nerve root or spinal cord compression.

On imaging studies, the leukemic deposits can be localized or may extend as sheets of tumor over many spinal segments. CT and myelographic studies are nonspecific, revealing an epidural mass. On MR, the epidural mass is isointense to neural tissue on noncontrast studies; homogeneous enhancement occurs after infusion of paramagnetic contrast (Fig. 10.21). An indication as to the etiology of the epidural mass or masses may be sug-

gested by abnormal signal in the bone marrow. In patients with leukemia and lymphoma, the normal high signal intensity of the bone marrow on short TR/TE images is often replaced by a lower signal intensity (Fig. 10.22). It is not clear whether this abnormal signal intensity results from actual leukemic infiltration of the vertebral bodies, from increased activity of the bone marrow, or from chemotherapeutic intervention. The reader should be aware that the absence of fat intensity within the bone marrow is not a reliable sign in children under the age of 5 years. The bone marrow of the vertebral bodies in young children may still be active in hematopoiesis and, therefore, is normally of low signal intensity on the T1-weighted images. Hematopoietic marrow will enhance variably after intravenous infusion of paramagnetic contrast (64). *Thus, the demonstration of vertebral enhancement in children does not imply infiltration by tumor.* Lymphoma (Fig. 10.23) and metastatic Ewing's sarcoma (Fig. 10.13) may appear identical to leukemia.

CONGENITAL SPINAL TUMORS

Congenital tumors of the spine include lipomas, dermoids, epidermoids, teratomas, hamartomas, and enterogenous cysts. These lesions, which represent 4% of spinal tumors in children (1), are discussed in Chapter 9.

REFERENCES

1. Steinbok P, Cochrane DD, Poskitt K. Intramedullary spinal cord tumors in children. In: Berger MS, ed. *Pediatric neurooncology. neurosurgery clinics of North America.* Philadelphia: WB Saunders, 1992:931–945.
2. Anderson FM, Carson JJ. Spinal cord tumors in children: a review of the subject and presentation of 21 cases. *J Pediatr* 1953;43:190–207.
3. Banna M, Gryspaerat GL. Review article: intraspinal tumors in children (excluding dysraphism). *Radiology* 1971;22:17–32.
4. Epstein F, Epstein N. Intramedullary tumors of the spinal cord. In: Shillito J Jr, Matson DD, eds. *Pediatric neurosurgery: surgery of the developing nervous system.* New York: Grune & Stratton, 1982:529–240.
5. Raffel C, Edwards MSB. Intraspinal tumors in children. In: Youmans JR, ed. *Neurological surgery,* 3rd ed. Philadelphia: WB Saunders, 1990:3574–3588.
6. Pascual-Castroviejo I. *Spinal cord tumors in children and adolescents.* New York: Raven, 1990.
7. Arseni C, Hrovath L, Iliescu D. Intraspinal tumors in children. *Psychiatr Neurol Neurochir* 1976;70:123–133.
8. Pool JL. The surgery of spinal cord tumors. *Clin Neurosurg* 1970;17:310–330.
9. Haft H, Ransohoff J, Carter S. Spinal cord tumors in children. *Pediatrist* 1959;23:1152–1159.
10. Coxe WS. Tumors of the spinal canal in children. *Am Surg* 1961;27:62–73.
11. Rifkinson-Mann S, Wisoff JH, Epstein F. The association of hydrocephalus with intramedullary spinal cord tumors: a series of 25 patients. *Neurosurgery* 1990;27:749–754.
12. Ucar S, Florez G, Garcia J. Increased intracranial pressure associated with spinal cord tumors. *Neurochirurgia (Stuttg)* 1976;19:265–268.
13. Messer HD, Brinker RA. Hydrocephalus and dementia complicating spinal tumor. Case reports. *J Neurosurg* 1980;53:544–547.
14. Ammerman BJ, Smith DR. Papilledema and spinal cord tumors. *Surg Neurol* 1975;3:55–57.

15. Di Lorenzo N, Giuffre R, Fortuna A. Primary spinal neoplasm in childhood: analysis of 1234 published cases (including 56 personal cases) by pathology, sex, age, and site. *Neurochirurgia* 1982;25: 153–164.

16. Okazaki H. *Fundamental of neuropathology.* New York: Igaku-Shoin, 1983.

17. Dillon WP, Norman D, Newton TH, et al. *Intradural spinal cord lesions: Gd-DTPA enhanced MR imaging.* 1989.

18. Goy AM, Pinto RS, Raghavenda BN, et al. Intramedullary spinal cord tumors: MR imaging with emphasis on associated cysts. *Radiology* 1986;161:381–386.

19. Parziel PM, Baleriaux D, Rodesch G, et al. Gd-DTPA enhanced MR imaging of spinal tumors. *Am J Neuroradiol* 1989;10:249–258.

20. Sze G, Krol G, Zimmerman RD, Deck MDF. Intramedullary disease of the spine: diagnosis using Gd-DTPA-enhanced MR imaging. *Am J Neuroradiol* 1988;9:847–858.

21. Valk J. Gd-DTPA in MR of spinal lesions. *Am J Neuroradiol* 1988;9:345–350.

22. Epstein FJ, Farmer J-P, Freed D. Adult intramedullary spinal cord ependymomas: the result of surgery in 38 patients. *J Neurosurg* 1993;79:204–209.

23. Sherman JL, Barkovich AJ, Citrin CM. The MR appearance of syringohydromyelia: new observations. *Am J Neuroradiol* 1986;7: 985–995.

24. Stein BM. Surgery of intramedullary spinal cord tumors. *Clin Neurosurg* 1979;26:529–542.

25. Nemoto Y, Inoue Y, Tashiro T, et al. Intramedullary spinal cord tumors: significance of associated hemorrhage at MR imaging. *Radiology* 1992;182:793–796.

26. Murovic J, Sundaresan N. Pediatric spinal axis tumors. In: Berger MS, ed. *Pediatric neuro-oncology. Neurosurgery clinics of North America.* Philadelphia: WB Saunders, 1992:947–958.

27. McLauren RL. Extramedullary spinal tumors. In: Shillito J Jr, Matson DD, eds. *Pediatric neurosurgery: surgery of the developing nervous system.* New York: Grune & Stratton, 1982:541–549.

28. Packer RJ, Siegel KR, Lutton L, Litman P, Bruce DA, Schut L. Leptomeningeal dissemination of primary CNS tumors of childhood. *Ann Neurol* 1985;18:217–221.

29. Lee Y-Y, Glass JP, van Eys J, Wallace S. Medulloblastoma in infants and children: CT follow-up after treatment. *Radiology* 1985;154:677–682.

30. George RE, Laurent JP, McCluggage CW, Cheek WR. Spinal metastasis in primitive neuroectodermal tumors of the posterior fossa: evaluation with CT myelography and correlation with patient age and tumor differentiation. *Pediatr Neurosci* 1986;12:157–160.

31. Kramer E, Rafto S, Packer R, Zimmerman RA. Comparison of myelography with CT follow-up versus gadolinium MRI for subarachnoid metastatic disease in children. *Neurology* 1991;41:46–50.

32. Stanley PO, Senac MO, Segall HD. Intraspinal seeding from intracranial tumors in children. *Am J Roentgenol* 1984;144:157–161.

33. Blews DE, Wang H, Kumar AJ, Robb PA, Phillips PC, Bryan RN. Intradural spinal metastases in pediatric patients with primary intracranial neoplasms: Gd-DTPA enhanced MR vs CT myelography. *J Comput Assist Tomogr* 1990;14:730–735.

34. Sze G, Abramson A, Krol G, et al. Gd-DTPA in the evaluation of intradural, extramedullary spinal disease. *Am J Neuroradiol* 1988;9:153–163.

35. Zimmerman RA, Bilaniuk L, Harris C, Phillips P. Use of 0.3 mmol/kg Gadoteridol in the evaluation of pediatric central nervous system diseases. *Radiology* 1993;189P:222.

36. Wiener MD, Boyko OB, Friedman HS, Hockenberger B, Oakes WJ. False positive spinal MR findings for subarachnoid spread of primary CNS tumor in postoperative pediatric patients. *AJNR* 1990;11:1100–1103.

37. Klein DM. Extramedullary spinal tumors. In: McLaurin RL, Schut L, Venes JL, et al, eds. *Pediatric neurosurgery: surgery of the developing nervous System,* 2nd ed. Philadelphia: WB Saunders, 1989:443–452.

38. Dahlin DC. *Bone tumors: general aspects and data on 6,221 cases.* Springfield, IL: Charles C Thomas, 1978.

39. Dorwart RH, LaMasters DL, Watanabe TJ. Tumors. In: Newton TH, Potts DG, eds. *Computed tomography of the spine and spinal cord.* San Anselmo, CA: Clavedel, 1983:115–147.

40. Clough JR, Price CHG. Aneurysmal bone cyst: pathogenesis and long term results of treatment. *Clin Orthop* 1973;97:52–63.

41. Beltran J, Noto AM, Chakeres DW, Christoforidis AJ. Tumors of the osseous spine: staging with MR imaging versus CT. *Radiology* 1987;162:565–569.

42. Lichtenstein L. Histiocytosis X. Integration of eosinophilic granuloma of bone, "Letterer-Siwe disease," and "Schüller-Christian disease" as related manifestations of a single nosologic entity. *Arch Pathol* 1953;56:84–102.

43. McGavran MH, Spady HA. Eosinophilic granuloma of bone: a study of 28 cases. *J Bone Joint Surg (Am)* 1960;42:979–992.

44. Green NE, Robertson WW Jr, Kilroy AW. Eosinophilic granuloma of the spine with associated neural deficit. *J Bone Joint Surg (Am)* 1980;62:1198–1202.

45. Zimmerman RD, Weingarten K, Johnson CE, et al. Neuroradiology of the spine. In: Youmans JR, eds. *Diagnostic procedures,* 3rd ed. In: Youmans JR, ed. *Neurological surgery.* Philadelphia: WB Saunders, 1990:364–404.

46. Sundaresan N, Schiller AL, Rosenthal DI. Osteosarcoma of the spine. In: Sundaresan N, Schmidek HH, Schiller AL, et al, eds. *Tumors of the spine: diagnosis and clinical management.* Philadelphia: WB Saunders, 1990:128–145.

47. Sundaresan N, Krol G, Hughes JEO. Primary malignant tumors of the spine. In: Youmans JR, ed. *Neurological surgery.* Philadelphia: WB Saunders, 1990:3548–3573.

48. Sypert GW. Osteoid osteoma and osteoblastoma of the spine. In: Sundaresan N, Schmidek HH, Schiller AL, et al, eds. *Tumors of the spine: diagnosis and clinical management.* Philadelphia: WB Saunders, 1990:117–127.

49. Nemoto O, Moser RP Jr, Van Dam BE, Aoki J, Gilkey FW. Osteoblastoma of the spine: a review of 75 cases. *Spine* 1990;15: 1272–1280.

50. Kroon HM, Schurmans J. Osteoblastoma: clinical and radiologic findings in 98 new cases. *Radiology* 1990;175:783–790.

51. Crim JR, Mirra JM, Eckardt JJ, Seeger LL. Widespread inflammatory response to osteoblastoma: the flare phenomenon. *Radiology* 1990;177:835–836.

52. Matson DD. *Neurosurgery of infancy and children,* 2nd ed. Springfield, IL: Charles C Thomas, 1969.

53. Naidich TP, McLone DG, Harwood-Nash DC. Arachnoid cysts, paravertebral meningoceles, and perineural cysts. In: Newton TH, Potts DG, eds. *Computed tomography of the spine and spinal cord.* San Anselmo, CA: Clavedel, 1983:383–388.

54. Nugent G, Odom G, Woodhall B. Spinal extradural cysts. *Neurology* 1959;9:397–406.

55. Nabors MW, Pait TG, Byrd EB, et al. Updated assessment and current classification of spinal meningeal cysts. *J Neurosurg* 1988;68:366–377.

56. Russell DS, Rubenstein LJ. *Pathology of tumors of the nervous system.* Baltimore: Williams and Wilkins, 1989.

57. Halliday A, Sobel RA, Martuza RL. Benign spinal nerve sheath tumors: their occurrence sporadically and in neurofibromatosis types 1 and 2. *J Neurosurg* 1991;74:248–253.

58. Burk DL, Brunberg JA, Kanal E, et al. Spinal and paraspinal neurofibromatosis: surface coil imaging at 1.5T. *Radiology* 1987;162: 797–801.

59. Massad M, Haddad F, Slim M, et al. Spinal cord compression in neuroblastoma. *Surg Neurol* 1985;23:567–572.

60. Punt J, Pritchard J, Pincott JR, Till K. Neuroblastoma: a review of 21 cases presenting with spinal cord compression. *Cancer* 1980;45: 3095–3101.

61. Pochedly C. *Neuroblastoma.* Acton, MA: PSG, 1976.

62. Stowens D. Neuroblastoma and related tumors. *Arch Pathol* 1957;63:451–459.

63. Feigin I, Cohen M. Maturation and anaplasia in neuronal tumors of the peripheral nervous system, with observations on the glial-like tissues in the ganglioneuroblastoma. *J Neuropathol Exp Neurol* 1977;36:748–763.

64. Sze G, Bravo S, Baierl P, Shimkin PM. Developing spinal column: gadolinium-enhanced MR imaging. *Radiology* 1991;180:497–502.

CHAPTER 11

Infections of the Nervous System

Although infections are common in children, involvement of the central nervous system by the infectious process is infrequent. Early recognition of CNS infections in children, especially infants, is extremely important, as the long-term effects upon the brain may be devastating. The manifestations of CNS infections on imaging studies are similar in children and adults. The epidemiology and the causative organisms, however, tend to be different. This chapter reviews the various infectious processes that involve the central nervous system in the pediatric age group. The characteristic features of these processes on imaging studies and how they may vary from the adult appearance will be stressed.

CONGENITAL INFECTIONS

Infections of the fetal nervous system differ from those of older children and adults in that they act on the nervous system while it is developing; the manifestations of the infection differ, depending upon the age of the fetus at the time. It is important to remember in this context that *the age of the fetus at the time of the insult is of greater importance than the nature of the insult*. In general, infections during the first two trimesters will result in congenital malformations, whereas those that occur during the third trimester are manifest as destructive lesions.

Another feature of prenatal infections is an *altered biological response to injury*. As described in Chapter 4, the immature brain does not respond to injury by a glial reaction; instead the immune response in the brain repairs the damage, removes abnormal cells, and compensates for missing tissue. The inflammatory response by the immune system, which contributes to the damage produced by viral infection at a later age, is absent or less marked in the fetus (1).

There are two main pathways for the transmission of infection to the fetus. Bacteria usually ascend from the cervix to the amniotic fluid. Toxoplasmosis, syphilis, rubella, cytomegalovirus, and other viruses generally are transmitted via the transplacental route (1).

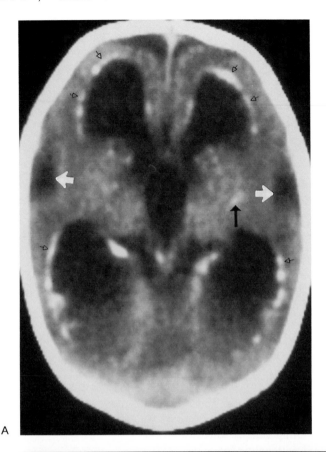

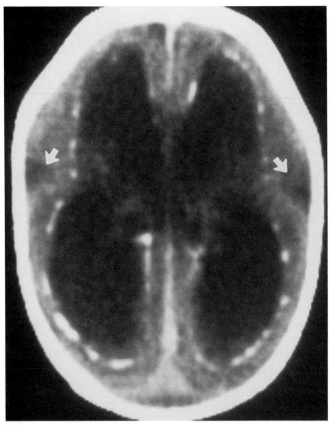

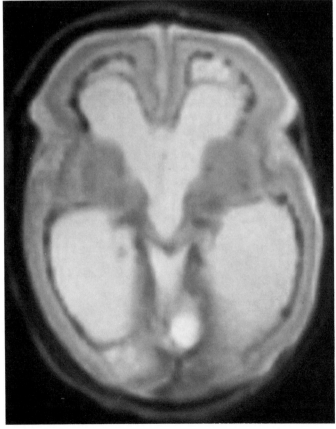

FIG. 11.1. Congenital cytomegalovirus infection in a neonate. **A:** Axial CT at the level of the third ventricle shows calcifications lining the walls of the lateral ventricles (*open black arrows*). Calcification is also seen in the basal ganglia (*closed black arrow*), although to a lesser extent. The shallow, vertical, Sylvian fissures (*white arrows*) suggest an accompanying neuronal migration anomaly, which are frequently seen in cytomegalovirus. **B:** Axial CT at the level of the bodies of the lateral ventricles shows even more extensive periventricular calcification surrounding the ventricles. The shallow, vertical Sylvian fissures are still present at this level (*arrows*). **C:** Axial SE 2500/100 image shows the periventricular calcifications as hypointense compared to neonatal brain tissue. Lissencephaly is more easily appreciated on this MR image than on the CT images.

Congenital brain malformations, caused by infections during the first two trimesters, have been discussed in Chapter 5. Therefore, this section will deal primarily with differences (if any) in the imaging appearance of malformations caused by infections from those caused by ischemia or chromosomal disorders and with infections that occur during the third trimester and result in destructive brain lesions.

Cytomegalovirus

Congenital cytomegalovirus (CMV) disease is the most common serious viral infection among newborns in the United States (2). Congenital CMV infection occurs in approximately 40,000 newborns each year, or approximately 1% of all births. Of these, 10% have the various hematologic, neurologic, and developmental symptoms and signs that define the disease, including hepatosplenomegaly, microcephaly, impaired hearing, and small head size. An additional 10% to 15% of infected infants subsequently develop neurologic or developmental abnormalities in the first year of life (3). In a large recent study from the congenital CMV disease registry (4), hepatosplenomegaly (52%) and petechiae (51%) were found to be the most common clinical signs among

affected children. Severe, permanent neurologic conditions were found in 55%, including intracranial calcifications (43%), microcephaly (27%), chorioretinitis (15%), and seizures (10%). "Less severe neurologic abnormalities" (not specified) were found in 31%, and hearing loss of variable degree was noted in 27%.

The cause of the CNS injury in congenital cytomegalovirus disease is disputed. Some speculated that the virus has an affinity for the rapidly growing cells of the germinal matrix, resulting in abnormalities of the cerebral and cerebellar cortices and a deposition of calcium in the periventricular region. Others postulate a primary vascular target for the virus, with resultant brain injury secondary to fetal brain ischemia (5). Whatever the underlying cause, affected patients typically are microcephalic with polymicrogyria, diminished and gliotic white matter, cerebral calcifications, delayed myelination, and cerebellar hypoplasia (6–10). Findings on cross-sectional imaging examinations are variable, depending upon the degree of brain destruction and the timing of the injury. Some patients, presumably infected during the first half of the second trimester, have complete lissencephaly, with a thin cortex, hypoplastic cerebellum, delayed myelination, marked ventriculomegaly, and significant periventricular calcification (Figs. 11.1, 11.2). Those injured later, presumably in the middle of the second tri-

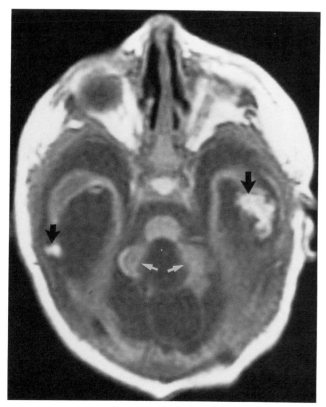

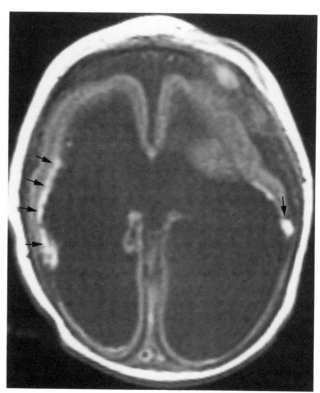

A   B

FIG. 11.2. Congenital cytomegalovirus infection in a neonate. **A, B:** Axial SE 600/20 images show the agyria, markedly hypoplastic cerebellar hemispheres (*white arrows*) and periventricular calcifications (*black arrows*) common in this disorder. (Reprinted with permission from ref. 6.)

mester, have more typical polymicrogyria (cortical dysplasia), less ventricular dilatation, and less consistent cerebellar hypoplasia (Figs. 11.3, 11.4). Patients infected near the end of gestation have normal gyral patterns, mild ventricular and sulcal prominence, and scattered periventricular calcification or hemorrhage (Fig. 11.5) (6). Calcifications can be seen on CT as foci of high attenuation. Although calcifications can also be detected on MR as foci of short T1 and T2 relaxation times, they are much more easily and reliably detected on CT than on MR. Differentiation of calcification from hemorrhage may be difficult by either modality (6). In general, the sensitivity of CT to calcification makes CT the most sensitive method for detection of congenital CMV of the brain. However, calcification is not specific by itself, as any injury to the brain, including those caused by ischemia and metabolic errors (11,12), can cause dystrophic calcification. MR can often be helpful in the detection of cortical dysplasia, which is far more common in CMV than in other causes of cerebral calcification.

Toxoplasmosis

Toxoplasmosis is caused by the protozoan *Toxoplasma gondii,* a parasite first found in North African rodents. It infects a wide range of birds and mammals. Pregnant women usually acquire the infection by ingestion of oocysts in uncooked meat (13,14). The incidence of congenital infections is estimated at 1 out of 1,000–3,500 live births; when stillborns are included, the incidence is as high as 1% of all pregnancies (13).

Symptoms may become apparent at birth or after several days to weeks. The infection may be generalized or concentrated primarily in the nervous system. The principal CNS findings are a chorioretinitis (bilateral in 85% of affected patients), abnormal cerebrospinal fluid, hydrocephalus, and seizures (15). Whether involvement is generalized or primarily limited to the CNS, the prognosis is quite poor. Overall mortality ranges from 11% to 14%. Survivors tend to be mentally retarded, with seizures and spasticity (16).

Pathologically, a diffuse inflammatory infiltration of the meninges is found, with large and small granulomatous lesions or a diffuse inflammation of the brain. Hydrocephalus is frequent, most often caused by an ependymitis occluding the aqueduct (12,17). Hydranencephaly may occur if the disease is severe and occurs in the second trimester (18).

The findings on cross-sectional imaging studies may be similar to those in cytomegalovirus infection. Calcifications are common; they are usually both periventric-

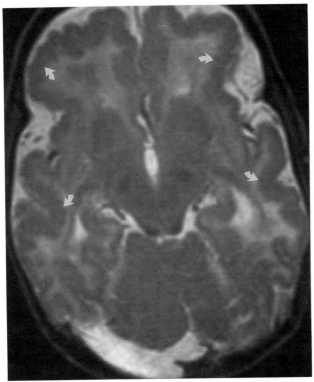 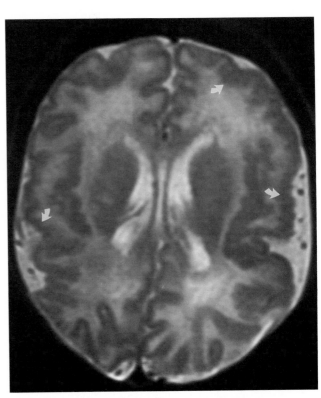

A   B

FIG. 11.3. An 8-month-old with congenital cytomegalovirus infection. **A, B:** Axial SE 3000/120 images show several foci of polymicrogyria (*arrows*), with cortical thickening and irregularity of the gray matter–white matter border. Myelination is delayed. (Reprinted with permission from ref. 6.)

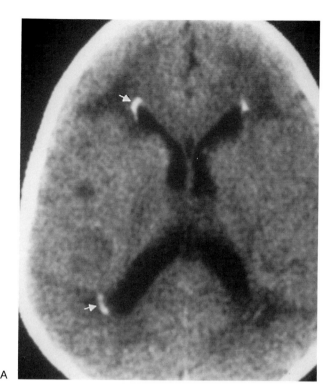

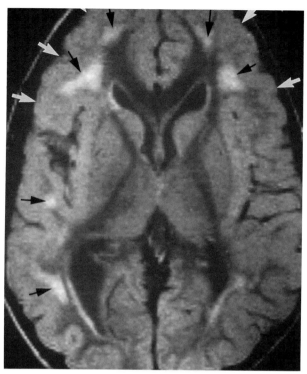

A

B

FIG. 11.4. An 8-year-old with congenital cytomegalovirus infection. **A:** Axial CT image shows calcifications (*white arrows*) and lucent white matter at the corners of the lateral ventricles. **B:** Axial SE 2000/25 image shows bilateral frontal cortical dysplasia (*white arrows*) and multiple foci of high signal intensity (*black arrows*) in the periventricular and subcortical white matter.

ular and cortical. Microcephaly, large ventricles, and hydrocephalus can be seen. As with cytomegalovirus, a spectrum is seen, from relatively mild disease, with a few periventricular calcifications and mild atrophy, to severe disease, with near total destruction of the cortex and brain accompanied by marked, diffuse cerebral calcification. Diebler and colleagues have related the severity of the brain involvement to the date of maternal infection (19). They found that early infection (before 20 weeks) is generally accompanied by severe neurologic signs, including microcephaly, hydrocephalus, tetra- or diplegia, seizures, mental retardation, and blindness. The CT scan in this group of patients reveals ventricular dilatation, areas of porencephaly, and extensive calcifications, particularly in the basal ganglia (Fig. 11.6). Infection between 20 and 30 weeks leads to a more variable outcome. On CT scan, multiple periventricular calcifications and ventricular dilatation are present. Infection after the 30th week is generally associated with mild clinical manifestations. The CT findings are those of small periventricular and intracerebral calcifications that are only rarely accompanied by ventricular dilatation (19). An important differentiating feature is the absence of cortical dysplasia, which is a common finding in congenital CMV infection; cortical dysplasia is rare in congenital toxoplasmosis.

Herpes Simplex Virus

Infection of the fetus with herpes simplex virus may result in a fatal generalized disease. Most cases result from exposure of the fetus to maternal type II herpetic genital lesions as the baby passes through the birth canal. The incidence of neonatal herpes simplex infections is estimated to be 1 per 2,000–5,000 deliveries per year (20). The brain is involved in approximately 30% of infected infants.

Symptoms usually develop within the first 2–4 weeks of life. The principal clinical findings may be (1) visceral disease with cyanosis, jaundice, fever, and respiratory distress, or (2) CNS meningoencephalitis with focal or generalized seizures; lethargy and fever are common (21). With CNS involvement, CSF studies will show a mononuclear pleocytosis with a negative Gram stain. Central nervous system involvement may result in mental retardation, severe neurologic deficits, or death (16). The outcome is usually poor (20).

Imaging studies in patients with neonatal herpes encephalitis show patchy, widespread areas of abnormal signal (low attenuation on CT, prolonged T1 and T2 on MR), primarily in the white matter, which rapidly progress in prominence and area of involvement during the course of the disease. Contrast enhancement, although

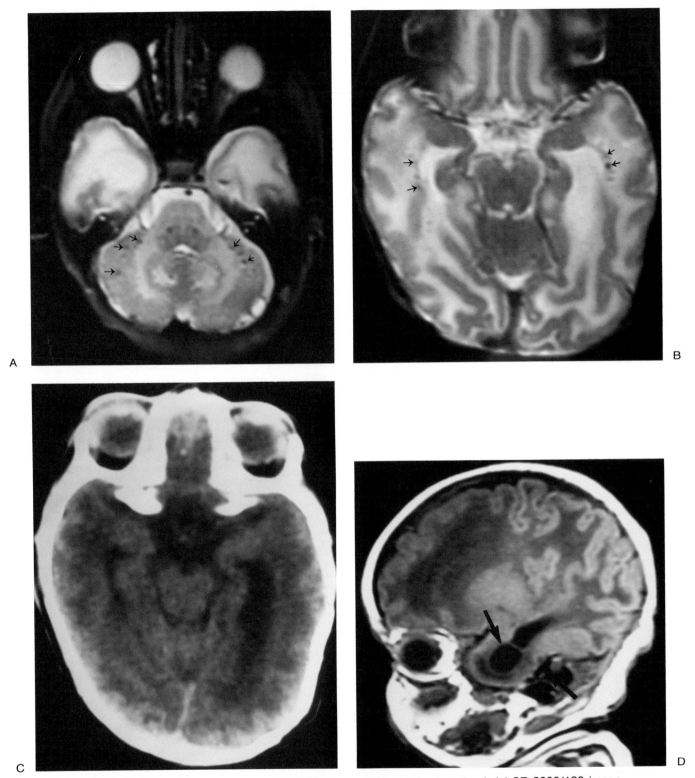

FIG. 11.5. Newborn infant with congenital cytomegalovirus infection. **A:**. Axial SE 3000/120 image shows multiple low-intensity foci (*arrows*) in the posterior fossa and edema in the right temporal lobe. **B:** Axial SE 3000/120 image at the level of the midbrain shows periventricular punctate hypointensities (*arrows*) around the temporal horns. **C:** Axial CT image shows that the areas of abnormal MR signal are not calcification. **D:** Parasagittal SE 550/15 image shows a cyst (*arrows*) anterior to the temporal horn. (Reprinted with permission from ref. 6.)

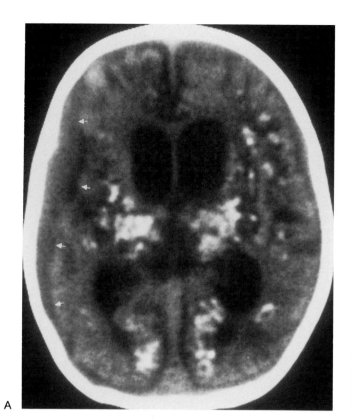

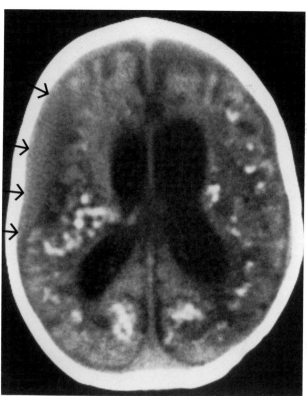

A

B

FIG. 11.6. Congenital toxoplasmosis. **A, B:** Axial CT images show extensive parenchymal damage. Calcifications are scattered throughout the brain but are most prominent in the basal ganglia. There is less periventricular calcification than is usually seen in cytomegalovirus. The brain is shrunken, falling away from the calvarium with a resultant subdural hematoma (*white arrows*). The cortical gyral pattern, seen best in B, appears normal.

minimal, occurs in a meningeal pattern, presumably reflecting meningeal involvement. As the disease progresses, the cortical gray matter undergoes a change in signal (increase in attenuation on CT, shortening of T1 and T2 on MR) that persists for weeks to months (21) (Fig. 11.7). Loss of brain substance occurs rapidly, often as early as the third week. Eventually, severe, diffuse cerebral atrophy evolves, with profound cortical thinning, encephalomalacia (often multicystic in nature) of white matter, and either punctate or gyriform calcification. The cerebellum is involved in about half of affected patients (21).

Although the white matter changes in neonatal herpes encephalitis are nonspecific, the meningeal pattern of enhancement and the increased attenuation/short T1/T2 of cortical gray matter that may persist for weeks to months should lead to a suggestion of the diagnosis of neonatal herpes simplex encephalitis. A clinical diagnosis requires isolation of the virus. It is preferable to isolate the virus from the cerebrospinal fluid or from skin lesions, but often brain biopsy is required. The reader should note that the clinical presentation and imaging appearance of herpes encephalitis in older children and

adults (usually caused by herpes simplex virus, type I) are quite different from those of the neonatal infection. Details are given in the section on viral encephalitis later in this chapter.

Congenital Rubella

Congenital rubella is now extremely rare in Western countries because of screening techniques now performed on pregnant women. This virus affects the fetus more commonly during the first and second trimesters; in fact, it is nearly benign when it occurs during the third trimester (22). Cataracts, glaucoma, and cardiac malformations occur when the infant is infected during the first 2 months of gestation; hearing loss and psychomotor retardation may follow infection that occurs any time during the first trimester and, occasionally, as late as 16 weeks postconceptional age (16). The clinical presentation at birth is usually one of lethargy, hypotonia, and a large or bulging fontanel. By the time they are 4 months old, affected patients are usually irritable, with vasomotor instability and photophobia. Seizures develop in approximately 25% (16,23).

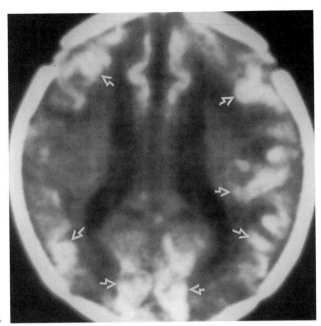
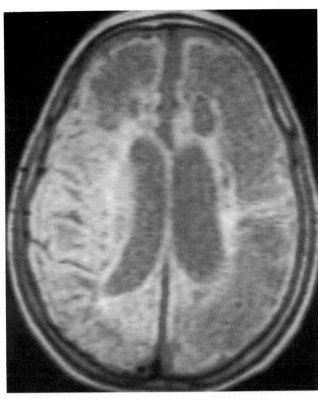

FIG. 11.7. Neonatal herpes encephalitis. **A:** Axial noncontrast CT scan shows abnormally low attenuation in the white matter. The cerebral cortex shows an abnormally high signal intensity (*arrows*), suggestive of neonatal herpes meningoencephalitis. **B:** Follow-up MR study at age 3 months shows severe macrocystic encephalomalacia involving most of the cerebrum.

On pathologic examination, brains of affected infants are micrencephalic, with ventriculomegaly secondary to marked loss of brain tissue. Microphthalmia, cataracts, glaucoma, and chorioretinitis are common. Multiple small areas of liquefactive necrosis and gliosis with calcification are seen in the periventricular white matter, the basal ganglia, and the brain stem. Encephalitis is usually not progressive after infancy.

The appearance of the brain on imaging studies varies, depending upon the time of the *in utero* infection. Early infection will result in congenital anomalies, whereas late infection will result in a nonspecific generalized edema or loss of brain tissue. CT typically shows calcification in the basal ganglia and cortex. In severe cases, nearly total brain destruction and microcephaly are present (24).

MENINGITIS

The most common form of central nervous system infection in children is meningitis. In general, meningitis is relatively benign, especially when viral in origin (25,26). Imaging studies are not performed routinely; they are indicated if the clinical diagnosis is unclear, if neurologic

deterioration occurs secondary to increased intracranial pressure, if the meningitis is associated with persistent seizures or focal neurologic deficits, or if patient recovery from the disease is slow (26,27).

Pathophysiology

Organisms reach the meninges by five routes: (1) direct hematogenous spread, (2) passage through the choroid plexus, (3) rupture of superficial cortical abscesses, (4) penetrating trauma, as from a knife wound (or sometimes a shunt), and (5) contiguous spread of an adjacent infection (26,28). Contiguous spread is particularly common in otitis media and in sinusitis.

Even when predisposing factors are present, meningitis is uncommon because the subarachnoid space tends to resist infection in normal children (1). Once the infection is established, however, meningeal infection can cause neurologic sequelae by a number of methods. The infection generally spreads along the leptomeningeal sheaths of penetrating cortical vessels in the Virchow-Robin spaces. The endothelial cells swell, proliferate, and crowd into the vessel lumen within 48–72 hours of the initial infection. Moreover, inflammatory cells infiltrate the vessel wall. Foci of necrosis develop in the arterial walls and occasionally induce arterial thrombosis (29). A similar process occurs in the veins; focal necrosis of the vessel wall and mural thrombi can partially or totally occlude the lumen. Venous thrombosis is more frequent than arterial thrombosis (1,27) and is particularly common when the meningitis is associated with a subdural empyema; the thrombus forms in the vein as it courses through the infected subdural space. Overall, cerebral infarctions (arterial and venous) can be seen in up to 30% of neonates with bacterial meningitis (30). Moreover, extension of the infectious process through obstructed vessels into brain parenchyma can result in cerebritis and abscess formation.

Large quantities of fibrinopurulent exudate can accumulate around the spinal cord, resulting in obstruction of the spinal subarachnoid space. Exudate in the foramina of Luschka and Magendie can cause a noncommunicating hydrocephalus. Communicating hydrocephalus develops when exudate accumulates in the basilar cisterns or over the cerebral convexity, interfering with normal flow and absorption of cerebrospinal fluid. Proliferation of ependymal or glial cells within the Sylvian aqueduct and involvement of the arachnoid villi exacerbate the imbalance between CSF production and absorption. The hydrocephalus may spontaneously resolve after resolution of the infection. Ventricular enlargement may also result from injury to and resorption of periventricular white matter, a process that evolves over several weeks.

An associated ventriculitis occurs in 30% of patients. This complication is especially common in neonates, with an incidence as high as 92% (31). Ependymal changes are minimal early in the course of the infection. In severe or prolonged meningitis, however, cellular infiltration of the subependymal perivascular spaces and glial proliferation may occur, resulting in overgrowth of the ependymal lining and obliteration of the aqueduct (1).

Clinical Presentation of Purulent Meningitis

Clinical presentation varies with the age of the patient. A history of preceding upper respiratory or gastrointestinal infection can often be elicited. Older children present with fever, headache, nausea, vomiting, nuchal and spinal rigidity, alterations of sensorium, convulsions, disturbances in vision, and, occasionally, papilledema (1). Later complications may include cranial nerve palsies, shock, disseminated intravascular coagulation, cerebral infarction, hydrocephalus, or respiratory failure. The cranial nerve involvement presumably results from local inflammation of the perineurium as well as impaired vascular supply to the nerves. Cranial nerves 6, 3, and 4 are most commonly affected.

The presentation of meningitis in neonates and young infants differs from that in older children; only nonspecific signs of sepsis may be present. Nuchal rigidity is rare; fever and a full fontanel may be absent. CSF findings are less useful than in older children because of the wide range of normal findings in neonates. Seizures are a presenting sign in up to 40% of affected neonates and, because of the high incidence of cerebral infarction in neonatal meningitis, hemiparesis may be present. A high index of suspicion is critical (26).

Imaging Manifestations of Meningitis

Uncomplicated Purulent Meningitis

CT and MR studies in uncomplicated cases of purulent meningitis are usually normal. Occasionally, some enhancement of the meninges will be seen on postcontrast scans (24). Contrast-enhanced MR is more sensitive than contrast-enhanced CT in detecting inflammatory changes in the meninges (32); however, enhancement of the meninges is only occasionally seen, even with MR. *Except for rare occasions, the diagnosis of meningitis is made from clinical signs and symptoms and the results of a lumbar puncture.* As stated earlier, *imaging is best reserved to look for complications of meningitis in patients with complicated clinical courses.*

Complications of Meningitis

Hydrocephalus as a sequel of meningitis is well evaluated by all imaging modalities; MR is the most effective at localizing the level of the obstruction (see Chapter 8).

Deep vein, cortical vein, and sinus thrombosis are uncommon complications of meningitis; they are more likely in the presence of dehydration. Sinus thrombosis is recognizable on CT by the so-called Delta sign, which is a triangle of decreased density in the posterior portion of the superior sagittal sinus on a contrast-enhanced scan. This sign is only visible after the clot becomes less dense than the contrast-enhanced blood flowing within it; in the acute phase (when the clot is dense), thrombus can be seen as high density in the sagittal sinus on a noncontrast scan (Fig. 11.8) (33,34).

Recent advances in MR angiography have greatly aided the diagnosis of venous sinus thrombosis by MR. Other than in the subacute phase, the MR diagnosis of sinus thrombosis is difficult. In the acute phase, the sinus is isointense to brain on T1-weighted images and hypointense on T2-weighted images. This appearance can be mistaken for slow flow or pseudogating (in which the sinus is always imaged during diastole). To establish a lack of blood flow, MR venography using a phase contrast technique with gradient timing set to detect a phase change of 180° at 20 cm/sec (V_{enc} = 20 cm/sec) is necessary. In the subacute phase, MR diagnosis of sinus

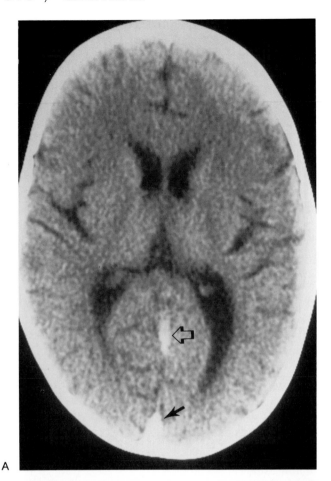

A

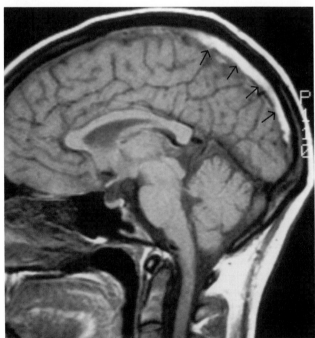

B

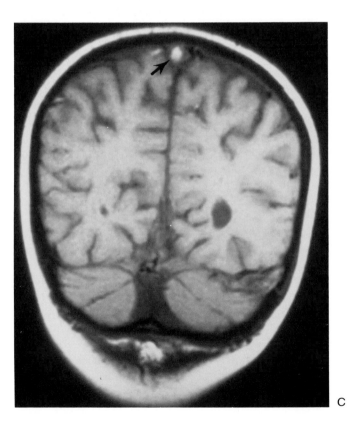

C

FIG. 11.8. Sagittal sinus thrombosis secondary to meningitis. **A:** Noncontrast CT scan shows high attenuation in the straight sinus (*open arrow*) and the superior sagittal sinus (*arrow*). The presence of such high signal intensity within vascular structures in a child beyond the first few months of life is extremely suspicious for sinus thrombosis. **B:** Sagittal SE 600/20 image shows high signal intensity in the posterior half of the superior sagittal sinus (*arrows*). **C:** Coronal SE 700/20 image using saturation pulses to eliminate entry flow phenomena shows high signal intensity within the superior sagittal sinus (*arrow*), supporting the diagnosis of sagittal sinus thrombosis.

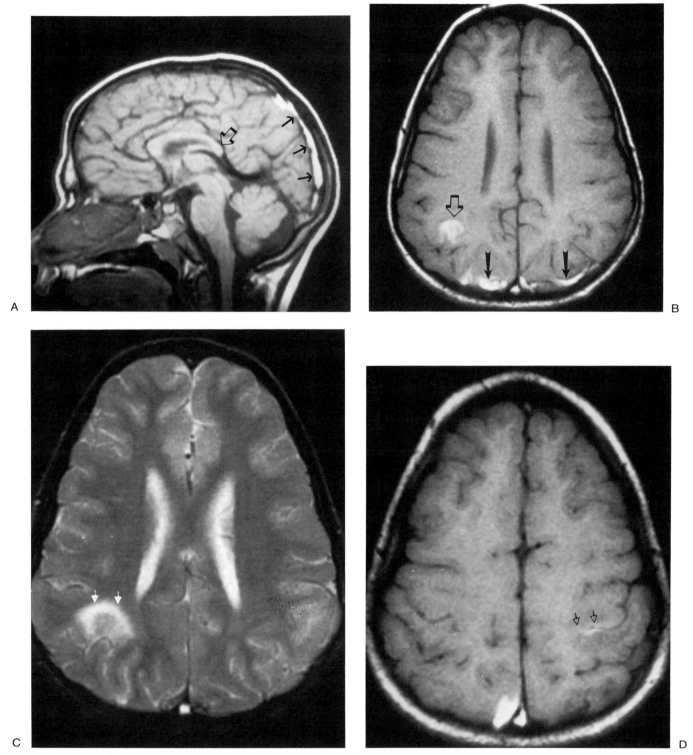

FIG. 11.9. Superior sagittal sinus thrombosis with venous infarcts. **A:** Sagittal SE 600/20 image shows high signal intensity in the posterior superior sagittal sinus (*arrows*). Note that the splenium of the corpus callosum is hypogenetic (*open arrow*) and the rostrum of the corpus callosum is absent, indicating that this patient has an underlying congenital brain anomaly. **B:** High signal intensity in the posterior parietal white matter (*open arrow*) represents a hemorrhagic venous infarct secondary to the sinus thrombosis. The high signal intensity in the occipital cortical veins (*arrows*) may represent entry flow phenomena or venous thrombosis. This illustrates the difficulty of diagnosing venous thrombosis using MR imaging. **C:** SE 2800/70 image shows that the hematoma is isointense with white matter. The high signal intensity (*arrows*) surrounding the hematoma represents edema. **D:** SE 600/20 image at the level of the cerebral convexities shows a curvilinear cortical hemorrhage (*open arrows*). This is another manifestation of a venous infarct. (This case courtesy of Dr. W. Peck.)

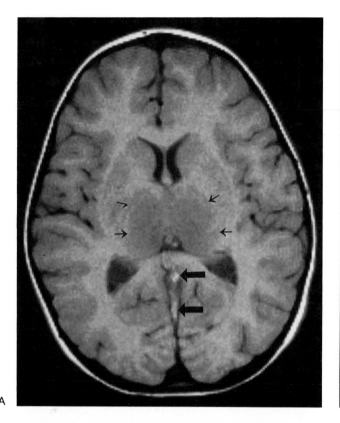

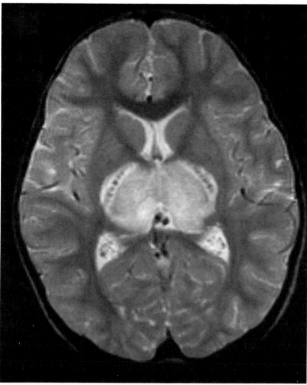

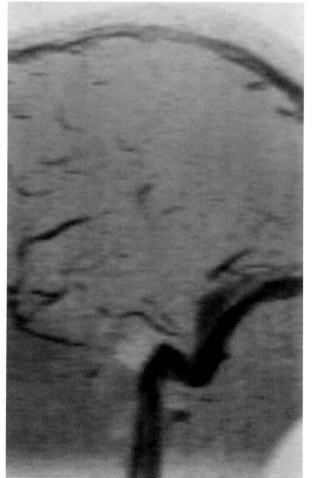

FIG. 11.10. Bilateral thalamic ischemia secondary to straight sinus thrombosis. **A:** Axial SE 600/16 image shows hypointensity in the thalami (*small arrows*). The straight sinus (*large arrows*) shows hyperintensity, suggesting thrombus. **B:** Axial SE 2500/90 image shows hyperintensity in the thalami, extending into the posterior limbs of the internal capsules. **C:** Phase contrast MR angiogram shows no signal from the vein of Galen or straight sinus.

thrombosis is straightforward, as high signal intensity is seen along most of the affected (superior sagittal or straight) sinus on a sagittal T1-weighted image (Figs. 11.8–11.10). Diagnosis of thrombosis of the transverse or sigmoid sinuses is nearly impossible without the use of MR venography, although the lack of flow void within the sinus on parasagittal views is helpful. Two-dimensional time of flight MR venography (with images acquired in the coronal plane; see Chapter 1) or phase contrast MR venography (with V_{enc} = 20 cm/sec) is necessary to make the diagnosis. The most reliable and cost-effective means of diagnosing venous sinus thrombosis is intravenous digital subtraction angiography. The serial angiographic images should be obtained in the AP oblique plane with the head turned 10° to one side.

Venous infarcts are diagnosed by their characteristic location and appearance. Typically, infarcts from sagittal sinus thrombosis are parasagittal (Fig. 11.9), infarcts from straight sinus/vein of Galen thrombosis involve the thalami (Fig. 11.10), and infarcts from vein of Labbé, transverse sinus, or sigmoid sinus thrombosis involve the temporal lobe (see discussion in Chapter 4). On CT, venous infarcts are usually poorly delimited, hypodense, or mixed attenuation areas involving the subcortical white matter and producing a slight mass effect on ventricular structures. The low attenuation is probably due to localized cerebral edema, whereas high-attenuation areas usually represent hemorrhage. Following contrast administration, linear or round gyral enhancement frequently overlies the hypodensity (35). On MR, the edematous areas have prolonged T1 and T2 relaxation times (Figs. 11.9, 11.10). Twenty-five percent of venous infarcts are hemorrhagic and have an imaging appearance that varies from large subcortical hematomas to petechial hemorrhages within edematous brain parenchyma (Fig. 11.9) (34,35). The hemorrhages are generally subcortical and often multifocal with irregular margins. They are occasionally linear in nature, indicating hematoma in and around the vein; this appearance is quite specific.

Periarteritis accompanying meningitis can be reliably diagnosed by CT or MR because of the resulting infarcts, which tend to be sharply marginated and confined to a specific arterial vascular territory. Large or small vessels can be affected. When major vessels, such as the middle or anterior cerebral arteries, are involved, large, usually cortical infarctions result (Fig. 11.11). Frequently, multiple lacunar-type infarcts are seen in the distribution

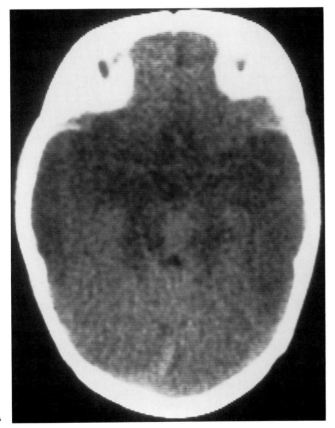
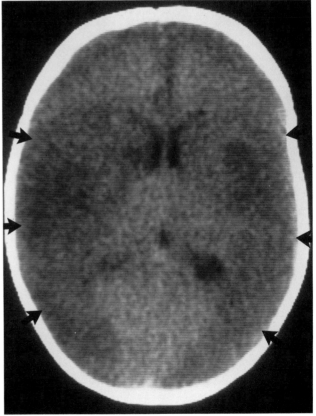

A   B

FIG. 11.11. Bilateral middle cerebral artery infarcts secondary to meningitis. **A:** Noncontrast CT shows low attenuation bilaterally in the distribution of the middle cerebral arteries. **B:** At a higher level, the low attenuation is seen to involve the entire middle cerebral artery distribution (*arrows*) bilaterally.

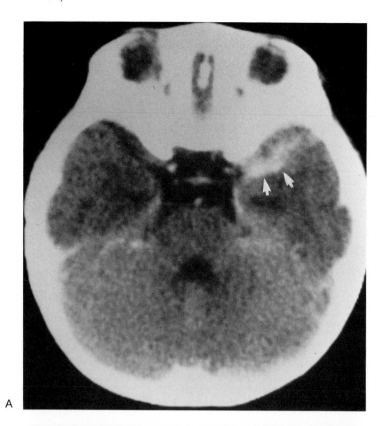

A

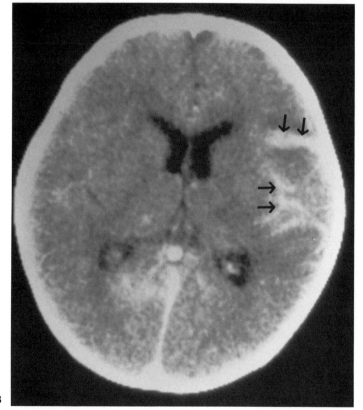

B

FIG. 11.12. Meningitis with infarctions as a result of periarteritis. **A-C:** Patient with tuberculous meningitis. **A:** Axial contrast-enhanced CT shows enhancement within the inferior left Sylvian fissure near the limen insula (*arrows*). **B:** At a slightly higher level, marked enhancement can be seen throughout the left Sylvian fissure (*arrows*).

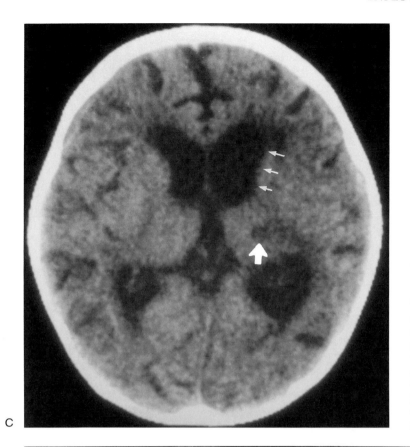

C

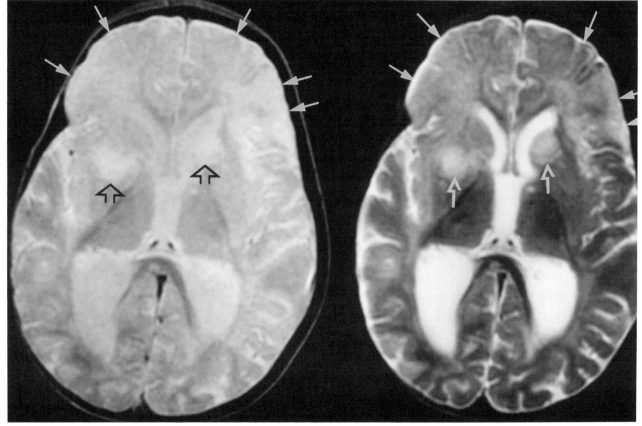

D
E

FIG. 11.12. (*Continued*.) **C:** Follow-up noncontrast scan taken 2 months later. There is marked atrophy with a prominent interhemispheric fissure and prominent cortical sulci. There is *ex vacuo* dilatation of the lateral ventricles. A lacunar infarct is seen in the left thalamus (*large arrow*). The left caudate head is poorly seen and the lateral border of the left frontal horn is straightened (*small arrows*), indicating infarction of the left caudate. **D, E:** Patient with *Haemophilus influenza* meningitis. Axial SE 3000/60 (D) and 120 (E) images show cortical (*solid arrows*) and basal ganglia (*open arrows*) infarcts.

of perforating vessels in the brain stem and basal ganglia (Fig. 11.12), presumably resulting from involvement of the basilar cisterns and vessels contained therein.

Infants with meningitis, particularly that due to *Hemophilus influenzae*, frequently develop *subdural effusions*, sterile fluid collections that develop within the subdural space. They are not empyemas and do not need to be surgically treated. Effusions are isointense to cerebrospinal fluid and located over the frontal and temporal regions of the brain. Occasionally, a portion of the medial surface (the cerebral surface) of an effusion will show enhancement, presumably from an inflammatory membrane or underlying cortical infarction (24,36). Subdural empyemas and their differentiation from hygromas will be discussed in a later section.

Cerebritis and abscesses can develop as a complication of meningitis when the infectious process travels through thrombosed venules into the cerebral parenchyma. Cerebritis and abscess formation are discussed in detail in following sections.

When *ventriculitis* is present, intense enhancement of the ependyma is seen following contrast administration on both CT and MR (Fig. 11.13). MR may have a greater sensitivity to the inflammatory process. The ventricles are nearly always dilated as a result of the obstruction of CSF flow that is typically present in meningitis. Loculations of cerebrospinal fluid within and external to the ventricles (Fig. 11.13) are fairly common. The loculations may result from obstruction of ventricular outlets, the formation of septations across the ventricles, or necrosis of periventricular brain tissue (37). The septations may arise from organization of exudate that forms on the damaged ependyma (38) or from incorporation of coalescent lakes of periventricular white matter edema into the ventricle (37). Septations are identified much better by ultrasound or MR than by CT.

Tuberculous Meningitis

Tuberculous meningitis remains a serious pediatric infectious disease, particularly in underdeveloped nations. Even in the United States, it causes more deaths than any other form of tuberculosis (1). Tuberculous meningitis is

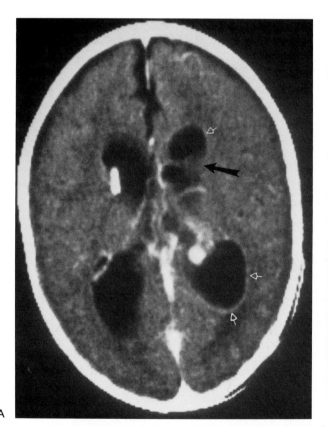
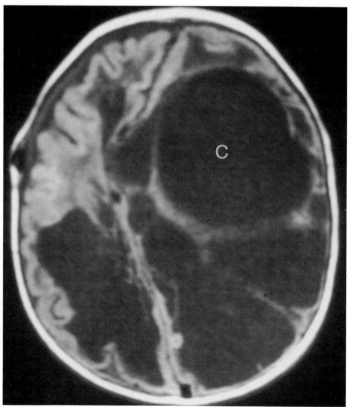

FIG. 11.13. Ventriculitis as a result of meningitis. **A:** Contrast-enhanced CT scan shows ventricular dilatation and enhancement (*open arrows*) of the ventricular wall. A glial septation (*closed black arrow*) is present in the left frontal horn. A ventriculostomy tube is in place because this patient developed hydrocephalus. **B:** Ventriculitis. Axial SE 600/20 image in a different patient shows a distorted brain with multiple intraventricular and extraventricular cysts. Multiple septations are present within and between the cysts. The cyst under the highest pressure **(C)** compresses adjacent cysts and ventricular structures.

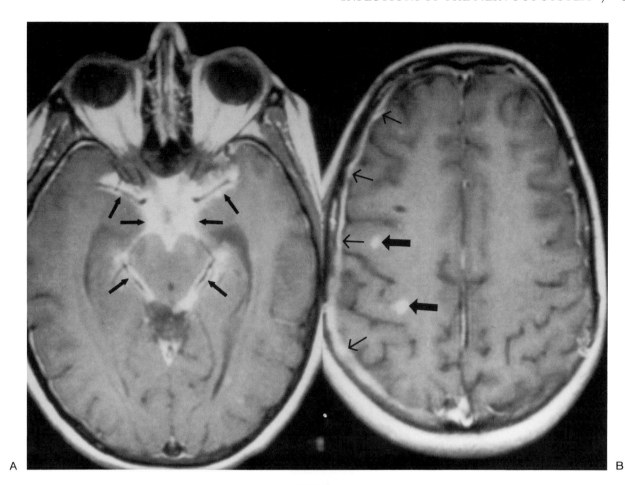

A

B

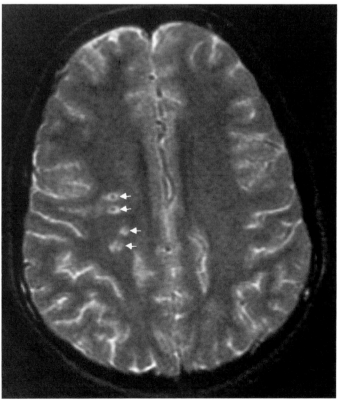

C

FIG. 11.14. Tuberculous meningitis. **A:** Axial SE 600/20 image after infusion of paramagnetic contrast shows marked enhancement of the basilar cisterns. Note how the suprasellar cistern, medial Sylvian fissures, interpeduncular cistern, and ambient cisterns all markedly enhance (*arrows*). **B:** On this image through the centrum semiovale, there is meningeal enhancement on the right (*narrow arrows*) and two enhancing tuberculomas (*large arrows*) at the gray–white junction of the parietal lobe. **C:** Axial SE 2800/70 image shows several tuberculomas in the parietal white matter of the right hemisphere (*arrows*).

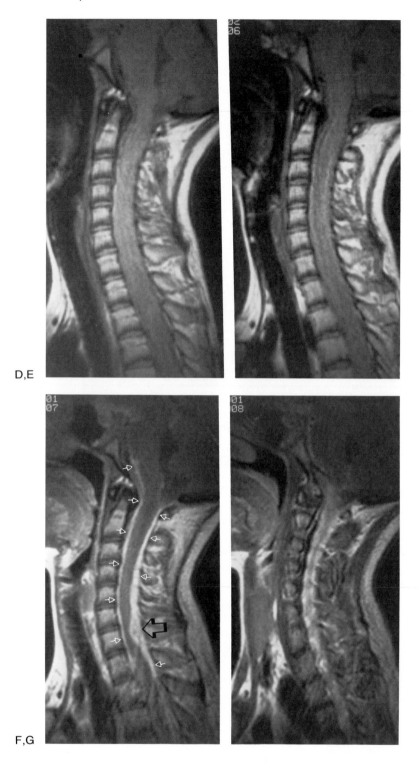

D,E

F,G

FIG. 11.14. (*Continued.*) **D, E:** Noncontrast SE 600/20 images through the cervical spine. A diffuse process in the subarachnoid space obscures the spinal cord, which is normally distinctly outlined by cerebrospinal fluid on T1-weighted images. **F, G:** After infusion of paramagnetic contrast, the subarachnoid space and meninges (*open white arrows*) diffusely enhance. A large tuberculoma is seen dorsal to the spinal cord at the C7 level (*open black arrow*).

often not readily recognized clinically because characteristic signs and symptoms of meningitis may be absent; tuberculous meningitis differs in clinical presentation and radiographic appearance from the pyogenic meningitides (26,28). Fever is present in less than half the patients, headache in 20%, nuchal rigidity in 75% (26,28). If tuberculous meningitis is not promptly recognized and treated, the results to the brain are devastating. Affected patients will develop hydrocephalus from blockage of the CSF pathways and severe brain atrophy resulting from multiple micro- and macroinfarctions. If untreated, tuberculous meningitis rapidly progresses to death, with an average disease duration of only 3 weeks (39).

Tuberculous meningitis in children almost always accompanies generalized miliary tuberculosis. Involvement of the meninges probably results from rupture of a small tuberculoma in the cortex, spinal cord, or leptomeninges; tuberculomas of the choroid plexus may be another source of infection (26,40). In tuberculous meningitis, a gelatinous exudate fills the basal cisterns, particularly the prepontine cistern. Small tubercles may lie over the convexity of the brain or in the periventricular area. The basal ganglia and thalamus in the region of the lenticulostriate and thalamo-perforating arteries are involved by a perivasculitis in almost half of all cases (26,28).

On imaging studies, ventriculomegaly, most often secondary to hydrocephalus, is present in 50% to 77% of affected patients (40,41). The basal cisterns are filled by the purulent tuberculous exudate, which can extend into the spinal subarachnoid space. On noncontrast CT or T1-weighted MR scans, the exudate appears as soft tissue density filling the cisterns. The exudate may be easily overlooked on T2-weighted images, because the high-intensity CSF signal will obscure the cisternal disease. Following contrast administration, the involved cisterns exhibit marked enhancement (Figs. 11.12, 11.14) (41–44).

Infarcts are seen in the basal ganglia and thalamus in the subacute phase in most patients as a result of infiltration of the meningeal infection into the Virchow-Robin spaces and the resulting vasculitis (41,45,46) (Fig. 11.12). They appear as low-density regions on CT and areas of prolonged T1 and T2 relaxation time on MR. Cortical infarctions can result from involvement of cortical vessels but are less common (39,41).

Multiple punctate or ring-enhancing foci of enhancement, representing tuberculomas, may be seen at the junction of the gray and white matter (Fig. 11.14). They may be single or multiple, with multiple lesions being more common above the tentorium and solitary lesions being more frequent below the tentorium (47). Tuberculomas are most often parenchymal but can occasionally be dural based (48). When they are less than 2 cm in diameter, tuberculomas usually show uniform enhancement (Fig. 11.14), whereas those greater than 2 cm in diameter tend to have a thick ring of enhancement with a center that is isointense to brain parenchyma (48). Tuberculomas uncommonly calcify or generate surrounding vasogenic edema. Calcified granulomas appear as small, ring-enhancing lesions on contrast-enhanced MR. Miliary tuberculosis appears as multiple small foci of high intensity on T2-weighted images, and enhancing after contrast administration, throughout the brain; the primary locations are at the cortical–white matter junction and in the distribution of perforating vessels (thalami, basal ganglia, brain stem) (49). Other granulomatous meningitides, such as cryptococcosis or coccidioidomycosis, are extremely rare in the pediatric age group. Their CT and MR appearances are similar to those of tuberculous meningitis.

BACTERIAL CEREBRITIS

Cerebritis is the earliest stage of purulent brain infection (17). It is a focal or multifocal suppurative process that may resolve, or evolve to frank abscess formation. A single site or multiple sites within the brain may become involved. The pyogenic organisms that cause cerebritis gain access to the brain by one of four routes: (1) hematogenous spread from a distant infection or generalized sepsis, (2) extension of contiguous infections (such as in the middle ear or paranasal sinuses) either directly or as a result of septic thrombophlebitis of bridging veins, (3) complications from a penetrating wound, and (4) cardiopulmonary malfunction, such as cyanotic congenital heart disease or a pulmonary arteriovenous malformation. Congenital defects of the overlying bone, such as in encephaloceles or dermal sinus tracts, can also be a source of infection (28,50). Pathologically, in cerebritis there is infiltration of the brain with inflammatory cells, the development of tissue necrosis, and frank edema. The surrounding edematous brain tissue has very similar consistency to the involved area of cerebritis.

It is difficult to distinguish cerebritis from frank abscess by clinical criteria. The distinction is important, however, because cerebritis frequently responds to appropriate antibiotic therapy; more important, surgery is contraindicated in cerebritis. Once cerebritis has evolved to an encapsulated abscess, antibiotic therapy may continue to be effective, but surgery is often a useful or indicated adjunct. During the early phases of cerebritis, both CT and MR will show evidence of increased water in the affected brain, that is, ill-defined areas of low density on CT and ill-defined regions of prolonged T1 and T2 relaxation time on MR (51). Ill-defined foci of enhancement may be seen after infusion of contrast (Fig. 11.15). Mild to moderate mass effect is usually present. Sequential imaging studies are imperative in determining whether the process responds to antibiotic therapy or whether it progresses to abscess formation.

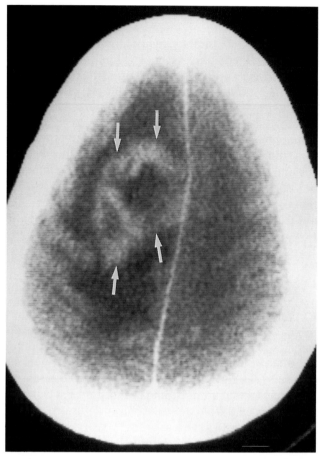

FIG. 11.15. Cerebritis. Contrast-enhanced CT shows an irregularly enhancing mass in the right frontal convexity (*arrows*) with surrounding vasogenic edema. Note the indistinct, irregular enhancement of the wall at this stage.

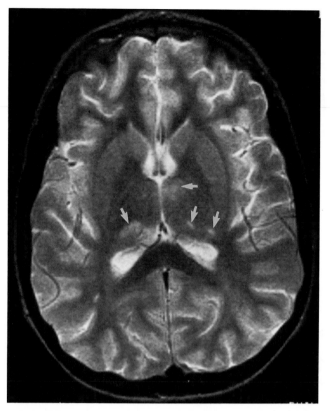

FIG. 11.16. Lyme disease. Axial SE 2800/80 image shows multiple foci of T2 prolongation (*arrows*) in the thalami. (Case courtesy Dr. William Kelly, Fairfield, CA.)

LYME DISEASE

Lyme disease is a multisystem disorder caused by *Borrelia burgdorferi*, an arthropod-borne spirochete. It is the most common tick-borne disease in the United States and Europe (52,53). Children are commonly affected by the disease; 23% of reported cases have been in children and adolescents (52). Lyme disease can involve the joints, skin, eyes, heart, and nervous system. Neurologic involvement is present in 15% to 22% of affected children, most commonly manifest as lymphocytic meningitis, meningoencephalitis, cranial neuropathy, or a pseudotumor cerebrilike syndrome (52). Most common presenting signs and symptoms are headache, behavioral changes, facial palsy, and papilledema.

CT scans are usually normal in Lyme disease, although focal areas of decreased attenuation have been reported (52,54). MR is positive in about 25% of affected patients, typically showing focal regions of T2 prolongation in the brain (Fig. 11.16) (52,55).

BRAIN ABSCESS

If cerebritis is not successfully treated medically, the affected portion of the brain liquefies and a surrounding capsule of granulation tissue and collagen forms, resulting in an abscess. Patients with intracranial abscesses present with headache, lethargy, obtundation, vomiting, or seizures. Fever may be present but is usually intermittent. Focal neurologic deficits, papilledema, or nuchal rigidity may develop (56).

Brain abscesses in infants and newborns are distinguished by two features: (1) They are relatively large and (2) capsule formation is relatively poor, resulting in rapid enlargement (57) (Fig. 11.17). The abscess cavities are usually located within the cerebral hemispheres and often involve several lobes, with the frontal lobe most commonly affected (56,58). Cerebellar abscesses, which are less frequent, most commonly develop from ear infections but can also be associated with dermal sinuses extending into the cerebellum from the occipital region (Fig. 11.18) (17).

Two major clinical syndromes have been described with neonatal brain abscesses. Most commonly, there is an acute to subacute evolution of signs of increased in-

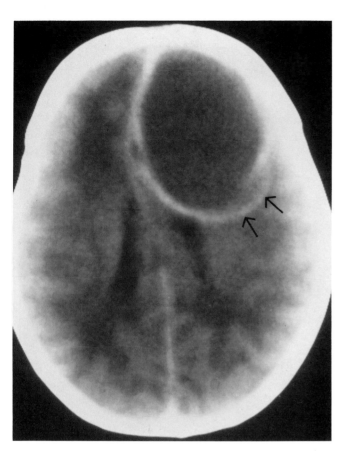

FIG. 11.17. Brain abscess in a neonate. In infants and newborns, abscesses are distinguished by their relatively large size and poor capsule formation. In this patient we see an enormous left frontal abscess. The capsule appears somewhat deficient in its posterolateral aspect (*arrows*).

tracranial pressure (vomiting, bulging anterior fontanel, separated sutures, and enlarging head). The initial diagnosis in these patients is often congenital hydrocephalus. Less commonly, the patients have an acute onset of a fulminating bacterial meningitis that differs little from other neonatal and infantile meningitis. The most common organisms involved in neonatal abscesses are *Citrobacter* and *Proteus*, both of which have the capacity to invade the nervous tissue and cause necrosis (1,56,58).

Pathologically, the abscess is a continually evolving lesion. Enzmann and colleagues (50,59) showed that there are four stages in the evolution of experimental brain abscesses: (1) early cerebritis, (2) late cerebritis, (3) early capsule formation, and (4) late capsule formation. In *stage 1 (early cerebritis)*, necrotic tissue becomes infiltrated by inflammatory cells; no capsule is present. Considerable edema is present in the surrounding white matter. In *stage 2 (late cerebritis)*, the necrotic area becomes much better defined. Encapsulation begins to occur, as vessels proliferate around the necrotic area and

deposit more inflammatory cells, reticulin, and a minimal amount of collagen. In *stage 3 (early capsule formation)*, increasing collagen and reticulin surround the necrotic center of the abscess, forming a wall that is much better defined than that in stage 2. Moreover, the surrounding area of cerebritis regresses, with corresponding regression of mass effect and edema. In *stage 4 (late capsule formation)*, the collagen capsule is essentially complete. The capsule is thicker and better developed on the cortical side than on the ventricular side, presumably because the increased vascularity on the cortical side of the abscess wall allows more collagen-producing fibroblasts to reach that side. Further maturation of the capsule results in continued reduction in the surrounding inflammatory infiltrate, the mass effect, and the edema. The evolution of cerebritis to abscess usually takes 7–14 days.

On noncontrast CT scans, abscesses appear as areas of low density with a thin wall of slightly increased density (Fig. 11.18). After contrast administration, a ring of enhancing tissue, representing the abscess wall and surrounding inflammatory tissue, encircles the low-density center. The enhancing wall is thin (usually around 5 mm), is most commonly located at or near the gray matter–white matter junction, and is surrounded by low-density edema. The inner margin of the ring tends to be smooth and regular. The capsule is thinner on its medial aspect in approximately 50% of patients, resulting from the decreased vascularity of the adjacent white matter as compared to gray matter laterally (50,59). The early cerebritis stage (stage 1), therefore, usually can be recognized by CT and treated with antibiotics. A late cerebritis (stage 2) has a CT appearance that cannot be distinguished from stages 3 and 4.

The MR characteristics of pyogenic brain abscesses are characteristic. On MR, *stage 1 cerebritis* appears as an area of heterogeneous hyperintensity on both T1- and T2-weighted images; patchy heterogeneous enhancement is seen after administration of paramagnetic contrast. In the *late stage 2 cerebritis/early abscess,* the abscess wall is hyperintense on T1-weighted sequences and slightly hypointense on T2-weighted sequences (Fig. 11.19); the center of the abscess is heterogeneous on both imaging sequences. The developing abscess wall is slightly thicker in stage 2 than in stages 3 and 4, when it is better defined. The abscess wall enhances dramatically in stage 2; on delayed images, the center of the abscess will enhance. In *stage 3 (subacute abscess),* the abscess wall is hyperintense on both T1- and T2-weighted images (Fig. 11.19) and enhances intensely after contrast administration. The abscess center is uniformly hypointense on T1-weighted images, uniformly hyperintense (similar to cerebrospinal fluid) on T2-weighted sequences, and does not enhance. In *stage 4 (the chronic phase)*, the abscess wall is isointense on T1-weighted se-

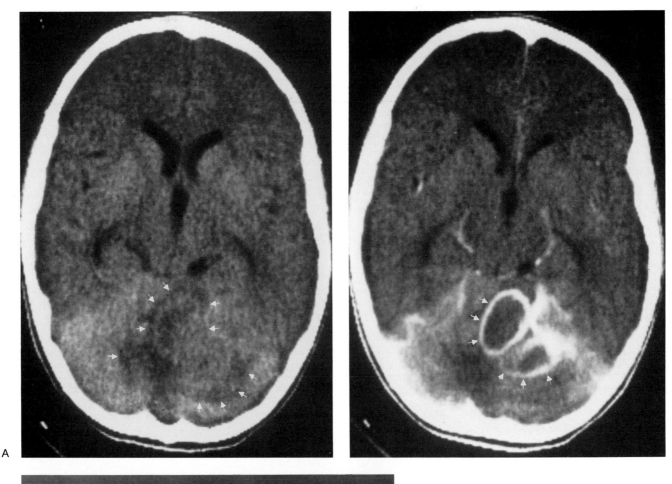

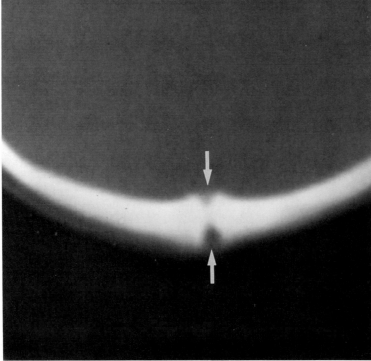

FIG. 11.18. Cerebellar abscess secondary to dermal sinus tract. **A:** Axial noncontrast CT image shows ill-defined mass (*arrows*) in the cerebellum. **B:** After administration of iodinated contrast, two distinct masses (*arrows*) with smooth, enhancing walls are seen. **C:** Examination of bone windows in the occipital bone shows a defect (*arrows*) secondary to the dermal sinus. After shaving the patient's head, the orifice of the sinus was found.

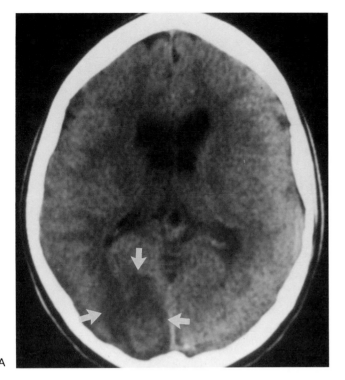

A

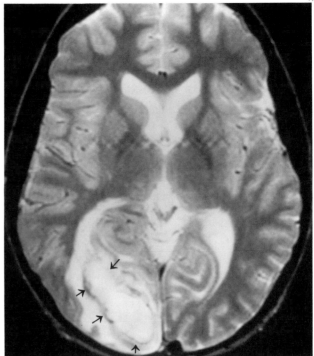

B

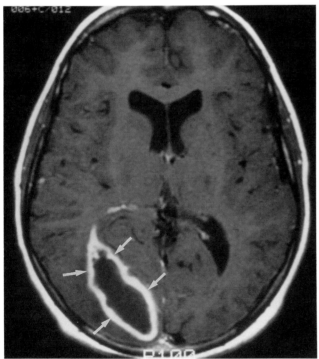

C

FIG. 11.19. Late cerebritis/early cerebral abscess. **A:** Axial noncontrast CT image shows hypodense mass (*arrows*) in the right occipital lobe. A well-defined dense rim cannot be seen. **B:** Axial SE 2800/70 image 2 days later shows a developing hypointense capsule (*arrows*) with surrounding vasogenic edema. **C:** Postcontrast SE 600/29 image shows intense smooth enhancement of the abscess capsule (*arrows*).

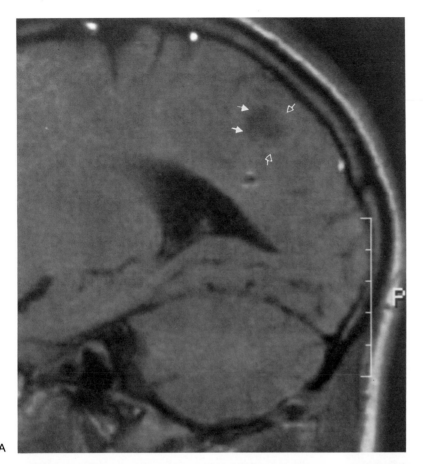

A

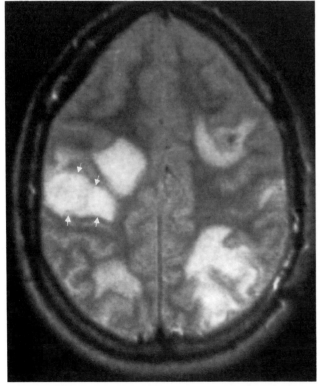

B

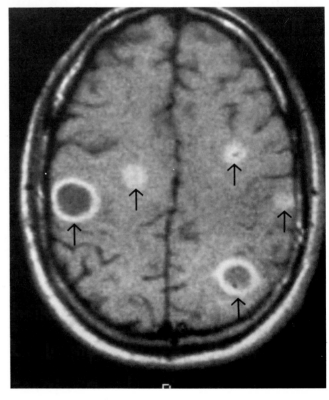

C

FIG. 11.20. Multiple cerebral abscesses. **A:** Sagittal SE 500/40 image shows a round area of low signal intensity in the posterior parietal lobe (*closed arrows*). A high-intensity capsule can be seen around the posterior aspect of the abscess cavity (*open arrows*). **B:** Axial SE 2500/80 image shows the same right parietal abscess as being uniformly isointense with surrounding vasogenic edema (*arrows*). The other areas of high signal intensity are the result of vasogenic edema from other abscesses. **C:** After intravenous infusion of paramagnetic contrast, multiple small abscesses (*arrows*) are seen.

quences and markedly hypointense on T2-weighted sequences; the abscess center is iso- to slightly hypointense on T1-weighted sequences and hyperintense on T2-weighted sequences. The low signal intensity of the capsule on T2-weighted images in stage 4 is thought to be secondary to enhanced T2 relaxation by decreased free water in the collagenous tissue of the capsule and perhaps a small amount of blood or free radicals (60). Although stages 2–4 all exhibit ring-type enhancement following paramagnetic contrast infusion, the enhancement of stage 2 lesions shows much better edge definition than those in stages 3 and 4.

As aspiration of abscess contents, gram stain, culture, and antibiotic sensitivity analysis with subsequent medical therapy now constitute the treatment of choice for patients with brain abscesses, CT or MR guidance of aspiration is very helpful in the management of affected patients. Moreover, serial CT or MR is valuable in assessing the response to medical therapy (61). Medical management is particularly indicated in patients with multiple abscesses (Fig. 11.20), those with abscesses in critical areas of brain, or those with severe underlying illnesses (26). Close monitoring with imaging is neces-

sary to ensure response; if the cavity has not decreased in size by the tenth day of treatment, repeat aspiration is indicated (57).

VIRAL ENCEPHALITIS

Many viral infections involve the central nervous system. Most of these reach neural tissues by hematogenous spread. Primary replication of the virus occurs at the site of inoculation, such as the skin and subcutaneous tissues, gastrointestinal tract, or nasopharyngeal lymphoid tissues. Viremia, with dissemination of virions to other organs, ensues in susceptible hosts. Secondary virus replication occurs in affected tissues, leading to organ system dysfunction. A few viral pathogens, such as rabies and herpes simplex virus type 1, reach the central nervous system via peripheral nerves (16,62).

All viruses affecting the central nervous system exhibit two major pathologic features: neuronal degeneration and inflammation. Although some viruses, such as polio virus, produce specific clinical symptoms, many other viruses can produce a number of different clinical syn-

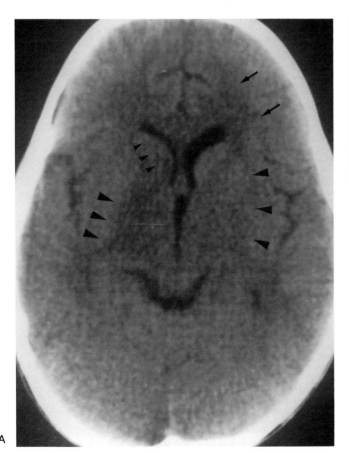
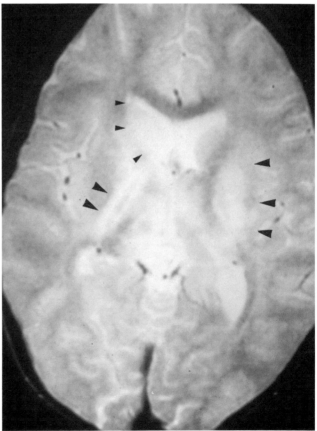

FIG. 11.21. Viral encephalitis. **A:** Axial CT scan shows hypodensity in both thalami, the bilateral lentiform nucleus (*large arrowheads*), right caudate head (*small arrowheads*), and left frontal white matter (*arrows*). **B:** Axial SE 2500/70 image shows T2 prolongation in the same areas identified in (A).

dromes that overlap with the syndromes produced by other viruses. The imaging findings overlap considerably as well. Therefore, it is very difficult to differentiate among most viral infections based on radiologic or clinical criteria. Some viruses produce meningitis, others result in encephalitis, and still others cause leukoencephalitis (16,63). Meningitis can be caused by mumps, nonparalytic polio, Coxsackie virus, and lymphocytic choriomeningitis. Encephalitis results from infection with herpes simplex type 1, arboviruses, and rabies. Leukoencephalitis (involving exclusively white matter) is caused by subacute sclerosing panencephalitis (SSPE), progressive multifocal leukoencephalitis (PML, caused by papovavirus), and western and eastern equine encephalitis (63,64).

Essentially all the viruses that affect the brain result in a nonspecific increase in water content of the affected area. Therefore, the imaging findings in these patients are patchy areas of hyperechogenicity on sonography, low density on CT, and prolonged T1 and T2 relaxation times on MR (Fig. 11.21). A few viral infections have fairly specific clinical or radiographic features and will be discussed in some depth.

Herpes Simplex Virus

Herpes simplex virus is a ubiquitous organism that commonly infects humans but rarely results in neurologic manifestations. Two distinct types of herpes simplex virus can be distinguished by serology or by culturing lesions. The type 1 virus, which is generally associated with orofacial herpes infections, is the cause of herpes simplex encephalitis in most patients 6 months of age or older. The type 2 virus is the cause of genital herpes and causes most of the congenital or perinatally acquired infections discussed earlier in this chapter. With either serotype, cerebritis may develop from a primary infection or reactivation of preexisting infection. In the type 2 infections that become symptomatic at 4 months of age or later, reinfection or reactivation of infection is the probable cause (16,20).

Herpes simplex encephalitis occurs in all age groups but is particularly common in the pediatric age group. Thirty-one percent of cases occur in patients under 20 years of age, with 12% involving those between 6 months and 10 years of age (1). Prodromal symptoms, such as fever and malaise, occur in about 60% of patients. Symp-

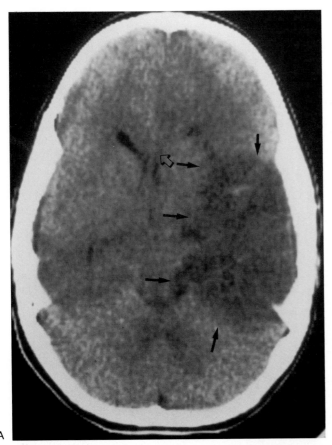
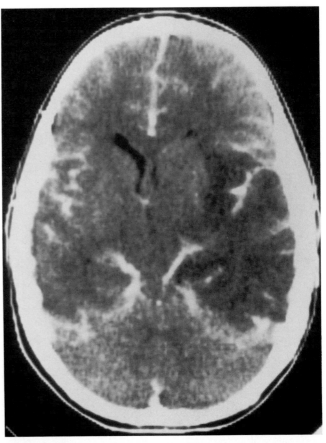

A   B

FIG. 11.22. Herpes simplex type I encephalitis. **A:** Noncontrast CT scan shows low signal intensity (*arrows*) involving the left temporal lobe with mass effect compressing the frontal horn of the left lateral ventricle (*open arrow*). **B:** After infusion of iodinated contrast, a gyral pattern of contrast enhancement is seen. This enhancement is accentuated by the low intensity within the temporal lobe.

toms of respiratory infection are present in approximately 30%. Within several days, alterations in consciousness, fever, seizures, vomiting, and hemiparesis ensue (65).

Pathologically, herpes encephalitis consists of a fulminating necrotic meningoencephalitis that usually begins in the temporal lobes. The disease tends to spread into the insular cortex and the orbital regions of the frontal lobes, particularly in the region of the cingulate gyri. The involved brain is diffusely softened and hemorrhagic, with a loss of neural and glial elements.

Imaging studies are insensitive early in the course of herpes encephalitis. CT is usually not positive before the fifth day. MR and SPECT studies are more sensitive than CT early in the course of the disease (66–69). MR has much greater spatial resolution than SPECT and should therefore be the imaging modality of choice when herpes encephalitis is suspected. The characteristic CT findings in herpes type I encephalitis are poorly defined areas of low density in the anteromedial portion of the temporal lobe (Fig. 11.22). Extension to the insular cortex is common but the lentiform nucleus tends to be spared. Occasionally, small foci of high density, representing hemor-

rhage, may be seen within the involved brain tissue. A gyral pattern of contrast enhancement is frequently seen in the involved areas of the brain; enhancement does not usually appear until the low density in the region can be identified (70,71) (Fig. 11.22). The MR appearance of herpes type I encephalitis is that of prolonged T1 and T2 relaxation time in the medial temporal lobe, the insular cortex, and the orbital surface of the frontal lobe, particularly the cingulate gyrus (Fig. 11.23) (66,67). The abnormalities are much more easily identified on T2-weighted sequences. Involvement is most commonly unilateral, but bilateral involvement (Fig. 11.23) is not rare. Sequential studies can show rapid changes as the disease process extends superiorly within the frontal lobes and into the parietal lobes. The diseased areas eventually become well demarcated as the tissue within them degenerates and atrophies.

Human Immunodeficiency Virus

Human immunodeficiency virus (HIV), causing pediatric acquired immunodeficiency syndrome (AIDS), re-

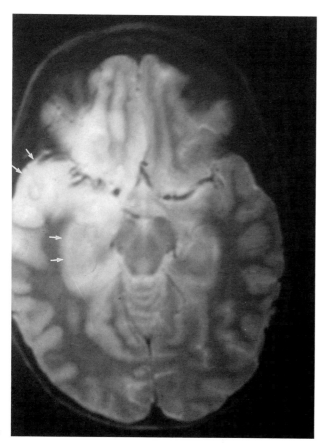

A

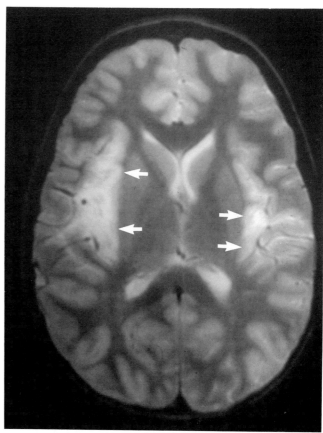

B

FIG. 11.23. Bilateral herpes simplex encephalitis. **A:** Axial SE 2800/70 image shows swelling and hyperintensity (*arrows*) of the anterior and medial temporal lobe with spread into the frontal lobe. **B:** At the level of the basal ganglia, swelling and hyperintensity (*arrows*) are seen in both insular cortices.

sults in neurologic manifestations in 50% to 90% and frank encephalopathy in 30% to 50% of affected children (72,73). Neurologic manifestations are most commonly the result of direct HIV infection of the nervous system; opportunistic infections and tumors are uncommon. Affected children typically present with developmental delay, cognitive impairment, or pyramidal signs, such as hyperreflexia, spasticity, ataxia, or frank paraparesis (73,74). The encephalopathy may be static, progressive, or haltingly progressive, with static periods (75,76).

On pathologic examination, brains of affected children typically show atrophy (decreased brain weight), infiltration of microglial nodules, multinucleated giant cells containing viral particles, and calcification. The calcium is found both in the cerebral parenchyma and in small and medium-sized blood vessels; inflammation is always present in the surrounding tissue (77).

The most common finding on imaging studies of affected patients is lymphadenopathy in the head and neck, found in more than 95%. The most prominent intracranial findings are prominence of the subarachnoid spaces and ventricles, most likely secondary to atrophy,

and calcification of the basal ganglia and subcortical white matter (Fig. 11.24) (74). The calcification is only seen in patients who were infected *in utero* (vertical transmission) and who are already encephalopathic from the disease (78). Subcortical calcification is most common in the frontal lobes (Fig. 11.24) but can occur in other areas of the cerebrum as well. MR and ultrasound are much less sensitive than CT for its detection.

Myelopathy is often present in children with AIDS, presenting with prominent signs of spasticity (72). Pathologic findings consist of corticospinal tract degeneration with myelin pallor and sparing of the posterior columns (79). The majority of affected patients have associated encephalopathy; therefore, imaging studies of HIV myelopathy in children are uncommon.

Of note is the rarity of intracranial neoplastic or infectious lesions in HIV-infected children (74,80). The most common intracranial mass lesion is lymphoma, reported in less than 5% of affected patients (72,73); the basal ganglia and thalami are the intracranial structures that are typically involved (76,80). Most affected patients have associated systemic lymphoproliferation (76). Infections

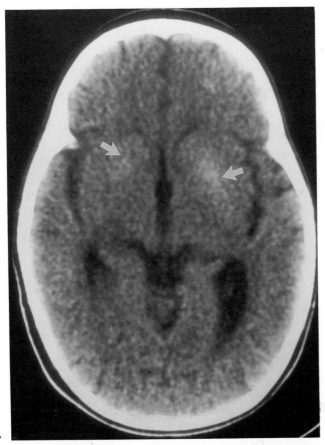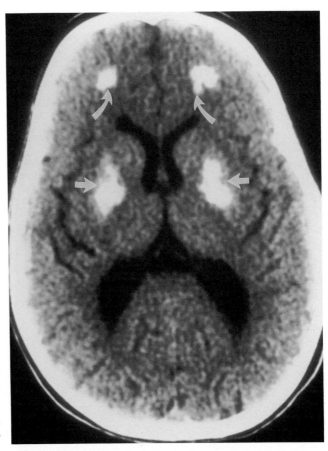

FIG. 11.24. Congenital HIV encephalitis. **A:** Axial CT image at age 1 year shows mild prominence of the ventricles and subarachnoid spaces with mildly increased attenuation in the basal ganglia (*arrows*). **B:** Follow-up CT image at age 2 years shows marked calcification of the lentiform nuclei (*straight arrows*) and subcortical frontal white matter (*curved arrows*).

are quite rare; toxoplasmosis, the most common infecting organism in adults with AIDS, is conspicuously uncommon in affected children. In our experience at UCSF, progressive multifocal leukoencephalopathy (PML) has been the most common opportunistic infection in pediatric AIDS.

Other intracranial pathology in pediatric AIDS includes intracranial hemorrhage (from immune thrombocytopenia) and infarction (from arteriopathy) (74, 76,81). The arteriopathies that result from HIV infection are varied (82) and may result from the HIV virus itself or from any of a number of superinfecting organisms, such as cytomegalovirus or varicella zoster. Of note is a condition of diffuse dilatation of the vessels of the circle of Willis that seems to predispose the affected patients to thrombosis and embolization (82).

Subacute Sclerosing Panencephalitis

Subacute sclerosing panencephalitis (SSPE) is predominantly a disease of children that is characterized by the insidious onset of behavior changes and mental deterioration, followed by myoclonus, ataxia, and sometimes seizures. Severe dementia, quadriparesis, and autonomic instability eventually ensue (63). The age of onset ranges from 1 to 30 years, with a mean of 7 years; most children are between 5 and 14 years of age at the time of onset (83). About half the patients are known to have had measles before the age of 2 years (16,63). This disease seems to be an infection caused by the measles virus that reactivates many years after the initial illness (84). A satisfactory explanation for the long latency and the slow evolution of the disease does not exist. It may be related to the fact that patients with SSPE have failed to produce antibody to a specific virus protein (63).

The CT findings in SSPE are nonspecific. Diffuse atrophy is accompanied by multifocal areas of low attenuation in the periventricular and subcortical white matter (84). No abnormal contrast enhancement is seen. Generalized cerebral atrophy ensues. MR scans show a similarly nonspecific picture of patchy regions of prolonged T2 relaxation (Fig. 11.25) in the cerebral and cerebellar white matter.

Progressive Multifocal Leukoencephalitis

Progressive multifocal leukoencephalopathy (PML) is caused by the JC polyomavirus, a member of the papovavirus family. It is an uncommon disorder that typically occurs in patients with abnormal cell-mediated immunity, such as AIDS, congenital immunodeficiency syndromes, and disorders requiring immunosuppressive therapy, such as leukemia, lymphoma, systemic lupus erythematosis, and renal transplantation (16). Patients typically present with slowly progressive mental deterio-

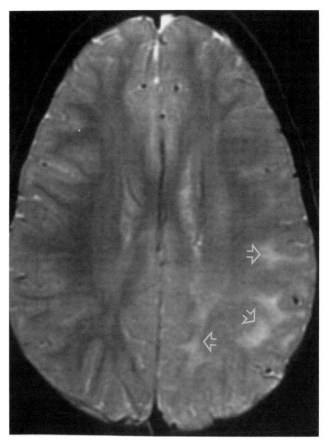

FIG. 11.25. Subacute sclerosing panencephalitis. Axial SE 2800/70 image shows patchy T2 prolongation (*arrows*) in the left parietal and occipital white matter.

ration, sensory deficits, visual loss, paralysis, and ataxia. Pathologic features are multifocal demyelination with intranuclear inclusion bodies in oligodendrocytes (85).

Imaging studies are characterized by single or multiple areas of decreased attenuation (CT) or prolonged T1 and T2 relaxation times (MR) in white matter; the lesions lack mass effect and do not enhance after administration of contrast material (86). The most common locations are the frontal and parieto-occipital regions, but any myelinated areas of the brain, including the corpus callosum, thalami, and basal ganglia, can be involved.

Rasmussen Encephalitis

Rasmussen encephalitis, or chronic localized encephalitis, is a disorder characterized by progressive hemiplegia, epilepsia partialis continua, and progressive psychomotor deterioration (87–89). (Epilepsia partialis continua is a condition characterized by clonic movements, usually localized to the face or upper extremities, that persists over long periods, either continuously or with only brief interruptions.) Pathologic examination of the affected brain shows inflammatory changes and atrophy in the cerebral cortex and white matter (90,91). Viruses have been demonstrated in the neurons, astrocytes, oligodendrocytes, and perivascular cells in affected brains, suggesting a viral etiology. Patients deteriorate progressively until death ensues unless the affected regions of brain are surgically resected (88–90).

On imaging studies, Rasmussen encephalitis is characterized by progressive atrophy and, on MR, T2 prolongation in the affected regions of the brain.

Reye Syndrome

Reye syndrome is a disease of unknown cause that predominantly affects children between the ages of 6 months and 16 years. Symptoms usually develop while the patient is recovering from a presumed viral illness. A profound illness suddenly develops, with severe vomiting and lethargy. Symptoms progress to major convulsions and coma, sometimes leading to death within a few days as a result of increased intracranial pressure (92). About half the patients have enlarged livers, and all show evidence of liver failure (elevated serum transaminases and ammonia). Mortality is about 20% (93). Toxic agents, such as salicylates, aflatoxin, and insecticides,

have been associated with the syndrome. Current theories postulate the interaction of viral infection and toxin as the cause of the syndrome (93).

Pathologically, examination reveals severe brain swelling; the white matter is soft and edematous without focal lesions. On imaging studies, mild cases show minimal ventricular compression and normal attenuation values of gray and white matter. More severe cases may show diffuse cerebral edema with low attenuation (CT) or prolonged T1 and T2 relaxation times (MR) of both cerebral hemispheres; the basal ganglia may or may not be spared (24,93,94).

Polio Virus Infections

Although rarely seen in Western countries, the imaging findings of poliomyelitis are distinctive enough to warrant discussion of the disease. The disease is transmitted among humans by direct contact with infected feces or oropharyngeal secretions. The incubation period is 1–3 weeks. Patients initially present with nonspecific complaints of sore throat, fever, and abdominal pain. In abortive infections, these symptoms resolve and patients completely recover. Neurologic complications

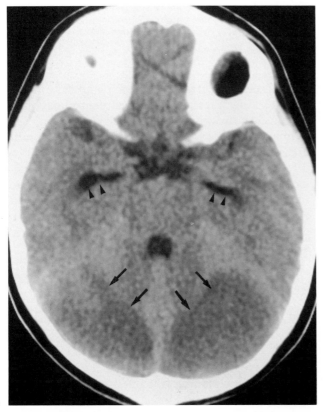
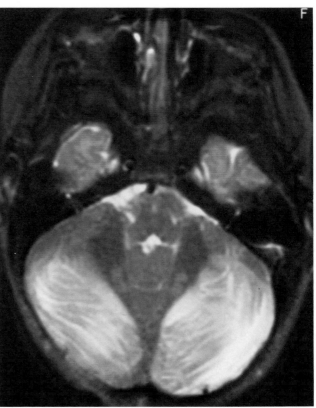

FIG. 11.26. Acute cerebellitis. **A:** Axial CT image shows hypodensity (*arrows*) in both cerebellar hemispheres. The temporal horns of the lateral ventricles (*arrowheads*) are enlarged, indicating hydrocephalus. **B:** Axial SE 3000/120 image shows hyperintensity and swelling of the cerebellar hemispheres.

ensue in 0.1% to 1% of patients and can consist of aseptic meningitis, poliomyelitis, bulbar polio, and encephalitis.

Spinal poliomyelitis is the most common form. Patients develop headache, vomiting, meningism, and muscle pain. Flaccid paralysis ensues within 1–2 days. MR studies show T2 prolongation of the ventral horns of the spinal cord (95). Bulbar polio is less common, only affecting 10% to 15% of neurologically symptomatic patients. It typically affects the 9th–11th cranial nerves, leading to hoarseness, difficulty in swallowing, or airway obstruction. Cranial nerves 5, 7, and 12 are less commonly affected (16). Imaging studies show T2 prolongation in the brain stem (96). Patients with encephalitis have nonspecific T2 prolongation involving the cerebral hemispheres.

Acute Cerebellitis

Acute cerebellitis is an uncommon syndrome characterized by cerebellar dysfunction of acute onset. Although the cause in many cases is unknown, most are attributed to viral infections (97–99). Patients typically present with abnormal spontaneous eye movements, myoclonic jerks, truncal ataxia, dysarthria, nausea, headaches, tremor, and altered mental status. A history of recent viral illness can often be elicited. Fever and meningismus may or may not be present. Symptoms usually resolve spontaneously over weeks to months, although permanent disability, and even death, may ensue in some cases (97–99).

Imaging findings reveal bilateral, symmetrical low attenuation (CT) or T1 and T2 prolongation (MR) in the cerebellar hemispheres (Fig. 11.26); both gray and white matter can be affected (98). Localized edema can cause decreased efflux of cerebrospinal fluid from the fourth ventricle, with resultant hydrocephalus. Contrast enhancement may be present in the subacute phase.

It is important to remember that *acute cerebellitis is a diagnosis of exclusion.* Many processes can lead to cerebellar inflammation and swelling, including lead intoxication (see Chapter 3), demyelinating processes, and vasculitis. Acute childhood illnesses—such as rubeola, pertussis, diphtheria, typhoid fever, Coxsackie virus, polio virus, varicella zoster, and Epstein-Barr virus—can also cause similar patterns of cerebellar inflammation and edema. Some cases may be a manifestation of acute disseminated encephalomyelitis (see Chapter 3) (98).

Postviral (Parainfectious) Leukoencephalopathies

Postviral (parainfectious) leukoencephalopathies are felt to be autoimmune and can follow infection by a large number of viral illnesses. They have been described in Chapter 3 under the subheading "Acute Disseminated Encephalomyelitis (ADEM)."

FUNGAL INFECTIONS

For practical purposes, fungal infections of the nervous system can be divided into two principal categories: those induced by pathogens and those produced by saprophytes in patients whose resistance to infection is lowered by such conditions as diabetes, leukemia, and lymphoma or by the prolonged use of antibiotics, corticosteroids, cytotoxic drugs, or immunosuppressive agents. The latter group of infections is referred to as *opportunistic.* Mycotic infections of the nervous system can lead to chronic granulomatous meningitis or abscesses. They are uncommon in children; moreover, their manifestations in children are identical to those in adults. Therefore, they will be reviewed only briefly here.

Candida

Candida may produce a mycosemia and subsequent meningitis in infants, especially those born with congenital anomalies, such as intestinal malrotation, meconium ileus, or hydrocephalus with shunt complications. Candidal meningitis can also be a complication of prolonged antibiotic or corticosteroid therapy, immune suppression, surgery, or extensive burns. When *Candida* invades the nervous system primarily, it usually progresses to gross abscess formation; in those patients in whom it is a secondary invader complicating antibiotic therapy, a diffuse cerebritis with widespread microabscesses more commonly develops (1,100,101). Meningeal inflammation may occur as well. As with other granulomatous meningitides, *Candida* can invade the walls of blood vessels, producing a vasculitis that results in thrombus formation with resultant infarction and hemorrhage.

Candidal meningitis resembles other granulomatous meningitides in that tissue fills the basilar cisterns and markedly enhances after infusion of intravenous contrast. Candidal abscesses differ somewhat from pyogenic abscesses in that the walls are thicker and less sharply defined.

Coccidioidosis

Coccidioidosis is endemic in the southwestern United States; infection rates are particularly high in the central valley of California, southern Nevada, central and southern Arizona, southern New Mexico, and western Texas. The central nervous system tends to be involved secondarily, after a systemic infection, usually hematogenous (100,102). The principal symptoms are headache, low-grade fever, weight loss, progressive obtundation, and minimal meningeal signs.

Pathologically, the leptomeninges are thickened and congested with formation of multiple granulomas, most frequently in the basal cisterns (100). The result of these processes is a communicating hydrocephalus. Noncommunicating hydrocephalus can result from ependymitis within the cerebral aqueduct or fourth ventricle. As with other basilar meningitides, a perivasculitis or true vasculitis may result in vessel occlusions and infarctions.

Imaging findings reflect the pathologic changes. Often the basilar cisterns are filled by granulomatous, opaque, thickened meninges. After contrast enhancement, the basal cisterns and other cisternal spaces enhance markedly. Hydrocephalus is almost always present. Parenchymal lesions are unusual (a differentiating point from tuberculosis). Rarely, infarcts are seen as a result of vasculitis (102,103).

Cryptococcosis

Cryptococcosis is one of the most common fungal infections of the nervous system; it is, however, unusual in children. Adults are more commonly affected because of greater exposure and because of the predilection of cryptococcal infection for immunocompromised individuals (1,101). Symptoms usually reflect meningeal involvement; occasionally, neurologic signs or alterations in mental status may predominate. Clinical diagnosis is usually accomplished by CSF analysis (104). Pathologically, most cases with cerebral involvement demonstrate a meningitis. As in other fungal and granulomatous infections, the exudate is found mainly in the basilar cisterns, although it may be diffuse (105). A predilection for the choroid plexus results in ventriculitis with occasional secondary trapping of the temporal horn(s) of the lateral ventricle(s) (106). Parenchymal mass lesions rarely occur.

Imaging studies in cryptococcosis most commonly show hydrocephalus, cortical atrophy, pseudocysts, and ischemic changes from the vasculitis. The pseudocysts appear as areas of low attenuation (CT) or prolonged T1 and T2 (MR) in the basal ganglia that do not enhance after administration of intravenous contrast (107). In the presence of a trapped temporal horn without an obvious associated mass, cryptococcosis should be a strong consideration. Following contrast administration, enhancement of the basal cisterns occurs. In rare cases, parenchymal mass lesions that enhance in either a ring or solid fashion can be visualized (104–106).

Other Fungal Infections

Other fungal infections that occur in children include histoplasmosis, blastomycosis, and mucormycosis (101). These disorders are rare in children in Western countries, and the imaging manifestations are not well described. Interested readers are referred to other texts that deal specifically with infectious diseases (108–110).

MISCELLANEOUS INFECTIONS

A number of protozoan and parasitic infections can involve the nervous system, including cysticercosis, toxoplasmosis, sparganosis, toxocariasis, schistosomiasis, paragonimiasis, echinococcosis, amebiasis, and coenurosis, among others (101). Aside from cysticercosis and toxoplasmosis, none of these organisms commonly invades the nervous system of North American or Western European children. Consequently, the author's experience with these diseases is limited. The reader is referred to references in the accompanying table (Table 11.1) or to infectious disease texts (108–110) for further information on these diseases.

TABLE 11.1. *Protozoan and parasitic infections of the nervous system*

Organism	Clinical features	References
Malaria (*Plasmodium falciparum*)	High fever, convulsions, focal neurologic signs	(137,138)
African trypanosomiasis (*Trypanosoma gambiense* or *T. rhodesiense*)	Fever, lymphadenopathy, hepatomegaly. Later: apathy, meningeal signs, seizures	(139)
American trypanosomiasis (*T. cruzi*)	Infants: convulsions, nuchal rigidity. Older children: spastic diplegia, choreoathetosis	(140)
Amebiasis (*Entamoeba histolytica*)	Meningoencephalitis, brain abscess	(141)
Amebiasis (*Naegleria fowleri*)	Meningoencephalitis	(142)
Visceral larva migrans (*Toxocara canis*)	Encephalitis, optic neuritis, transverse myelitis, seizures	(100)
Schistosomiasis (*Schistosoma japonicum, S. mansoni, S. hemotobium*)	Transverse myelitis, radiculitis, encephalitis, meningeal signs, granulomata of spinal cord	(143,144)
Paragonimiasis	Meningoencephalitis, seizures, visual disturbances, dementia	(100,145,146)
Hydatidosis (*Echinococcosis*)	Focal neurologic findings from intracranial cysts	(147,148)

Cysticercosis

Cysticercosis of the central nervous system is rare in the United States. It is not unusual in Latin America and is seen fairly frequently in immigrants from Latin America, Asia, India, and Africa. The condition is almost always caused by the encysted form of *Taenia solium*. Humans are an intermediate host, acquiring the organism by accidental ingestion of tapeworm eggs from feces-contaminated substances. The eggs hatch in the small intestine, burrow into the mucosa, and penetrate the venules. Mature larvae, or cysticerci, develop after 60–70 days (111,112).

Clinically, the expression of the disease is variable, although seizures have been reported in as many as 92% of cases (113). Hydrocephalus develops from obstruction within the ventricles or basilar cisterns by multiple cysts or by leptomeningitis associated with the disease. Vasculitis can occur, resulting in infarction (111,112).

Pathologically, four forms of cysticercosis have been described: (1) leptomeningitis, (2) parenchymal cysticerci, (3) intraventricular cysticerci, and (4) racemose cysts (111,112). Each form has its own particular appearance on CT and MR.

Parenchymal cysticerci, the most common form, produce a variety of symptoms and signs that develop when the death of the parasite elicits an inflammatory reaction. The cysts may be located anywhere in the brain, most commonly in the cerebral gray matter, followed by the brain stem cerebellum, and spinal cord (101,112). Intraparenchymal cysticerci can be either solid or cystic. Solid lesions are often associated with punctate calcifications, whereas cystic foci commonly have a rim of enhancement (114–118) (Figs. 11.27, 11.28). When the cysticercus dies, it sets up an antigenic stimulus resulting in a local inflammatory process and breakdown of the blood-brain barrier; as a consequence, contrast enhancement is seen. Both calcified and cystic foci tend to be located in the gray matter and will usually have surrounding vasogenic edema when visualized on T2-weighted MR scans prior to the initiation of therapy (Figs. 11.27, 11.28). The edema resolves during treatment (Fig. 11.29). Although the calcifications within the lesions are seen better by CT, MR more clearly demonstrates those lesions in the cortex, adjacent to the skull, because of the lack of beam-hardening artifact (117,118). The completely calcified lesions of cysticercosis represent the dead cysticercus larvae and do not enhance or elicit edema (116). It is esti-

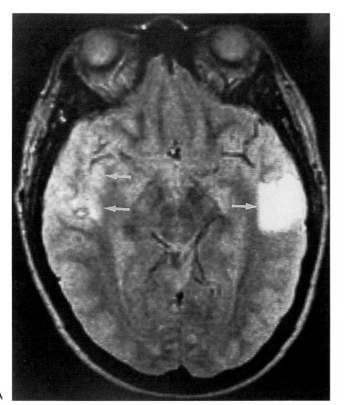

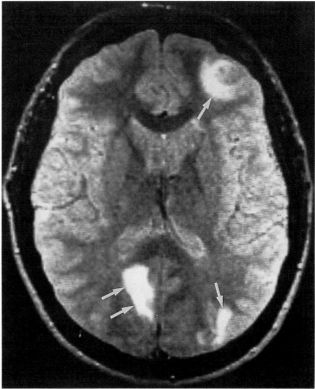

A B

FIG. 11.27. Parenchymal cysticercosis. **A:** Axial SE 2500/30 image shows areas of prolonged T2 relaxation (*arrows*), consistent with vasogenic edema, bilaterally in the temporal lobes. **B:** Image at the level of the frontal horns shows additional lesions (*arrows*) in the left frontal lobe and bilaterally in the occipital lobes. Multiple areas of involvement are common in cysticercosis.

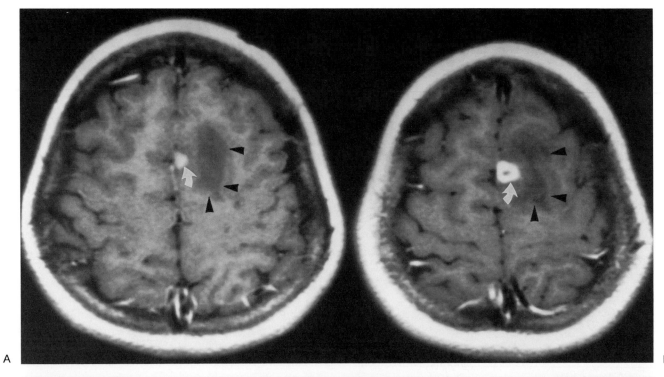

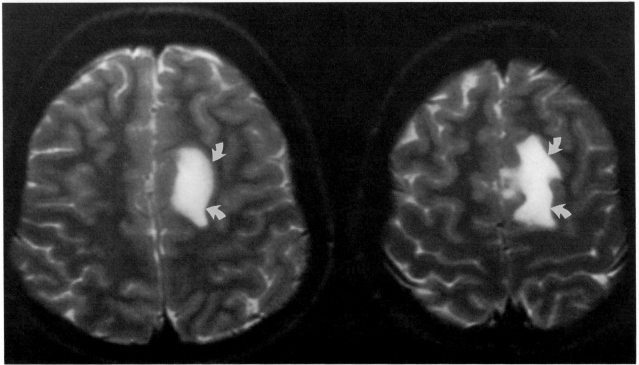

FIG. 11.28. Parenchymal cysticercosis. **A, B:** Postcontrast axial SE 600/15 images show a ring-enhancing lesion (*curved white arrows*) with surrounding vasogenic edema (*black arrowheads*). **C, D:** Axial SE 2800/70 images do not clearly show the cysticercal lesion but clearly show the surrounding vasogenic edema (*curved white arrows*).

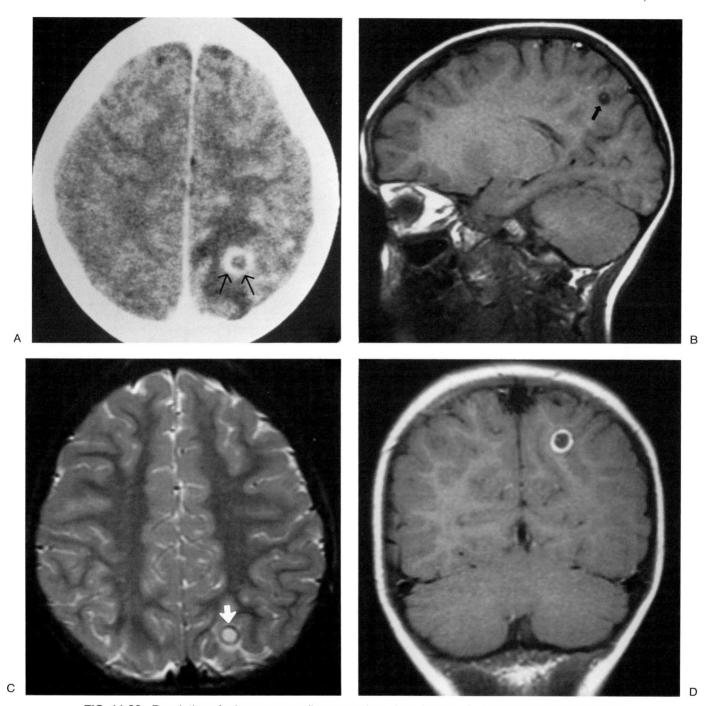

FIG. 11.29. Resolution of edema surrounding parenchymal cysticercus. **A:** Axial contrast-enhanced CT shows a rim-enhancing lesion (*arrows*) in the left parieto-occipital cortex with surrounding vasogenic edema. **B:** Sagittal SE 600/20 image after 1 week of treatment again shows the lesion (*arrow*) in the left parieto-occipital region. The week of treatment has diminished the amount of vasogenic edema. Before the lesions die and calcify, they have round, high-signal-intensity capsules (prolonged T1 relaxation) and are similar in appearance to abscesses. **C:** Axial SE 2500/70 image shows the parenchymal cysticercus as a region of prolonged T2 relaxation with a rim (*arrow*) of shortened T2 relaxation. **D:** After infusion of intravenous paramagnetic contrast, the parenchymal cysticercus is seen as a rim-enhancing lesion.

mated that it takes 4–7 years for the dead larvae to calcify, which may explain why calcification is much less commonly seen in the pediatric age group than in adult patients with cysticercosis (115). In fact, the only significant differences in the imaging findings between adults and children with cysticercosis are the following: (1) Calcifications are more commonly seen in adults, and (2) diffusely homogeneously enhancing lesions are more commonly seen in children (115).

The *leptomeningitis form* is seen on both CT and MR as soft tissue filling the basilar cisterns on noncontrast scans. With contrast, as with other granulomatous meningitides, there will be marked enhancement of the subarachnoid space in the involved area (see Figs. 11.12, 11.14, and 11.30) (119). Granulomas, which may calcify (Fig. 11.30), are commonly present within the subarachnoid space. The enhancement characteristics of these granulomas are similar to those of parenchymal granulomas. Hydrocephalus (Fig. 11.30) and vasculitis (with resulting infarction) are common when leptomeningitis is present.

Intraventricular cysticerci are especially important to identify because affected patients can die from acute ventricular obstruction. Intraventricular cysts are difficult to identify on CT unless water-soluble contrast is introduced into the ventricular system. MR is superior in identification of intraventricular cysts because the scolex (head) of the parasite can be identified within the ventricle as a soft tissue intensity nodule (Fig. 11.31) (117,118). T1-weighted sections 3 mm or less in thickness optimize detection of the scolex. Moreover, imaging in the coronal plane allows better appreciation of the degree and nature of the ventricular distortion. If surgical removal of an intraventricular cyst is contemplated, imaging should be performed in close temporal proximity to the surgery, since these cysts can migrate through the ventricular system (120).

Racemose cysts are multilobular, nonviable (therefore lacking a scolex) cysts located in the cisterns. They are often quite large, ranging up to several centimeters in size. Although sterile, these lesions can grow by proliferation of the wall and, consequently, may be amenable to praziquantel therapy. Chronic meningitis can accompany these cysts (112). Racemose cysts are most common in the cerebellopontine angle, the suprasellar region, the Sylvian fissures, and the basilar cisterns. On CT, large cystic lesions are seen (Fig. 11.32) that may enhance after intravenous contrast infusion; the multiple inner septations are not easily seen (115). On MR, multiple cysts of varying size, clustered together like grapes within the basilar, suprasellar, or Sylvian cisterns, are seen (Fig. 11.32) (119). The morphologic detail is more specific. Patients usually experience multiple exposures to the organism, so that more than one form of this disease can be seen within the central nervous system at any one time (117–119).

When the symptoms suggest intraspinal involvement, MR is the preferred diagnostic procedure. Thin-section studies will demonstrate the scolex within the cyst and the mass effect upon the cord. Myelography will show intradural, extramedullary masses that move with tilting of the patient in the head-up and head-down positions (121). Arachnoiditis may be present as well, resulting in a partial or complete block to contrast flow within the subarachnoid space.

SARCOIDOSIS

Sarcoidosis is a granulomatous disease of unknown etiology. Although it occurs worldwide, the disease is particularly common in the southeastern portions of the United States and has a much higher incidence among blacks (1). Sarcoid involves the nervous system in 5% to 10% of affected individuals, both adult and pediatric (122,123). The disease is unusual in children, with about 6% of all cases involving the pediatric age group (122). The age of onset in adults is usually the third and fourth decades of life. Most affected children are between 9 and 15 years old.

Sarcoidosis is characterized pathologically by widely disseminated noncaseating granulomas. The most frequently involved tissues are the lymph nodes, lungs, skin, eyes, and bone. In adults, any part of the nervous system may be affected. Basal or diffuse granulomatous leptomeningitis is the most common form of the disease; the infundibulum and the floor and anterior walls of the third ventricle are frequently involved (28). Granulomas can form in the extradural and subdural spaces, leptomeninges, brain parenchyma, spinal cord, optic nerves, or peripheral nerves (122).

In descending order of frequency, clinical manifestations are cranial neuropathy (most commonly VII, II, and VIII), aseptic meningitis, hydrocephalus, hypothalamic dysfunction, hydrocephalus, focal neurologic signs secondary to intracranial masses at other sites, intraspinal masses, encephalopathy or vasculopathy, seizures, peripheral neuropathy, and myelopathy (124). A review of 23 published cases of neurologic involvement in children with sarcoid found that the disease does not differ significantly from the disease in adults (123). The most common finding was transient paralysis of the seventh cranial nerve; hypothalamic-pituitary involvement was quite common as well.

The imaging findings in neurosarcoidosis include hydrocephalus, parenchymal nodules that enhance homogeneously with contrast medium, increased water in periventricular white matter (manifest as low density on CT and prolonged T1 and T2 on MR), and diffuse enhancement of the basal meninges and tentorium (125,126). Extraparenchymal masses may mimic meningiomas (126,127). The smoothly marginated paren-

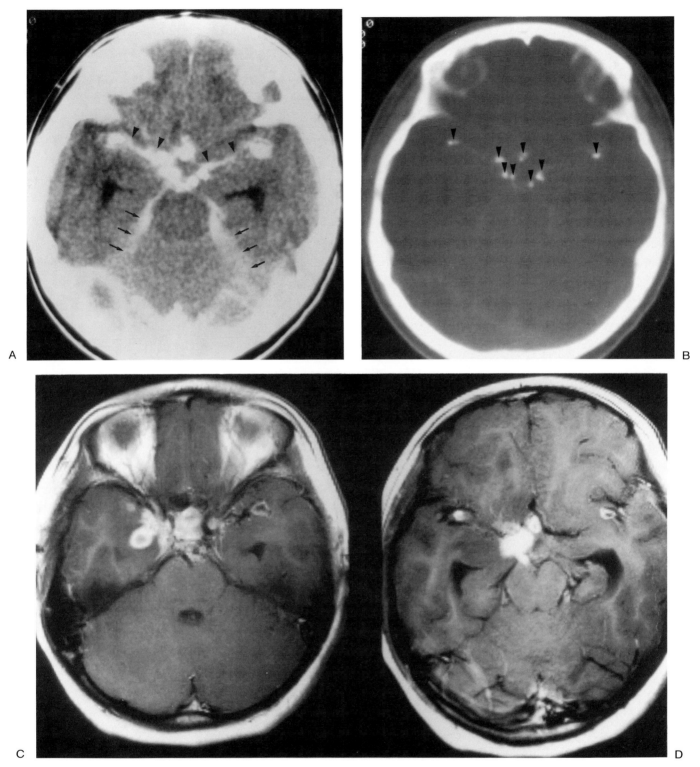

FIG. 11.30. Meningeal cysticercosis. **A:** Postcontrast CT image shows enhancement in the suprasellar and Sylvian cisterns (*arrowheads*) and along the tentorium (*arrows*). The temporal horns of the lateral ventricles are dilated secondary to hydrocephalus. **B:** Bone window CT image shows multiple punctate calcifications (*arrows*) within the suprasellar and Sylvian cisterns. **C, D:** Postcontrast axial SE 600/16 images show multiple enhancing nodules in the suprasellar cistern, temporal lobe, and inferior Sylvian cisterns.

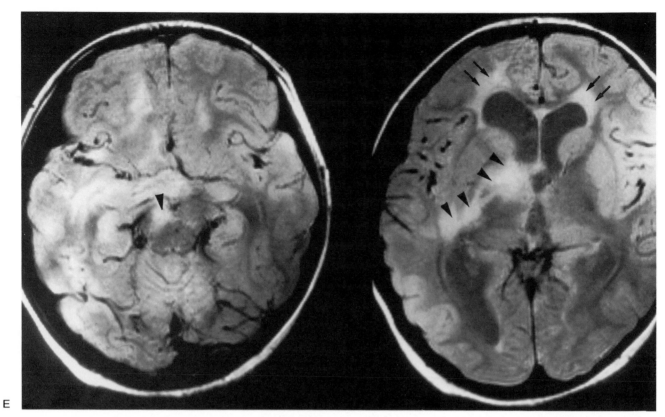

FIG. 11.30. (*Continued.*) E, F: Axial SE 2800/20 images show multiple areas of T2 prolongation in the brain parenchyma secondary to edema from adjacent cysticerci (*arrowheads*) and transependymal CSF resorption (*arrows*).

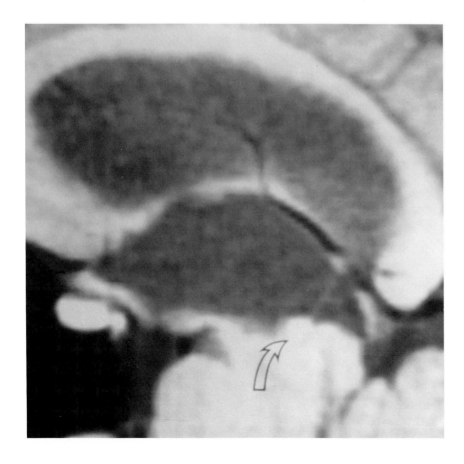

FIG. 11.31. Intraventricular cysticercus. Sagittal SE 600/20 image shows the scolex of the cysticercus (*arrow*) at the rostral opening of the aqueduct.

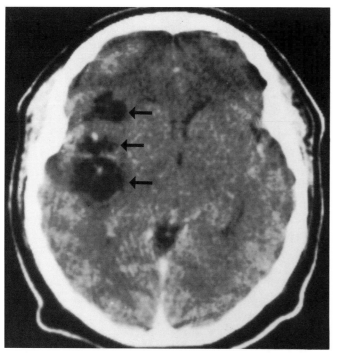

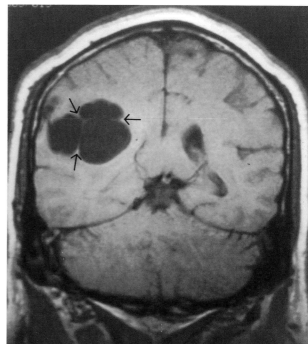

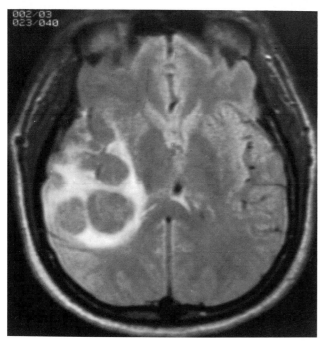

FIG. 11.32. Racemose cerebral cysticercosis. **A:** Axial contrast-enhanced CT shows several cystic lesions (*arrows*) in the region of the right Sylvian fissure. **B:** Sagittal SE 800/ 20 image shows the cystic lesions to be multiple adjacent loculations with intervening septae (*arrows*). **C:** Axial SE 2500/30 image shows a moderate amount of edema surrounding the cysticercal cysts within the Sylvian fissure. This degree of edema was not appreciated on either the CT or the short TR/TE MR image.

chymal nodules lack peripheral edema, may be single or multiple, and may be located at the base of the brain or scattered throughout the hemispheres. They are isodense with gray matter prior to contrast infusion on CT; on MR, they are isointense to gray matter on T1-weighted images and iso- to hyperintense on T2-weighted images (126). The granulomas enhance uniformly after administration of intravenous contrast (125,128). Imaging studies are valuable not only in the diagnosis of intra-

cranial sarcoid, but also in its follow-up. The sarcoid granulomas can be seen to diminish in size or resolve completely following steroid therapy.

INTRACRANIAL EMPYEMAS

Subdural and epidural empyemas will be discussed collectively, as differentiation of the two by CT or MR is extremely difficult unless the lesion is parafalcine (necessarily subdural) in location. The most common source of intracranial empyema is a direct extension of otitis media or sinusitis into the epidural or subdural spaces. In children, extension of pneumococcal meningitis from the subarachnoid to the subdural or epidural space is another common source. Other, less common causes are osteomyelitis, orbital cellulitis, direct penetrating trauma, congenital osseous defects (such as dorsal dermal sinuses and encephaloceles), sepsis with metastatic infection, and contamination of a subdural effusion (1,28,36).

Affected patients initially present with evidence of meningismus, such as fever, stiff neck, headache, and lethargy. They subsequently develop symptoms of a space-occupying lesion with blurred vision, focal neurologic findings, and focal seizures (26,129). When these symptoms are seen in association with a head wound, otitis media, or sinusitis, an empyema should be suspected and work-up should be directed toward finding the collection of pus.

Pathology studies have shown that the pus in these patients is commonly both intra- and extradural (130). As a result, differentiating intradural from extradural abscesses is impractical, even if the collection of pus is predominantly in one compartment or the other. Convexity empyemas are the most common and outnumber parafalcine empyemas by two to one (36). Tentorial collections are less common and are usually the result of an extension of a preexisting empyema. Empyemas can be accurately localized to the extradural space if they are bilateral (extending across the midline) or if they displace the falx from the inner table of the skull (Fig. 11.33). In the more common lateral convexity empyema, these signs are not useful, and localization is less accurate.

On imaging studies, empyemas are seen as a widening of the extracerebral space with compression of adjacent sulci (Fig. 11.34). There are no signal characteristics of the fluid collections that are helpful in distinguishing them from nonpurulent collections. On MR, empyemas are slightly hyperintense to cerebrospinal fluid on both T1- and T2-weighted images (131). Loculation within the collections is seen in approximately 50% of affected patients (Fig. 11.35). Vasogenic edema does not occur in association with empyemas. If low density (CT) or T1 and T2 prolongation (MR) is seen in the adjacent parenchyma (Fig. 11.35), it is usually the result of associated cerebritis, which is concurrent with empyemas in approximately 20% of patients (36,131). Less commonly, low density or T1 and T2 prolongation can occur in the brain substance from ischemia. After infusion of intravenous contrast, enhancement is unusual in the early stages of the empyema. A rim of contrast enhancement central to the collection becomes apparent after about 1–

3 weeks; it is not certain whether the enhancement represents a capsule around the pus or cortical enhancement secondary to ischemic cortical damage.

When an extra-axial fluid collection is seen in a pediatric patient, it is important to seek a source of infection in the sinuses, middle ear and mastoid air cells, orbit, and skull (132) (Figs. 11.33, 11.35). The empyema is frequently contralateral to the infected sinus; it can even be contralateral to an infected middle ear cavity or mastoid (36). *If extra-axial collections are seen in association with sinusitis, otitis, or orbital cellulitis, an empyema should be highly suspected.* It is difficult to differentiate an empyema from subdural effusions, such as those that occur during the course of a *Hemophilus influenzae* meningitis, by imaging. Reactive effusions from *H. influenzae* meningitis are almost always bilateral; the bilaterality is useful because empyemas are rarely bilateral (28,36,133).

EMPYEMAS OF THE SPINE

Although extremely rare in childhood, infections of the spinal epidural space (spinal empyemas) are important to recognize because a delay in diagnosis can result in devastating neurologic injury. The clinical course of spinal empyemas may be acute and rapidly progressive or chronic. The acute course is more common in children and is usually the result of a blood-borne, metastatic infection; chronic empyemas are most often caused by direct extension of a spinal osteomyelitis. Classically, hematogenous spinal epidural abscesses follow a typical clinical pattern (1). Approximately 1–2 weeks after an infection, a backache develops; the back pain is enhanced by jarring or straining and is accompanied by local spinal tenderness. Within a few days, radicular pain develops, followed by symptoms of spinal cord compression, including weakness and impaired sphincter control. Paraplegia may be complete within a few hours or days.

Pathologically, the infection is usually limited to the dorsal aspect of the canal in blood-borne empyemas, whereas the ventral canal is initially affected when infection extends from the vertebral body. The anatomy of the epidural space limits extension to vertical spread and results in the extradural compression (1). If compression of the spinal cord persists long enough, thrombosis of spinal vessels may develop, leading to spinal cord infarct and permanent paraplegia (28).

When the abscess is the result of metastatic infection, the results of imaging are not specific, although the MR findings are very suggestive in the proper clinical setting. A mass is seen extending rostrally and caudally in the

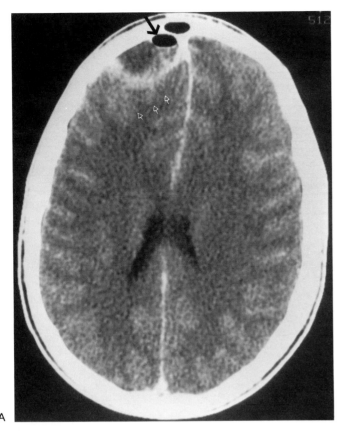

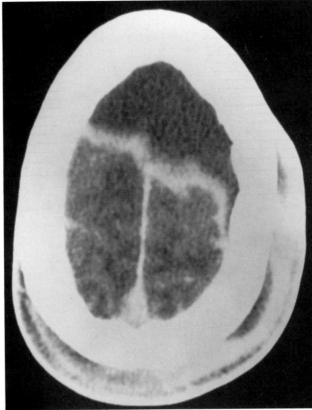

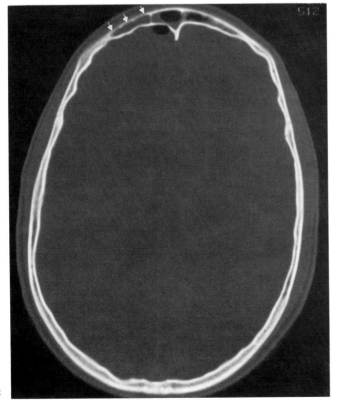

FIG. 11.33. Extradural empyema. **A:** Axial contrast-enhanced CT shows a collection of fluid in the right frontal region that contains a focus of air (*black arrow*). The gray–white junction (*open white arrows*) is displaced posteriorly by this collection, indicating it is extra-axial. **B:** At a higher level, the extra-axial collection is seen to extend across the midline and displace the falx from the inner table of the skull. These findings localize the collection to the extra-dural space. **C:** It is important to look at the paranasal sinuses in all patients with extra-axial fluid collections. Soft tissue density is present within the frontal sinuses, suggestive of sinusitis (*arrows*). If extra-axial collections are seen in association with sinusitis, otitis, or orbital cellulitis, an empyema should be highly suspected.

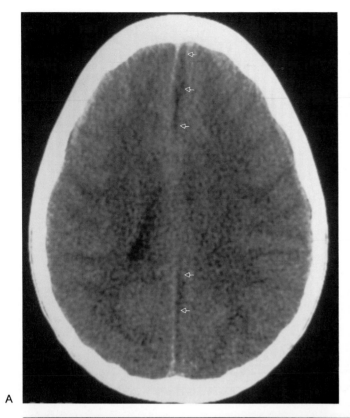

A

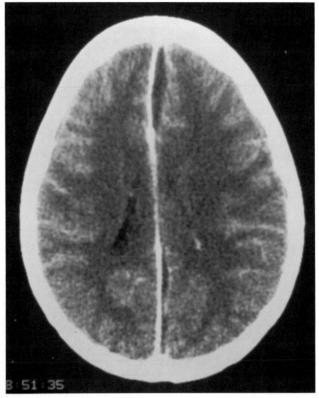

B

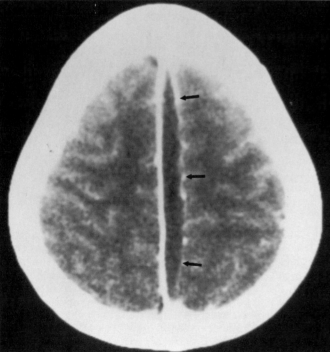

C

FIG. 11.34. Subdural empyema. **A:** Noncontrast CT scan shows widening of the interhemispheric fissure (*arrows*) with compression of adjacent sulci. **B:** After infusion of iodinated contrast, the interhemispheric collection and the displacement of the adjacent gyri are more clearly seen. **C:** Near the vertex, the interhemispheric subdural empyema (*arrows*), which in this case was a consequence of sinusitis, is easily appreciated.

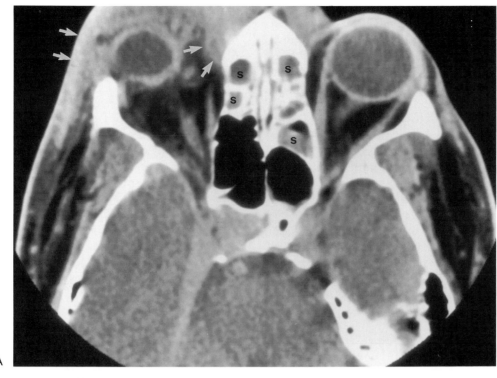

A

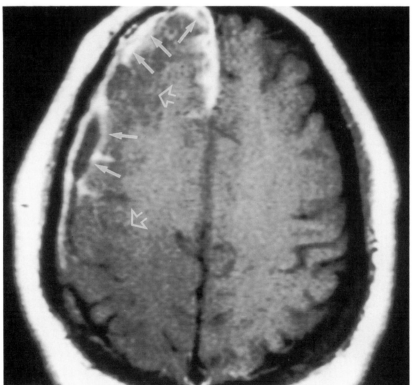

B

FIG. 11.35. Orbital cellulitis and empyema secondary to sinusitis. **A:** Axial CT image shows soft tissue density(s) filling the ethmoid sinuses. Soft tissue swelling (*arrows*) is seen around the right orbit. **B:** Postcontrast MR image shows several loculations of extraparenchymal fluid (*arrows*) and meningeal enhancement. The low-intensity regions (*open arrows*) in the cerebral parenchyma may represent cerebritis or ischemia.

dorsal epidural space, compressing the thecal sac. The mass is usually of soft tissue or liquid density on CT. On MR, the epidural collection has a variable appearance on T1-weighted images. Most commonly, it appears as heterogeneous hypointensity in the dorsal epidural fat that uniformly enhances after administration of paramagnetic contrast (Fig. 11.36). Less commonly, the empyema may be homogeneously isointense or slightly hyperintense compared to cerebrospinal fluid on precontrast T1-weighted images. Identification and diagnosis are facilitated by the use of fat suppression pulses on the postcontrast sequences. The empyema is isointense to cerebrospinal fluid on T2-weighted images.

When the abscess is the result of adjacent osteomyelitis, the adjacent disc space is usually narrowed and pus often extends ventral to the vertebral bodies as well as into the ventral spinal canal. The abscess is generally isointense to the cord on T1-weighted images and hyperintense to the cord but iso- to slightly hypointense to ce-

rebrospinal fluid on T2-weighted images (134,135) (Figs. 11.37, 11.38). Although CT better demonstrates erosion of the endplates of the bone by the inflammatory process, MR demonstrates prolonged T1 and T2 relaxation time within the disc and adjacent vertebral bodies, because of increased water content (resulting from the inflammatory process). T1-weighted images after intravenous administration of paramagnetic contrast will show enhancement of infected bone and constitute the most sensitive method for detecting vertebral osteomyelitis (136). Thus, MR is the imaging modality of choice for empyemas of the spine. The sagittal images show the rostral to caudal extent of the abscess and are invaluable in localizing associated discitis or osteomyelitis. MR is more specific than CT or myelography because of the increased sensitivity to enhancement of the empyema and to the involvement of adjacent bone. Moreover, the danger of entering the abscess by a lumbar puncture is removed.

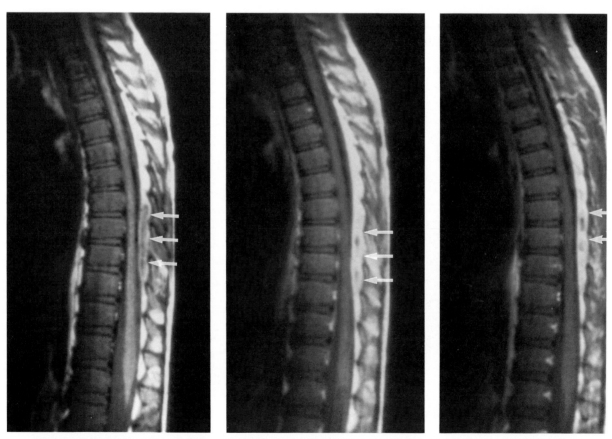

A,B   C

FIG. 11.36. Spinal epidural empyema. **A:** Sagittal SE 600/20 images show a soft tissue intensity mass (*arrows*) dorsal to the spinal cord in the mid-thoracic level. This patient developed back pain and local spinal tenderness 10 days after a bacterial pharyngitis. **B, C:** Postcontrast images show heterogeneous enhancement of the epidural collection (*arrows*).

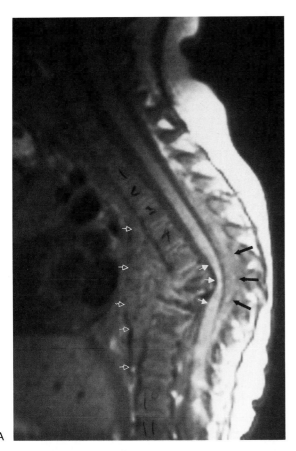

A

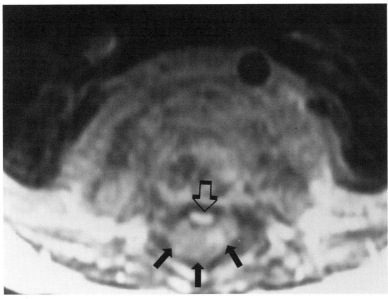

B

FIG. 11.37. Epidural empyema secondary to vertebral osteomyelitis. **A:** Sagittal SE 600/20 image shows destruction of the T6 and T7 vertebral bodies. There is a large soft tissue mass anterior to the mid-thoracic spine (*open white arrows*) that at surgery was found to be purulent material. A gibbous deformity is seen at the site of the collapsed vertebral bodies, and a retropulsed bony fragment is seen to compress the spinal cord (*closed white arrows*). A collection of pus was also present dorsal to the spinal cord within the spinal canal (*closed black arrows*). **B:** Axial SE 1000/20 image through the middle of the gibbous deformity. The dorsal epidural empyema (*closed arrows*) can be seen dorsal to the spinal cord (*open arrow*). Anterior to the spinal cord is the destroyed vertebral body and the surrounding abscess. (This case courtesy of Dr. Wallace Peck, Irvine, CA.)

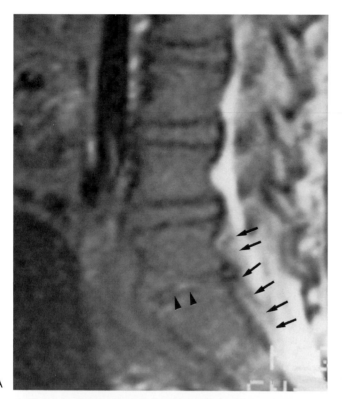

A

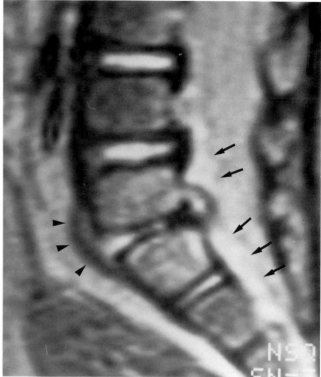

B

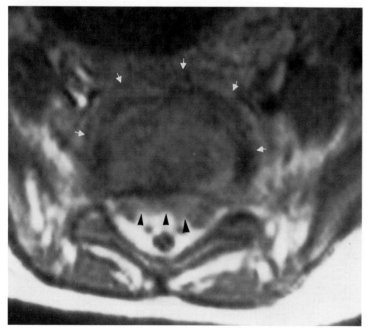

C

FIG. 11.38. Spinal epidural abscess secondary to vertebral osteomyelitis. **A:** Sagittal SE 700/33 image shows narrowing of the L5–S1 disc space (*arrowheads*) and soft tissue intensity dorsal to the L5 and S1 vertebral bodies (*arrows*). **B:** Sagittal SE 2000/80 image shows a slight increased signal intensity of the L5 vertebral body and sacrum. The disc space is narrowed, and there is purulent material extending ventrally under the anterior longitudinal ligament (*arrowheads*) and posteriorly into the epidural space (*arrows*) at the L5 and S1 levels. The pus is of high signal intensity on this long TR/TE image. **C:** Axial SE 800/33 image at the L5–S1 disc space shows indistinct anterior margins of the disc (*white arrows*) as a result of the infection extending anteriorly and obscuring fat planes. Posterior extension of the infection into the ventral epidural space can be seen effacing epidural fat (*arrowheads*).

REFERENCES

1. Weil ML. Infections of the nervous system. In: Menkes JH, ed. *Textbook of child neurology.* Philadelphia: Lea and Feibiger, 1985:316–431.
2. Alford CA, Stagno S, Pass RF, Britt WJ. Congenital and perinatal cytomegalovirus infections. *Rev Infect Des* 1990;12 (Suppl 7): S745–S753.
3. Yow MD. Congenital cytomegalovirus disease: a now problem. *J Infect Dis* 1989;159:163–167.
4. Dobbins JG, Stewart JA, Demmler GJ. Surveillance of congenital cytomegalovirus disease, 1990–1991. Collaborating Registry Group. *Mmwr Cdc Surveill Summ* 1992;41:35–39.
5. Marques-Dias MJ, Harmant-van Rijckevorsel G, Landrieu C, et al. Prenatal cytomegalovirus disease and cerebral microgyria; evidence for perfusion failure, not disturbance of histogenesis, as the major cause of fetal cytomegalovirus encephalopathy. *Neuropediatrics* 1984;15:18–24.
6. Barkovich AJ, Linden CL. Congenital cytomegalovirus infection of the brain: imaging analysis and embryologic considerations. *Am J Neuroradiol* (in press).
7. Boesch CH, Issakainen J, Kewitz G, Kikinis R, Martin E, Boltshauser E. Magnetic resonance imaging of the brain in congenital cytomegalovirus infection. *Pediatr Radiol* 1989;19:91–93.
8. Hayward JC, Titelbaum DS, Clancy RR, Zimmerman RA. Lissencephaly-pachygyria associated with congenital cytomegalovirus infection. *J Child Neurol* 1991;6:109–114.
9. Perlman JM, Argyle C. Lethal cytomegalovirus infection in preterm infants: clinical, radiological, and neuropathological findings. *Ann Neurol* 1992;31:64–8.
10. Sugita K, Ando M, Makino M, Takanashi J, Fujimoto N, Niimi H. Magnetic resonance imaging of the brain in congenital rubella virus and cytomegalovirus infections. *Neuroradiology* 1991;33: 239–242.
11. Banker BQ, Larroche JC. Periventricular leukomalacia of infancy. *Arch Neurol* 1962;7:386–410.
12. Friede RL. *Developmental neuropathology,* 2nd ed. Berlin: Springer-Verlag, 1989.
13. Robertson JS. Toxoplasmosis. *Dev Med Child Neurol* 1962;4: 507–512.
14. Desmonts G, Couvreur J. Congenital toxoplasmosis. *N Engl J Med* 1974;290:1110–1112.
15. Eichenwald HF, ed. *Human toxoplasmosis.* Baltimore: Williams and Wilkins, 1956.
16. Bale JF Jr. Viral infections. In: Berg BO, ed. *Neurologic aspects of pediatrics.* Boston: Butterworth-Heinemann, 1992:227–256.
17. Alvord EC Jr, Shaw CM. Infectious, allergic and demyelinating diseases of the nervous system. In: Newton TH, Potts DG, eds. *Anatomy and pathology.* St Louis: CV Mosby, 1977:3088–3172.
18. Altschuler G. Toxoplasmosis as a cause of hydranencephaly. *Am J Dis Child* 1973;125:251–252.
19. Diebler C, Dusser A, Dulac O. Congenital toxoplasmosis: clinical and neuroradiological evaluation of the cerebral lesions. *Neuroradiology* 1985;27:125–130.
20. Whitley RJ, Hutto C. Neonatal herpes simplex virus infections. *Pediatr Rev* 1985;7:119–126.
21. Noorbehesht B, Enzmann DR, Sullinder W, Bradley JS, Arvin AM. Neonatal herpes simplex encephalitis: correlation of clinical and CT findings. *Radiology* 1987;162:813–819.
22. Miller E, Craddock-Watson JE, Pollock TM. Consequences of confirmed maternal rubella at successive stages of pregnancy. *Lancet* 1982;2:781–782.
23. Cooper LZ, Ziring PR, Ockerse AB, Fedun BA, Kiely C, Krugman.S. Rubella: clinical manifestations and management. *Am J Dis Child* 1969;118:18–23.
24. Fitz CR. Inflammatory diseases. In: Gonzalez CF, Grossman CB, Masden JC, eds. *Head and spine imaging.* New York: Wiley, 1985:537–554.
25. Fee WE, Marks MI, Kardash S, et al. The long term prognosis of aseptic meningitis in childhood. *Dev Med Child Neurol* 1970;12: 321–329.
26. Snyder RD. Bacterial infections of the nervous system. In: Berg BO, ed. *Neurologic aspects of pediatrics.* Boston: Butterworth-Heinemann, 1992:195–226.
27. Dunn DW, Daum RS, Weisberg L, Vargas R. Ischemic cerebrovascular complications of *Haemophilus influenza* meningitis. *Arch Neurol* 1982;39:650–652.
28. Harriman DGF. Bacterial infections of the central nervous system. In: Adams JH, Corsellis JAN, Duchen LW, eds. *Greenfield's neuropathology,* 4th ed. New York: Wiley, 1984:236–259.
29. Yumashima T, Kashihara K, Ikeda K, et al. Three phases of cerebral arteriopathy in meningitis: vasospasm and vasodilatation followed by organic stenosis. *Neurosurgery* 1985;16:546–553.
30. Friede RL. Cerebral infarcts complicating neonatal leptomeningitis. *Acta Neuropathol* 1973;23:245–251.
31. Berman PH, Banker BQ. Neonatal meningitis: a clinical and pathological study of 29 cases. *Pediatrics* 1966;38:6–11.
32. Mathews VP, Kuharik MA, Edwards MK, et al. Gd-DTPA enhanced MR imaging of experimental bacterial meningitis: evaluation and comparison with CT. *Am J Neuroradiol* 1988;9:1045–1050.
33. Virapongse C, Cazenave C, Quisling R, Sarwar M, Hunter S. The empty delta sign: frequency and significance in 76 cases of dural sinus thrombosis. *Radiology* 1987;162:779–785.
34. Rao KCVG, Knipp HC, Wagner EJ. The findings in cerebral sinus and venous thrombosis. *Radiology* 1981;140:391–398.
35. Chiras J, Dubs M, Bories J. Venous infarctions. *Neuroradiology* 1985;27:593–600.
36. Moseley IF, Kendall BE. Radiology of intracranial empyemas, with special reference to computed tomography. *Neuroradiology* 1984;26:333–345.
37. Naidich TP, McLone DG, Yamanouchi Y. Periventricular white matter cysts in a murine mode of gram-negative ventriculitis. *Am J Neuroradiol* 1983;4:461–465.
38. Schultz P, Leeds NE. Intraventricular septations complication neonatal meningitis. *J Neurosurg* 1973;38:620–626.
39. Lincoln E, Sordillo SVR, Davies PA. Tuberculous meningitis in children: a review of 167 untreated and 74 treated patients with special reference to early diagnosis. *J Pediatr* 1960;57:807–823.
40. Rich AR, McCordock HA. The pathogenesis of tuberculous meningitis. *Bull Johns Hopkins Hosp* 1933;52:5–9.
41. Wallace RC, Burton EM, Barrett FF, Leggiadro RJ, Gerald BE, Lasater OE. Intracranial tuberculosis in children: CT appearance and clinical outcome. *Pediatr Radiol* 1991;21:241–246.
42. Casselman ES, Hasso AN, Ashwal S, et al. CT of tuberculous meningitis in infants and children. *J Comput Assist Tomogr* 1980;4:211–216.
43. Chang KH, Han MH, Roh JK, et al. Gd-DTPA enhanced MR imaging in intracranial tuberculosis. *Neuroradiology* 1990;32: 19–25.
44. Offenbacher H, Fazekas F, Schmidt R, et al. MRI in tuberculous meningoencephalitis: report of four cases and review of the neuroimaging literature. *J Neurol* 1991;238:340–344.
45. Tang PS, Low LC. Radiological and clinical features of basal ganglia infarction in tuberculous meningitis. *Aust Paediatr J* 1989;25:361–362.
46. Hsieh FY, Chia LG, Shen WC. Locations of cerebral infarctions in tuberculous meningitis. *Neuroradiology* 1992;34:197–199.
47. Bhargava S, Tandon PN. Intracranial tuberculomas: a CT study. *Br J Radiol* 1980;53:935–945.
48. Welchman JM. CT of intracranial tuberculomata. *Clin Radiol* 1979;30:567–579.
49. Gee GT, Bazan C III, Jinkins JR. Miliary tuberculosis involving the brain: MR findings. *Am J Roentgenol* 1992;159:1075–1076.
50. Enzmann DR, Britt RH, Placone R. Staging of human brain abscess by computed tomography. *Radiology* 1983;146:703–708.
51. Liston TE, Tomasovic JJ, Stevens EA. Early diagnosis and management of cerebritis in a child. *Pediatrics* 1979;65:484–487.
52. Belman A. Neurologic complications of Lyme disease in children. *Int Pediatr* 1992;7:136–143.
53. Miller GL, Craven R, Bailey M, Tsai T. The epidemiology of Lyme disease in the United States, 1987–1988. *Lab Med* 1990;21:285–289.
54. Feder H, Zalneraitis E, Reik L Jr. Lyme disease: acute focal meningoencephalitis in a child. *Pediatrics* 1988;82:931–934.
55. Belman AL, Coyle PK, Roque C, Cantos E. MRI findings in chil-

dren infected by *Borrelia burgdorferi. Pediatr Neurol* 1992;8:428–431.

56. Jadavji T, Humphreys RP, Prober CG. Brain abscesses in infants and children. *Pediatr Infect Dis J* 1985;4:394–398.

57. Krajewski R, Stelmasiak Z. Brain abscess in infants. *Childs Nerv Syst* 1992;8:279–280.

58. Renier D, Flandin C, Hirsch E, Hirsch J-F. Brain abscesses in neonates: a study of 30 cases. *J Neurosurg* 1988;69:877–882.

59. Enzmann DR, Britt RH, Yeager AS. Experimental brain abscess evolution: CT and neuropathologic correlation. *Radiology* 1979;133:113–120.

60. Haimes AB, Zimmerman RD, Mrogello S, et al. MR imaging of brain abscesses. *Am J Neuroradiol* 1989;10:279–291.

61. Ferriero DM, Derechin M, Edwards MSB. Outcome of brain abscess treatment in children: reduced morbidity with neuroimaging. *Pediatr Neurol* 1987;3:148–152.

62. Johnson RT, Mims CA. Pathogenesis of viral infections of the nervous system. *N Engl J Med* 1968;278:54–92.

63. Johnson RT. *Viral infections of the nervous system.* New York: Raven, 1982.

64. Weiner LP, Fleming JV. Viral infections of the nervous system. *J Neurosurg* 1984;61:207–224.

65. Whitley RJ. Herpes simplex encephalitis. Clinical assessment. *JAMA* 1982;247:317–320.

66. Neils EW, Lukin R, Tomsick T, Twe JM. MR imaging and CT scanning of herpes simplex encephalitis. *J Neurosurg* 1987;67:592–594.

67. Schroth G, Gawehn J, Thron A, et al. Early diagnosis of herpes simplex encephalitis by MRI. *Neurology* 1987;37:179–183.

68. Launes J, Nikkinen P, Lindroth L, Brownell AL, Liewendahl K, Iivanainen M. Diagnosis of acute herpes simplex encephalitis by brain perfusion single photon emission computed tomography. *Lancet* 1988;1:1188–1191.

69. Gasecki AP, Steg RE. Correlation of early MRI with CT scan, EEG, and CSF: analyses in a case of biopsy-proven herpes simplex encephalitis. *Eur Neurol* 1991;31:372–375.

70. Kaufmann D, Zimmerman RD, Leeds NE. CT in herpes simplex encephalitis. *Neurology* 1979;29:1392–1395.

71. Enzmann DR, Ranson B, Norman D, Talberth E. CT of herpes simplex encephalitis. *Radiology* 1978;129:419–425.

72. Koch TK. AIDS in children. In: Berg BO, ed. *Neurologic aspects of pediatrics.* Boston: Butterworth-Heinemann, 1992:531–549.

73. Epstein LG, Sharer LR, Goudsmit J. Neurological and neuropathological features of human immunodeficiency virus infection in children. *Ann Neurol* 1988;23 (suppl):S19–S23.

74. Kauffman W, Sivit CJ, Fitz CR, Rakusan TA, Herzog K, Chandra RS. CT and MR evaluation of intracranial involvement in pediatric HIV infection: a clinical-imaging correlation. *Am J Neuroradiol* 1992;13:949–957.

75. Chamberlain MC, Nichols SL, Chase CH. Pediatric AIDS: comparative cranial MRI and CT scans. *Pediatr Neurol* 1991;7:357–362.

76. Civitello LA. Neurologic complications of HIV infection in children. *Pediatr Neurosurg* 1991–1992;17:104–112.

77. Joshi VV, Powell B, Connor E, et al. Arteriopathy in children with AIDS. *Pediatr Pathol* 1987;7:261–268.

78. DeCarli C, Civitello L, Brouwers P, Pizzo P. The prevalence of CT abnormalities of the cerebrum in 100 consecutive children symptomatic with the human immune deficiency virus. *Ann Neurol* 1993;34:198–205.

79. Dickson DW, Belman A, Kim TS, et al. Spinal cord pathology in pediatric acquired immunodeficiency syndrome. *Neurology* 1989;39:227–235.

80. Price DB, Inglese CM, Jacobs J. Pediatric AIDS, neuroradiologic and neurodevelopmental findings. *Pediatr Radiol* 1988;18:445–448.

81. Kugler SL, Barzilai A, Hodes DS, et al. Acute hemiplegia associated with HIV infection. *Pediatr Neurol* 1991;7:207–210.

82. Park YD, Belman AL, Kim T-S, et al. Stroke in pediatric acquired immunodeficiency syndrome. *Ann Neurol* 1990;28:303–311.

83. Modlin J, Jabbour J, Witte J, et al. Epidemiologic studies of measles, measles vaccine, and subacute sclerosing panencephalitis. *Pediatrics* 1977;59:505–512.

84. Krawiecki NS, Dyken PR, El Gammal T, DuRant RH, Swift A. CT of the brain in subacute sclerosing panencephalitis. *Ann Neurol* 1984;15:489–493.

85. Walker DL. Progressive multifocal leukoencephalopathy: an opportunistic viral infection of the central nervous system. In: Vinken PJ, Bruyn GW, eds. *Infections of the nervous system.* Amsterdam: North-Holland, 1978:307–329.

86. Whiteman MLH, Post MJD, Berger JR, Tate LG, Bell MD, Limonte LP. Progressive multifocal leukoencephalopathy in 47 HIV-seropositive patients: neuroimaging with clinical and pathologic correlation. *Radiology* 1993;187:233–240.

87. Rasmussen T, Andermann F. Update on the syndrome of "chronic encephalitis" and epilepsy. *Clev Clin J Med* 1989;56(Suppl 2):S181–S184.

88. Rasmussen T. Further observations on the syndrome of chronic encephalitis and epilepsy. *Appl Neurophysiol* 1978;41:1–12.

89. Rasmussen T, McCann W. Clinical studies of patients with focal epilepsy due to "chronic encephalitis." *Trans Am Neurol Assoc* 1968;93:89–95.

90. Farrell MA, DeRosa MJ, Curran JG, et al. Neuropathologic findings in cortical resections (including hemispherectomies) performed for the treatment of intractable childhood epilepsy. *Acta Neuropathol* 1992;83:246–259.

91. Gray F, Serdaru M, Baron H, et al. Chronic localized encephalitis (Rasmussen's) in an adult with epilepsia partialis continua. *J Neurol Neurosurg Psychiatry* 1987;50:747–751.

92. Reye RDK, Morgan D, Baral J. Encephalopathy and fatty degeneration of the viscera: a disease entity in childhood. *Lancet* 1963;2:749–752.

93. Trauner D. Reye syndrome. In: Berg BO, ed. *Neurologic aspects of pediatrics.* Boston: Butterworth-Heinemann, 1992:309–316.

94. Russell E, Zimmerman RA, Leeds N. Reye syndrome: CT documentation of disordered intracerebral structure. *J Comput Assist Tomogr* 1979;3:217–220.

95. Malzberg MS, Rogg JM, Tate CA, Zayas V, Easton JD. Poliomyelitis: hyperintensity of the anterior horn cells on MR images of the spinal cord. *Am J Roentgenol* 1993;14:863–865.

96. Wasserstrom R, Mamourian AC, McGary CT, Miller G. Bulbar poliomyelitis: MR findings with pathologic correlation. *Am J Neuroradiol* 1992;13:371–373.

97. Weiss S, Carter S. Course and prognosis of acute cerebellar ataxia in children. *Neurology* 1959;9:711–721.

98. Horowitz MB, Pang D, Hirsch W. Acute cerebellitis: case report and review. *Pediatr Neurosurg* 1991–1992;17:142–145.

99. King G, Schwarz G, Slade H. Acute cerebellar ataxia of childhood. Report of nine cases. *Pediatrics* 1958;21:731–745.

100. Scaravelli F. Parasitic and fungal infections of the nervous system. In: Adams JH, Corsellis JAN, Duchen LW, eds. *Greenfield's neuropathology.* New York: Wiley Medical, 1984:304–337.

101. Bebin EM, Gomez MR. Mycotic and parasitic infections. In: Berg BO, ed. *Neurologic aspects of pediatrics.* Boston: Butterworth-Heinemann, 1992:257–284.

102. Dublin A, Phillips H. CT of disseminated cerebral coccidioidomycosis. *Radiology* 1980;135:361–365.

103. Post M, Huffman T. Cerebral inflammatory disease. In: Rosenberg R, Heinz ER, ed. *The clinical neurosciences,* vol. 4. *Neuroradiology.* New York: Churchill-Livingstone, 1984:525–594.

104. Tan C, Kuan B. Cryptococcal meningitis: clinical–CT considerations. *Neuroradiology* 1987;29:43–46.

105. Cornell S, Jacoby C. The varied CT appearance of intracranial cryptococcosis. *Radiology* 1982;143:703–707.

106. Penar P, Kim J, Chyatte D, Sabshin JK. Intraventricular cryptococcal granuloma: report of two cases. *J Neurosurg* 1988;68:145–148.

107. Tien R, Chu P, Hesselink J, et al. Intracranial cryptococcus in immunocompromised patients: CT and MR findings in 29 cases. *Am J Roentgenol* 1991;156:1245–1252.

108. Mandell G, Douglas R, Bennett J. *Principles and practice of infectious disease.* New York: Wiley, 1985.

109. Booss JM, Thorton GF. *Infectious diseases of the central nervous system.* Philadelphia: WB Saunders, 1986.

110. Vinken P, Bruyn G. *Infections of the nervous system.* Amsterdam: North-Holland, 1978.

111. Hernandez AL, Garaizer C. Analysis of 89 cases of infantile cerebral cysticercosis. In: Flisser A, ed. *Cysticercosis: present state of knowledge and perspectives.* New York: Academic, 1982:334.
112. Trelles J, Trelles L. Cystercosis. In: Vinken P, Bruyn G, ed. *Infections of the nervous system.* Amsterdam: Elsevier, 1978:291–320.
113. Carbajal J, Palacios E, Azar-Kia B, et al. Radiology of cysticercosis of the CNS including computed tomography. *Radiology* 1977;125:127–133.
114. Barkovich AJ, Citrin CM, Klara P, Wippold F, Kattah J. MR imaging of cysticercosis. *West J Med* 1986;145:687–690.
115. Byrd S, Locke G, Biggers S, Percy A. The CT appearance of cerebral cysticercosis in adults and children. *Radiology* 1982;144:819–823.
116. Kramer LD, Locke G, Byrd S, Daryabagi J. Cerebral cysticercosis: documentation of natural history with CT. *Radiology* 1989;171:459–462.
117. Suss R, Maravilla K, Thompson J. MR imaging of intracranial cysticercosis: comparison with CT and anatomopathologic features. *Am J Neuroradiol* 1986;7:235–242.
118. Titelbaum G, Otto R, Lin M, et al. MR imaging of neurocysticercosis. *Am J Neuroradiol* 1989;10:709–718.
119. Suh D, Chang K, Han M, Lee S, Han M, Kim C. Unusual MR manifestations of neurocysticercosis. *Neuroradiology* 1989;31:396–402.
120. Zee C-S, Segall H, Apuzzo M, Ahmadi J, Dobkin W. Intraventricular cysticercal cysts: further neuroradiologic observations and neurosurgical implications. *Am J Neuroradiol* 1984;5:727–730.
121. Zee C-S, Segall H, Ahmadi J, Tsai F, Apuzzo M. CT myelography in spinal cysticercosis. *J Comput Assist Tomogr* 1986;10:195–198.
122. Dyken PR. Neurosarcoidosis. In: Berg BO, ed. *Neurologic aspects of pediatrics.* Boston: Butterworth-Heinemann, 1992:299–308.
123. Weinberg S, Bennett H, Weinstock I. CNS manifestations of sarcoidosis in children. *Clin Pediatr* 1983;22:447–481.
124. Delaney P. Neurologic manifestations of sarcoidosis. *Ann Int Med* 1977;87:336–345.
125. Brooks BS, El Gammal T, Hungerford G, et al. Radiologic evaluation of neurosarcoidosis: role of computed tomography. *Am J Neuroradiol* 1982;3:513–521.
126. Hayes W, Sherman J, Stern B, Citrin C, Pulaski P. MR and CT evaluation of intracranial sarcoidosis. *Am J Neuroradiol* 1987;8:841–847.
127. Clark W, Acker J, Dohan F Jr, Robertson J. Presentation of central nervous system sarcoidosis as intracranial tumors. *J Neurosurg* 1985;63:851–856.
128. Williams D III, Elster A, Kramer S. Neurosarcoidosis: gadolinium-enhanced MR imaging. *J Comput Assist Tomogr* 1990;14:704–709.
129. Luken MG, Whelan MA. Recent diagnostic experience with subdural empyema. *J Neurosurg* 1980;52:764–767.
130. Courville CB. Subdural empyema secondary to purulent frontal sinusitis. *Arch Otolaryngol* 1944;39:211–230.
131. Weingarten K, Zimmerman RD, Becker R, Heier S, Haimes A, Deck MDF. Subdural and epidural empyemas: MR imaging. *Am J Neuroradiol* 1989;10:81–87.
132. Carter B, Bankhoff M, Fisk J. CT detection of sinusitis responsible for intracranial and extracranial infections. *Radiology* 1983;147:739–742.
133. Zimmerman RD, Leeds N, Danzinger A. Subdural empyema: CT findings. *Radiology* 1984;150:417–422.
134. Numaguchi Y, Rigamonti D, Rothman MI, Sato S, Mihara F, Sadato N. Spinal epidural abscess: evaluation with gadolinium-enhanced MR imaging. *Radiographics* 1993;13:545–559.
135. Kricun R, Shoemaker E, Chovanes G, Stephens H. Epidural abscess of the cervical spine: MR findings in five cases. *Am J Roentgenol* 1992;158:1145–1149.
136. Morrison WB, Schweitzer ME, Bock GW, et al. Diagnosis of osteomyelitis: utility of fat-suppressed contrast-enhanced MR imaging. *Radiology* 1993;189:251–257.
137. Wyler D. Malaria: resurgence, resistance, research. *N Engl J Med* 1983;308:875–879.
138. Blount R. Acute falciparum malaria. *Ann Int Med* 1969;70:142–145.
139. Van Boghert L, Janssen P. Contribution à l'étude de la neurologie et neuropathologie de la trypanosominiase humaine. *Ann Soc Belg Med Trop* 1957;37:379–391.
140. Laranja F, Dias E, Bobrega G, Miranda A. Chagas' disease: a clinical, epidemiologic, and pathologic study. *Circulation* 1956;14:1035–1060.
141. Becker G, Knep S, Lance K, Kaufman L. Amebic abscess of the brain. *Neurosurgery* 1980;6:192–194.
142. Cain AR, Wiley P, Brownell B, Warhurst D. Primary amebic meningoencephalitis. *Arch Dis Child* 1981;56:140–143.
143. Pitella J, Lana-Piexoto M. Brain involvement in hepatosplenic shistosomiasis. *Brain* 1981;104:621–632.
144. Brown W, Voge M. *Neuropathology of parasitic infections.* Oxford: Oxford University Press, 1982.
145. Udaka F, Okuda B, Okada M, Tsuji T, Kameyama M. CT findings of cerebral paragonimiasis in the chronic state. *Neuroradiology* 1988;30:31–34.
146. Shim J, Park C. Cerebral paragonimiasis. *Proc Austr Assoc Neurol* 1968;5:361–365.
147. McCorkell S, Lewall D. CT of intracerebral echinococcal cysts in children. *J Comput Assist Tomogr* 1985;9:514–518.
148. Boles D. Cerebral echinococcus. *Surg Neurol* 1981;16:280–285.

CHAPTER 12

Anomalies of Cerebral Vasculature

Van V. Halbach and A. James Barkovich

Cerebrovascular disease is uncommon in children and adolescents. In one study of children under the age of 15, the average annual incidence of cerebrovascular disease unrelated to trauma or infection was 2.5 per 100,000 population (1). The disease processes can be grossly divided into occlusive vascular disease and causes of intracranial hemorrhage. A partial list of these disease processes is included (Table 12.1). The CT manifestations of embolic events in children are quite similar to those in adults and will not be discussed. Chapter 4 analyzes the MR appearance of infarction in neonates. Venous thrombosis was discussed in Chapter 11. This chapter considers cerebrovascular anomalies and those cerebrovascular disorders that are amenable to neuroradiologic intervention.

V. V. Halbach: Professor of Radiology and Neurological Surgery, Department of Radiology, University of California, San Francisco, California 94143.

VEIN OF GALEN MALFORMATIONS

Malformations involving the vein of Galen are rare congenital connections occurring between intracranial vessels (usually thalamoperforator, choroidal, and anterior cerebral arteries) and a vein in the region of the vein of Galen (2,3). These connections can be large direct fistulas, numerous small connections, or a combination of the two. The cause of these connections is unknown; however, some investigators have noted a strong association with venous anomalies (absent straight sinus, persistent falcine, and occipital sinuses) and suggested that intrauterine straight sinus thrombosis with recanalization is responsible (2). Recent embryologic studies have shown that the large venous structure that receives the arteriovenous shunt is not the vein of Galen but the midline prosencephalic vein. The usual outflow of this persistent fetal structure is to the falcine sinus or straight sinus. Occasionally, both a falcine and straight sinus can drain the prosencephalic vein (Fig. 12.1). This midline

TABLE 12.1. *Occlusive vascular disease*

Arterial thrombosis
  Congenital heart disease
  Fibromuscular dysplasia
  Homocystinuria
  Infection
  Moyamoya syndrome
  Radiation arteritis
  Trauma
  Vasculitis
  Hypercoagulable disorders
    Protein S or C deficiency
    Antithrombin 3 deficiency
    Anticardiolipin antibody
    Thrombocytosis
Venous thrombosis
  Congenital heart disease
  Dehydration
  Hematologic disorders (leukemia, sickle cell disease)
  Infection
  Lead encephalopathy
  Trauma
  Hypercoagulable disorders
    Protein S or C deficiency
    Antithrombin 3 deficiency
    Anticardiolipin antibody
    Thrombocytosis
Embolism
  Air (from cardiac/thoracic surgery)
  Cardiac (arrhythmias, right-to-left shunts, rheumatic heart disease)
  Fat (from long bone fractures)
  Septic (from pneumonia, bacterial endocarditis)
Intracranial hemorrhage
  Vascular malformations
  Aneurysms
  Hematologic
  Hypertension
  Trauma

structure drains only the arteriovenous shunt, and the normal venous drainage of the brain has been rerouted to collaterals. This explains why procedures that occlude the recipient vein, such as transvenous embolization, do not produce venous infarction.

The clinical presentation can be categorized into three groups: the neonate presenting with intractable congestive heart failure (CHF) and loud intracranial bruit, the infant presenting with hydrocephalus and/or seizures, and the older child or young adult presenting with hemorrhage (4). More than 90% of the vein of Galen malformations fall into the first group; they have the largest amount of arteriovenous shunting (5,6), have the poorest prognosis, and are usually fatal without treatment.

Classifications

Several classifications based on the angioarchitecture and anatomy have been developed (7,8). The most widely utilized scheme is from Yasargil's experience (8). In his classification there are four subtypes of vein of Galen malformations. Type I lesions are direct arteriovenous shunts to the medial prosencephalic vein supplied by choroidal, pericallosal, and superior cerebellar arteries. Type II lesions have similar shunts supplied by transmesencephalic and transdiencephalic perforators. Type III lesions are combinations of types I and II. Type IV consists of an arteriovenous shunt distant from the vein of Galen but drains to it, producing dilatation. Ironically, this is not a true vein of Galen malformation but is the only type where a vein of Galen exists.

Another useful and practical classification has arisen from the endovascular group at Bicêtre Hospital in Paris (9). They subdivide true vein of Galen malformations into choroidal and mural types. The *choroidal type* is an arteriovenous connection in the anterior wall of the prosencephalic vein supplied by a plethora of vessels, usually numerous choroidal, pericallosal, and thalamoperforator vessels. The choroidal type is most common and usually presents with intractable congestive heart failure in the newborn. Figure 12.2 is an example of a newborn with severe intractable heart failure successfully treated with transvenous embolization techniques. If a severe downstream venous obstruction exists, there is less arteriovenous shunting and the presentation may be delayed. This usually results in development delay or seizures occurring in infancy rather than in congestive heart failure in the newborn. The less common type of vein of Galen malformations is the *mural type,* where fewer (usually one to four) but larger-caliber connections exist between the posterior choroidal or collicular arteries and the prosencephalic vein. Children with the mural type may have cardiomegaly but usually are not in severe congestive heart failure. These patients usually present in infancy with developmental delay, seizure, or increasing head circumference. In our experience the mural type consists of 10% of vein of Galen malformations. These are technically easier to treat and all were completely cured by transarterial embolization alone or in combination with transvenous techniques in our series. Figure 12.3 is an example of a patient with a mural type of malformation treated by endovascular transarterial occlusion with complete cure.

Imaging

On imaging studies these malformations appear as large masses in the posterior incisural region, sometimes extending rostrally and anteriorly displacing the third ventricle (Fig. 12.4). On sonography, the varix will appear mildly echogenic (Fig. 12.4B); it is important to demonstrate continuity with the straight sinus or a persistent falcine sinus. On CT, the varix will be iso- to hyperdense to brain prior to contrast administration.

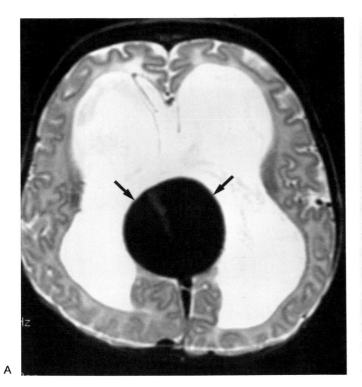

A

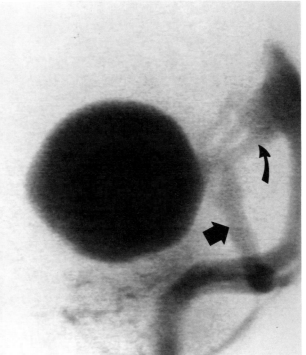

C

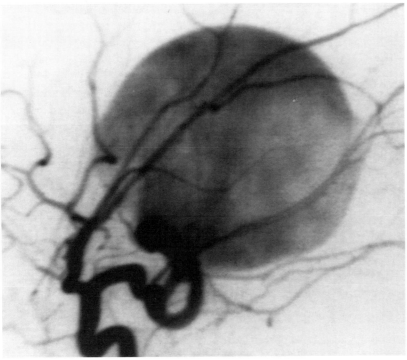

B

FIG. 12.1. A 4-month-old neonate presents with increasing head circumference. **A:** Axial T2-weighted image demonstrates hydrocephalus produced by a large spherical flow void (*arrows*). **B, C:** Left internal carotid injection, lateral projection, demonstrates a mural-type vein of Galen malformation that drains both to a straight sinus (*straight arrow*) and to a falcine sinus (*curved arrow*).

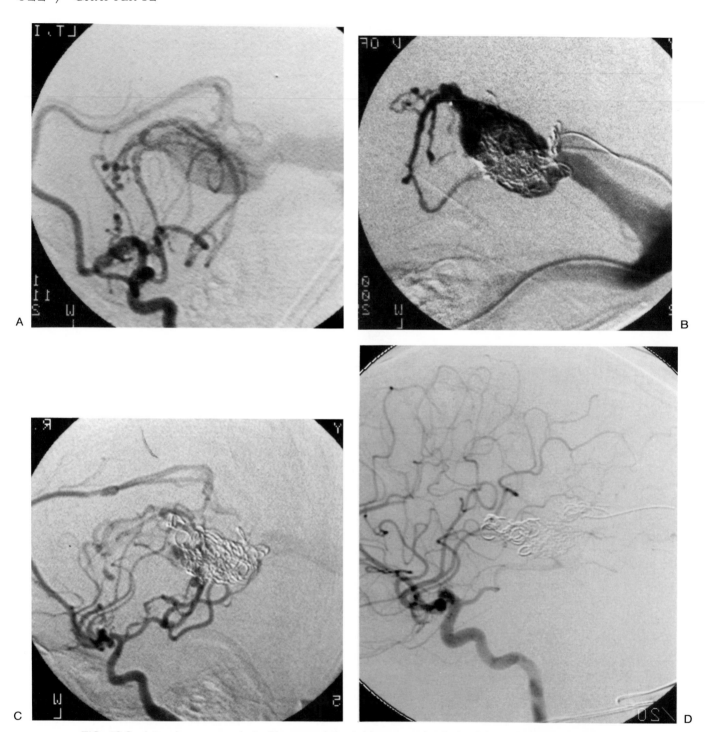

FIG. 12.2. A newborn presented with severe intractable congestive heart failure. **A:** Right internal carotid injection, lateral projection, demonstrates a choroidal type vein of Galen malformation draining to a falcine sinus. **B:** From a transfemoral venous access a microcatheter has been navigated into the medial prosencephalic vein and multiple coils are deposited. Notice retrograde filling of the numerous thalamoperforator feeding arteries. **C:** Postembolization arteriogram demonstrates multiple coils producing markedly reduced flow in the fistula. The patient was discharged several days later with dramatically improved cardiac function.

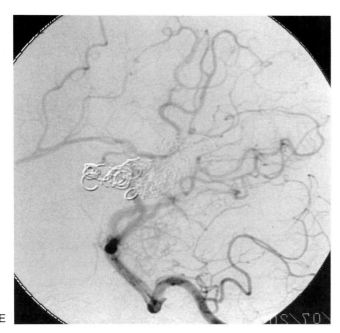

E

FIG. 12.2. (*Continued*.) **D, E:** Right internal carotid injection, lateral projection (D) and left vertebral artery injection, lateral projection (E) at 4 years of age demonstrate complete thrombosis of the vein of Galen malformation. The patient is neurologically and developmentally normal. Note the distal anterior cerebral artery is collateralized from the posterior circulation.

Mixed attenuation may be seen if the varix is partially thrombosed. Areas of low attenuation (infarct) and high attenuation (hemorrhage in the neonate and young infant, calcification in the older infant and child) are sometimes present in the brain parenchyma. On MR, the varix will be hypointense, resulting from a loss of phase coherence of the mobile protons (Fig. 12.1A). Areas of acute thrombosis will usually be isointense to brain on short TR/TE sequences and hypointense on T2-weighted spin echo or on gradient echo sequences, whereas subacute thrombus will have a high intensity on both short TR and long TR spin echo sequences. Thrombus of varying age sometimes lines the wall of the varix.

Therapy

Aggressive medical management of the cardiac failure is an essential adjunct to surgery or endovascular procedures, but medical management alone can rarely control the failure. Johnston's review of neonates presenting with CHF revealed a mortality of 95%, and none were stabilized without surgical intervention (6). Surgical ligations of the anomalous connections have been described, but the results have been disappointing. In a recent review of 60 neonates treated by surgery there were only six survivors; half had neurologic deficits (6). Sev-

eral recent series have reported the efficacy of endovascular procedures as a palliative or definitive treatment (9–20). The earliest reported endovascular treatments consisted of free-particle embolization. Although the majority of these emboli would lodge in the fistulous connections, the risk of an errant embolus occluding a normal cerebral blood vessel was inversely proportional to the flow in the fistula, and the majority of these procedures were palliative. With the development of newer microcatheter delivery systems and embolic agents [such as platinum coils (15,16,21), silk sutures, and liquid adhesives (9,11)] superselective embolization of the fistula connections alone can be achieved. Mickle and colleagues have developed a technique where the torcula is surgically exposed, a small catheter is placed transvenously through the straight or falcine sinus into the involved prosencephalic vein, and stainless steel coil emboli are deposited to diminish the arteriovenous shunting (18,22). We have developed techniques to deliver platinum coils emboli into the recipient's draining vein from a transfemoral venous access (15,16). The advantages of this approach are that the need for the craniotomy is eliminated and the platinum coils are compatible with MRI imaging, whereas the ferromagnetic stainless steel coils are not.

The current recommendation for treatment of vein of Galen malformations presenting with severe congestive failure follows: If the diagnosis is established prenatally with ultrasound, the delivery should be performed at an institution offering both surgical and radiologic techniques to palliate the patient should intractable congestive heart failure develop. Severe fetal heart failure *in utero* can result in polyhydramnios and hydrops fetalis, which can be detected by ultrasound and be an indication for induced delivery. Close coordination among the obstetricians, neurosurgeons, neonatologists, and endovascular team is essential to optimize prenatal planning. In the newborn, baseline ultrasonography (Fig. 12.4) of the heart and brain with color flow Doppler should be performed to serve as a standard in evaluating the results of the interventional techniques. Large vein of Galen malformations often have elevated right heart pressure and will have right-to-left shunting at the level of the foramen ovale (persistent fetal circulation) and may have a patent ductus arteriosus. We have found quantification of retrograde diastolic aortic flow useful in following patients treated with endovascular techniques (13). If possible, an umbilical arterial line should be placed. This allows repeated vascular access using exchange wires for both diagnostic and therapeutic procedures, thus obviating the necessity for repeated femoral arterial punctures. A baseline CT scan and/or ultrasound (Fig. 12.2) should be performed to assess any ischemic damage already produced by the congenital fistula; to disclose hydrocephalus, which may require ventriculoperitoneal shunting;

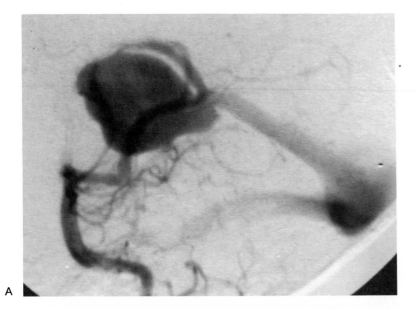

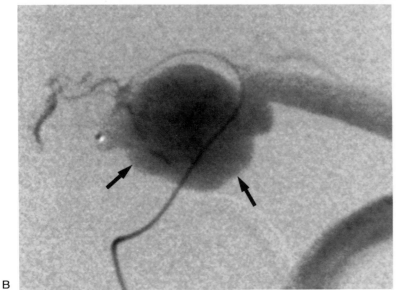

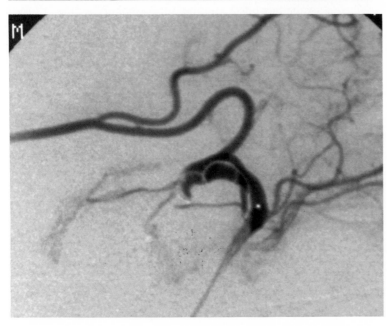

FIG. 12.3. A 3-month-old infant presents with Parinaud's syndrome (paralysis of upward gaze) and an enlarging head circumference. **A:** Left vertebral artery injection, lateral projection, demonstrates a mural type vein of Galen malformation with two large-caliber connections. **B:** A small microcatheter has been navigated into the fistula site and contrast material injected delineating the draining prosencephalic vein (*arrows*). **C:** Superselective injection following embolization with microcoils demonstrates complete occlusion of the fistula. Note preservation of all normal vessels, including the choroidal vessels, parieto-occipital branches, and connection to the distal splenial and pericallosal artery.

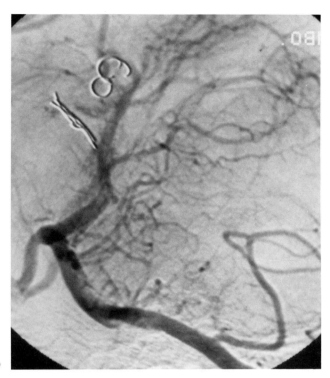
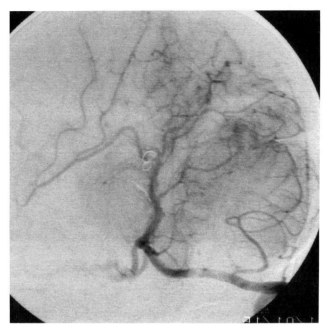

FIG. 12.3. (*Continued.*) **D:** Left vertebral artery injection, lateral projection, postembolization, demonstrates complete obliteration of the vein of Galen malformation. **E:** Same injection and projection as D, 1-year follow-up arteriogram confirms persistent and complete obliteration of the malformation. Patient is neurologically normal with complete resolution of his partial third nerve dysfunction.

and to serve as a baseline for comparison. Hydrocephalus can be produced by mechanical compression of the aqueduct by the prosencephalic vein or impairment of CSF absorption produced by elevated venous pressure in the draining sinuses. Shunting procedures in patients with vein of Galen malformations can be hazardous because of shunt catheter damage of venous collateral that exist lining the ventricle (8).

If intractable congestive failure persists despite aggressive medical management, arteriography should be performed to delineate the vascular anatomy. Biplane digital subtraction arteriography is best to minimize the amount of contrast utilized for the diagnostic study. Palliative arterial embolization can be performed at this time, preferably with superselective catheterization of each feeding pedicle to reduce the risk of ischemic damage to normal surrounding brain. The embolization procedures may be repeated soon thereafter if congestive failure persists. If the congestive failure continues and further arterial embolization is considered risky or technically impossible, a transvenous embolization is performed. Transvenous embolization is usually done from a transfemoral venous access (15) or internal jugular venous access (11), but occasionally it is done via direct surgical access through a burr hole (2, 9). For a transtor-

cular approach an angiogram or ultrasound is performed to localize the draining venous sinuses. A small burr hole is made over the draining falcine or straight sinus (Fig. 12.1). A direct needle puncture is made into the sinus, a small catheter is advanced into the midline prosencephalic vein, and steel or platinum coils are deposited. These techniques are usually palliative, but generally they alleviate the congestive failure and allow the child to develop normally until a definitive treatment can be performed with further radiologic or surgical techniques. MRI scanning, contraindicated in patients with ferromagnetic emboli, has been useful in our experience to assess brain development and demonstrate subtotal thrombosis in the fistula site.

Many endovascular teams have published the results of therapy of vein of Galen malformations, and the angiographic cure rates range from 40% to 60% (9–12,16, 17). The cure rates for mural-type vein of Galen malformations that present in the infant or young child are higher than those for the choroidal type, which presents mostly in a newborn with severe heart failure. Our results with a group of newborns in severe congestive failure have shown an angiographic cure rate of 50%, with the vast majority having no or minimal neurologic deficits on long-term follow-up [up to 5 years after the last ther-

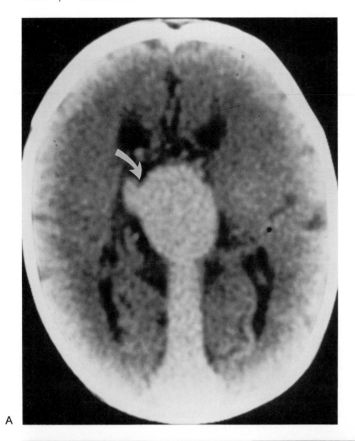

A

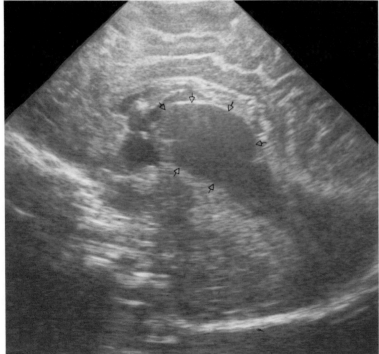

B

FIG. 12.4. Newborn with severe intractable congestive failure. **A:** Contrast-enhanced CT reveals the vascular structure and confirms a vein of Galen malformation. A fistula is seen (*arrow*) entering the right side of the varix. **B:** Transfontanelle ultrasound, sagittal plane, shows hypoechoic region (*arrows*) compressing the third ventricle.

apy (16)]. Twenty-five percent of the neonatal group died of severe cardiac decompensation within the first few weeks of life despite maximal endovascular and medical management. Lylyk (18,19) reported similar angiographic cure rates (46%) and mortality (18%), with 61% of patients enjoying a good long-term clinical outcome. Garcia-Monaco and colleagues (9) achieved anatomic occlusion in 61% of their 39 patients using transarterial embolization techniques, in a population with relatively fewer neonates. Our cure rate for the less common mural type vein of Galen malformations in infants is 100%.

Although the endovascular management of this disease has resulted in tremendous improvements over both the natural history of the disease and other medical and surgical treatments, many complications can accompany this innovative treatment. Despite aggressive endovascular and medical treatment, the patient may succumb to high output failure. One of our neonates that had complete angiographic obliteration of the fistula by transvenous embolization expired from severe right heart failure attributed to the pulmonary hypertension produced from the previously existing large-volume shunt. Transarterial embolization techniques can occasionally result in femoral artery thrombosis, resulting in subsequent leg length discrepancy. Stroke can occur, with inadvertent embolization of arteries that supply functional tissue. Perforation of an artery or venous structure can result in hemorrhage. If promptly recognized and occluded, a good outcome can ensue (23). Embolic material can pass through a large-caliber connection and lodge in the lungs, further compromising oxygenation, or it can pass through a right-to-left shunt and produce a paradoxical arterial embolus. Volume overload from the saline flushes and contrast can aggravate the heart failure. Contrast can also produce or aggravate renal failure in rare instances. Successful embolization can produce thrombosis in the prosencephalic vein and use up available coagulation factors and platelets that may require replenishment. Despite the plethora of potential complications from this new therapy, the results of treatment have been quite promising. Advances in technique and improved understanding of this complex disease will undoubtedly improve the outcome in the future.

CAROTID CAVERNOUS FISTULAS

Carotid cavernous fistulas are solitary connections between the cavernous internal carotid artery and cavernous sinus; most often they result from trauma (24,25). The most common clinical presentations are bruit, headaches, proptosis, chemosis, and diplopia (24,26,27). Rarely, hydrocephalus, neurologic deficits, severe visual loss, blindness, or hemorrhage can occur (24,28). The

CT and MR findings in carotid cavernous fistulas consist of dilatation of the affected cavernous sinus and the venous structures that normally drain into or from it, most commonly the ipsilateral superior orbital vein and the petrosal sinuses (Fig. 12.5). Not infrequently, both cavernous sinuses and the adjacent venous structures will be enlarged as a result of shunting of blood through intracavernous connections. Rarely, only the contralateral venous pathways will enlarge because of pressure gradients within the venous system. Depending upon the pattern of venous drainage, proptosis may be present in the ipsilateral and/or contralateral orbit (Fig. 12.5). Rarely can the venous structures be normal in caliber with enlargement of ocular muscles.

Surgical techniques of trapping or proximal ligation are usually ineffective at fistula closure and have been largely supplanted by more recent techniques of balloon embolization (29,30). In the vast majority of cases, a balloon can be guided through the carotid artery and into the fistula (Fig. 12.6). The balloon is then inflated in the cavernous sinus, occluding the fistula and preserving the parent artery in the majority of cases. The balloon is usually inflated with a solidification agent to prevent deflation and delayed pseudoaneurysm formation. Rarely, the balloon cannot be navigated into the fistula site from an arterial route and transvenous pathways must be utilized (22,31). In the rare instances where proximal carotid occlusion has occurred and venous pathways are unavailable, direct puncture of the carotid (32) or surgical exposure of the cavernous sinus and placement of embolic material into the sinus can be curative (33). With smaller fistulas complete cure can sometimes be achieved by intermittently compressing the internal carotid artery and jugular vein to induce thrombosis within the fistula (34). In some instances intimal damage occurs as the result of the initial trauma and carotid occlusion is performed to eliminate the risk of distal thromboembolic events. With all these procedures there is usually dramatic resolution in clinical symptoms of bruit, headache, proptosis, and chemosis. There is often a transient exacerbation in the diplopia resulting from mechanical compression of the cranial nerves by the balloon, which resolves within 1 or 2 months.

Rarely, trauma can result in a basal skull fracture that damages the carotid artery without the development of a carotid cavernous fistula. The resulting carotid injury can give rise to a pseudoaneurysm that can project medially into the sphenoid sinus and produce massive epistaxis (35). Intimal damage can be a source for embolic stroke. Any basal skull fracture that involves the carotid canal should prompt angiographic evaluation of that carotid artery. Traumatic monocular blindness should also raise the suspicion for associated carotid artery injury as the fracture that crosses the optic canal, producing the blindness, frequently damages the adjacent carotid artery (36).

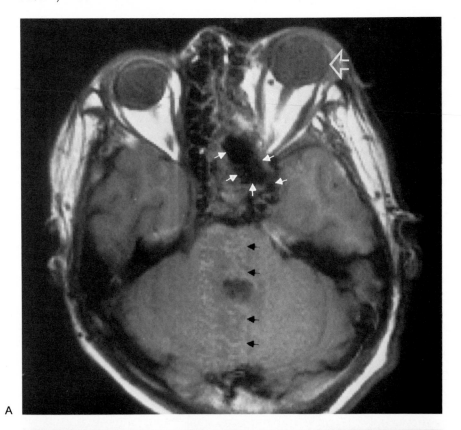

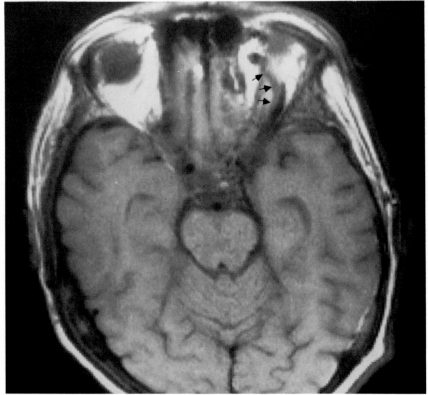

FIG. 12.5. Carotid-cavernous fistula. **A:** Axial SE 700/25 image shows a large, low-intensity mass in the region of the cavernous sinus (*white arrows*). There is misregistration artifact (*black arrows*) dorsal to this area in the phase-encoding direction, indicating flowing blood within the structure. The left globe is proptotic (*open arrow*). **B:** Axial SE 700/25 image shows an enlarged superior orbital vein in the left orbit (*black arrows*).

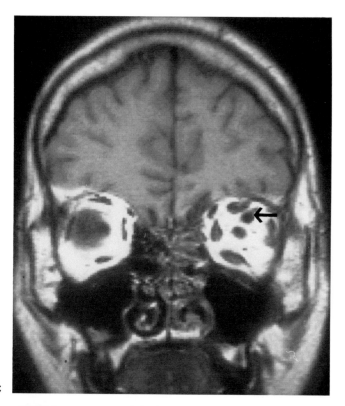

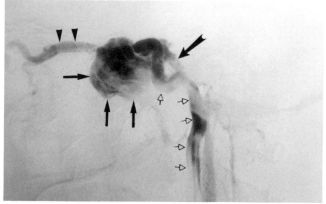

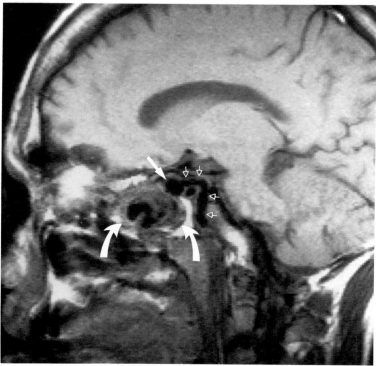

C

D

E

FIG. 12.5. (*Continued.*) **C:** Coronal SE 700/25 image also shows the enlarged superior orbital vein on the left (*arrow*). The extraocular muscles are also enlarged on the left side. **D:** Parasagittal SE 700/25 image shows the internal carotid artery (*open arrows*) emptying into the cavernous sinus at the site of the fistula (*straight arrow*). The enlarged cavernous sinus is seen as a large area of mixed signal intensity (*curved arrows*). **E:** Lateral film from an internal carotid angiogram shows the internal carotid artery (*open arrows*) emptying into the cavernous sinus (*small closed arrows*). The venous blood is seen to drain through an enlarged superior orbital vein (*arrowheads*) and inferior petrosal sinus (*flared arrow*).

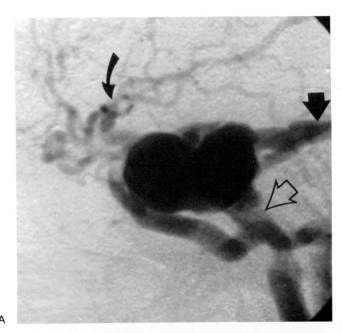

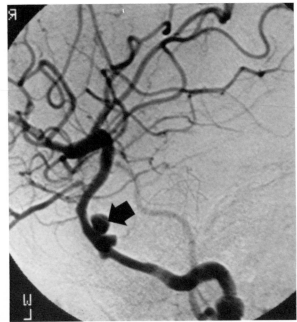

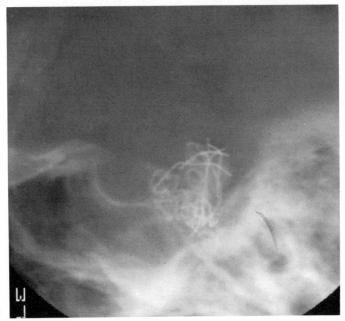

FIG. 12.6. Eighteen-year-old who sustained a basal skull fracture during a motor vehicle accident and developed a loud bruit, proptosis, and visual loss in the right side. **A:** Right internal carotid angiogram, lateral projection, demonstrates a large carotid cavernous fistula with venous drainage to cortical veins (*curved arrow*), superior petrosal sinus (*thick arrow*), and interior petrosal sinus (*open arrow*). **B:** Same injection and projection, postembolization, shows complete closure of the fistula and reestablishment of intracranial flow. A small pseudoaneurysm exists marking the fistula site (*arrow*). **C:** Plain skull x-ray, lateral projection, shows the balloons and platinum coils utilized to produce fistula closure.

VERTEBRAL FISTULAS

Vertebral fistulas are usually solitary connections between the vertebral artery and surrounding paravertebral plexus. Although most result from penetrating (37,38) or blunt trauma (39), congenital vertebral fistulas are not uncommon (40,41). The most common presenting symptoms are bruit and neck pain. Rarely, neurologic deficits (42,43) can result from steal phenomenon away from the intracranial vessels into the fistula, especially with large congenital fistulas. If the venous drainage is to the epidural or medullary venous system, the patient may present with radiculopathy or subarachnoid hemorrhage, respectively (40,41). It must be remembered that congenital fistulas can have an exceptionally loud bruit that is totally unnoticed by the child, since they accept the pulse synchronous noise as normal. These anomalies are diagnosed angiographically.

Surgical techniques have been described, including proximal ligation (37), trapping procedures, and direct surgical repair. Trapping procedures, as elsewhere in the body, are often ineffective at producing fistula closure,

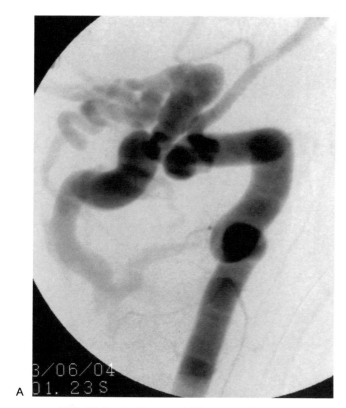
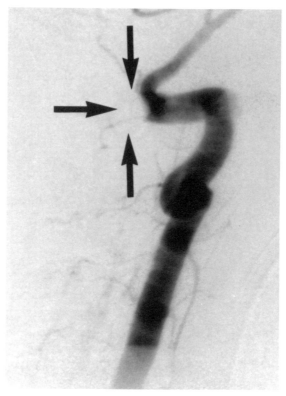

FIG. 12.7. A 13-year-old female suffered blunt trauma to the upper cervical spine at age 6 and subsequently developed a loud bruit and severe headaches. **A:** Left vertebral injection, lateral projection, demonstrates a vertebral fistula at the C2 level. Note the tremendous hypertrophy of the vertebral artery proximal to the fistula site. **B:** Same injection and projection as A, postembolization, with a single detachable balloon (*arrows*) demonstrates complete closure of the fistula with preservation of the vertebral artery. The patient's headaches and bruit abated immediately after closure of the fistula.

and proximal ligation can increase steal away from the cerebral vasculature, producing neurologic deficits. Direct surgical approaches to the fistula are often effective in fistula obliteration, but maintaining patency of the parent vertebral artery is difficult, and surgical exposure through the surrounding bone and arterialized veins is difficult. Endovascular treatment of vertebral fistulas can be performed by fluoroscopically guiding a detachable balloon through the involved vertebral artery and into the fistula (41–43). The balloon is inflated and, if properly positioned in the fistula, detached. Figure 12.7 is an example of a traumatic vertebral fistula treated with endovascular occlusion with a detachable balloon. In some instances of traumatic fistulas the vertebral artery is completely transected. These injuries require placement of balloons or coils in both severed ends to ensure fistula closure. Rarely, with long-standing congenital vertebral fistulas, the steal away from the brain into the fistula impairs the brain's ability to autoregulate blood flow. When the fistula is abruptly closed, reestablishing perfusion to chronically ischemic brain, overperfusion can occur, resulting in neurologic deficits or hemorrhage (40). These cases require slow, staged closure to allow for the gradual recovery of autoregulation.

The vertebral artery can be injured by blunt or direct trauma without the development of a fistula. A cervical spine fracture that involves the foramen transversarium deserves prompt angiographic evaluation of the ipsilateral vertebral artery to rule out intimal damage, dissection, or occlusion.

INTRACEREBRAL VASCULAR MALFORMATIONS

Intracerebral vascular malformations (AVMs) are congenital malformations involving the vascular development of the fetal brain that include abnormalities in arteries, capillaries, or venous structures. Although there have been a few reports of familial association (44), the majority are sporadic.

Pathologically, vascular malformations can be subdivided into four groups: arteriovenous malformations, venous malformations, cavernous malformations, and capillary telangiectasias (45).

Arteriovenous Malformations

Arteriovenous malformations (AVMs) are defined as a compact collection of abnormal thin-walled vessels connecting dilated arteries to veins without intervening capillaries. The absence of the capillaries produces a low-resistance shunt that results in rapid arteriovenous shunting within the malformation. These malformations can increase in size with age and result in progressive dilation of the feeding arteries and draining veins. Because of the rapid flow, there is a tendency to develop feeding arterial aneurysms in the same distribution as classic berry aneurysms (circle of Willis) and in the feeding arteries close to the malformation. The high-pressure turbulent flow can produce vascular changes in the draining veins, resulting in stenosis or occlusion, particularly where the veins enter a dural sinus. Proximal to the stenosis, venous aneurysms (varices) can develop and may hemorrhage. Contrary to earlier descriptions, AVMs can have mass effect unassociated with hemorrhage. Although this group does not constitute the most common form of vascular malformations, it is responsible for most AVM patients who present with neurologic deficits other than seizures.

Clinically, these lesions usually present with seizures, recurrent headaches, progressive neurologic deficits, hydrocephalus, and hemorrhage. Approximately 20% of AVMs become symptomatic before the patient is 20 years of age (3). Hemorrhage most often occurs in the substance of the cerebral parenchyma; however, rupture of a superficial malformation can result in subarachnoid hemorrhage. Rarely, deep-seated malformations can present with intraventricular hemorrhage. The mortality associated with the initial rupture of an AVM is 10%, with a morbidity between 30% and 50% (3,46). The morbidity and mortality increase with each subsequent hemorrhage. Symptomatic vasospasm and rebleeding are relatively rare unless the source of hemorrhage has been rupture of an associated aneurysm. The risk of rehemorrhage from an AVM has been estimated to be higher in children than in adults (46). In children less than 15 years of age, AVMs are the most common cause of spontaneous intracranial hemorrhage and account for 20% of all strokes (47). Seizures occur in approximately 70% of patients with AVMs, with one-half of the seizures being generalized (48); the majority are well controlled with anticonvulsants. Chronic recurrent headaches may be the presenting symptoms in some malformations, presumably caused by hypertrophied dural vessels that develop in peripheral AVMs and in those that develop narrowing or occlusion of draining cerebral veins. AVMs located in the occipital region are associated with an increased frequency of migraines that have visual symptoms during the migrainous episodes. Progressive neurologic deficit can occur in a small percentage of children with AVMs, particularly the large AVMs located close to the motor cortex; presumably, there is steal of blood away from the normal surrounding brain into the malformation (49,50). Other possible etiologies of neurologic deficit include the development of venous hypertension where increased venous pressure is transmitted through the AVM, impairing the venous drainage of normal adjacent brain sharing the same venous drainage pathway. This has long been understood as a mechanism for neurologic deficit in the spinal cord, but it has only recently been recognized in the brain. Rarely, the venous hypertension is so marked that it impairs the reabsorption of cerebrospinal fluid, producing hydrocephalus that results in neurologic dysfunction. Lastly, with the advent of newer noninvasive screening techniques of the brain, such as CT scanning and MR imaging, asymptomatic AVMs are frequently discovered.

Cavernous Malformations

Cavernous malformations are spherical collections of sinusoidal (cavernous) vascular spaces (51). The caliber of feeding arteries and draining veins is normal and there is no arteriovenous shunting. These malformations can produce seizures and, rarely, clinical hemorrhage, although many are discovered incidentally. Multiple cavernous hemangiomas are common and are associated with a familial predisposition.

Venous Malformations

Venous malformations consist of a radially oriented collection of dilated medullary or subcortical veins that drain into a single dilated venous structure (52). There is no arteriovenous shunting. The dilated medullary or subcortical veins are separated by normal surrounding brain parenchyma. Venous malformations located in the cerebral hemispheres rarely cause symptoms and are most commonly incidental findings disclosed on diagnostic studies obtained for other reasons. Venous malformations located in the brain stem or cerebellum do have a slightly increased incidence of hemorrhage (53).

Capillary Telangiectasias

Capillary telangiectasias are collections of dilated capillaries separated by normal parenchyma. These lesions are commonly found in the pons, rarely hemorrhage, and are usually discovered incidentally at autopsy.

Diagnostic Work-Up

The diagnostic work-up of vascular malformations usually includes computed tomography (CT), magnetic

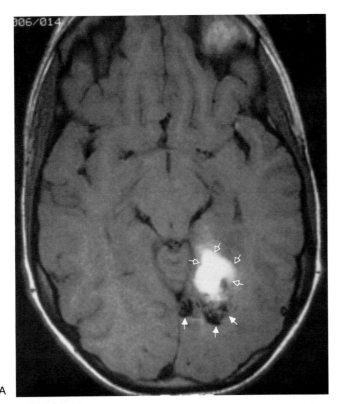

A

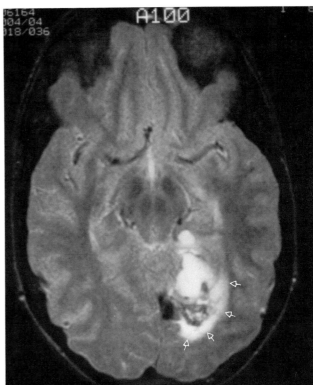

B

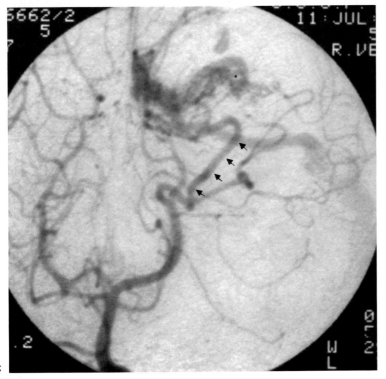

C

FIG. 12.8. AVM with hemorrhage. **A:** Axial SE 600/20 image shows an area of high signal intensity in the left temporo-occipital region (*open arrows*). This subacute hematoma lies directly ventral to a tangle of vessels (*closed arrows*), which presumably represents the nidus of the AVM. **B:** Axial SE 2800/70 image shows the tangle of vessels and hematoma. The area of high signal intensity (*arrows*) dorsal and lateral to the tangle of vessels represents a small amount of edema. **C:** AP image from a left vertebral artery angiogram shows the vascular malformation being fed by the left posterior temporal artery (*arrows*).

resonance imaging (MR), and angiography. Although plain films occasionally reveal enlargement of the vascular grooves of the skull or associated calcifications, this yield is too low to justify their routine use. CT, with and without intravenous contrast, is an effective screening technique to study patients with suspected intracranial hemorrhage in the acute phase (less than 2 weeks). With intravenous contrast, the malformation may appear as an enhancing region adjacent to a high-density hematoma. A noncontrast CT scan may reveal high density of the associated acute hematoma or calcifications within the interstices of the AVM. In addition, CT may show subarachnoid hemorrhage that sometimes accompanies rupture of a superficial AVM or an associated aneurysm. After approximately 2 weeks, the hematoma becomes isointense with brain with a rim of peripheral enhancement following intravenous contrast; this appearance is nonspecific and can be confused with other pathologic processes, such as tumors and abscesses. MR is evolving as an excellent initial screening modality for the evaluation of intracranial AVMs (54,55). Fast-flowing intraluminal blood in arteriovenous malformations appears as regions of decreased signal on routine spin echo images. A tangle of curvilinear foci of flow-void represents the nidus of the malformation (Fig. 12.8). The multiplanar capabilities of MRI can delineate the location of the malformation in relation to adjacent critical structures. Associated parenchymal hematomas evolve through a recognizable and often specific pattern of signal charac-

teristics (Fig. 12.8) (see Chapter 4 and refs. 24 and 45). The residua of previous hemorrhages adjacent to malformations can be detected many years after hemorrhage as areas of very low intensity on long TR/TE or gradient-echo images. In addition, MR can often yield specific information about the type of intracranial malformation. For example, the CT appearance of a cavernous hemangioma is nonspecific, often showing calcifications, variable degrees of contrast enhancement following intravenous contrast, and (sometimes) mass effect. Although these findings are suggestive of a cavernous hemangioma, slow-growing tumors can exhibit the same CT appearance. The MR appearance is often quite characteristic, showing regions of both recent and old hemorrhage with a circumferential rim of hypointensity on long TR/TE images (Fig. 12.9) (56). (Although hemorrhagic tumors can rarely mimic this appearance in adults, the appearance seems quite specific in children.) The specificity of MR, without the necessity for intravenous iodinated contrast, makes MR the imaging modality of choice in patients with suspected cavernous hemangiomas. The MR appearance of venous malformations is also quite specific; a "tuft" of small vessels is seen to coalesce to form a single large vessel that drains into a venous sinus (Figs. 12.10 and 12.11). The addition of gadolinium can aid in the detection of these venous structures. In the subacute and chronic phases of intraparenchymal hemorrhage, MR is more sensitive and specific than CT. However, CT remains the imaging

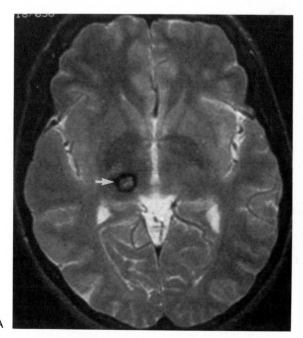

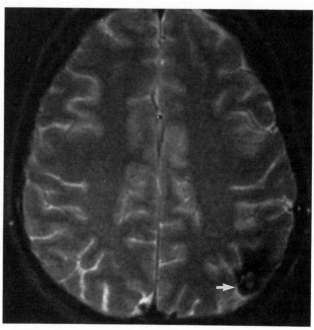

A

B

FIG. 12.9. Cavernous malformation. A: Axial SE 2800/70 image shows an area of mixed signal intensity surrounded by a low-intensity rim (arrow) in the right thalamus. This is the classic appearance for an occult vascular malformation, most of which are cavernous malformations. B: A second cavernous malformation is seen in the parieto-occipital cortex (arrow). These malformations are frequently multiple.

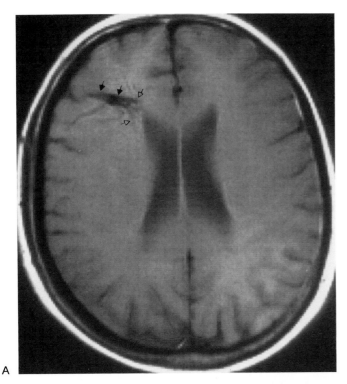

A

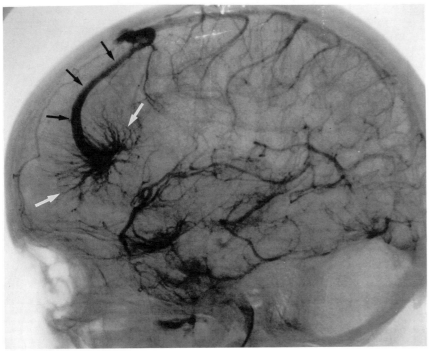

B

FIG. 12.10. Venous malformation. **A:** Axial SE 700/33 image shows a tuft of vessels (*open arrows*) feeding into a curvilinear vascular channel (*closed arrows*) that drains into the superior sagittal sinus (not seen on this image). This appearance is characteristic of venous malformations. **B:** Venous phase angiogram, lateral projection, from a right internal carotid artery injection. The tuft of vessels (*white arrows*) is seen to form a curvilinear venous channel (*black arrows*) that drains into the superior sagittal sinus. The findings are identical to what was seen on the MR study.

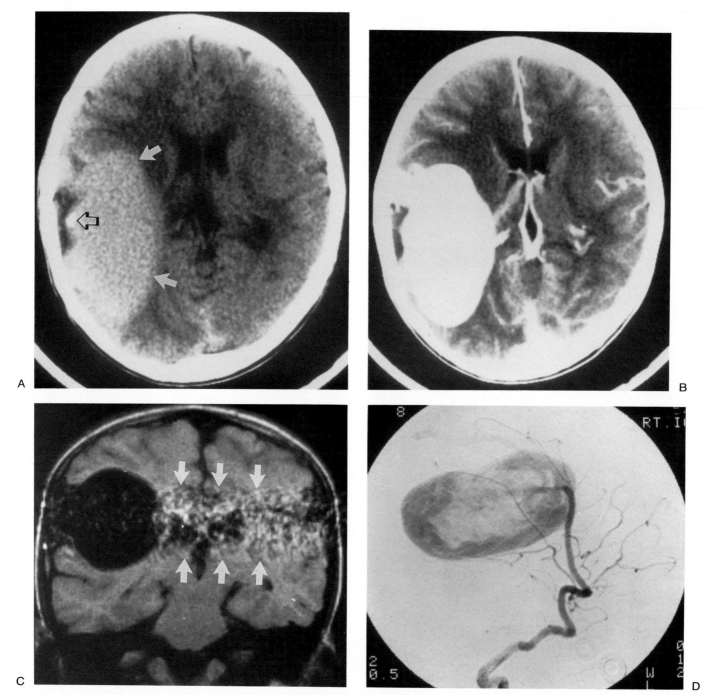

FIG. 12.11. A solitary arteriovenous connection (fistula). **A:** Axial noncontrast CT scan shows a large mass in the right Sylvian area (*arrows*) that is hyperdense compared with brain parenchyma. A small focus of calcification (*open arrow*) is present within the mass. **B:** After infusion of iodinated contrast, the mass uniformly enhances. **C:** Coronal SE 500/30 image shows a large amount of signal misregistration (*arrows*) from the mass in the phase-encoding direction. This phase misregistration artifact is essentially pathognomonic for a vascular lesion. **D:** Arterial phase image from a right internal carotid arteriogram, lateral projection, shows an enlarged Rolandic branch of the middle cerebral artery emptying into a large venous varix at the site of the solitary A-V connection.

modality of choice for both acute intraparenchymal and acute subarachnoid hemorrhage. In patients with arteriovenous malformations, conventional arteriography should be performed to delineate any associated feeding arterial aneurysms or venous occlusive disease that would be affiliated with a poorer natural history.

Therapy

The decision to undertake treatment for symptomatic arteriovenous malformations should consider the natural history of the disease and the projected risks and benefits of the therapy. A complete discussion of the natural history and current therapeutic options is beyond the scope of this book, and the reader should consult a more complete text for the discussion of management. Briefly, the therapeutic options fall into three categories: surgical excision, radiosurgery, and endovascular techniques. Often combinations of these techniques are utilized for the treatment of complex malformations.

With the improvement in *microneurosurgical techniques*, even large and complex malformations can be excised with relatively low morbidity and mortality. The nidus or core of the malformation infrequently contains cerebral parenchyma, and if the surgical excision is performed along the margins of the malformation with attention to preserving the surrounding brain, an excellent outcome can often be achieved. Total excision of the malformation is the goal of surgery, as prior studies have shown that subtotal resection or ligation of feeding vessels does not provide protection from subsequent hemorrhage (57,58). The surgical results of the treatment of AVMs in the pediatric age group have shown that complete excision can often be achieved with relatively low morbidity and mortality (59).

Radiation therapy has been utilized to produce proliferative changes in the blood vessel wall that can result in complete AVM obliteration in selected cases. To minimize the risk of radiation-induced damage to adjacent normal parenchyma, only focused techniques are utilized today, such as the Bragg-peak proton beam therapy or intersecting beam techniques. The results with smaller AVMs have been quite encouraging; angiographic obliteration is present in 80% of patients with small malformations 2 years after treatment (60). The major disadvantage of radiosurgical techniques at the present time is the difficulty in treating larger lesions and the 1- to 2-year interval that is often required to produce the proliferative changes, during which the patient is at continued risk of hemorrhage.

Endovascular techniques have emerged as a third technique for the treatment of symptomatic intracranial malformations. Complete angiographic obliteration following embolization of large malformations is unusual; however, complete obliteration can occur with smaller lesions (14). Endovascular embolization can palliate patients whose symptoms do not warrant more aggressive therapy or where the size or location of the malformation preclude more traditional forms of therapy. Patients who present with intractable unilateral headache frequently have recruitment of dural vascular supply to the malformation (14,61). These dural vessels can be subselectively catheterized and embolized, often resulting in total alleviation of the headache. In addition, patients who demonstrate severe venous occlusion can have improvement in their headaches following embolization of their malformation. Patients with progressive neurologic decline from arterial steal or venous hypertension can have improvement following partial embolization of their malformation. Preoperative adjuncts constitute the vast majority of endovascular techniques performed at our institution. By occluding the deep or inaccessible feeders to the malformation, surgical excision can be facilitated (62). Preoperative embolization can reduce the size and pressure within the nidus, making subsequent surgical excision easier and reducing intraoperative hemorrhage (62). In larger malformations where the adjacent brain parenchyma can lose its ability to autoregulate, staged palliative embolization can reestablish the microcirculation's regulatory control and prevent the development of normal perfusion pressure breakthrough (62). In reducing the size and speed of flow through a malformation, improved obliteration of AVMs following radiosurgery may be achieved.

Recently, we have identified an unusual group of patients with solitary arteriovenous connections (Figs. 12.12, 12.13). These patients presented in childhood with hemorrhage or neurologic deficit. All ten patients were treated by transvascular embolization techniques with placement of either platinum coils or balloons at the fistula site. Nine of the ten patients were completely cured, and the tenth underwent surgical excision without incident.

INTRACRANIAL ANEURYSMS

Saccular Aneurysms

Intracranial saccular aneurysms rarely present in the pediatric population. In the cooperative study of 6,368 patients with intracranial aneurysms and subarachnoid hemorrhage, only 41 (0.6%) were less than 19 years of age (63). Aneurysms in the pediatric population are more commonly of the large ("giant") type and arise peripheral to the circle of Willis more often than in the adult population. The distribution of aneurysms within the circle of Willis also differs slightly from that in adults. One study reported 50% arising from the internal carotid bifurcation, 25% from the anterior cerebral artery, and 12.5% from the posterior cerebral artery (64).

Clinically, patients present most commonly with subarachnoid hemorrhage that results in severe headache,

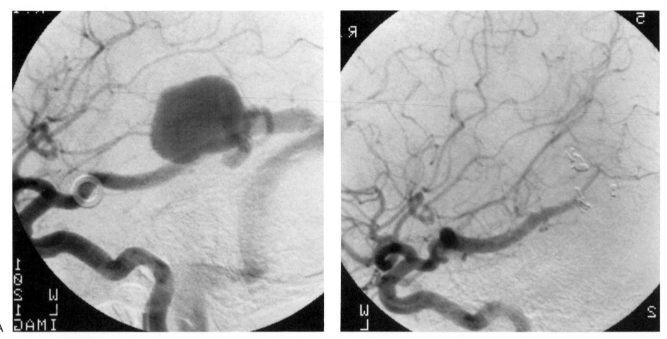

FIG. 12.12. Fourteen-year-old girl with severe unilateral headaches. **A:** Left internal carotid angiogram, lateral projection, shows a solitary fistula arising from the posterior temporal branch of the posterior cerebral artery. **B:** Same injection and projection, status after coil embolization, confirms complete closure of the fistula.

vomiting, and obtundation, which may progress to coma. About 20% of patients have a history of recurrent headaches. Those patients with giant aneurysms (20% to 40% of pediatric patients with aneurysms) present with focal neurologic symptoms and signs as a result of compression of the surrounding brain by the aneurysm sac. Although aneurysms can sometimes be detected by CT and MR as blood-filled saccular dilatations arising from major intracerebral vessels (Fig. 12.14), angiography is essential to define the neck of the aneurysm and search for multiplicity.

The vast majority of pediatric aneurysms can be managed by surgical techniques. When surgical techniques fail or the aneurysm has no definable neck, endovascular obliteration of the aneurysm can be performed (65). A detachable balloon can be navigated into the aneurysm occluding the neck and dome (Fig. 12.13). The balloon contents can be solidified and the balloon detached. More recently, electrolytically detachable coils have supplanted the use of balloon for the treatment of saccular aneurysms and some fusiform aneurysms. The infant in Figure 12.14 has a fusiform aneurysm arising from the posterior inferior cerebellar artery that failed a surgical attempt at obliteration. The patient was successfully treated with electrolytically detachable coils. If the aneurysm has no definable neck, then a test occlusion of the parent vessel is performed. If tolerated, the parent artery and the aneurysm are occluded by either proximal occlusion or trapping with detachable balloons. Of the 361 endovascular procedures performed for intracranial an-

eurysms at our institution, only 19 occurred in the pediatric age group. Of these, the majority were giant fusiform aneurysms, that is, larger than 2.5 cm.

Mycotic Aneurysms

The term *mycotic aneurysm* refers to those aneurysms resulting from any infectious process and includes bacterial and protozoan infections as well as fungal ones. The most common cause of mycotic aneurysms is an underlying bacterial endocarditis from which infectious thrombi are embolized into the intracranial circulation. The emboli cause a focal arteritis with degeneration of the elastic lamina and muscularis, resulting in a fusiform aneurysmal dilatation. Rupture of a mycotic aneurysm is, in fact, often the presenting sign of subacute bacterial endocarditis (66). Groups at risk for endocarditis in the pediatric population include those with congenital heart disease (especially right-to-left shunts) and those with rheumatic heart disease. Another important cause of mycotic aneurysms in children is invasion of intracranial vessels by adjacent infections (i.e., middle ear/sinus infection, meningitis, osteomyelitis of the skull, septic cavernous thrombophlebitis). In these patients, the adventitia is involved first, followed by the muscularis and the internal elastic lamina (66).

The most common presenting symptom in patients with mycotic aneurysms caused by bacterial endocarditis is subarachnoid or intracerebral hemorrhage resulting from aneurysmal rupture (67)(Fig. 12.15). Less com-

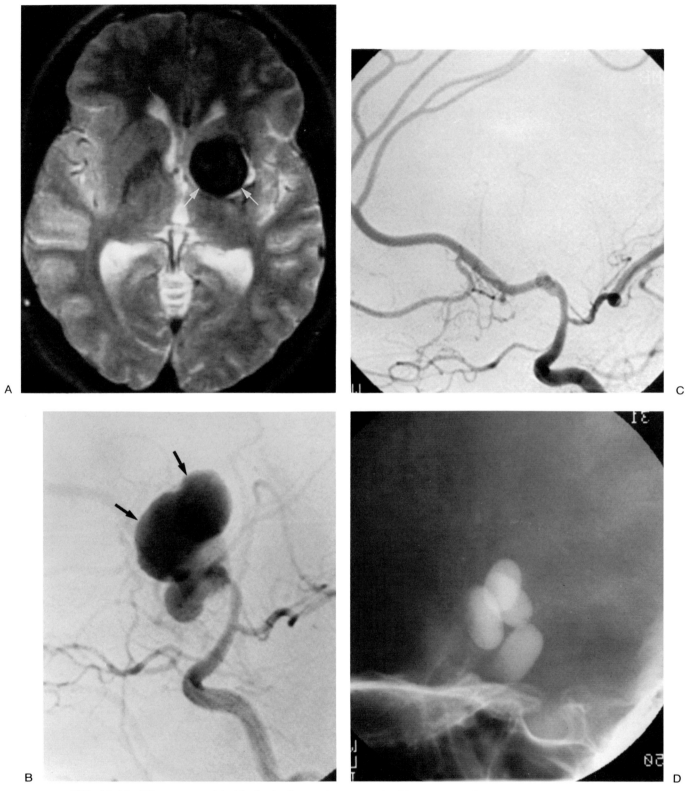

FIG. 12.13. Fifteen-year-old girl who had a stroke at age 4 with recovery who now presents with progressive weakness. **A:** T2-weighted axial MR scan demonstrates an area of decreased signal (*arrows*) in the left basal ganglia. **B:** Left internal carotid angiogram, lateral projection, demonstrates a giant aneurysm (*arrows*) arising from the distal internal carotid. The middle cerebral artery is occluded, presumably coincident with the stroke at age 4. **C:** Same injection and projection, after balloon embolization, shows occlusion of aneurysm. **D:** Plain film, lateral skull, shows four balloons within the aneurysm. The patient had complete recovery in neurologic function and remains intact.

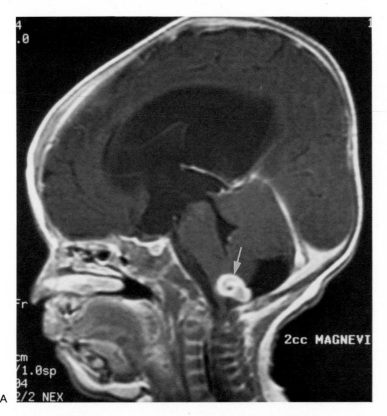

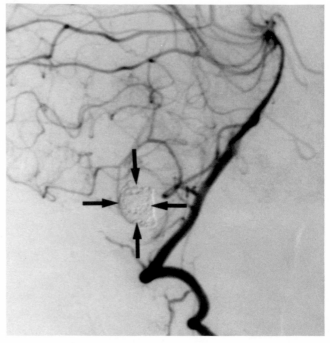

FIG. 12.14. A 3-month-old infant suffered repeated subarachnoid hemorrhages. **A:** Sagittal T1-weighted MRI, status after gadolinium enhancements, demonstrates a spherical region of enhancement (*arrow*) near the foramen of Luschka, producing severe hydrocephalus. A surgical exploration revealed a vascular structure that was unable to be clipped. **B:** Right vertebral injection, lateral projection, demonstrates a fusiform aneurysm (*arrow*) arising from the posterior inferior cerebellar artery. A small microcatheter was navigated into the aneurysm cavity and multiple electrolytically detachable coils were deposited. **C:** Same injection and projection, follow-up arteriogram demonstrates multiple platinum coils (*arrows*) producing complete occlusion of the aneurysm. The distal PICA is filled from SCA and AICA collaterals.

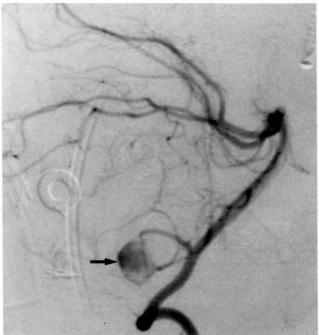

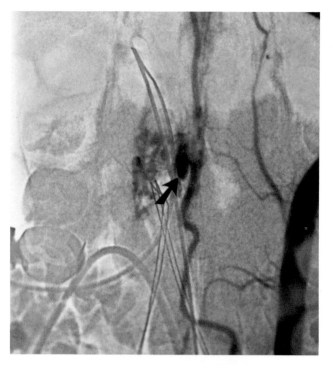

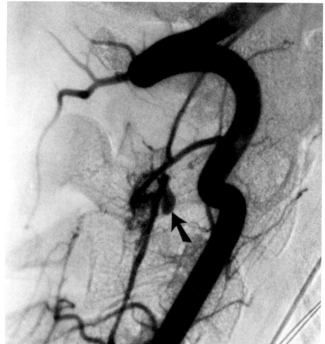

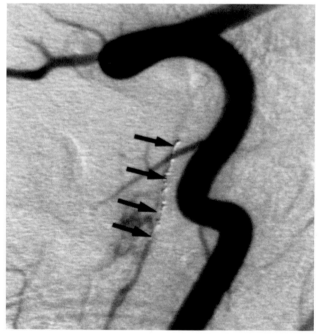

FIG. 12.15. A 13-year-old girl presented with a repeated subarachnoid hemorrhages. **A, B:** Left vertebral artery injection, AP (A) and lateral (B) projections demonstrate an arteriovenous malformation located in the right anterior spinal cord at C-2. A fusiform pseudoaneurysm arises from the mid-anterior spinal artery projecting anteriorly (*oblique arrow*). Subselective catheterization of the anterior spinal artery was performed with particulate embolization of the AVM and coil deposition across the zone of the aneurysm. **C:** Left vertebral artery injection, 1 month follow-up, lateral projection, demonstrates marked diminished vascularity to the arteriovenous malformation and persistent obliteration of the anterior spinal artery aneurysm and pseudoaneurysm by small platinum coils (*short straight arrows*). The patient remained neurologically intact.

monly, symptoms of cerebral ischemia may precede hemorrhage (38,66). Those patients with mycotic aneurysm within the cavernous sinus present with symptoms of septic cavernous sinus thrombophlebitis, including fever, orbital edema, venous engorgement, proptosis, chemosis, and ophthalmoplegia.

CT or MR may help to localize the aneurysm by demonstrating adjacent intraparenchymal hemorrhage or by directly visualizing the lesion, especially in the case of intracavernous aneurysms. Moreover, associated cerebritis, abscess, edema, or infarction may be identified. Cerebral angiography is necessary for definitive diagnosis. The aneurysms appear as fusiform dilatations of the vessel and tend to be located peripherally, most frequently in the distribution of the middle cerebral artery (38,66), in contrast to the saccular congenital aneurysms, which tend to be located on the circle of Willis. New mycotic aneurysms can develop on appropriate antibiotic therapy; therefore, follow-up arteriography should include all cerebral vessels.

SPINAL CORD ARTERIOVENOUS MALFORMATIONS

Spinal vascular malformations can be subdivided into separate categories based on anatomic localization of the vascular pathology.

Intramedullary Arteriovenous Malformations

Intramedullary arteriovenous malformations are tangles of abnormal connections between artery and veins that occur in the spinal cord substance and usually present with abrupt neurologic decline often related to hemorrhage. The onset of symptoms occurs most commonly in the first two decades of life, with 65% of patients under 25 years of age at presentation (68). Most reported cases show a male predominance (68).

Two separate types have been described (68). The less common *glomus type*, where the arteriovenous connections are tightly packed within the spinal cord substance, most often presents with hemorrhage (70% in a recently reported series), which results in an abrupt neurologic decline (68). The hemorrhage may occur into the spinal cord substance, from rupture of the nidus, and may produce an acute myelopathy. Spinal subarachnoid hemorrhage can also occur from dysplastic aneurysms that develop in arteries that supply the arteriovenous malformation. Figure 12.16 shows the arteriograms of a 13-year-old female who presented with subarachnoid hemorrhage. Initial evaluation at an outside hospital consisted of a CT scan that revealed hemorrhage in the basal cisterns. A subsequent four-vessel cerebral arteriogram was performed and interpreted as normal. She was dis-

charged and had a second subarachnoid hemorrhage 1 week later. Repeat evaluation at our institution revealed an intramedullary arteriovenous malformation at C-2 with a dysplastic aneurysm arising from the feeding anterior spinal artery. A small microcatheter was navigated through the vertebral artery into the radicular artery to the aneurysm site. Small-fibered platinum microcoils were delivered in the aneurysm and adjacent anterior spinal artery. Particulate embolization was also performed with 80% reduction of the AVM and elimination of the aneurysm. She had no change in her neurologic status, and subsequent surgery reduced the malformation further.

The more common *juvenile type* of intramedullary arteriovenous malformation involves a tangle of abnormal arteriovenous connections that fills up the entire spinal cord and has neural parenchyma within the nidus of the malformation. These juvenile malformations usually present with progressive weakness. The initial work-up should include a MRI examination. The abnormal tangle of vessels creates signal voids, which are outlined by the adjacent spinal cord parenchyma. Any associated parenchymal hemorrhage can be appreciated. Selective spinal arteriography is needed to delineate the feeding medullary arteries and draining veins. Plain films and myelography are rarely helpful in this disorder.

The treatment depends on the presenting symptoms and the anatomy of the malformation. Glomus-type malformations that are located posteriorly in the spinal cord substance, especially those that touch the surface of the spinal cord, can be surgically resected in some instances. Figure 12.16 shows an example of a glomus-type malformation that presented with spinal cord hemorrhage and was treated with superselective embolization and surgical excision. Superselective arteriography and preoperative embolization can be beneficial in many instances. Juvenile-type malformations are usually not amenable to surgical resection because of the intervening neural parenchyma. Palliative embolization often results in improvement in symptoms in these difficult lesions.

Perimedullary Arteriovenous Fistulas

Perimedullary arteriovenous fistulas are abnormal arteriovenous connections, sometimes referred to as direct AV fistulas, where the transition from artery to vein occurs without an intervening nidus (68,69). They usually occur on the surface of the spinal cord and are supplied by medullary arteries. The connection can be quite small, resulting in only slight increase in size of the feeding medullary arteries and veins, or they can be gigantic, with massively dilated medullary veins. The clinical presentation is usually progressive radiculomedullary signs and, if untreated, a gradual progression to spinal cord

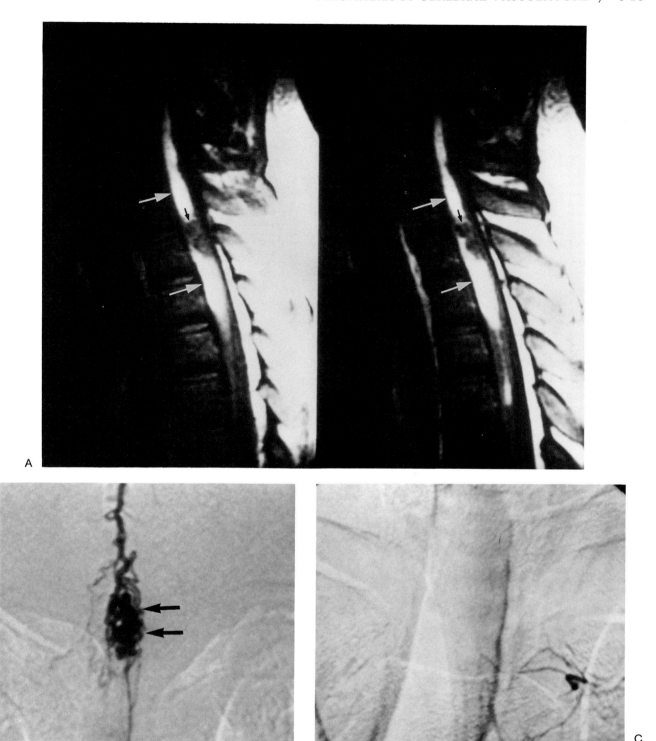

FIG. 12.16. A 17-year-old male presented with acute quadriparesis. **A:** Sagittal T1-weighted images demonstrated hematomyelia (*white arrows*) surrounding an area of signal void (*black arrows*) consistent with an intramedullary AVM. **B:** Left T4 intercoastal injection demonstrates a glomus-type arteriovenous malformation (*arrows*) located in the posterior aspect of the spinal cord. **C:** Same injection and projection as B, status postembolization, demonstrates complete obliteration of the malformation. Subsequent surgery was performed, resulting in complete cure of the malformation. The patient made a remarkable recovery with only mild residual arm weakness.

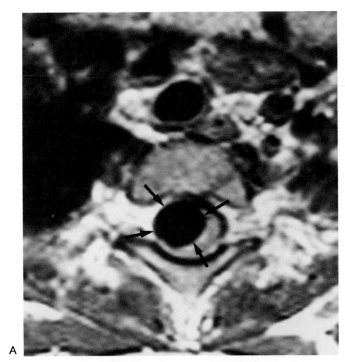
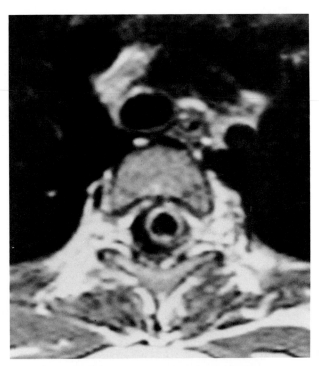

FIG. 12.17. A previously healthy 7-year-old female developed acute dense paraparesis over a 2-hour period. **A, B:** Axial T1-weighted images (TR500, TE30) at the cervical-thoracic junction demonstrate a large signal void (*arrows*) displacing the spinal cord to the right. At a slightly inferior level (B) a signal void is noted within the spinal cord substance.

transection. Less commonly, spinal subarachnoid hemorrhage can occur. Abrupt paraplegia can occur secondary to mechanical compression of the cord by the enlarged varix. Figure 12.17 shows an example of a 7-year-old girl who presented with a rapidly progressive paraparesis, treated with endovascular occlusion of the fistula with subsequent dramatic recovery. In our experience with ten giant perimedullary fistulas (70), half presented in the pediatric age. In these five cases, two were associated with Osler-Weber-Rendu syndrome and one had Cobb's syndrome. The majority of perimedullary fistulas can be detected with high-quality MRI imaging of the spine, which should be the initial examination when a perimedullary malformation is suspected. A supine myelogram may rarely be necessary to detect smaller fistulas. Smaller fistulas are optimally managed by surgical clipping, and large and giant fistulas can often be treated by endovascular techniques (69–71).

Epidural Fistulas

Epidural fistulas are rare, large-caliber connections that occur outside of the thecal sac, but because of their proximity, they can drain into medullary veins. They can present with subarachnoid hemorrhage or progressive myelopathy.

DURAL ARTERIOVENOUS MALFORMATIONS

Both adults and children with dural arteriovenous malformations can present with a wide clinical spectrum of signs and symptoms, depending on the location, size, and venous drainage of the malformation (54). Recent evidence has shown that some fistulas located in the transverse and sigmoid sinus region are acquired following dural sinus thrombosis (72). Children with dural arteriovenous malformations tend to have larger connections and increased flow compared to their adult counterparts. They can present with macrocephaly, heart murmur, cardiac failure, distended scalp veins, increased intracranial pressure, and hemorrhage (73) (Figs. 12.18, 12.19).

The radiographic evaluation usually involves selective angiography of the internal and external carotid artery and both vertebral arteries. CT and MR can elucidate hemorrhage secondary to the fistula but are not sensitive enough to screen for this elusive disease. An important angiographic feature associated with a high risk of hemorrhage is cortical venous drainage from the fistula site, which is generally a result of dural sinus occlusion (54) (Fig. 12.19).

Treatment can include transarterial embolization (74), transvenous embolization (75,76), or surgical excision (77). Often the larger dural malformations necessitate combined therapy.

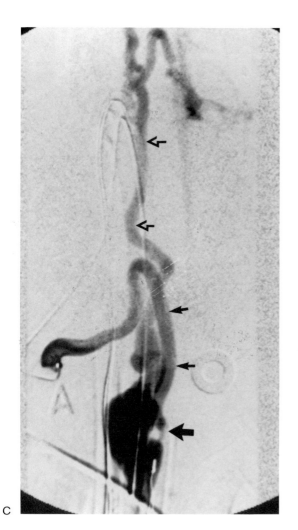

C

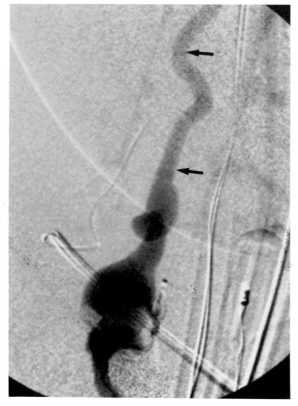

D

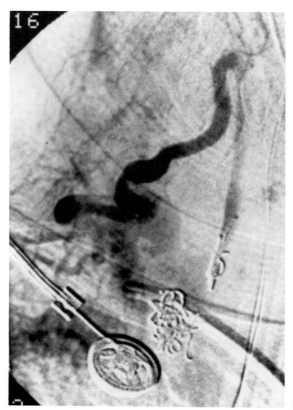

E

FIG. 12.17. (*Continued.*) **C:** Right costicervical injection, AP projection, demonstrates a large perimedullary fistula (*large arrow*) supplied by the anterior spinal artery (*small arrows*). Open arrows point to superiorly draining vein. **D:** Superselective injection through a microcatheter placed through the anterior spinal artery into the draining varix demonstrates the superiorly draining vein (*arrows*). Multiple platinum coils were delivered within the varix and distal anterior spinal artery. **E:** Right costicervical injection, AP projection, demonstrates obliteration of the flow to the varix. Over the ensuing 3 months the patient made a dramatic recovery, regained full strength in her left leg and sufficient strength in the right leg to ambulate with an ankle orthosis. Her physical examination was consistent with Osler-Weber-Rendu syndrome.

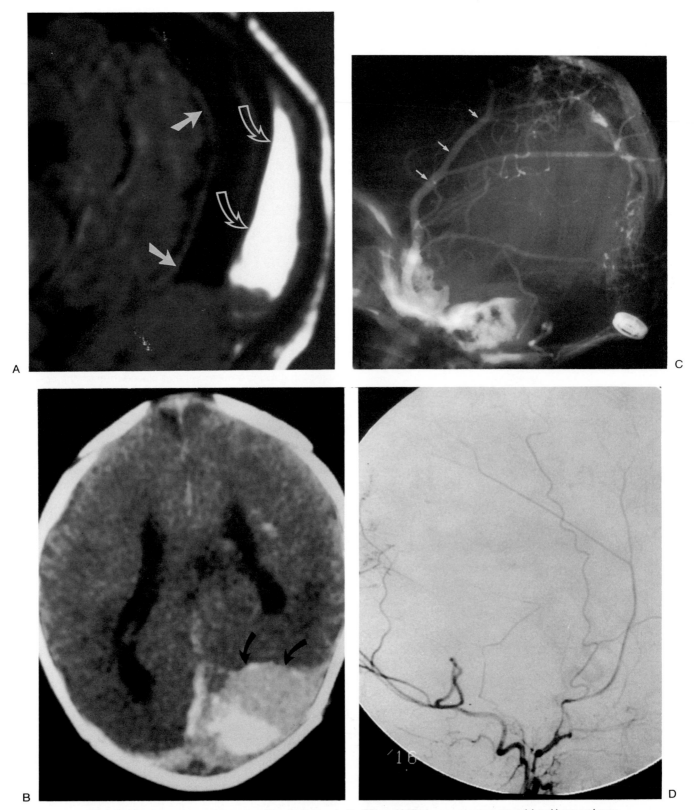

FIG. 12.18. A newborn presents with a seizure. **A, B:** CT and MR demonstrates an epidural hemorrhage (*open arrows*) displacing the superior sagittal sinus (*closed arrows*) anteriorly. **C:** Left external carotid injection, demonstrates a giant middle meningeal artery (*arrows*) shunting to a congenital dural fistula. **D:** The middle meningeal artery was embolized at 4 months with liquid adhesives. Follow-up arteriogram, lateral projection, demonstrates near complete obliteration of the fistula.

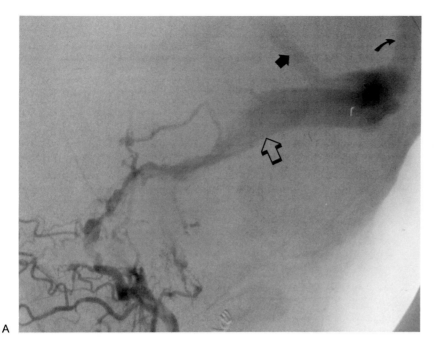

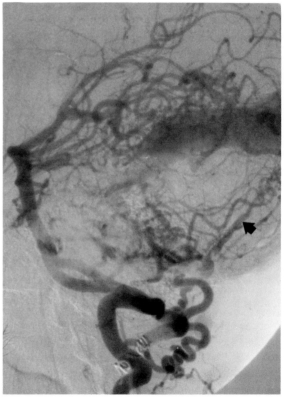

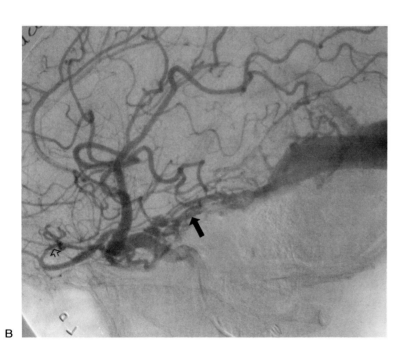

FIG. 12.19. A 13-year-old with hemorrhage secondary to a transverse sinus dural fistula. **A:** External carotid injection, lateral view, shows supply to transverse sinus (*open arrow*) that drains retrograde into superior sagittal (*curved arrow*) sinus and cortical veins (*straight arrow*). **B:** Left internal carotid injection, lateral projection, shows supply from meningohyposal trunk (*arrow*) and recurrent meningeal branches of ophthalmic artery (*open arrow*) to the same fistula. **C:** Vertebral artery injection, lateral view, shows enlarged meningeal supply (*arrow*) to the same fistula.

A

B

C

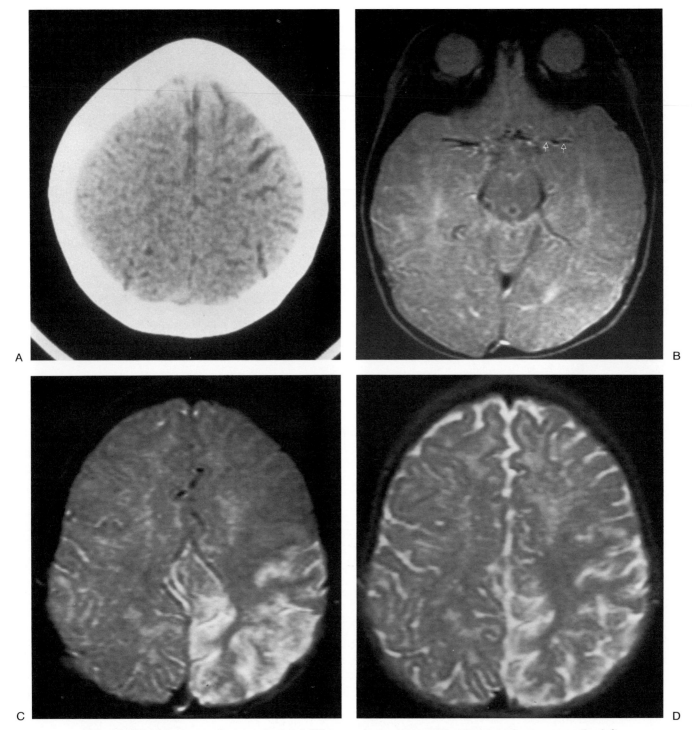

FIG. 12.20. Moyamoya disease. **A:** Axial CT scan shows increased sulcal prominence over the left cerebral hemisphere as compared with the right. **B:** Axial SE 2800/30 image at the level of the circle of Willis shows a small left middle cerebral artery (*arrows*). **C:** Axial SE 2800/30 image at the level of the centrum semiovale shows high cortical signal intensity in the left parietal and occipital regions, indicating ischemia or infarction of the cortex in those regions. **D:** Axial SE 2800/70 image is less sensitive to the cortical damage because the high-signal-intensity cortex is now isointense with cerebrospinal fluid. The appearance is that of sulcal prominence.

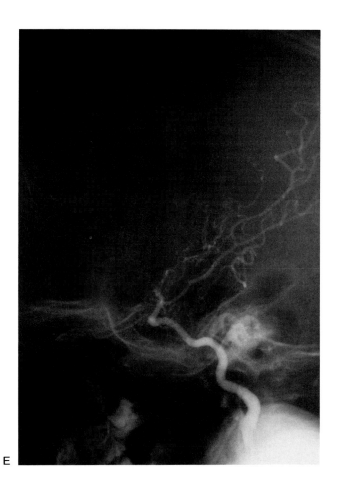

E

FIG. 12.20. (*Continued.*) **E:** Lateral projection from left internal carotid arteriogram shows occlusion of the supraclinoid internal carotid artery with multiple enlarged perforating vessels coursing dorsally through the region of the basal ganglia.

MOYAMOYA SYNDROME

Moyamoya syndrome is characterized by slowly progressive stenosis involving the proximal intracranial vessels (66,78). The collateral vessels (most commonly lenticulostriates and thalamoperforators) that hypertrophy to compensate for the slowly progressive occlusions resemble a "puff of smoke" on angiography, an appearance from which the disease derives its name (79). The cause is unknown, although associations have been described between this syndrome and neurofibromatosis, Down's syndrome, sickle cell disease, radiation therapy, and genetic factors (80). Approximately 70% of the reported cases occur in patients less than 20 years of age, and 50% occur in those less than 10 years of age (81). In contradistinction to adults, who typically present with subarachnoid or intraparenchymal hemorrhage, children usually have recurrent transient ischemic attacks with progressive neurologic impairment. Partial and secondary generalized seizures are common in younger children, whereas recurrent headache is more frequent in older children.

The radiographic evaluation includes angiography, which defines the extent of the disease as well as the adequacy of the compensatory collaterals. The typical angiographic appearance is that of narrowing of the supraclinoid internal carotid artery, proximal anterior cerebral artery, and proximal middle cerebral artery (Figs. 12.20, 12.21). The posterior circulation is uncommonly involved. The lenticulostriate arteries hypertrophy to compensate for narrowing of the major vessels.

CT and MR can be of benefit to define regions of cerebral infarction. CT may show focal regions of frank infarction or diffuse atrophy, depending upon the adequacy of collateral flow. MR is more sensitive in the demonstration of ischemic and infarcted regions of brain (see Chapter 4) and often reveals narrowing of intracranial vessels (Fig. 12.20). Moreover, enlarged lenticulostriate collateral vessels can be seen on MR as small flow voids in the basal ganglia (Fig. 12.21). MR angiography is not sensitive to flow in small vessels and will only detect lenticulostriate collaterals after they have become markedly enlarged (Fig. 12.21). In addition, MRA does not accurately assess the size of the superficial temporal artery, a crucial factor in surgical planning for these patients. As a result, MRA cannot, at present, replace catheter angiography in the preoperative evaluation of affected patients. However, MRA can sometimes be used to follow patients after surgical therapy by encephaloduralarterial synangiosis, as the superficial temporal artery markedly enlarges after successful treatment (82).

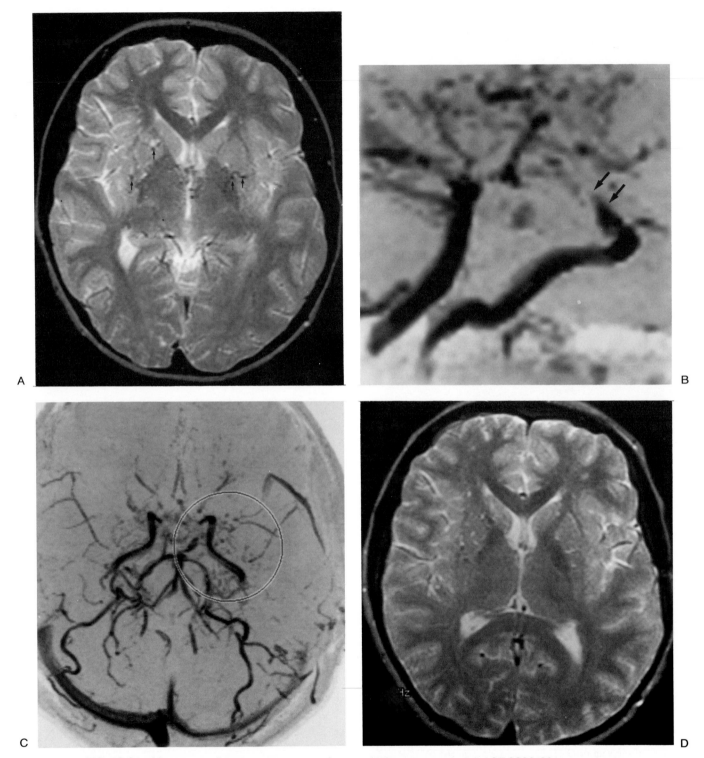

FIG. 12.21. Moyamoya disease: appearance after surgical treatment. **A:** Axial SE 2800/80 image shows dilated lenticulostriate vessels as curvilinear flow voids (*arrows*) in the basal ganglia. **B:** Maximum intensity projection image from a 3D TOF MRA shows narrowing (*arrows*) of the supraclinoid carotid artery and multiple dilated lenticulostriate collaterals. **C:** Collapsed view from 3D TOF MRA. Circle shows area from which image in B was reformatted. Note that the superficial temporal artery is not seen. Compare with E. **D:** Axial SE 2800/80 image after surgery shows marked regression of the lenticulostriate vessels. Compare with A.

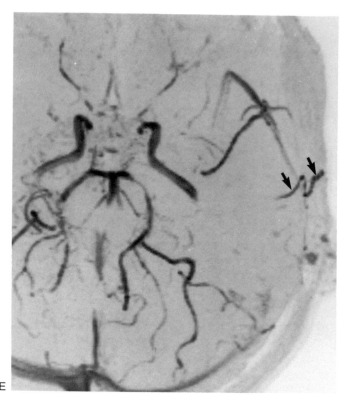
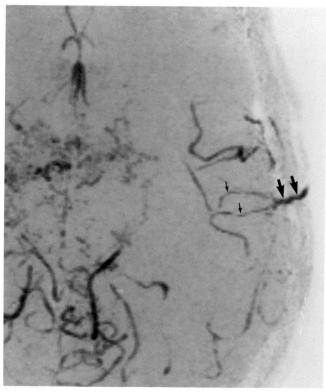

E

F

FIG. 12.21. (*Continued.*) **E:** Collapsed view from 3D TOF MRA shows an enlarging superficial temporal artery (*arrows*) compared with the preoperative study in C. **F:** Collapsed view from MRA at a superior level shows filling of middle cerebral artery vessels (*small arrows*) from the superficial temporal artery (*large arrows*).

REFERENCES

1. Schoenberg BS, Schoenberg DG. Spectrum of pediatric cerebrovascular disease. In: Rose FC, ed. *Clinical neuroepidemiology.* New York: State Mutual Books, 1980:151–162.

2. Lasjaunias P, Ter Brugge K, Lopez Ibor L, et al. The role of dural anomalies in vein of Galen aneurysms: report of six cases and review of the literature. *Am J Neuroradiol* 1987;8:185–92.

3. Perret G, Nishioka H. Report on the cooperative study of intracranial aneurysms and subarachnoid hemorrhage. Section VI. Arteriovenous malformations. An analysis of 545 cases of craniocerebral arteriovenous malformations and fistulae reported to the cooperative study. *J Neurosurg* 1966;25:467–90.

4. Gold AP, Ransohoff JR, Carter S. Vein of Galen malformation. *Acta Neurol Scand* 1964;40(suppl 11):5–31.

5. Amacher AL, Shillito J Jr. The syndromes and surgical treatment of aneurysms of the great vein of Galen. *J Neurosurg* 1973;39:89–98.

6. Hoffman HJ, Chuang S, Hendrick EB, Humphreys RP. Aneurysms of the vein of Galen. Experience at the Hospital for Sick Children, Toronto. *J Neurosurg* 1982;57:316–322.

7. Raybaud CA, Strother CM, Hald JK. Aneurysms of the vein of Galen: embryonic considerations and anatomical features relating to the pathogenesis of the malformation. *Neuroradiology* 1989;31: 109–128.

8. Yarsargil MG. *Microneurosurgery.* New York: Thieme, 1988.

9. Garcia-Monaco R, Lasjaunias P, Berenstein A. Therapeutic management of vein of Galen aneurysmal malformations. In: Viñuela F, Halbach VV, Dion JE, eds. *Interventional neuroradiology: endovascular therapy of the central nervous system.* New York: Raven, 1992:113–127.

10. Berenstein A, Epstein F. Vein of Galen malformations: combined neurosurgical and neuroradiological intervention. In: McLaurin RL, Schut L, Venes, eds. *Pediatric neurosurgery.* New York: Grune and Stratton, 1982:637–647.

11. Casasco A, Lylyk P, Hodes JE, Kohan G, Aymard A, Merland JJ. Percutaneous transvenous catheterization and embolization of vein of galen aneurysms. *Neurosurgery* 1991;28:260–266.

12. Ciricillo SF, Edwards MS, Schmidt KG, et al. Interventional neuroradiological management of vein of Galen malformations in the neonate. *Neurosurgery* 1990;27:22–27.

13. Ciricillo SF, Schmidt KG, Silverman NH, et al. Serial ultrasonographic evaluation of neonatal vein of Galen malformations to assess the efficacy of interventional neuroradiological procedures. *Neurosurgery* 1990;27:544–548.

14. Debrun G, Vinuela F, Fox A, Drake CG. Embolization of cerebral arteriovenous malformations with bucrylate. *J Neurosurg* 1982;56:615–627.

15. Dowd CF, Halbach VV, Barnwell SL, Higashida RT, Edwards MS, Hieshima GB. Transfemoral venous embolization of vein of Galen malformations. *Am J Neuroradiol* 1990;11:643–648.

16. Dowd CF, Halbach VV, Higashida RT, Fraser KW, Smith TP, Hieshima GB. Endovascular management of vein of Galen malformations. In: DaPian R, Pasqualin A, eds. *New trends in management of cerebrovascular malformations.* Berlin: Springer-Verlag, in press.

17. Edwards MSB, Hieshima GB, Higashida RT, Halbach VV. Management of vein of Galen malformations in the neonate. *Interven Pediatr* 1988;3:184–188.

18. Lylyk P, March AD, Kohan G, Viñuela F. Alternative therapeutic approaches in intravascular embolization of vein of Galen malformations. In: Viñuela F, Halbach VV, Dion JE, eds. *Interventional neuroradiology: endovascular therapy of the central nervous system.* New York: Raven, 1992:129–139.

19. Lylyk P, Viñuela F, Dion JE, et al. Therapeutic alternatives for vein of Galen vascular malformations. *J Neurosurg* 1993;78:438–445.

20. Mickle JP, Quisling RG. The transtorcular embolization of vein of Galen aneurysms. *J Neurosurg* 1986;64:731–735.

21. Yang PJ, Halbach VV, Higashida RT, Hieshima GB. Platinum wire: a new transvascular embolic agent. *Am J Neuroradiol* 1988;9:547–550.

22. Manelfe C, Berenstein A. Treatment of carotid cavernous fistulas by venous approach. Report of one case. *J Neuroradiol* 1980;7:13–19.

23. Halbach VV, Higashida RT, Dowd CF, Barnwell SL, Hieshima GB. Management of vascular perforations that occur during neurointerventional procedures. *Am J Neuroradiol* 1991;12:319–327.

24. Dandy WE. Carotid cavernous aneurysms (pulsating exophthalmos). *Zentralbl Neurochir* 1937;2:77–113, 165–204.

25. Delens E. De la communication de la carotide interne et du sinus caverneux (anéurysme artérioveineux). *Thèse de Paris. A Parent* 1870;.

26. Hamby WB. *Carotid cavernous fistula.* Springfield, IL: Charles C Thomas, 1966.

27. Sattler CH. *Pulsierender Exophthalmus. Handbuch der Gesamten Augenheikunde.* Berlin: Springer-Verlag, 1920.

28. Halbach VV, Hieshima GB, Higashida RT, Reicher M. Carotid cavernous fistulae: indications for urgent treatment. *Am J Roentgenol* 1987;149:587–593.

29. Debrun G, Lacour P, Viñuela F, Fox A, Drake CG, Caron JP. Treatment of 54 traumatic carotid-cavernous fistulas. *J Neurosurg* 1981;55:678–692.

30. Norman D, Newton TH, Edwards MS, De Caprio V. Carotid-cavernous fistula: closure with detachable silicone balloons. *Radiology* 1983;149:149–157.

31. Halbach VV, Higashida RT, Hieshima GB, Hardin CW, Yang PJ. Transvenous embolization of direct carotid cavernous fistulas. *Am J Neuroradiol* 1988;9:741–747.

32. Halbach VV, Higashida RT, Hieshima GB, Hardin CW. Direct puncture of the proximally occluded internal carotid artery for treatment of carotid cavernous fistulas. *Am J Neuroradiol* 1989;10:151–154.

33. Batjer HH, Purdy PD, Neiman M, Samson DS. Subtemporal transdural use of detachable balloons for traumatic carotid-cavernous fistulas. *Neurosurgery* 1988;22:290–296.

34. Higashida RT, Hieshima GB, Halbach VV, Bentson JR, Goto K. Closure of carotid cavernous sinus fistulae by external compression of the carotid artery and jugular vein. *Acta Radiol Suppl (Stockh)* 1986;369:580–583.

35. Halbach VV, Higashida RT, Dowd CF, Hieshima GB. Traumatic vascular injuries of the head and neck: clinical presentation, angiographic assessment and endovascular therapy. In: Margulis AR, Gooding CA, eds. *Diagnostic radiology.* San Francisco: University of California Printing Services, 1992:479–490.

36. King MA, Barkovich AJ, Halbach VA, Hieshima GB, Edwards MS. Traumatic monocular blindness and associated carotid injuries. *Pediatrics* 1989;84:128–132.

37. Matas R. Traumatisms and traumatic aneurysms of the vertebral artery and their surgical treatment with the report of a cured case. *Ann Surg* 1893;18:477–521.

38. Weinberg PE, Flom RA. Traumatic vertebral arteriovenous fistula. *Surg Neurol* 1973;1:162–167.

39. Hayes P, Gerlock AJ Jr, Cobb CA. Cervical spine trauma: a cause of vertebral artery injury. *J Trauma* 1980;20:904–905.

40. Halbach VV, Higashida RT, Hieshima GB, Norman D. Normal perfusion pressure breakthrough occurring during treatment of carotid and vertebral fistulas. *Am J Neuroradiol* 1987;8:751–756.

41. Halbach VV, Higashida RT, Hieshima GB. Treatment of vertebral arteriovenous fistulas. *Am J Roentgenol* 1988;150:405–412.

42. Debrun G, Legre J, Kasbarian M, Tapias PL, Caron JP. Endovascular occlusion of vertebral fistulae by detachable balloons with conservation of the vertebral blood flow. *Radiology* 1979;130:141–147.

43. Reizine D, Laouiti M, Guimaraens L, Riche MC, Merland JJ. Vertebral arteriovenous fistulas. Clinical presentation, angiographical appearance and endovascular treatment: a review of twenty-five cases. *Ann Radiol (Paris)* 1985;28:425–438.

44. Aberfeld DC, Rao KR. Familial arteriovenous malformation of the brain. *Neurology* 1981;31:184–186.

45. McCormick WF. Pathology of vascular malformations of the brain. In: Wilson CB, Stein BM, eds. *Intracranial arteriovenous malformation.* Baltimore: Williams and Wilkins, 1984:44–63.

46. Celli P, Ferrante L, Palma L, Cavedon G. Cerebral arteriovenous malformations in children. Clinical features and outcome of treatment in children and in adults. *Surg Neurol* 1984;22:43–49.

47. Schoenberg BS, Mellinger JF, Schoenberg DG. Cerebrovascular disease in infants and children: a study of incidence, clinical features, and survival. *Neurology* 1978;28:763–768.

48. Parkinson D, Bachers G. Arteriovenous malformations. Summary of 100 consecutive supratentorial cases. *J Neurosurg* 1980;53:285–299.

49. Gerosa MA, Cappellotto P, Licata C, Iraci G, Pardatscher K, Fiore DL. Cerebral arteriovenous malformations in children (56 cases). *Childs Brain* 1981;8:356–371.

50. So SC. Cerebral arteriovenous malformations in children. *Childs Brain* 1978;4:242–250.

51. McCormick WF. The pathology of vascular ("arteriovenous") malformations. *J Neurosurg* 1966;24:807–816.

52. Fierstien SB, Pribram HW, Hieshima G. Angiography and computed tomography in the evaluation of cerebral venous malformations. *Neuroradiology* 1979;17:137–148.

53. Rothfus WE, Albright AL, Casey KF, Latchaw RE, Roppolo HM. Cerebellar venous angioma: "benign" entity? *Am J Neuroradiol* 1984;5:61–66.

54. Lasjaunias P, Chiu M, ter Brugge K, Tolia A, Hurth M, Bernstein M. Neurological manifestations of intracranial dural arteriovenous malformations. *J Neurosurg* 1986;64:724–730.

55. Schorner W, Bradac GB, Treisch J, Bender A, Felix R. Magnetic resonance imaging (MRI) in the diagnosis of cerebral arteriovenous angiomas. *Neuroradiology* 1986;28:313–318.

56. Lemme Plaghos L, Kucharczyk W, Brant Zawadzki M, et al. MRI of angiographically occult vascular malformations. *Am J Roentgenol* 1986;146:1223–1228.

57. Drake CG. Cerebral arteriovenous malformations: considerations for and experience with surgical treatment in 166 cases. *Clin Neurosurg* 1979;26:145–208.

58. Forster DM, Steiner L, Hakanson S. Arteriovenous malformations of the brain. A long-term clinical study. *J Neurosurg* 1972;37:562–570.

59. Martin NA, Edwards M, Wilson CB. Management of intracranial vascular malformations in children and adolescents. *Concepts Pediatr Neurosurg* 1983;4:264–290.

60. Steiner L. Treatment of arteriovenous malformations by radiosurgery. In: Wilson CB, Stein BM, eds. *Intracranial arteriovenous malformations.* Baltimore: Williams and Wilkins, 1984:295–313.

61. Kusske JA, Kelly WA. Embolization and reduction of the "steal" syndrome in cerebral arteriovenous malformations. *J Neurosurg* 1974;40:313–321.

62. Halbach VV, Higashida RT, Yang P, Barnwell S, Wilson CB, Hieshima GB. Preoperative balloon occlusion of arteriovenous malformations. *Neurosurgery* 1988;22:301–308.

63. Locksley HB. Natural history of subarachnoid hemorrhage, intracranial aneurysms and arteriovenous malformations. Based on 6368 cases in the cooperative study. *J Neurosurg* 1966;25:219–239.

64. Heiskanen O, Vilkki J. Intracranial arterial aneurysms in children and adolescents. *Acta Neurochir (Wien)* 1981;59:55–63.

65. Halbach VV, Higashida RT, Hieshima GB. Treatment of intracranial aneurysms by balloon embolization therapy. *Semin Interven Radiol* 1987;4:261–268.

66. Suzuki J, Kodama N. Cerebrovascular "Moyamoya" disease. Collateral routes to forebrain via ethmoid sinus and superior nasal meatus. *Angiology* 1971;22:223–236.

67. Turner DM, Vangilder JC, Mojtahedi S, Pierson EW. Spontaneous intracerebral hematoma in carotid-cavernous fistula. Report of three cases. *J Neurosurg* 1983;59:680–686.

68. Rosenblum B, Oldfield EH, Doppman JL, Di Chiro G. Spinal arteriovenous malformations: a comparison of dural arteriovenous fistulas and intradural AVMs in 81 patients. *J Neurosurg* 1987;67:795–802.

69. Gueguen B, Merland JJ, Riche MC, Rey A. Vascular malforma-

tions of the spinal cord: intrathecal perimedullary arteriovenous fistulas fed by medullary arteries. *Neurology* 1987;37:969–979.

70. Halbach VV, Higashida RT, Dowd CF, Fraser KW, Edwards MS, Barnwell SL. Treatment of giant intradural perimedually spinal fistulas. *Neurosurgery* 1993;33:972–980.

71. Riche MC, Modenesi Freitas J, Djindjian M, Merland JJ. Arteriovenous malformations (AVM) of the spinal cord in children. A review of 38 cases. *Neuroradiology* 1982;22:171–180.

72. Chaudhary MY, Sachdev VP, Cho SH, Weitzner I Jr, Puljic S, Huang YP. Dural arteriovenous malformation of the major venous sinuses: an acquired lesion. *Am J Neuroradiol* 1982;3:13–19.

73. Albright AL, Latchaw RE, Price RA. Posterior dural arteriovenous malformations in infancy. *Neurosurgery* 1983;13:129–135.

74. Lasjaunias P, Halimi P, Lopez Ibor L, Sichez JP, Hurth M, De Tribolet N. Endovascular treatment of pure spontaneous dural vascular malformations. Review of 23 cases studied and treated between May 1980 and October 1983. *Neurochirurgie* 1984;30: 207–223.

75. Halbach VV, Higashida RT, Hieshima GB, Hardin CW, Pribram H. Transvenous embolization of dural fistulas involving the cavernous sinus. *Am J Neuroradiol* 1989;10:377–383.

76. Halbach VV, Higashida RT, Hieshima GB, Mehringer CM, Hardin CW. Transvenous embolization of dural fistulas involving the transverse and sigmoid sinuses. *Am J Neuroradiol* 1989;10:385–392.

77. Barnwell SL, Halbach VV, Higashida RT, Hieshima G, Wilson CB. Complex dural arteriovenous fistulas. Results of combined endovascular and neurosurgical treatment in 16 patients. *J Neurosurg* 1989;71:352–358.

78. Suzuki J, Takaku A. Cerebrovascular "moyamoya" disease. Disease showing abnormal net-like vessels in base of brain. *Arch Neurol* 1969;20:288–299.

79. Kudo T. Juvenile occlusion of the circle of Willis. *Clin Neurol* 1965;5:607.

80. Rajakulasingam K, Cerullo LJ, Raimondi AJ. Childhood moyamoya syndrome. Postradiation pathogenesis. *Childs Brain* 1979;5: 467–475.

81. Harwood-Nash DC, Fitz CR. *Neuroradiology in infants and children.* St Louis: CV Mosby, 1976.

82. Maas K, Barkovich AJ, Dong L, Edwards MSB, Piecuch R, Charlton V. Selected indications for and applications of magnetic resonance angiography in children. *Pediatr Neurosurg* 1994;20:113–125.

Subject Index

Page numbers followed by f refer to figures.